PEARSON CUSTOM FOR

NURSING

NSG 482

Pathophysiological and Pharmacological
Evidence Based Care
University of North Carolina-Wilmington

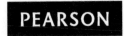 **PEARSON**   ISBN 10: 1-269-66525-1
ISBN 13: 978-1-269-66525-4

Table of Contents

Introduction to Pharmacology: Concepts and Connections

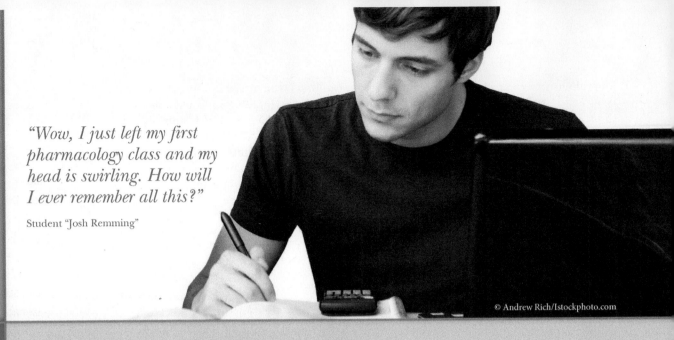

> "Wow, I just left my first pharmacology class and my head is swirling. How will I ever remember all this?"
>
> Student "Josh Remming"

© Andrew Rich/Istockphoto.com

Introduction to Pharmacology: Concepts and Connections

Learning Outcomes

After reading this chapter, the student should be able to:

1. Identify key events in the history of pharmacology.
2. Compare and contrast the terms *drug*, *pharmacology*, and *pharmacotherapy*.
3. Explain the importance of pharmacotherapy to clinical nursing practice.
4. Using specific examples, explain the difference between the pharmacologic and therapeutic methods of classifying drugs.
5. Identify the advantages of using prototype drugs to study pharmacology.
6. Classify drugs by their chemical, generic, and trade names.
7. Compare the advantages and disadvantages of a pharmaceutical company being granted exclusivity for the development of a new drug.
8. Analyze possible differences between generic drugs and their brand-name equivalents.
9. Assess the responsibilities of the nurse in drug administration.

Chapter Outline

Brief History of Pharmacology

Pharmacology: The Study of Medicines

Characteristics of an Ideal Drug

Classification of Drugs

Drug Prototypes

Naming Drugs

Connecting Pharmacology to Clinical Nursing Practice

More drugs are being administered to consumers than ever before. Over 3.6 billion prescriptions are dispensed each year in the United States, and the number is rapidly approaching 4 billion. The applications of pharmacology to medicine have evolved over the centuries and the nurse now serves a key role in ensuring the success of pharmacotherapy. The purpose of this chapter is to introduce fundamental concepts of pharmacology and to emphasize the connections between drug therapy and clinical nursing practice.

PharmFACT

According to the National Association of Chain Drug Stores (2010), the average cost of a prescription drug was $76.94 in 2009. The average brand name drug cost was $155.45, whereas the average generic drug cost was $39.73.

Brief History of Pharmacology

1 The practice of applying products to relieve suffering has been recorded throughout history by virtually every culture.

The story of pharmacology is rich and exciting, filled with accidental discoveries and landmark events. Its history likely began when a human first used a plant to relieve symptoms of disease. One of the oldest forms of health care, herbal medicine has been practiced in virtually every culture dating to antiquity. The Babylonians recorded the earliest surviving "prescriptions" on clay tablets in 3000 BC, although magic and the art of reading omens were probably considered as legitimate to healing as the use of drug remedies. At about the same time, the Chinese recorded the *Pen Tsao* (Great Herbal), a 40-volume compendium of plant remedies dating to 2700 BC. The Egyptians followed in 1500 BC by archiving their remedies on a document known as the Eber's papyrus, which contains over 700 magical formulas and remedies. Galen, the famous Greek physician, described over 1,000 healing preparations using plant products before his death in AD 201.

Little is known about pharmacology during the Dark Ages. Although it is likely that herbal medicine continued to be practiced, especially in monasteries and in centers of Arabic culture, few historical events related to drug therapy were recorded. Pharmacology, and indeed medicine, could not advance until the discipline of science was eventually viewed differently than magic and superstition.

The first recorded reference to the word *pharmacology* was found in a text titled "Pharmacologia sen Manuductio and Materiam Medicum" by Samuel Dale in 1693. Before this date, the study of herbal remedies was called "Materia Medica." Indeed, the term *Materia Medica* likely originated from a Latin term meaning "medical matters" in the Roman Empire that continued into the early 20th century.

Although the exact starting date is obscure, modern pharmacology is thought to have begun in the early 1800s. At that time, chemists were making remarkable progress in separating specific substances from complex mixtures. This enabled chemists to isolate the active agents morphine, colchicine, curare, cocaine, and other early drugs from their natural plant products. Pharmacologists could then study their effects in animals more precisely, using standardized amounts. Some of the early researchers even used themselves as test subjects. Friedrich Sertürner, who first isolated morphine from opium in 1805, injected himself and three of his friends with a huge dose of 100 mg of his new product. He and his cohorts suffered acute morphine intoxication for several days afterward.

Pharmacology as a distinct discipline was officially recognized when the first Department of Pharmacology was established in Estonia in 1847. John Jacob Abel, who is considered the father of American pharmacology due to his many contributions to the field, founded the first pharmacology department in the United States at the University of Michigan in 1890.

In the 20th century, the pace of change in all areas of medicine became exponential. Pharmacologists no longer needed to rely on the slow, laborious process of isolating active agents from scarce natural products. They could synthesize drugs "from scratch" in the laboratory. Hundreds of new drugs could be synthesized and tested in a relatively short time span. More importantly, it became possible to understand how drugs produced their effects, right down to their molecular mechanism of action.

The current practice of pharmacology is extremely complex and has progressed far beyond its early, primitive history. The nurses and other health professionals who practice it, however, must never forget its early roots: the application of products to relieve human suffering. Whether a substance is extracted from the Pacific yew tree, isolated from a fungus, or created totally in a laboratory, the central purpose of pharmacology is focused on the patient and improving the quality of life.

CONNECTION Checkpoint 1.1

Opium, colchicine, and cocaine are drugs obtained from natural products that were used hundreds, and perhaps thousands, of years ago. Are any of these products still used as drugs today? Use a drug guide or encyclopedia to determine the modern names of these drugs and what they are used to treat. *See Answer to Connection Checkpoint 1.1 on student resource website.*

Pharmacology: The Study of Medicines

2 Pharmacology is the study of medicines.

The word *drug* has already been used numerous times in this text. What exactly is a drug? Is everything a drug, including water, vitamin C, or perhaps a can of cola? What about substances

Key Terms

bioavailability

chemical names

combination drugs

drug

exclusivity

generic name

indications

pharmacologic classification

pharmacology

pharmacotherapy

prototype drug

therapeutic classification

trade name

naturally found in the body, such as estrogen or testosterone? Is it even possible to define a drug?

The definition of a drug is indeed difficult but is nevertheless important to the health care profession. There are many definitions, but perhaps the clearest is that a **drug** is any substance that is taken to prevent, cure, or reduce symptoms of a medical condition. Considering the substances listed earlier, which, then, are drugs? Although it may seem vague, the correct answer is "it depends."

- The caffeine consumed in a cup of coffee is not considered a drug. Yet caffeine is included in several therapies for headache pain, including Excedrin and Fioricet. For the patient trying to get pain relief, caffeine is a drug.

- Vitamin C, if ingested as part of an orange or tomato, is food. Food is not a drug. However, someone with a vitamin C deficiency may be administered vitamin C to cure scurvy. For this patient, vitamin C is then considered a drug.

- A can of cola is certainly not listed in any drug guide. However, if a patient with diabetes is experiencing a hypoglycemic reaction, the glucose in a can of soda may raise the patient's blood sugar and prevent a coma; thus the glucose in the cola may be considered a drug in this example.

- Substances normally found in the body are not considered drugs unless they are administered to treat a condition. For example, the hormone estrogen circulating in the blood is

not a drug. However, if it is taken as an oral contraceptive to prevent a condition (pregnancy), estrogen is considered a drug.

Once the meaning of the term drug is understood, the next essential term is pharmacology. The word pharmacology is derived from two Greek words, *pharmakon,* which means "medicine" or "drug," and *logos,* which means "study." Thus, **pharmacology** is most simply defined as the study of medicines. Pharmacology is an expansive subject, ranging from understanding how drugs are administered, to where they travel in the body, to the actual responses they produce. **Pharmacotherapy**, or pharmacotherapeutics, is the application of drugs for the purpose of disease prevention and treatment of suffering.

Drugs are a form of medical intervention given to improve a patient's condition or to prevent harm. Pharmacotherapy often begins when the patient experiences signs or symptoms that cause dissatisfaction with current or future health status. A major role of the nurse is to design interventions that meet the desired health goals of the patient. Pharmacotherapy is a critical intervention for many conditions. The rationale for pharmacotherapy is illustrated in Figure 1.

Over 11,000 brand-name and generic drugs and combination agents are currently available for pharmacotherapy. Each has its own characteristic set of therapeutic applications, interactions, adverse effects, and mechanism of action. Many

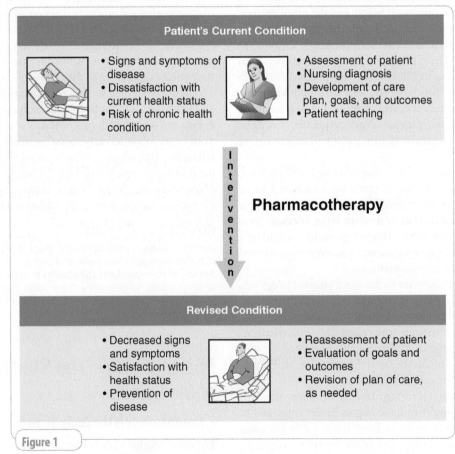

Figure 1

Rationale for pharmacotherapy: a partnership between the patient and the health care provider.

drugs are prescribed for more than one disease and most produce multiple effects on the body. Further complicating the study of pharmacology is the fact that drugs may elicit different responses depending on individual patient factors such as age, gender, race, body mass, health status, and genetics. Indeed, learning the applications of existing medications and staying current with new drugs introduced every year are an enormous challenge for the nurse. The task, however, is a critical one for both the patient and the health care provider. If applied properly, drugs can dramatically improve patients' quality of life. If applied improperly, the consequences of drug action can cause permanent disability and even death.

There are important exceptions to the drug definition mentioned earlier. What about crack cocaine, ecstasy, LSD, or the fumes in glues and paint thinners? These are certainly drugs, but they are not taken "to prevent, cure, or reduce symptoms of a medical condition." In fact, they are taken to produce a biologic effect viewed as desirable or pleasurable by the user. There are a few exceptions to the drug definition, and these will become apparent as the student studies pharmacology.

Characteristics of an Ideal Drug

3 The perfect drug is safe and effective.

As they begin their journey in mastering pharmacology, nurses should start with a notion of the ideal or "perfect drug." Learning the characteristics of an ideal drug gives a basis for comparison to "real drugs." It is always the goal of pharmacotherapy to select the perfect or ideal drug for the patient. Just what is a perfect drug? It is one that:

- Effectively treats, prevents, or cures the patient's condition.
- Produces a rapid, predictable response at relatively low doses.
- Produces no adverse effects or long-term adverse effects.
- Can be taken conveniently, usually by mouth.
- Can be taken infrequently, usually once a day, and for a short length of time.
- Is inexpensive and easily accessible.
- Is quickly eliminated by the body after it produces its beneficial effect.
- Does not interact with other medications or food.

The student should recognize that there is no such thing as a perfect drug. Some drugs meet most of the preceding criteria, whereas others meet very few. At the very least, it is expected that all prescription drugs have some degree of effectiveness at treating or preventing a health condition. The conditions for which a drug is approved are its **indications**. Every prescription drug has at least one indication, and most have multiple indications. Some drugs are used for conditions for which they have not been approved; these are called unlabeled or off-label indications.

As a general rule, the more a medicine strays from the "perfect drug" profile, the less commonly it is used. This is because

whenever possible, health care providers strive to prescribe the most effective, safest, and most convenient medication for the patient. In the home care setting, drugs that cause annoying adverse effects, have inconvenient dosing schedules, or are expensive are often not taken by patients, potentially worsening their condition and causing failure of treatment outcomes. Of course, some essential drugs do produce serious adverse effects or must be given by invasive routes, such as intravenously. In these cases, the drug is either administered in a clinical setting by a licensed nurse, or the patient receives careful instructions and regular monitoring on an outpatient basis.

Classification of Drugs

4 Drugs may be organized by their therapeutic classification or pharmacologic classification.

The U.S. Food and Drug Administration (FDA, 2011) document *Approved Drug Products with Therapeutic Equivalence Evaluations,* informally called the "Orange Book," lists over 11,000 approved drugs. With the vast number of drugs available, it is essential that methods be used to group similar agents to aid in their study and understanding. The two basic classifications of drugs are therapeutic and pharmacologic. Both categories are widely used in classifying prescription and nonprescription drugs. The key difference is that the **therapeutic classification** describes what is being treated by the drug, whereas the **pharmacologic classification** describes how the drug acts.

Drugs are placed into therapeutic classes based on their usefulness in treating a specific disease. Table 1 shows the method of therapeutic classification, using cardiovascular

---

CONNECTIONS

Lifespan Considerations
Cost of Prescription Medications

Older adults are affected more than any other age group by the high cost of prescription drugs. Americans over age 65 comprise only 13% of the population but account for about 34% of all prescriptions dispensed and 40% of all over-the-counter (OTC) medications. More than 80% of all older adults take at least one prescribed drug each day. The average older person is taking more than four prescription medications at once, plus two OTC medications. Many of these medicines, such as those for hypertension and heart disease, are taken on a permanent basis and not all medications are available in a cheaper generic version.

Even with Medicare insurance coverage, the cost of prescription medications may exceed the amount Medicare will cover. A gap in coverage begins after approximately $3,000 has been spent on medications and only after spending over $6,000 does coverage resume, a gap termed the "doughnut hole." While some older adults may purchase additional private-plan coverage, not all plans fill this gap. Older adults should be encouraged to review their private supplemental insurance plans annually to be sure appropriate coverage is maintained.

TABLE 1 Organizing Drug Information by Therapeutic Classification

THERAPEUTIC FOCUS: DRUGS AFFECTING CARDIOVASCULAR DISEASE

Therapeutic Usefulness	Therapeutic Classification
Influence blood clotting	Anticoagulants
Lower blood cholesterol	Antihyperlipidemics
Lower blood pressure	Antihypertensives
Restore normal cardiac rhythm	Antidysrhythmics
Treat angina	Antianginals

TABLE 2 Organizing Drug Information by Pharmacologic Classification

FOCUS ON HOW A DRUG WORKS: PHARMACOTHERAPY OF HYPERTENSION

Mechanism of Action	Pharmacologic Classification
Lowers plasma volume	Diuretic
Blocks heart calcium channels	Calcium channel blocker
Blocks hormonal activity	Angiotensin-converting enzyme inhibitor
Blocks physiological reactions to stress	Adrenergic antagonist (or blocker)
Dilates peripheral blood vessels	Vasodilator

CONNECTION Checkpoint 1.2

State whether each of the following classifications for aspirin is therapeutic or pharmacologic: anticoagulant, salicylate, central nervous system agent, analgesic, antipyretic. Use a drug guide, if needed. *See Answer to Connection Checkpoint 1.2 on student resource website.*

Drug Prototypes

5 A prototype drug is the agent to which all other drugs in a class are compared.

drugs as an example. Many different types of drugs affect cardiovascular function. Some drugs influence blood coagulation, whereas others lower cholesterol levels or prevent the onset of stroke. Drugs may be used to treat hypertension, heart failure, abnormal cardiac rhythm, chest pain, myocardial infarction (MI), or circulatory shock. Thus, drugs that treat cardiovascular disorders may be placed in several therapeutic classes, for example, anticoagulants, antihyperlipidemics, and antihypertensives. The key to therapeutic classification is to simply state what condition is being treated by the particular drug. Other examples of therapeutic classifications include antidepressants, antipsychotics, drugs for erectile dysfunction, and antineoplastics. Notice how the prefix *anti-* often refers to a therapeutic classification.

The pharmacologic classification addresses a drug's mechanism of action or how a drug produces its effect in the body. Table 2 illustrates the use of pharmacologic classification, using hypertension as an example. A diuretic treats hypertension by lowering plasma volume. Calcium channel blockers treat this disorder by decreasing the force of cardiac contractions. Other drugs block components of the renin-angiotensin system. Notice that each example describes how hypertension might be controlled. A drug's pharmacologic classification is more specific than its therapeutic classification and requires an understanding of biochemistry and physiology. Pharmacologic classifications may use a drug's chemical name.

Although classifications help to organize drugs, the process is by no means easy or standardized. Most drugs have multiple classifications. For example, the drug epinephrine is classified as a vasoconstrictor, an autonomic nervous system agent, an adrenergic agonist, a sympathomimetic, a bronchodilator, an agent for anaphylaxis, an ocular mydriatic, an antiglaucoma agent, a catecholamine, and a topical hemostatic. This is clearly a mix of therapeutic (e.g., antiglaucoma) and pharmacologic (e.g., catecholamine) classifications. Which one(s) should the student remember? Unfortunately for beginning students of pharmacology, the answer is all of them. The classification chosen primarily depends on the specific clinical use of the drug (What condition of the patient is the nurse treating?). Sometimes it is simply a preference of the attending nurse or health care provider. Although challenging, remembering the different classifications will pay dividends as the student's pharmacology course progresses.

As discussed in Section 4 learning thousands of drugs is simplified, at least somewhat, by grouping similar drugs together into broad classifications. Just knowing its therapeutic or pharmacologic classification can reveal important information about a drug. An additional strategy is helpful when learning pharmacology. It is a common and useful practice to select a single drug from a class and compare all other medications in the class to this representative medication. This is called a **prototype drug**. By learning about the prototype drug in depth, the actions and adverse effects of other drugs in the same class may be predicted. For example, by learning the actions and effects of penicillin V, students can extend this knowledge to all other drugs in the penicillin class of antibiotics. In this text, the drug prototypes are clearly identified, and detailed information regarding their therapeutic effects, mechanism of action, adverse effects, contraindications, precautions, and nursing responsibilities, including patient and family education, is presented.

Selecting a drug to serve as the prototype for a class is not always a simple matter; health care providers and textbooks sometimes disagree. The traditional prototype approach uses the oldest and best understood drug in the class. Sometimes, however, newer drugs are developed in the same class that are more effective or have a more favorable safety profile. Over time, an older prototype drug may be infrequently prescribed and a different, more clinically useful prototype may be chosen for the class. This text uses a practical approach to drug prototypes, selecting a combination of traditional drugs and those most widely used. Regardless of the approach, the student must remember that the prototype is the drug to which all others in a class are compared.

Naming Drugs

6 Drugs have chemical, generic, and trade names.

Despite the utility of using drug classes and prototypes when studying pharmacology, learning thousands of drug names remains a challenge. Adding to this difficulty is that most drugs have multiple names. The three basic types of drug names are chemical, generic, and trade names.

Chemical names are assigned using standard nomenclature established by the International Union of Pure and Applied Chemistry (IUPAC). A drug has only one chemical name. This chemical name is sometimes helpful in predicting a drug's physical and chemical properties. Although chemical names convey a clear and concise meaning about the nature of a drug to the chemist, these names are often complicated and difficult to remember or pronounce. For example, it is unlikely that the nurse would remember that the chemical name for alprazolam (Xanax) is 8-chloro-1-methyl-6-phenyl-4H-5-triazolo[4,3-α][1,4]-benzodiazepine. In only a few cases, usually when the name is brief and easily remembered, will nurses use chemical names. Examples of easy to remember chemical names of common drugs include lithium carbonate, calcium gluconate, and sodium chloride.

Drugs are sometimes named and classified by a portion of their chemical structure, known as the chemical group name. In the Xanax example, a portion of the chemical name, benzodiazepine, is used as a drug class. Other examples include the fluoroquinolones, aminoglycosides, phenothiazines, and thiazides. Although these names may seem complicated when first encountered, knowledge of chemical group names will become invaluable as the nursing student begins to learn and understand the actions of the drugs in the major drug classes.

The **generic name** of a drug is assigned by the United States Adopted Name Council. With few exceptions, generic names are less complicated and easier to remember than chemical names. Many organizations, including the FDA, the *United States Pharmacopeia,* and the World Health Organization routinely describe a medication by its generic name. Because there is only one generic name for each drug, health care providers often use this name, and students must memorize it. Fortunately, sometimes components of a generic name can help a student recognize other drugs in that same class. For example, the ending -*lol* is used in the generic name of beta-adrenergic blockers and the ending -*statin* denotes a lipid-lowering drug.

A drug's **trade name**, sometimes called the proprietary, product, or brand name, is assigned by the pharmaceutical company marketing the drug. The trade name is intentionally selected to be short and easy to remember so that patients will remember it (and ask for it by name). The term *proprietary* suggests ownership. In the United States, the FDA grants the pharmaceutical company exclusive rights to name and market a drug for a certain number of years after it approves a new drug application. During the period of **exclusivity**, competing companies are not allowed to market generic versions of the product. The rationale for exclusivity is that the developing pharmaceutical company needs sufficient time to recoup the millions of dollars in research and development costs involved in designing and testing the new drug. Without the guarantee of exclusivity, there is little incentive to pharmaceutical companies to develop new and unique drugs. When exclusivity expires, competing companies may sell a generic equivalent drug, sometimes using a different name, which the FDA must approve. The typical length of exclusivity for a new drug is 5 years; however, this may be extended by 3 additional years if the drug is determined to have a new indication, can be delivered by a different route, or is made available in a different dosage form. If, for example, the pharmaceutical company completes pediatric studies and determines the dosage and safety of a drug in this population, the FDA adds 6 months of exclusivity. Orphan drugs have 7 years of exclusivity. Pharmaceutical companies can make millions of dollars in sales from exclusivity; thus they usually make great efforts to receive extensions from the FDA. Expiration dates for the exclusivity of specific drugs are listed by the FDA in the *Approved Drug Products with Therapeutic Equivalence Evaluations.*

Trade names are a challenge for students to learn because there may be dozens of product names containing the same drug. In addition, many products contain more than one active ingredient. Drugs with more than one active generic ingredient are called **combination drugs**. This poses a problem in trying to match one generic name with one product name. As an example, refer to Table 3 and consider the drug diphenhydramine (generic name), also called Benadryl (one of many trade names). Low doses of diphenhydramine may be purchased OTC. Higher doses require a prescription. If the nurse is looking for diphenhydramine, it may be listed under many trade names such as Benadryl, Nytol QuickCaps, Sominex, and Unisom, formulated alone or in combination with other active ingredients. Acetaminophen and aspirin are additional examples of agents that appear in many combination drugs with dozens of different trade names. To avoid this confusion, generic names should be used when naming the active ingredients in a combination drug. When referring to a drug, it is conventional to write the generic name in lowercase first, followed by the trade name in parentheses with the first letter capitalized. Examples include alprazolam (Xanax) and acetaminophen (Tylenol).

TABLE 3 Examples of Generic Drugs Contained in Brand-Name Products	
Generic Drugs	**Brand Names**
aspirin	Acetylsalicylic Acid, Acuprin, Anacin, Aspergum, Bayer, Bufferin, Ecotrin, Empirin, Excedrin, Maprin, Norgesic, Salatin, Salocol, Salsprin, Supac, Talwin, Traphen-10, Vanquish, Verin, ZORprin
diphenhydramine	Allerdryl, Benadryl, Benahist, Bendylate, Caladryl, Compoz, Diahist, Diphenadril, Eldadryl, Fenylhist, Fynex, Hydramine, Hydril, Insomnal, Noradryl, Nordryl, Nytol, Tusstat, Wehdryl
ibuprofen	Advil, Amersol, Apsifen, Brufen, Haltran, Medipren, Midol 200, Motrin, Nuprin, Pamprin-IB, Rufen, Trendar

7 Generic drugs are less expensive than brand-name drugs, but they may differ in bioavailability.

During the years of exclusivity for a new drug, the pharmaceutical company determines the price of the medication. Because there is no competition, the price is generally quite high. Once the exclusive rights end, competing companies market the generic equivalent drug for less money, and consumer savings may be considerable. In some states, pharmacists may routinely substitute a generic drug when the prescription calls for a brand name. In other states, the pharmacist must dispense drugs directly as written by a health care provider or obtain approval before providing a generic substitute.

PharmFACT

In a recent study, almost 50% of the physicians surveyed expressed negative perceptions about the quality of generic drugs, and more than a quarter preferred not to use generics as first-line drugs for themselves or their family (Shrank et al., 2011).

Pharmaceutical companies marketing brand-name drugs often lobby aggressively against laws that might restrict the routine use of certain brand-name drugs. The lobbyists claim that there are significant differences between a trade name drug and its generic equivalent and that switching to the generic drug may be harmful for the patient. Consumer advocates on the other hand argue that generic substitutions should always be permitted because of the cost savings to patients.

Are there really significant differences between a brand-name drug and its generic equivalent? The answer is unclear. Despite the fact that the dosages may be identical, drug formulations are not always the same. The two drugs may have different inert ingredients. If in tablet form, the active ingredients may be more tightly compressed in one of the preparations. Liquid drugs may use different solvents such as water or alcohol.

The key to comparing brand-name drugs and their generic equivalents lies in measuring the **bioavailability** of the two agents. Bioavailability is defined by the Federal Food, Drug and Cosmetic Act as the rate and extent to which the active ingredient is absorbed from a drug product and becomes available at the site of drug action to produce its effect. Bioavailability may be affected by many factors, including inert ingredients and tablet compression. Anything that affects the absorption of a drug or its travel to the target cells can certainly affect drug action. Measuring how long a drug takes to exert its effect (onset time) gives pharmacologists a crude measure of bioavailability. If the trade and generic products have the same rate of absorption and have the same onset of therapeutic action, they are said to be bioequivalent.

The importance of bioavailability differences between a trade name drug and its generic equivalent depends on the specific circumstances of pharmacotherapy. For example, if a patient is in circulatory shock and the generic equivalent drug takes 5 minutes longer to produce its effect, that may indeed be significant. However, if a generic medication for arthritis pain relief takes 45 minutes to act, compared to the brand-name drug, which takes 40 minutes, it probably does not matter which drug is used, and the inexpensive product should be prescribed to provide cost savings to the consumer. As a general rule, bioavailability is of most concern when using

critical care drugs and those with a narrow safety margin. In these cases, the patient should continue taking the brand name drug and *not* switch to a generic equivalent, unless approved by the health care provider. For most other drugs, the generic equivalent may be safely substituted for the trade name drug.

In the age of Internet pharmacies, the issue of exclusive marketing rights has drastically changed. Other countries are not bound by U.S. drug laws, and it is easy for patients to obtain brand-name drugs through the mail at a fraction of what they cost in the United States. For example, a pharmaceutical company may have exclusivity for selling Cialis in the United States but companies in India and China sell the identical drug through Internet pharmacies and ship it to customers in the United States. In some cases, they even sell the drug to consumers without a prescription. Other countries do not have the same quality control standards as the United States, and the patient may be purchasing a useless or even harmful product. Furthermore, although Internet sites may appear to be based in the United States, they may instead be obtaining their medications from unreliable sources. Nurses must strongly urge their patients not to purchase drugs from overseas pharmacies because there is no assurance that the drugs are safe or effective.

Connecting Pharmacology to Clinical Nursing Practice

8 Pharmacology is intimately connected to nursing practice and is a key intervention in relieving and preventing human suffering.

The importance of pharmacology to nursing clinical practice cannot be overstated. As nursing students progress toward their chosen specialty, pharmacology is at the core of patient care and is integrated into the nursing process. Indeed, pharmacology would not be an important science without its connections to nursing practice.

Whether administering medications or supervising drug use, the nurse is expected to understand the pharmacotherapeutic principles for all medications received by each patient. Given the large number of different drugs and the potential consequences of medication errors, this is indeed an enormous task. The nurse's responsibilities include knowledge and understanding of the following:

- What drug is ordered:
  - Name (generic and trade) and drug classification
  - Intended or proposed use
  - Effects on the body
  - Contraindications
  - Special considerations, such as how age, weight, body fat distribution, and pathophysiologic states affect pharmacotherapeutic response
  - Expected and potential adverse events

- Why the drug has been prescribed for this particular patient
- How the drug is supplied by the pharmacy
- How the drug is to be administered, including dose ranges
- What nursing process considerations related to the drug apply to this patient

A major goal in studying pharmacology is to eliminate medication errors and to limit the number and severity of adverse drug events. Many adverse effects are preventable. Professional nurses can routinely avoid many serious adverse drug effects in their patients by applying their experience and knowledge of pharmacotherapeutics to clinical practice. Some adverse effects, however, are not preventable. It is vital that the nurse be prepared to recognize and respond to potential adverse effects of medications.

Before any drug is administered, the nurse must obtain and process pertinent information regarding the patient's medical history, physical assessment, disease processes, and learning needs and capabilities. Growth and developmental

factors must always be considered. It is important to remember that a large number of variables influence a patient's response to drugs throughout the life span. Having a firm understanding of these variables can increase treatment success. For a nurse, knowledge of pharmacology is an ongoing, lifelong process that builds as a nurse is in practice and chooses specific clinical areas. It may seem daunting at first, but learning prototypes, recognizing key similarities in generic names, and always looking up unknown or new drugs will help build this knowledge base.

Despite its essential nature, the study of pharmacology should be viewed in the proper perspective. Drugs are just one of many tools available to the nurse for preventing or treating human suffering. Although pharmacology is a key intervention in many cases, nurses must use all the healing sciences in treating their patients. The effectiveness of a drug in treating disease can never substitute for skilled, compassionate nursing care. Too much reliance on drug therapy can diminish the importance of the nurse–patient relationship.

UNDERSTANDING THE CHAPTER

Key Concepts Summary

1 The practice of applying products to relieve suffering has been recorded throughout history by virtually every culture.

2 Pharmacology is the study of medicines.

3 The perfect drug is safe and effective.

4 Drugs may be organized by their therapeutic classification or pharmacologic classification.

5 A prototype drug is the agent to which all other drugs in a class are compared.

6 Drugs have chemical, generic, and trade names.

7 Generic drugs are less expensive than brand-name drugs, but they may differ in bioavailability.

8 Pharmacology is intimately connected to nursing practice and is a key intervention in relieving and preventing human suffering.

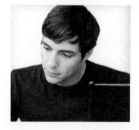

Making the PATIENT Connection

Remember the student "Josh Remming" at the beginning of the chapter? Now read the remainder of the case study. Based on the information presented within this chapter, respond to the critical thinking questions that follow.

Josh Remming, a 23-year-old student, is in his first semester of nursing school. He thought that nursing would provide him with a great career and lots of opportunity. He enjoys helping people and has always been fascinated with health care. However, after the first pharmacology class, Josh is worried because there seems to be an overwhelming amount of content to learn in just one semester.

At the end of the class, Josh talks with other students who are concerned and a bit anxious. Much of the conversation centers around lecture content provided by the professor. Following are some of the questions from Josh's classmates. How would you respond?

Critical Thinking Questions

1. What is the difference between therapeutic classification and pharmacologic classification?

2. What classification is a barbiturate? macrolide? birth control pills? laxatives? folic acid antagonist? antianginal agent?

3. What is a prototype drug, and what advantages does a prototype approach to studying pharmacology offer?

4. Why do nurses need to know all this pharmacology?

See Answers to Critical Thinking Questions on student resource website.

NCLEX-RN® Review

1 The nurse is using a drug handbook to determine the indications for the drug furosemide (Lasix). The term *indications* is defined as the:
   1. Way a drug works on the target organs.
   2. Amount of the drug to be administered.
   3. Conditions for which a drug is approved.
   4. Reason that the drug should not be given.

2 While completing the health history, the nurse asks the client, "What medications do you take regularly?" Which drug name would the nurse expect the client to use in providing the answer?
   1. Chemical
   2. Generic
   3. Trade
   4. Standard

3 When providing nursing care for the client, the nurse understands that drugs are:
   1. One of many tools available to prevent or treat human suffering.
   2. The most important part of the therapeutic treatment plan.
   3. Primarily the concern of the health care provider and not included in nursing care.
   4. Substances that should be relied on for health and wellness.

4 Which client characteristics, if noted in the client's medical record, would the nurse consider important information that may affect the physiological response to various types of drug therapy? Select all that apply.
   1. 82-year-old and female
   2. Asian and obese
   3. Past medical history of kidney disease
   4. Mother and sister with diabetes
   5. Has no medical insurance

5 The nurse is looking up a drug that has been prescribed and wants to know the therapeutic classification for the drug. Which of the following would indicate a therapeutic classification?
   1. Beta-adrenergic antagonist
   2. Antihypertensive
   3. Diuretic
   4. Calcium channel blocker

6 The nurse is asked by a family member: "They're giving mom Motrin and she takes Advil. Hasn't the wrong drug been ordered?" The nurse will respond, knowing that:
   1. There has been an error in the order and the nurse will contact the health care provider.
   2. There may be a reason for the health care provider to order a different drug.
   3. Not all health care agencies buy the same generic drugs and that may account for the difference.
   4. Motrin and Advil are trade names for the same generic drug, ibuprofen.

Additional Case Study

Sarah Hawkins, an elderly woman who lives on a fixed income, is on multiple medications. She says that all her friends are taking the generic form of their medications. While you are visiting her, she asks you, "What do you think of generic medicines? Are they safe? Are they as good? Are they worth it?"

1. How do generic equivalent drugs differ from a proprietary (trade name) drug?

2. What would you recommend that Sarah do about accepting generic drugs?

See Answers to Additional Case Study on student resource website.

Pearson Nursing Student Resources

Find additional review materials at
nursing.pearsonhighered.com

Prepare for success with additional NCLEX®-style practice
questions, interactive assignments and activities, web links,
animations, videos, and more!

References

National Association of Chain Drug Stores. (2010) *Industry facts-at-a-glance.* Retrieved from http://www.nacds.org/wmspage.cfm?parm1=6536

Shrank, W. H., Liberman, J. M., Fischer, M. A., Girdish, C., Brennan, T. A., & Choudry, N. K. (2011). Physician perceptions about generic drugs. *The Annals of Pharmacotherapy, 45*(1), 31–38. doi:10.1345/aph.1P389

U.S. Food and Drug Administration (FDA). (2011). *Electronic orange book: Approved drug products with therapeutic equivalence evaluations.* Washington, DC: U.S. Department of Health and Human Services. Retrieved from http://www.accessdata.fda.gov/scripts/cder/ob/default.cfm

Selected Bibliography

Duncan, D. (2010). Generic prescribing and substitution: The big issues. *British Journal of Community Nursing, 15*(5), 248–249.

Gandey, A. (2007). Drug costs pushing companies to abandon promising therapies. *Medscape Medical News.* Retrieved from http://www.medscape.com/viewarticle/554048

Howland, R. H. (2010). Are generic medications safe and effective? *Journal of Psychosocial Nursing Mental Health Services, 48*(3), 13–16. doi:10.3928/02793695-20100204-01

Kazmi, S. Z. (2007). Controversies in drug substitution. *Medscape Pharmacists.* Retrieved from http://www.medscape.com/viewarticle/563959

Kesselheim, A. S., Misono, A. S., Lee, J. L., Stedman, M.R., Brookhart, M.A., Choudhry, N. K., & Shrank, W. H. (2008). Clinical equivalence of generic and brand-name drugs used in cardiovascular disease: A systematic review and meta-analysis. *Journal of the American Medical Association, 300*(21), 2514–2526. doi:10.1001/jama.2008.758

Openshaw, M. (2006). The economics of prescription drug prices, government intervention, and the importation of drugs from Canada. *Nursing Economics, 23*(6), 307–311.Sarah Hawkins, an elderly woman who lives on a fixed income, is on multiple medications. She says that all

Answers to NCLEX-RN® Review

1 Answer: 3 Rationale: Indications are the conditions for which a particular drug is approved. Options 1, 2, and 4 are incorrect. A description of how a drug works on its target organs and cells is called the mechanism of action. The dosage is the amount of the drug that is given. The conditions whereby the drug should be avoided are contraindications. Cognitive Level: Applying; Client Need: Safe and Effective Care Environment; Nursing Process: Implementation

2 Answer: 3 Rationale: Trade names or proprietary names are designed to help the client remember the name of the drug. Options 1, 2, and 4 are incorrect. The chemical name refers to the chemical substances that comprise the drug. A drug's generic name is assigned by the U.S. Adopted Name Council, and each drug has only one generic name. There is no category that is referred to as "standard" in the categories of drug names. Cognitive Level: Applying; Client Need: Health Promotion and Maintenance; Nursing Process: Implementation

3 Answer: 1 Rationale: Drugs are only tools that are part of the overall therapeutic treatment plan. Other treatment options and the nurse–client relationship are also important to the care of the client as an individual. Options 2, 3, and 4 are incorrect. Drug therapy alone is usually insufficient to correct and cure human illness. Nurses play a major role in the drug therapy of clients by administering, educating, monitoring, and assessing the response to drugs. Too much reliance on drug therapy can diminish the importance of the nurse–client relationship. Cognitive Level: Applying; Client Need: Physiological Integrity; Nursing Process: Implementation

4 Answer: 1, 2, 3, 4 Rationale: Physiological responses to drug therapy are affected by a client's age, gender, race, body mass, and health status. Many diseases such as diabetes have genetic origins. Familial history of disease conditions may reflect potential problems in the client. Option 5 is incorrect because not having medical insurance is not a physiological variable that would affect drug therapy. Cognitive Level: Applying; Client Need: Physiological Integrity; Nursing Process: Evaluation

5 Answer: 2 Rationale: Antihypertensive indicates the therapeutic classification of the drug by describing its usefulness in lowering blood pressure. Options 1, 3, and 4 are incorrect. Beta-adrenergic antagonists, diuretics, and calcium channel blockers all focus on how the drug works, rather than on what therapeutic effects occur. Cognitive Level: Applying; Patient Need: Physiological Integrity; Nursing Process: Implementation

6 Answer: 4 Rationale: Motrin and Advil are trade names for the generic drug ibuprofen. Options 1, 2, and 3 are incorrect. No error is noted because "ibuprofen" is the generic name for Advil and Motrin, both trade names. Each drug has only one generic name but may have different trade names, depending on the company that manufactures the drug. Cognitive Level: Applying; Patient Need: Health Promotion and Maintenance; Nursing Process: Implementation

Drug Regulations

From Chapter 2 of *Pharmacology: Connections to Nursing Practice*, Second Edition. Michael Patrick Adams, Carol Quam Urban. Copyright © 2013 by Pearson Education, Inc. All rights reserved.

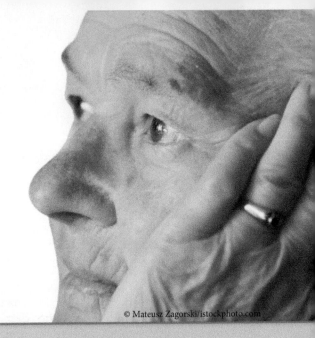

"This headache medicine I bought at the grocery store must be safe because I didn't need a prescription."

Patient "Gertrude Stone"

© Mateusz Zagorski/istockphoto.com

Drug Regulations

Learning Outcomes

After reading this chapter, the student should be able to:

1. Explain the role of patent medicines in the history of pharmacology and the legislation of drugs.

2. Outline the key U.S. drug regulations and explain how each has contributed to the safety and effectiveness of medications.

3. Describe how the *United States Pharmacopeia-National Formulary* (USP-NF) controls drug purity and standards.

4. Evaluate the role of the U.S. Food and Drug Administration in the drug approval process.

5. Categorize the four stages of new drug approval.

6. Explain the role of a placebo in new drug testing.

7. Discuss how recent changes to the approval process have increased the speed at which new drugs reach consumers.

8. Compare and contrast prescription and over-the-counter drugs.

9. Explain how scheduled drugs are classified and regulated.

10. Describe the Canadian drug approval process and identify similarities to the drug approval process in the United States.

Chapter Outline

Patent Medicines

Brief History of Drug Legislation

Drug Standards

The U.S. Food and Drug Administration

Drug Approval

Changes to the Drug Approval Process

Prescription and Over-the-Counter Drugs

Drug Schedules

Canadian Drug Standards

Laws govern all aspects of the drug approval, labeling, marketing, manufacturing, and distribution process. The purpose of this legislation is to inform the public and to protect it from unsafe and ineffective products. This chapter examines standards and legislation regulating drugs in the United States and Canada.

Patent Medicines

1 Early American history saw the rise of patent medicines and the lack of adequate drug regulations.

People have an expectation that the drug they are taking is effective at treating their condition, whether it is asthma, diabetes, or a headache. They expect the label to contain clear and accurate instructions on how the product should be taken. They expect that the drug will be safe if the instructions are correctly followed. Are these reasonable assumptions? In the United States and Canada, the answer is yes. But Americans have not always had this reassurance. Although drugs have been used for thousands of years, it was not until the 20th century that extensive standards and regulations were developed to protect the public from unsafe and ineffective products.

In early America, there were few attempts to regulate drugs. This period saw the rise of **patent medicines**. Although the term *patent* implies a legal right to manufacture or sell a drug, this was not the case. Patent medicines contained a brand name that clearly identified the product, such as William Radam's Microbe Killer, Stanley's Snake Oil, Dr. Kilmer's Swamp Root, or Dr. Moore's Indian Root Pills. Because there were no laws to the contrary, these products claimed to cure just about any symptom or disease. Dr. William's Pink Pills for Pale People, which contained iron oxide and magnesium sulfate, claimed to cure rheumatism, nervous headache, palpitations, grippe, neuralgia, locomotor ataxia, partial paralysis, sallow complexion, and all forms of weakness in men or women. A typical advertisement from this era is shown in Figure 1.

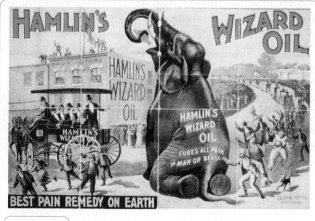

Patent medicines contained a name brand that clearly identified the product and claimed to cure just about any symptom or disease.
Source: Calvert Litho. Co./Corbis

Patent medicines were often harmless (and ineffective), containing coloring, flavoring, and an aromatic substance that "smelled like medicine." At their worst, some contained hazardous levels of dangerous or addictive substances. In fact, cocaine, heroin, and morphine were freely distributed in patent medicines; some elixirs contained up to 50% morphine, which indeed caused many painful disorders to "disappear." Addictive ingredients were purposely added to guarantee repeat customers for their products. (Note the similarity with nicotine added to tobacco and caffeine added to soft drinks.) In the late 1800s, the familiar Coca-Cola soft drink was a patented beverage that contained an estimated 9 mg of cocaine per serving and was claimed to cure headache, dyspepsia, hysteria, morphine addiction, and impotence. The need for stricter regulation became more apparent in the 1860s as cocaine was synthesized, and the use of opiates as painkillers during the Civil War caused thousands of soldiers to become addicted.

Although the marketing and use of patent medicines may seem humorous and even unbelievable to modern consumers, a few of these products are still available over the counter (OTC). Examples of patent medicines that survived the drug regulations of the 1900s include Smith Brothers Throat Drops, Fletcher's Castoria, Doan's Pills, Vick's VapoRub, and Phillip's Milk of Magnesia. Of course, the ingredients of these products have changed over time so that they conform to modern regulations regarding labeling, safety, and effectiveness.

Brief History of Drug Legislation

2 In the 1900s, drug legislation was enacted to make drugs safer and more effective.

Although individual states attempted to regulate drugs, the first national law was the Drug Importation Act, passed in 1848, which attempted to stop the entry of unsafe drugs into the United States. In the early 1900s, the United States began to develop and enforce tougher drug legislation to protect the public. This was, in part, spurred by the tragic deaths of 13 children in St. Louis in 1901 who were given diphtheria antitoxin that was contaminated with tetanus. In 1902, the Biologics Control Act was passed to standardize the quality of sera, antitoxins, and other blood-related products. Passed shortly thereafter, the Pure Food and Drug Act (PFDA) of

1906 was a significant and powerful piece of drug legislation that gave the government authority to control the labeling of medicines. Essentially, this law required that drug labels accurately reflect the contents. Prior to this date, many labels did not contain any indication of the active ingredient within the bottle or its amount.

Unfortunately, the PFDA did not address false therapeutic claims because although the ingredients had to be labeled accurately, a drug could still be marketed for any disease. In 1912, the Sherley Amendment to the PFDA prohibited the sale of drugs labeled with false therapeutic claims that were intended to defraud the consumer. A major weakness, as borne out in subsequent legal battles, was the difficulty of proving that the false claim made by the seller was intentional.

It is surprising that up to this point in American history there was no attempt to legislate the use of addictive drugs. The Harrison Narcotic Act of 1914 was passed to require prescriptions for high doses of narcotic drugs and to mandate that pharmacists and health care providers keep narcotic records. Since 1914, hundreds of additional state and federal laws have been passed to regulate drugs with abuse potential, including the landmark Comprehensive Drug Abuse Prevention and Control Act (see Section 8).

Unfortunately there were still two essential components missing from the regulation of drugs in the early 20th century. Although the PFDA and other legislation required that ingredients be listed on the label and prohibited intentional false claims, manufacturers did not have to prove that the drug was effective. Furthermore, product safety did not have to be tested before the drug was marketed. Bringing the issue to the forefront was an incident in 1937 in which an elixir of sulfanilamide containing a poisonous chemical (diethylene glycol) killed 107 persons, mostly children.

In 1938, Congress passed the landmark Food, Drug, and Cosmetic Act (FDCA), which corrected certain loopholes in previous laws. This was the first law preventing the sale of newly developed drugs that had not been thoroughly tested for safety before marketing. Drug labels were required to contain instructions for safe use. The FDCA was also the first attempt at regulating cosmetics and medical devices. Unfortunately, the FDCA did not clearly define "prescription" or specify which drugs required a prescription. Most drugs, including many addictive and harmful substances, were sold by the corner druggist, sometimes legally, other times illegally. In 1951, the Durham-Humphrey Amendment to the FDCA delineated the difference between safer drugs, which may be sold OTC, and more dangerous drugs, which require prescriptions.

In the late 1950s, the drug thalidomide was found to produce severe birth defects in the children of women taking the drug as a sleeping pill and to treat morning sickness during pregnancy. Although the drug was not approved in the United States, it is estimated that over 20,000 Americans received the drug, because it was widely distributed to health care providers without FDA approval. As with other drug legislation, it took a tragedy to convince Congress to pass tougher regulations. Passage of the Kefauver-Harris Amendment to the FDCA in 1962 mandated that manufacturers prove their

drugs were effective for specific purposes, as well as safe, through the conduct of "adequate and well-controlled" studies. This law was applied retroactively to all drugs introduced since the passage of the FDCA. This amendment also required all significant adverse reactions to be reported to the FDA and that complete information about adverse effects be included in literature distributed to health care providers. For the first time, informed consent was required from patients participating in experimental drug research.

The emphasis on effectiveness continued as the FDA contracted with the National Academy of Sciences and the National Research Council in 1966 to evaluate the effectiveness of 4,000 drugs that were approved between 1938 and 1962 based only on their safety. Approximately 40% of all drugs introduced between 1938 and 1962 were found to be ineffective and were subsequently removed from the market. In 1972, a review of OTC drugs began to examine the safety and effectiveness of these products.

In the 1980s, the public placed considerable political pressure on the FDA to find drugs to treat rare or unusual disorders. Pharmaceutical companies were reluctant to develop drugs for these disorders because there would not be enough sales to recoup their research and development costs. To encourage development of such drugs, the Orphan Drug Act became law in 1983. An **orphan disease** is defined as a serious, although rare, disease that affects fewer than 200,000 people in the United States. With the passage of this legislation, drug manufacturers are now offered development grants, tax credits for clinical investigation expenses, and 7 years of exclusivity to market an orphan drug. Over 700 medications have been approved as orphan drugs since the passage of this act.

A major focus in the 1990s was to speed the drug approval process, which could be prolonged for many years. The Prescription Drug User Fee Act (PDUFA) of 1992 assessed fees from drug manufacturers to be used specifically for reducing the review time for new drug applications. From 1992 to 2002, the fees collected exceeded a billion dollars and the number of full-time equivalent employees examining new drug applications at the FDA increased from 1,277 to 2,337. The PDUFA was reauthorized in 1997 with the passage of the Food and Drug Administration Modernization Act, which also included provisions to accelerate the review of medical devices, regulate the advertising of unapproved uses of drugs, and regulate health claims for foods.

In reaction to the rising popularity of dietary supplements, Congress passed the Dietary Supplement Health and Education Act of 1994 to control misleading industry claims. Due in part to intense lobbying from the dietary supplement industry, the regulation of these products remains less stringent than that for prescription or OTC drugs.

In early 2000, the focus of drug regulation turned to access. Advocacy groups claimed that the high cost of drugs caused unequal access to adequate health care for the poor, the uninsured/underinsured, and the elderly. After lengthy debate, the Medicare Prescription Drug Improvement and Modernization Act of 2003 was passed. This legislation provides for a standard benefit that pays 75% of prescription

TABLE 1 Historical Time Line of Regulatory Acts, Standards, and Organizations

Year	Regulatory Acts, Standards, and Organizations
1820	Physicians establish the first comprehensive publication of drug standards, the *United States Pharmacopeia* (USP).
1848	The Drug Importation Act requires that all drugs (as defined by the newly established pharmacopeia) entering the United States be inspected and analyzed for "quality, purity, and fitness for medical purposes."
1852	Pharmacists found the American Pharmaceutical Association (APhA). The APhA establishes the *National Formulary* (NF), a standardized publication focusing on pharmaceutical ingredients. The USP continues to catalog all drug-related substances and products.
1862	The Federal Bureau of Chemistry, established under the administration of President Lincoln, eventually becomes the Food and Drug Administration (FDA).
1902	The Biologics Control Act controls the quality of sera and other blood-related products.
1906	The Pure Food and Drug Act prohibits the manufacture and sale of adulterated or misbranded foods, drugs, and medications.
1912	The Sherley Amendment makes medicines safer by prohibiting the sale of drugs labeled with false therapeutic claims.
1914	The Harrison Narcotics Act requires those who dispense opium, cocaine, and related substances to keep records of the drugs they dispense and makes it illegal to possess narcotics without a prescription. This act allows physicians to prescribe narcotics only for treatment, not to addicts.
1938	The Food, Drug, and Cosmetic Act is the first law preventing the marketing of drugs not thoroughly tested.
1944	The Public Health Service Act is enacted and covers many health issues, including biologic products and the control of communicable diseases.
1970	The Comprehensive Drug Abuse Prevention and Control Act (also known as the Controlled Substances Act) organizes regulated drugs (including opiates, cocaine, cannabis, stimulants, depressants, and hallucinogens) into five schedules and imposes restrictions and penalties.
1975	The *United States Pharmacopeia* and *National Formulary* become a single standardized publication, the USP-NF.
1986	The Anti-Drug Abuse Act increases sentences and imposes mandatory minimum sentences for those convicted of illegal drug activity based on the type and quantity of drug involved.
1986	The Childhood Vaccine Act authorizes the FDA to acquire information about patients taking vaccines, to recall biologics, and to recommend civil penalties if guidelines regarding biologic use were not followed.
1988	The FDA is officially established as an agency of the U.S. Department of Health and Human Services.
1992	The Prescription Drug User Fee Act requires that nongeneric drug and biologic manufacturers pay fees to be used for improvements in the drug review process.
1994	The Dietary Supplement Health and Education Act requires clear labeling of dietary supplements and gives the FDA the power to remove supplements that cause a significant public risk.
1997	The FDA Modernization Act reauthorizes the Prescription Drug User Fee Act, representing the largest reform effort of the drug review process since 1938.
2002	The Best Pharmaceuticals for Children Act improves the safety and efficacy of medicines for children and continues the exclusivity provisions for pediatric drugs as mandated under the Food and Drug Administration Modernization Act of 1997.
2003	The Medicare Prescription Drug Improvement and Modernization Act provides seniors and those with disabilities a prescription drug benefit and better benefits under Medicare.
2007	The Food and Drug Administration Amendments Act (FDAAA) of 2007 reauthorized and expanded the Prescription Drug User Fee Act, the Modernization Act, the Best Pharmaceuticals for Children Act, and the Pediatric Research Equity Act.

drug spending up to the first $2,250. Those qualifying for the low-income criteria may have their premiums and cost subsidized by the government. Participants are protected against catastrophic costs at $3,600 per year with most beneficiaries paying a 5% copay amount. A brief time line of major events in U.S. drug regulation is shown in Table 1.

Drug Standards

3 The standardization of drug purity and strength is specified by the *United States Pharmacopeia-National Formulary*.

Until the 1800s, drugs were prepared from plants that were available in the natural environment. The strength and purity of the products varied considerably because they were entirely dependent on the experience (and integrity) of the druggist preparing the product and the quality of the local ingredients. Potency and safety varied from region to region and, indeed, from batch to batch. Consider the simple analogy of baking. If 100 people across the world were asked to bake a loaf of bread, the final products would vary considerably in size, taste, and nutritional value. It is likely that no two loaves would be the same. It is obvious that a standard recipe must be followed. Similarly, to obtain consistency in the preparation and potency of drugs, standards (recipes) are needed.

Among the first standards used by pharmacists was the **formulary,** or list of pharmaceutical products and drug recipes. In the United States, the first comprehensive publication of drug standards, the *United States Pharmacopeia* (USP), was established in 1820. A **pharmacopeia** is a medical reference summarizing standards of drug purity, strength, and directions for synthesis. From 1852 until 1975, two major compendia maintained drug standards in the United States, the USP and

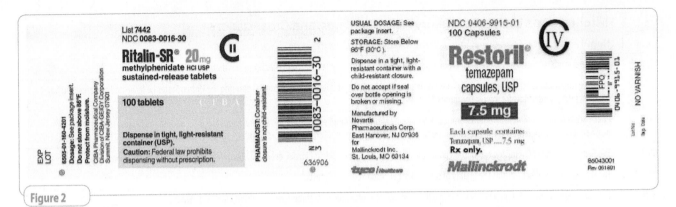

the *National Formulary* (NF), which were established by the American Pharmaceutical Association (APhA). All drug products were covered in the USP, whereas the NF focused on non-drug ingredients. In 1975, the two were merged into a single publication named the *United States Pharmacopeia-National Formulary* (USP-NF). The current document consists of about 2,400 pages and contains 3,777 drug monographs in more than 164 chapters. The USP-NF is published annually, with two supplements being issued throughout the year. Today, the USP label can be found on many medications verifying the purity and exact amounts of ingredients found within the container. Drugs marketed in the United States must conform to USP-NF standards to avoid possible charges of adulteration and misbranding. Sample labels are illustrated in Figure 2. The USP also provides a voluntary program for verifying the label accuracy of dietary supplements.

The U.S. Food and Drug Administration

4 The regulatory agency responsible for ensuring that drugs and medical devices are safe and effective is the U.S. Food and Drug Administration.

The establishment of a regulatory agency for food and drugs in the United States began with a single chemist appointed by President Lincoln in 1862. The **U.S. Food and Drug Administration (FDA)** was established by the PFDA of 1906 and later expanded to carry out the provisions of the FDCA of 1938. It is one of the oldest drug regulatory agencies in the world. The FDA states its mission as follows:

- Protecting the public health by ensuring the safety, efficacy, and security of human and veterinary drugs, biologic products, medical devices, the nation's food supply, cosmetics, and products that emit radiation

- Advancing the public health by helping to speed innovations that make medicines and foods more effective, safer, and more affordable

- Helping the public get the accurate, science-based information they need to use medicines and foods to improve their health

With such an important and vast mission, the FDA is organized around six branches, as shown in Figure 3. The Center for Drug Evaluation and Research (CDER) states its mission as facilitating the availability of safe, effective drugs; keeping unsafe or ineffective drugs off the market; improving the health of Americans; and providing clear, easily understandable drug information for safe and effective use. All new drugs must be approved by the CDER before they can be marketed. This includes prescription drugs, OTC drugs, and all generic equivalents. After marketing, the CDER is responsible for continued monitoring of safety and may issue additional warnings to health care providers or consumers as additional information becomes available.

The Center for Biologics Evaluation and Research (CBER) regulates the use of biologics (drugs derived from living sources), including sera, vaccines, and blood products. One historical achievement involving biologics is the 1986 Childhood Vaccine Act. This act authorizes the FDA to acquire information about patients taking vaccines, to recall biologics, and to recommend civil penalties if guidelines regarding biologics are not followed. The mission of the CBER was recently expanded to include the regulation of gene therapy and treatment with human cells or tissue-based products.

The FDA also oversees the administration of herbal products, dietary supplements, and cosmetics through the Center for Food Safety and Applied Nutrition (CFSAN). Although it does not require testing of herbal or dietary supplements prior to marketing, the CFSAN is responsible for taking action against any supplement that is deemed to be unsafe.

The CFSAN also regulates cosmetics, which are legally defined by the FDCA of 1938 as "articles intended to be rubbed, poured, sprinkled, or sprayed on, introduced into, or otherwise applied to the human body . . . for cleansing, beautifying, promoting attractiveness, or altering the appearance." Examples of products considered cosmetics are skin moisturizers, perfumes, lipsticks, fingernail polishes, eye and facial makeup preparations, shampoos, toothpastes, and deodorants. Can a product be both a cosmetic and a drug? In most cases, cosmetics are not drugs; however, it depends on a product's intended use. For example, if a shampoo is marketed to treat a condition such as dandruff, the active ingredient is considered a drug. If a skin cream claims to provide sunscreen protection, it may be considered a drug. Cosmetics do not require approval by the CFSAN

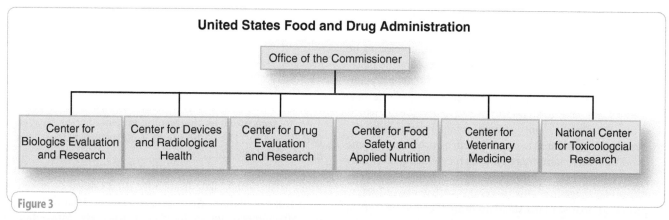

United States Food and Drug Administration

Office of the Commissioner

| Center for Biologics Evaluation and Research | Center for Devices and Radiological Health | Center for Drug Evaluation and Research | Center for Food Safety and Applied Nutrition | Center for Veterinary Medicine | National Center for Toxicologcial Research |

Figure 3

Organization of the Food and Drug Administration showing the six centers that regulate human and veterinary drugs, biologic products, medical devices, the nation's food supply, cosmetics, and products that emit radiation.

prior to marketing, and regulations are much less restrictive compared to drug approval. Manufacturers of cosmetics are generally careful not to promote unwarranted therapeutic claims, such as that a product prevents or treats a condition or disease. This would cause the product to be considered a drug by the FDA, and it would be subject to tighter regulations.

Drug Approval

5 The drug approval process established by the Food and Drug Administration ensures that drugs sold in the United States are safe and effective.

Drugs are discovered in any number of ways. Penicillin was discovered purely by accident while the scientist was studying an unrelated topic. Many drugs have been isolated from natural substances, including plants and bacteria. Some drugs are "me too" drugs, whereby the pharmacologist simply took a well-known drug and slightly modified the chemical structure to produce a very similar agent. As molecular biology and genetics have progressed into the modern era, drugs have been purposefully designed to fit into specific receptor sites on enzymes or cells.

Regardless of the path to discovery, all drugs must be approved by the FDA before they can be sold in the United States. The FDA drug review and approval process follows a well-developed and organized plan, as summarized in Figure 4.

The first stage of drug development is **preclinical research**, which involves extensive laboratory testing by the pharmaceutical company. Scientists perform testing on human and microbial cells cultured in the laboratory. Studies are performed in several species of animals to examine the drug's effectiveness at different doses and to look for adverse effects. The goals of this extensive testing on cultured cells and in animals are to determine drug action and to predict whether the drug will cause harm to humans. Because laboratory tests do not accurately reflect the precise way the human body will respond to the drug, preclinical research results are always inconclusive. Most drugs do not proceed past the preclinical research stage because they are either too toxic or simply not effective. The FDA does not regulate preclinical testing.

If a drug appears promising, the pharmaceutical company submits an **Investigational New Drug (IND)** application to the FDA that contains all the animal and cell testing data. Scientists at the FDA study the data and must be convinced that the drug is safe enough to allow human testing. Approval from the FDA is necessary before the next stage can begin.

Clinical investigation, the second stage of drug testing, takes place in three different stages termed **clinical phase trials**. These clinical trials are the longest part of the drug approval process and occur in sequential stages.

• **Phase 1.** Testing is conducted on 20 to 80 healthy volunteers for several months to determine proper dosage and to assess for adverse effects. The focus of the phase 1 trial

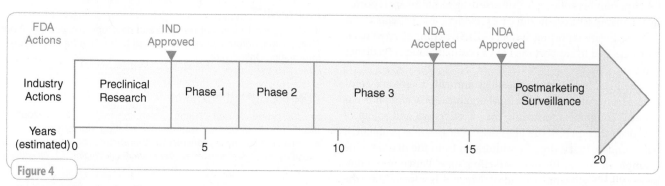

Figure 4

Drug development time line.

is on safety. If unacceptable levels of toxicity are noted, the clinical trials are stopped.

- **Phase 2.** Several hundred patients with the disease to be treated are given the drug. The primary focus of the phase 2 trial is on effectiveness, although safety data continue to be recorded. In most cases, the effectiveness of the new drug is compared to an inert substance, or **placebo**, which serves as a control "nontreatment" group. In other cases the new drug is compared to a standard drug used for the same condition. For example, a new drug for reducing fever may be compared to acetaminophen (Tylenol). If the new drug is found to have the same (or less) effectiveness and safety profile compared to the standard drug, the pharmaceutical company may stop the clinical trials. This phase may take several years.

- **Phase 3.** Large numbers of patients with the disease are given the drug to determine patient variability. Potential drug–drug interactions are examined. Patients with chronic conditions such as cardiac, renal, or hepatic impairment are given the drug to determine safety in these important populations. Assessment of effectiveness and safety continues for several years, and thousands of patients may be given the new drug during phase 3.

If the drug continues to show promise through the clinical phase trials, a **New Drug Application (NDA)** is submitted to the FDA. The NDA signals that the pharmaceutical company is ready to sell the new drug. During the NDA review, the FDA examines all preclinical and clinical data to assess whether the proposed new drug is safe and effective. By law, the CDER is obligated to act on at least 90% of the NDAs for standard drugs within 10 months of submission. For priority drugs, the benchmark is 6 months. If the NDA is approved, the manufacturer may begin selling the new drug. If the NDA is rejected, the FDA indicates whether the drug is "approvable" or "not approvable." "Approvable" means that the drug will likely be approved if the pharmaceutical company conducts additional testing or addresses specific issues identified by the FDA. A designation of "not approvable" indicates that the drug has significant barriers to approval.

Postmarketing surveillance, stage 4 of the drug approval process, begins after the NDA review has been completed. The purpose of stage 4 testing is to survey for harmful drug effects in a larger population. Some adverse effects are very subtle, take longer to appear, and are not identified until a drug is prescribed for large numbers of people. Adverse drug reactions are reported by the manufacturers, health care providers, and patients to the Adverse Event Reporting System (AERS), a computerized database designed to support the FDA's postmarketing surveillance program.

The FDA holds public meetings annually to receive comments from patients, professional organizations, and pharmaceutical companies regarding the effectiveness and safety of new drug therapies. If the FDA discovers a serious problem, it will mandate that a drug be withdrawn from the market. One example of successful postmarketing surveillance is the diabetes drug troglitazone (Rezulin), which was approved by the FDA in 1997. In 1998, Britain banned its use after discovering at least one death and several cases of liver failure in patients with diabetes taking the drug. The FDA became aware of a number of cases in the United States in which Rezulin was linked with liver failure. Consumer advocates also claimed that the drug caused several cases of heart failure. Rezulin was recalled in March 2000 after health professionals asked the FDA to reconsider its therapeutic benefits versus its identified risks. The FDA withdrew 11 prescription drugs from the market from 1997 to 2000.

The drug approval process has several important limitations. Historically, drug trials have used Caucasian males as their test population. Because gender and racial differences may affect how drugs are handled by the body, data obtained during clinical trials may not be representative of the population as a whole. Pharmaceutical companies are now including a more diverse population in their clinical trials. Most drugs have not been tested in children: Pediatric doses and responses are often based on experience rather than research data. Although clinical trials test drugs in pregnant laboratory animals and examine for possible birth defects, these data may not be representative of how drugs affect pregnant women or their fetuses. Finally, adverse effects may occur at such a low level that they are statistically insignificant in clinical trials using a few thousand patients. Several million patients may need to take the drug before these effects can be identified.

Another limitation of the drug approval process relates to off-label uses. When a new drug is tested by a pharmaceutical company it is for a specific indication; FDA approval is based on this indication. After several years of clinical experience, however, health care providers may find that the drug is also useful for indications not approved by the FDA. Once initially approved by the FDA for any indication, health care providers may prescribe the drug for other indications they feel appropriate, despite the fact that the drug was never tested or approved for these additional conditions. How widespread is off-label prescribing? It is estimated that over 20% of prescriptions are for indications not approved by the FDA. The use of off-label drugs is particularly prevalent in cancer treatment and in pediatric patients. Although the FDA does not regulate off-label uses of drugs, laws prohibit pharmaceutical companies from advertising or promoting their drugs for off-label uses. It has not been clearly established whether or not off-label prescriptions increase risks to patients.

PharmFACT

It takes about 12 years of research and development, costing about $350 million, before a drug is submitted to the FDA for review (Drug Information Online, n.d).

CONNECTION Checkpoint 2.1

In 2009, dronendarone (Multaq), an antidysrhythmic, and pazopanib (Votrient), a monoclonal antibody for treating kidney cancer, were approved. Are these considered therapeutic or pharmacologic classifications? *See Answer to Connection Checkpoint 2.1 on student resource website.*

Changes to the Drug Approval Process

6 The U.S. Food and Drug Administration has sped up the process of drug review.

The process of synthesizing a new drug and testing it in cells, experimental animals, and humans takes many years. The NDA can include dozens of volumes of experimental and clinical data that must be examined during the FDA drug review process. Some NDAs contain over 100,000 pages of data. Even after all experiments have been concluded and clinical data have been gathered, the FDA review process can take several years.

Expenses associated with development of a new drug can cost the drug developer millions of dollars. Recent studies estimate the cost of bringing a new drug to market at over $802 million. Pharmaceutical companies are often critical of the regulatory process and are anxious to get the drug marketed to recoup their high research and development expenses. The public is also anxious to receive new medications, particularly for diseases that have a high mortality rate. Although the criticisms of government regulatory agencies are certainly understandable, and sometimes justified, the fundamental priority of the FDA is to ensure the safety of medications. Without an exhaustive review of scientific data, the public could be exposed to dangerous or ineffective drugs.

In the early 1990s, due to pressures from organized consumer groups and various drug manufacturers, government officials began to plan how to speed up the drug review process. Reasons identified for the delay in the FDA drug approval process included outdated guidelines, poor communication, and not enough staff to handle the workload.

In 1992, the PDUFA was passed, requiring drug and biologic manufacturers to provide yearly product user fees. This added income allowed the FDA to hire more employees and to restructure its organization to more efficiently handle the processing of a greater number of drug applications. The result of restructuring was a resounding success. The average NDA review time for new medications approved in 2002 was 12.5 months: less than half the time it took for approval in the early 1990s. Although the approval time has decreased, the actual number of new drugs approved each year has declined from 110 (1996–1999) to 58 (2002–2004), a 47% decline.

As part of the FDA modernization, priority drugs now receive accelerated approval. These are drugs intended to treat serious and life-threatening conditions, such as cancer and AIDS, that lack effective treatments. In some cases, the FDA may grant accelerated approval before the drug has completed phase 3 trials. The FDA usually requires the pharmaceutical company to file subsequent reports confirming the effectiveness of the drug.

PharmFACT

The number of new drugs approved in recent years has been fairly stable: 18 in 2007, 24 in 2008, 25 in 2009, and 21 in 2010 (Drug Information Online, 2011).

Prescription and Over-the-Counter Drugs

7 Over-the-counter drugs are usually safe and effective when used according to label instructions.

The 1951 Durham-Humphrey Amendment to the FDCA clearly established the difference between prescription and OTC drugs. To obtain a prescription drug, an order must be given authorizing the patient to receive the medication. Prescription medications are judged by the FDA to be potentially addictive or too harmful for self-administration. In some cases, they are used to treat conditions too complex for self-diagnosis by the consumer or the drug may require a skilled nurse or health care provider to administer it.

The advantages of requiring a prescription are numerous. The health care provider has an opportunity to examine the patient and determine a specific diagnosis. The prescriber can maximize therapy by ordering the proper drug for the patient's condition and by controlling the amount and frequency of the drug to be dispensed. In addition, the health care provider has an opportunity to teach the patient proper use of the drug and its expected adverse effects.

In contrast to prescription drugs, OTC drugs do not require an order from a health care provider. In most cases, patients may treat themselves safely if they carefully follow instructions included with the medication. A key point to remember is that no drug is without risk; if patients do not follow the guidelines on the label, serious adverse effects may result.

Patients prefer to take OTC medications for many reasons. OTC drugs may be obtained more easily than prescription drugs. No appointment with a health care provider is required, thus saving time and money. Without the assistance of a health care provider, however, choosing the proper medication for a specific problem can be challenging for a patient. OTC drugs may interact with foods, herbal products, prescription drugs, or other OTC drugs. Patients may not be aware that some OTC medications can impair their ability to function safely. Self-treatment is sometimes ineffective, and the potential for harm may increase if the disease is allowed to progress.

During the past decade, consumer groups have pushed for the reclassification of certain drugs from prescription to OTC in cases whereby a high margin of safety exists with the medicines. For example, prior to 1996, substances that were used to assist in smoking cessation, such as nicotine patches and gum, were available by prescription only but are now available OTC. Other recent switches from prescription to OTC include famotidine (Pepcid AC), cimetidine (Tagamet HB), omeprazole (Prilosec), cetirizine (Zyrtec), and loratadine (Claritin). Over the past 20 years, 700 products have been changed from prescription to OTC. The decision to reclassify a drug may be initiated by the manufacturer or mandated by the FDA during its review process.

Herbal products and dietary supplements are also widely available OTC. Herbal products and dietary supplements are not considered drugs; they are not marketed to treat any disease, and they are not subject to the same regulatory process as drugs.

Some of these products can, however, cause adverse effects and interact with medications. Nurses should always inquire about their patients' use of herbal products and dietary supplements and caution them that the FDA has not tested these products for effectiveness or safety. In some cases, herbal products are contraindicated. For example, St. John's wort should not be taken concurrently with antidepressant medications.

PharmFACT

Over 900 emergency department visits each year involve the nonmedical use of prescription or OTC pharmaceuticals or dietary supplements. About half of these visits involve multiple drugs, and 18% involve alcohol (Drug Abuse Warning Network, 2011).

Drug Schedules

8 Drugs with a potential for abuse are categorized into schedules.

Dependence is a powerful physiological or psychological need for a substance. Some drugs are frequently abused or have a high potential for dependence; thus the selling and distribution of these drugs are highly restricted. Drugs that have a significant potential for abuse are placed into five categories called *schedules*. These **scheduled drugs** are classified and regulated according to their potential for abuse.

In the United States, **controlled substances** are drugs whose use is restricted by the Comprehensive Drug Abuse Prevention and Control Act of 1970 and its later revisions. Hospitals and pharmacies must register with the Drug Enforcement Administration (DEA) and use their registration numbers to purchase scheduled drugs. They must maintain complete records of all quantities purchased and sold. Drugs with the highest abuse potential have additional restrictions. For example, providers must use a special order form to obtain Schedule II drugs, and orders must be written and signed by the provider. Telephone orders to a pharmacy are not permitted. Refills for Schedule II drugs are not permitted; patients must visit their health care provider first. Health providers convicted of unlawful manufacturing, distributing, and dispensing of controlled substances face severe penalties.

CONNECTION Checkpoint 2.2

Once a new drug is approved, it is assigned names. What are the two basic types of drug names and who assigns them? *See Answer to Connection Checkpoint 2.2 on student resource website.*

Canadian Drug Standards

9 Canadian regulations ensure safe and effective drug use in the provinces and territories.

There are many similarities between how drugs are regulated in Canada and in the United States. In Canada, as in the United States, drug testing and risk assessment are major priorities. The steps in the Canadian drug approval process are shown in Table 2.

Health Canada is the federal department working in partnership with provincial and territorial governments. The Health Products and Food Branch (HPFB) of Health Canada is responsible for ensuring that health products and foods approved for sale to Canadians are safe and of high quality. The HPFB regulates the use of therapeutic products through directorates. The Therapeutic Products Directorate (TPD) authorizes marketing of a pharmaceutical drug or medical device, once a manufacturer presents sufficient scientific evidence of the product's safety, efficacy, and quality as required by the Food and Drugs Act and Regulations. The Biologics and Genetic Therapies Directorate (BGTD) regulates biologic drugs and radiopharmaceuticals. Products regulated by the BGTD include blood products, vaccines, tissues, organs, and gene therapy products. The Natural Health Products Directorate (NHPD) is the regulating authority for natural health products for sale in Canada.

The Canadian Food and Drugs Act is an important regulatory document specifying that drugs cannot be marketed without a Notice of Compliance (NOC) and Drug Identification Number (DIN) from Health Canada. Foods, drugs, cosmetics, and therapeutic devices must follow established guidelines for approval. Any drug that does not comply with standards established by recognized pharmacopeias and formularies in the United States, Europe, Britain, or France cannot be labeled, packaged, sold, or advertised in Canada.

TABLE 2	Steps of Approval for Drugs Marketed Within Canada
Step 1	Preclinical studies or experiments in culture, living tissue, and small animals are performed, followed by extensive clinical trials or testing done on humans.
Step 2	A drug company completes a drug submission to Health Canada. This report details important safety and effectiveness information, including testing data, how the drug product will be produced and packaged, and expected therapeutic benefits and adverse reactions.
Step 3	A committee of drug experts, including medical and drug scientists, reviews the drug submission to identify potential benefits and drug risks.
Step 4	Health Canada reviews information about the drug product and passes on important details to health providers and consumers.
Step 5	Health Canada issues a Notice of Compliance (NOC) and Drug Identification Number (DIN). Both permit the manufacturer to market the drug product.
Step 6	Health Canada monitors the effectiveness of the drug and any concerns after it has been marketed. This is done by regular inspection, notices, newsletters, and feedback from consumers and health care providers.

UNDERSTANDING THE CHAPTER

Key Concepts Summary

1 Early American history saw the rise of patent medicines and the lack of adequate drug regulations.

2 In the 1900s, drug legislation was enacted to make drugs safer and more effective.

3 The standardization of drug purity and strength is specified by the *United States Pharmacopeia-National Formulary.*

4 The regulatory agency responsible for ensuring that drugs and medical devices are safe and effective is the U. S. Food and Drug Administration.

5 The drug approval process established by the Food and Drug Administration ensures that drugs sold in the United States are safe and effective.

6 The U.S. Food and Drug Administration has sped up the process of drug review.

7 Over-the-counter drugs are usually safe and effective when used according to label instructions.

8 Drugs with a potential for abuse are categorized into schedules.

9 Canadian regulations ensure safe and effective drug use in the provinces and territories.

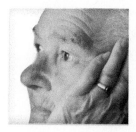

Making the PATIENT Connection

Remember the patient "Gertrude Stone" at the beginning of the chapter? Now read the remainder of the case study. Based on the information presented within this chapter, respond to the critical thinking questions that follow.

Gertrude Stone lives alone in the same house she has owned for 46 years. Although she is seldom sick, when she needs to see a health care provider she must ride the public bus system. The trip requires two bus transfers and can be tiring.

Because Gertrude lives only one block from a grocery store, she often self-medicates using OTC drugs. She strongly believes in the use of herbs, vitamins, and home remedies.

As a parish nurse, you assist with the health fair at a church where Gertrude is an active member.

Critical Thinking Questions

1. How would you respond to Gertrude about the safety of OTC drugs?
2. What are the advantages and disadvantages of OTC medications?
3. How can Gertrude be certain that OTC medications are safe for her?

See Answers to Critical Thinking Questions on student resource website.

NCLEX-RN® Review

1 The nurse knows that governmental drug legislation requires the drug manufacturer to prove that a drug is both safe and:
1. Free of adverse effects and potential reactions.
2. Effective for a specified purpose.
3. Reasonable in cost and easily accessible.
4. Beneficial to various population groups.

2 The drug research participant with a particular disease is taking part in an investigative study to examine the effects of a new drug. Previously, this drug was tested using healthy volunteers. In which phase of the clinical trial investigation is this client participating?
1. Phase 1
2. Phase 2
3. Phase 3
4. Phase 4

3 When considering various drug therapies, the nurse knows that most drug testing and approval occurs with which population?
1. Multiple population types and is usually safe for all clients
2. Caucasian males and may not be safe for other populations
3. The elderly and may be harmful to children and adolescents
4. Animals, which verifies the drug's effectiveness in humans

4 The client requests that a refill prescription of a schedule II controlled substance be telephoned to the drug store. When responding to the client, the nurse would consider which factor? Refills of schedule II drugs:

1. Are less costly than the original prescription.
2. Must be listened to by at least two people.
3. Are verified through the local DEA office.
4. Are not permitted under federal law.

5 The nurse knows that drugs that are subject to stricter regulations are those:

1. With a high potential for abuse or dependency.
2. That are most costly and difficult to produce.
3. With adverse effects and high occurrence of drug or food interactions.
4. That have taken years to be proven effective in the laboratory.

6 A nurse notes that multiple clients had a reaction to the same medication, a drug that has been available for several years. Which action should the nurse take? Select all that apply.

1. File an Adverse Event Report with the FDA.
2. Note the reaction in the client's chart.
3. Notify the health care provider who ordered the drug.
4. Wait until the FDA sends a notification of the drug's recall before informing the client.
5. Compare each client's reaction to determine if it is the same.

Additional Case Study

Your 12-year-old nephew is preparing a report for school about the FDA and the drug approval process. You, the nurse in the family, are often called on by family members to answer questions about anything health related. Below are his questions. How would you respond?

1. What is the role of the FDA?
2. What role does the FDA play in regulating herbal and dietary supplements?
3. How quickly can a new drug be approved by the FDA?

See Answers to Additional Case Study on student resource website.

Pearson Nursing Student Resources

Find additional review materials at
nursing.pearsonhighered.com

Prepare for success with additional NCLEX®-style practice questions, interactive assignments and activities, web links, animations, videos, and more!

References

Drug Abuse Warning Network, 2008. (2011). *National estimates of drug-related emergency department visits.* Retrieved from http://www.oas.samhsa.gov/DAWN/2K8/ED/DAWN2k8ED.htm

Drug Information Online. (n.d.). *New drug approval process.* Retrieved from http://www.drugs.com/fda-approval-process.html

Drug Information Online. (2011). *FDA approval down in 2010.* Retrieved from http://www.drugs.com/news/fda-s-approval-down-2010-28669.html

Selected Bibliography

Berger, M. M., Eck, S., & Ruberg, S. J. (2010). Raising the bar of efficacy for drug approval requires an understanding of patient diversity. *Journal of Clinical Oncology, 28*(20), e343–e344. doi:10.1200/JCO.2010.28.2475

DiMasi, J. A., Feldman, L., Seckler, A., & Wilson, A. (2010). Trends in risks associated with new drug development: Success rates for investigational drugs. *Clinical Pharmacology & Therapeutics, 87*, 272–277. doi:10.1038/clpt.2009.295

Goldberg, N. H., Schneeweiss, S., Kowai, M. K., & Gagne, J. J. (2010). Availability of comparative efficacy data at the time of drug approval in the United States. *Journal of the American Medical Association, 305*(17), 1786–1789. doi:10.1001/jama.2011.539

Lowes, R. (2010). FDA vows to bring its "Regulatory Science" into the 21st century. *Medscape Medical News,* Retrieved from http://www.medscape.com/viewarticle/730061

Marshall, V., & Baylor, N. W. (2011). Food and drug administration regulation and evaluation of vaccines. *Pediatrics, 127*, S23–S30. doi:10.1542/peds.2010-1722E

Radley, D. C., Finkelstein, S. N., & Stafford, R. S. (2006). Off-label prescribing among office-based physicians. *Archives of Internal Medicine, 166*, 1021–1026. doi:10.1001/archinte.166.9.1021

Tsuji, K., & Tsutani, K. (2010). Approval of new drugs 1999–2007: Comparison of the US, the EU and Japan situations. *Journal of Clinical Pharmacy and Therapeutics, 35*, 289–301. doi:10.1111/j.1365-2710.2009.01099.x

Wellman-Labadie, W. (2010). The U.S. orphan drug act: Rare disease research stimulator or commercial opportunity? *Health Policy, 95*(2), 216–228. doi:10.1016/j.healthpol.2009.12.001

Wertheimer, A. (2011). Off label prescribing of drugs for children. *Current Drug Safety, 6*(1), 44–48. doi:10.2174/157488611794479973

Answers to NCLEX-RN® Review

1 Answer: 2 Rationale: The FDA requires that drug manufacturers demonstrate both the safety and effectiveness of pharmaceutical products. Options 1, 3, and 4 are incorrect. All drugs have potential reactions and adverse effects. Many factors determine the cost of a drug and newly approved drugs may be the most expensive and not fully covered by health care insurance plans. Not all drugs have been tested in diverse populations and women, minority ethnic groups, children, and the older adults are often underrepresented in drug research studies. Cognitive Level: Applying; Client Need: Safe and Effective Care Environment; Nursing Process: Implementation

2 Answer: 2 Rationale: Phase 2 of the clinical investigation relies on studying clients with the disease to be treated. Options 1, 3, and 4 are incorrect. Phase 1 studies use small groups of healthy subjects. Phase 3 studies use large numbers of subjects with the condition being treated by the drug. Phase 4 is considered postmarketing surveillance after the drug has been approved. Cognitive Level: Applying; Client Need: Safe and Effective Care Environment; Nursing Process: Implementation

3 Answer: 2 Rationale: Most drug testing occurs using Caucasian males which may limit the generalization of the results to other populations. Options 1, 3, and 4 are incorrect. Drug testing is seldom performed on children, women, or older adults. Although many drugs are tested using animals, effectiveness in animals does not always verify that the drug will be effective in humans. Cognitive Level: Applying; Client Need: Safe and Effective Care Environment; Nursing Process: Implementation

4 Answer: 4 Rationale: Telephone orders are not permissible under federal law for schedule II controlled substances. Options 1, 2, and 3 are incorrect. Refill prescriptions are usually not any more or less expensive than the original prescription. The number of listeners is irrelevant. Prescriptions are not confirmed or verified by the DEA. Cognitive Level: Applying; Client Need: Safe and Effective Care Environment; Nursing Process: Implementation

5 Answer: 1 Rationale: The more likely a drug's potential for abuse and dependency, the stricter the regulation to control access to the substance. Options 2, 3, and 4 are incorrect. The cost and production difficulty do not influence the degree of regulation. Adverse effects and drug or food interactions do not dictate the level of regulatory control. The length of time taken to confirm that a drug is effective does not affect the degree of regulation. Cognitive Level: Applying; Client Need: Safe and Effective Care Environment; Nursing Process: Implementation

6 Answer: 1, 2, 3 Rationale: Adverse drug reactions may continue to be discovered well after the FDA approval process as larger groups of clients take the drug. Any reaction should be noted in the client's chart, the provider notified, and an Adverse Event Report filed with the FDA when adverse reactions are noted. Options 4 and 5 are incorrect. Health care providers are responsible for reporting adverse reactions as they occur and should not wait for the FDA to send a recall notice. Many factors influence a client's reaction to medications and each client may not have the same exact reaction to the medication. Cognitive Level: Applying; Client Need: Safe and Effective Care Environment; Nursing Process: Implementation

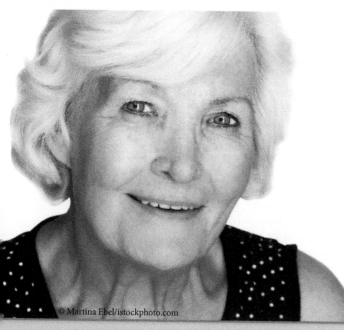

© Martina Ebel/istockphoto.com

"I always save some of my medicines, like antibiotics, just in case I need them later."

Patient "Lavenia Deberry"

Principles of Drug Administration

Chapter Outline

Learning Outcomes

After reading this chapter, the student should be able to:

1. Outline a plan for improving patient adherence to the medication regimen.
2. Describe how the storage of drugs can affect their effectiveness.
3. Describe the components of a legal prescription and the abbreviations associated with drug orders.
4. Relate the importance of dosing schedules to successful pharmacotherapeutic outcomes.
5. Compare and contrast the three systems of measurement used in pharmacology.
6. Explain the importance of properly documenting medication administration.
7. Compare and contrast enteral, topical, and parenteral drug administration.

A primary role of the nurse in drug administration is to ensure that medications are taken in a safe manner according to the instructions of the prescriber or as indicated on the label. In the course of drug administration, nurses will collaborate closely with physicians, pharmacists, other health care providers, and, of course, their patients. The purpose of this chapter is to introduce fundamental principles relating to drug administration that will help nurses to deliver medications safely and effectively.

Drug Administration and Patient Adherence

1 Achieving patient adherence with pharmacotherapy can be a major challenge for the nurse.

In a hospital setting, the pharmacist, nurse, and physician collaborate to ensure that the patient is receiving the correct drug in the manner designated by the prescriber. In the home setting, the focus shifts to self-administration of medications by the patient. For prescription drugs, health care providers provide the patients with verbal and written instructions on how and when to take the medication. For over-the-counter (OTC) medications, herbal products, and dietary supplements, labels clearly indicate the correct way to take the agent.

Adherence is a major factor affecting pharmacotherapeutic outcomes. As it relates to pharmacotherapy, **adherence**, or *compliance*, is defined as taking medications in the manner prescribed by the health care provider. In the case of OTC products, adherence means correctly following the instructions on the label. Patient nonadherence (noncompliance) ranges from not taking the medication at all to taking it at the wrong time or at the wrong dose. Research has confirmed that nonadherence is a major problem in health care, affecting 50% to 75% of patients, and that it is responsible for a significant number of unnecessary hospitalizations and deaths. Studies suggest that about half of all prescriptions never get filled by the patient. Of those that are picked up, about 50% are not taken correctly.

Many factors can influence patient adherence with pharmacotherapy. One of the most common sources of nonadherence is simply forgetting a dose of medication, which occurs frequently when the drug must be taken more than twice daily. Another source of nonadherence is that the drug may be too expensive or not approved by the patient's health insurance plan. Patients often discontinue the use of drugs that have annoying adverse effects or those that impair major lifestyle choices. Adverse effects that often prompt nonadherence are headache, dizziness, nausea, diarrhea, and impotence.

Patients often take medications in an unexpected manner, sometimes self-adjusting their doses. Some feel that if one tablet is good, two must be better. Others believe that they will become dependent on the medication if it is taken as prescribed; thus they only take half the necessary dose. Still others simply stop taking the medication when they start feeling better. Patients are usually reluctant to admit or report nonadherence to the nurse for fear of being reprimanded or feeling embarrassed. Because reasons for nonadherence are many and varied, the nurse must be vigilant in questioning patients about taking their medications. When pharmacotherapy fails to produce the expected treatment outcomes, nonadherence should always be considered as a possible explanation.

There are steps that the nurse can take to increase the potential for patient adherence to the therapeutic regimen. All of these steps focus on effective teaching. Before administering a drug, the nursing process should be used to formulate a personalized care plan that will best enable the patient to become an active participant in the treatment. This allows the patient to better understand and accept the recommended course of pharmacotherapy based on accurate information that is presented in a manner that addresses individual learning styles in terms that the patient can understand.

In the plan of care, it is important to address essential information that the patient must know regarding the prescribed medications. This includes factors such as the name of the medication, why it has been ordered, expected drug actions, associated adverse effects, and information regarding interactions with other medications, foods, herbal supplements, or alcohol. Patients need to be reminded that they share an active role in ensuring the effectiveness of their medication and their own safety.

For patients receiving outpatient therapy or those being released from a hospital, the nurse must carefully assess patients' ability to take their medications in a safe and effective manner. If the nurse believes that a patient may have difficulty in properly administering the medications, caregivers should be consulted and other arrangements made to ensure that the patient receives the correct drugs using the proper dosing schedule. During follow-up visits, the nurse should reinforce this drug education and assess whether the patient is taking or receiving the drugs correctly.

It is imperative to remember that, unless diagnosed as mentally incompetent, a well-informed adult always has the legal option of refusal to take any medication. It is the nurse's responsibility, however, to ensure that the patient has all the necessary information to make an informed decision.

Lifespan Considerations

Challenges of Pediatric Medication Administration

Administering medication to infants and young children requires special knowledge and techniques. Nurses must have knowledge of growth and development patterns and be certain that the prescribed dosages match each child's age and weight.

Children, like adults, want to have choices and control over decisions. Whenever possible, give children a choice of the use of a spoon, cup, dropper, or syringe. Approach children with a matter-of-fact attitude and avoid any dishonesty or threats. Allow time and give medications in a calm environment. Depending on a child's age, oral medications may need to be crushed so that the child can swallow them. Sometimes mixing medications with jelly, honey, flavored syrup, or fruit puree can make their taste more palatable for children. One caution is to avoid mixing medications with needed nutrients or foods such as milk or fruit juice because it may cause some children to dislike these foods in the future.

When children get upset or a medication is distasteful, nausea can be averted by allowing sips of cold carbonated beverages or drinks poured over crushed ice. Offer children crackers or dry cereal before medication administration. Encourage cooperation with praise or a reward system suited to the children's ages and interests.

Drug Storage and Expiration Dates

2 Drugs should be stored properly and never used past their expiration date.

Drugs, like most chemicals, degrade over time. As they deteriorate, drugs tend to lose their potency and their ability to produce a therapeutic effect. All drugs are packaged with an **expiration date**, which is an approximation as to when the medications will begin to lose their effectiveness. Drugs do not totally lose their effectiveness or become toxic immediately upon expiration. A large study conducted by the U.S. Food and Drug Administration (FDA) regarding expiration dates examined the potency of over 100 prescription and OTC drugs being stored by the military. The results showed that 90% of them were safe and effective even when 15 years past their expiration date.

Although it is likely that drugs retain some effectiveness beyond their expiration date, the nurse should never administer outdated medications. In clinical agencies, nurses and pharmacists rotate their drug stocks so that drugs are less likely to pass their expiration date.

A large number of storage factors can influence drug effectiveness. Some general principles are:

- **Temperature.** Most drugs should be stored at room temperature because high temperatures encourage faster degradation of the drugs. Some medications require lower temperatures and must be refrigerated or frozen. Drugs should always be administered at room temperature unless otherwise specified by the prescriber.

- **Light.** Because some chemicals are degraded by exposure to light, medications should be stored in cabinets away from direct light. Light-sensitive drugs are often supplied in amber-colored containers to prevent light entry. Some drugs are so light sensitive that their containers must be covered with foil during an intravenous (IV) infusion.

- **Moisture and air.** Drugs sometimes interact with atmospheric gases or with water vapor; thus they should be stored with tightly capped lids. Storage in areas with high humidity will enhance deterioration.

Scheduled drugs are stored in narcotics lockers or boxes. Access to these substances is restricted to protect these drugs from theft or misuse. These boxes have special locks or computerized operating systems and the drugs have additional recording and reporting requirements.

Nurses should become familiar with the specific colors and smells of each medication, because improper storage can sometimes cause changes in the physical characteristics of drugs. A change in color of a liquid drug could indicate contamination or loss of effectiveness. Likewise, for solid drugs, unusual odors, colors, or textures are a cause for concern. Nurses should never administer a drug that appears different from normal without checking with the pharmacist, even if it is within its expiration period. The old adage "when in doubt, throw it out" applies to medicines.

The nurse should teach patients to discard the drugs in their homes that are past their expiration date. Patients tend to keep drugs long past their usefulness, usually in bathroom medicine cabinets. This is an especially dangerous habit in households with small children and is responsible for a large number of accidental poisonings each year. In addition, unused controlled substances are targets for thieves or may be used for intentional overdoses in patients with suicidal ideation. A useful strategy is to encourage a general household review of all drug expiration dates twice yearly when the time changes to, or off of, Daylight Saving Time. Drugs should always be disposed of properly, as listed in Table 1.

Unused cancer drugs (chemotherapy) should never be disposed of in the trash or by flushing down the toilet. Consult the oncology provider or pharmacist about returning the drugs for appropriate disposal.

Prescription Writing

3 Prescriptions must be clearly written and include a heading, a body, and a closing.

An order for a prescription drug follows a standard format, which is designed to ensure that the correct drug is taken by the right patient in the prescribed dose. Each state has specific requirements for what must be included on a legal prescription. Although there are different methods of describing a prescription, all formats must include the following three elements, as shown in Figure 1.

- Heading
- Body
- Closing

TABLE 1 Federal Guidelines for Drug Disposal

Follow any specific disposal instructions on the label or patient information that accompanies the medication.
Take advantage of community drug take-back programs that allow the public to bring unused drugs to a central location for proper disposal. Some communities have pharmaceutical take-back programs or community solid-waste programs that allow the public to bring unused drugs to a central location for proper disposal. Where these exist, they are a good way to dispose of unused pharmaceuticals.
If no instructions are given on the drug label and no take-back program is available, throw the drugs in the trash. Take the drugs out of their original containers and mix them with an undesirable substance, such as used coffee grounds or kitty litter. This will make the drugs less appealing to children and pets, and unrecognizable to people who may go through the trash looking for drugs. Place them in a sealable bag, empty can, or other container to prevent the medication from leaking or breaking out of the garbage bag.
Before throwing out a medication container, scratch out all identifiable information on the label to make it unreadable.
Flush prescription drugs down the toilet only if the label or accompanying patient information specifically instructs doing so. Some states (e.g., California) have environmental laws prohibiting the disposal of drugs into the water system by flushing. Consult a local pharmacist if there are questions about proper disposal.

Source: From "How to Dispose of Unused Medications," U.S. Food and Drug Administration, 2011. Retrieved from http://www.fda.gov/ForConsumers/ConsumerUpdates/ucm101653.htm

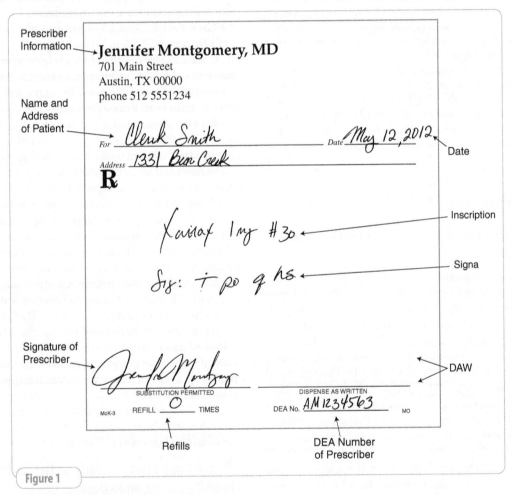

Figure 1

Sample prescription.
Source: From *Fundamentals of Pharmacy Practice* (p. 129), by M. Johnston, 2006, Upper Saddle River, NJ: Pearson Education.

At the top of a prescription, the heading includes the prescriber's name, address, and phone number. This information is essential should the pharmacist need to contact the prescriber for questions about the drug order. The patient's name, and sometimes the phone number and address, are required. The prescription is always dated. Pharmacies have policies that allow them to refuse a prescription if the order is more than a few months old.

The body of the prescription includes the drug name, dosage, and amount to be dispensed. Tablets or capsules usually include the # symbol, which indicates the number to be dispensed. The body also includes patient instructions on the label, including how and when to take the drug. Abbreviations are usually used when prescribing drugs. Common abbreviations associated with medication administration are shown in Table 2. Certain abbreviations are to be avoided because they have been shown to cause frequent medication errors.

The most important feature of the closing of a prescription is the prescriber's signature. A Drug Enforcement

TABLE 2 Medication Administration Abbreviations

Abbreviation	Meaning
ac	before meals
ad lib	as desired/as directed
AM	morning
bid	twice per day
cap	capsule
gtt	drop
h or hr	hour
IM	intramuscular
IV	intravenous
no	number
pc	after meals; after eating
PO	by mouth
PM	afternoon
prn	when needed/necessary
q	every
qh	every hour
qid	four times per day
q2h	every 2 hours
q4h	every 4 hours
q6h	every 6 hours
q8h	every 8 hours
q12h	every 12 hours
Rx	take
stat	immediately; at once
tab	tablet
tid	three times per day

Note: The Institute for Safe Medication Practices recommends that the following abbreviations be avoided because they can lead to medication errors: qd: instead use "daily" or "every day"; qhs: instead use "nightly"; qod: instead use "every other day."

Administration (DEA) number is required if the prescription is for a controlled substance. The closing may also include blanks or boxes, which indicate the number of refills permitted and whether the drug must be dispensed as written (DAW) or a generic equivalent may be substituted.

PharmFACT

From 1997 to 2007, the number of prescriptions purchased increased 72% (from 2.2 billion to 3.8 billion), compared to a U.S. population growth of only 11%. The average number of prescriptions per capita increased from 8.9 to 12.6 (Henry J. Kaiser Family Foundation, 2008).

CONNECTION Checkpoint 3.1

Explain why patients often prefer to take OTC drugs over prescription medications. *See Answer to Connection Checkpoint 3.1 on student resource website.*

Dosing Intervals

4 For maximum effectiveness, drugs must be administered at the proper dosing intervals.

Drugs are administered by a dosing schedule that is largely determined by the physical and biologic characteristics of the drug. As a general rule, drugs that remain longer in the body are administered less frequently than those that are quickly metabolized or eliminated by the body. Normal dosing intervals for oral drugs range from one to four times daily. For the past 20 years, the trend has been to develop drugs that require less frequent dosing because it is more convenient to take a drug once daily and adherence is increased. Patients tend to forget doses when they must be taken more than twice daily, which leads to lower and less consistent levels of the drug in the bloodstream. Dosing intervals are very important to pharmacotherapy.

In the hospital setting, drugs are often administered at specific times of the day, set by agency protocol, that are convenient for the patient and nurse. Some drugs are administered at specific times because this improves their effectiveness or reduces the risk of adverse effects. For example, if a drug causes stomach upset, it is often administered with meals to reduce epigastric pain, nausea, or vomiting. Certain other medications should be administered between meals because food interferes with their absorption. Some central nervous system (CNS) drugs and antihypertensives are best taken at bedtime, because they may cause daytime drowsiness. Drugs such as sildenafil (Viagra) are unique in that they should be taken 30 to 60 minutes prior to expected sexual intercourse in order to achieve an effective erection. Patients must be taught the importance of proper dose scheduling to enhance the potential for therapeutic success.

Medications that are given on a regular schedule are called *standing orders*. Standing orders may be continued indefinitely or they may have a date upon which they terminate. Some medications are given only once or by irregular scheduling. For example, a *stat order* refers to a medication that is needed immediately, usually because of an emergency or life-threatening situation. A *prn order* (Latin: *pro re nata*) is administered as required by the patient's condition. The nurse makes the judgment, based on patient assessment, as to when such a medication is to be administered. The prescriber may qualify the time frame of prn orders. For example, prn q4h would direct the nurse to administer the drug only once every 4 hours.

When self-administering medications, it is not unusual for a patient to forget a dose. This is especially true for patients taking multiple prescription drugs and those who have some degree of mental impairment. In most cases, taking a missed dose several hours late will not affect the outcomes of pharmacotherapy; thus patients should be urged to take their medication as soon as they discover the error. Some drugs, however, have a more rigid dosing schedule and forgetting a dose can result in serious effects. For example, taking multiple doses of the anticoagulant warfarin (Coumadin) too close together can cause bleeding. If the omission is discovered at a time very close to when the next dose is to be taken, the patient should skip the missed dose. Patients should be reminded never to take a double dose (or skip a dose), unless advised to do so by their health care provider. Some drugs, such as oral contraceptives, come with very specific patient instructions on the procedure to follow if a dose is missed.

Measurement of Drug Doses

5 The primary system of measurement used in pharmacology is the metric system.

Every OTC drug label and prescription must indicate the dose to be administered. Dosages are labeled and dispensed according to their weight (for solid drugs) or volume (for liquid drugs). Three systems of measurement are used in pharmacology: metric, household, and apothecary. Although health care providers and pharmacies primarily use the metric system, the apothecary and household systems are still encountered. Until the metric system totally replaces these other systems, the nurse must recognize dosages based on all three systems of measurement. Approximate equivalents between metric, apothecary, and household units of volume and weight are listed in Table 3.

By far, the most common system of drug measurement in pharmacology uses the **metric system of measurement**. The volume of a medication is expressed in terms of the liter (L) or milliliter (mL). The cubic centimeter (cc) is a common measurement of volume that is equivalent to 1 milliliter of fluid. Although cc is commonly used in clinical practice, note that mL is preferred because it results in fewer medical errors (see Table 2). The metric weight of a drug is stated in terms of kilograms (kg), grams (g), milligrams (mg), or micrograms (mcg or μg). Although scientists use the symbol μ for "micro," it is strongly recommended that mcg be used in prescription writing: When poorly written (as many prescriptions are), the symbol μ can be misinterpreted as "m" and cause medication errors.

Although not used very frequently in the health care setting, the **household system of measurement** is familiar to most Americans. Because patients understand the teaspoon, tablespoon, and cup, it is important for the nurse to be able to convert between the household and metric systems of measurement. For example, an 8-ounce glass of water is 240 mL. If a patient being discharged is ordered to drink 2,400 mL of fluid per day, the nurse may instruct the patient to drink 10 eight-ounce glasses or 10 cups of fluid per day. Likewise, when a child is to be given a drug that is administered in elixir form, the nurse should explain that 5 mL of the drug is the same as 1 teaspoon. The nurse should encourage the use of accurate medical dosing devices at home, such as oral dosing syringes, oral droppers, cylindrical spoons, and medication cups. These are preferred over the traditional household measuring spoon because they are more accurate. Eating utensils that are commonly referred to as teaspoons or tablespoons often do not hold the volume that their names imply.

The **apothecary system of measurement** was developed in ancient Greece. The system became popular in England in the 1600s and came to America with the colonists. In early U.S. history, apothecaries performed many of the same duties as physicians, including preparing and administering drugs and performing medical procedures, including surgery. Until the 1970s, apothecary units were still widely used when measuring pharmaceuticals. The basic unit, the grain (gr), was defined as the weight of one grain of wheat. It is now rare to find the apothecary system in use, although occasionally an aspirin tablet is referred to as being 5 grains (325 mg).

Dosage calculation is a skill that may seem less necessary today than in previous times because many drugs are dispensed in doses that are packaged by the pharmacy or manufacturer for unit dispensing, making dosage calculations unnecessary. Doses of solid drugs are often ordered in multiples of the prescribed dose, such as one or two pills per dose. The most complex dosage calculations, flow rates for IV medications, are simplified by the use of modern delivery devices. Correctly calculating the dose of a medication, however, is a key responsibility of the nurse because errors in simple calculations can have devastating consequences for the patient and bring litigation against the nurse. The nurse is responsible for checking that the dose packaged by the pharmacy is correct and for maintaining proficiency in dosage calculation.

Documenting Drug Administration

6 Medication administration should be properly recorded as soon as possible after the drug is administered.

Once a drug is administered, the nurse must correctly document on the **medication administration record (MAR)** that it has been given to the patient. Delay in documentation could result in a second dose being administered. It is not permissible to document medication before it is administered, because an emergency or other distraction could result in the medication not being given. Because the patient's chart is a medico-legal

TABLE 3 Metric, Apothecary, and Household Approximate Measurement Equivalents

Metric	Apothecary	Household
1 mL	15–16 minims	15–16 drops
4–5 mL	1 fluid dram	1 teaspoon or 60 drops
15–16 mL	4 fluid drams	1 tablespoon or 3–4 teaspoons
30–32 mL	8 fluid drams or 1 fluid ounce	2 tablespoons
240–250 mL	8 fluid ounces (1/2 pint)	1 glass or cup
500 mL	1 pint	2 glasses or 2 cups
1 L	32 fluid ounces or 1 quart	4 glasses or 4 cups or 1 quart
1 mg	1/60 grain	—
60–64 mg	1 grain	—
300–325 mg	5 grains	—
1 g	15–16 grains	—
1 kg	—	2.2 pounds

Note: To convert grains to grams, divide grains by 15 or 16. To convert grams to grains, multiply grams by 15 or 16. To convert minims to milliliters, divide minims by 15 or 16.

document, any errors, falsifications, or omissions in documenting drug administration could have legal consequences.

It is necessary to include on the MAR the drug's name, dosage, time administered, any assessments related to drug administration, and the nurse's signature. Drugs that are refused or omitted must be recorded on the appropriate form within the MAR. It is customary to document the reason for the nonmedication whenever possible. Patient concerns or complaints about the drug are also included. Documentation includes the signature or initials of the nurse who administered the drug. As health care agencies transition to the use of electronic medical records (EMRs), these tasks will be automated but will still be required to maintain patient safety in medication administration.

Routes of Drug Administration

The three broad categories of routes of drug administration are enteral, topical, and parenteral. Each route has characteristics that offer both advantages and disadvantages. Whereas some drugs are formulated to be given by several routes, others are specific to only one route. Certain general protocols and techniques common to all methods of drug administration are shown in Table 4.

7 Enteral drugs are administered by the oral route or through gastrostomy or nasogastric tubes.

The **enteral route** includes drugs delivered to the gastrointestinal (GI) tract, either orally or through nasogastric or gastrostomy tubes. Oral medication administration is the most common, most convenient, and usually the least costly of all

routes. It is also considered the safest route because the skin barrier is not compromised. In cases of overdose, drugs remaining in the stomach can be retrieved by inducing vomiting or by pumping out the stomach contents.

Most medications administered by the enteral route are intended for absorption to the general circulation, taking advantage of the combined absorptive surfaces of the oral mucosa, stomach, and small intestine. A few enteral medications are administered for local effects, such as infections of the GI tract. Oral preparations are available in tablet, capsule, and liquid forms.

Tablets and Capsules

Tablets and capsules are the most common forms of oral medications. Most patients prefer tablets or capsules because of their ease of use. In some cases, tablets may be scored, allowing for one-half or one-quarter dosing.

The body's strongly acidic stomach contents can present a destructive obstacle to some medications. To overcome this barrier, tablets may have a hard, waxy coating that enables them to resist acidity. These **enteric-coated** tablets are designed to dissolve in the alkaline environment of the small intestine. Some drugs are enteric coated because the agents will irritate the stomach mucosa if they dissolve in the stomach.

Studies have clearly demonstrated that patient adherence declines as the number of doses per day increases. **Extended release** (XR, XL) tablets or capsules are designed to dissolve very slowly, resulting in a longer duration of action for the medication. Also called long-acting (LA) or sustained release (SR) medications, these forms allow for the convenience of once or twice a day dosing.

Some patients, particularly children, have difficulty swallowing tablets and capsules. Crushing tablets or opening capsules and sprinkling the medication over food or mixing it with juice may make the drug more palatable and easier to swallow. The nurse should not crush tablets or open capsules, however, unless the manufacturer specifically states this is permissible. The following type of drugs should not be chewed, crushed, or opened:

- **Extended release formulations.** These drugs contain a high amount of medication that is intended to be released over an extended period. Opening the capsule or crushing the tablet will release the entire drug immediately, possibly resulting in a toxic effect.
- **Enteric-coated drugs.** When crushed or opened, these drugs are exposed to stomach acid, which may destroy them. In addition, the drugs may irritate the stomach mucosa and cause nausea or vomiting.
- **Oral cavity effects.** Drugs that have a bitter taste are often coated with a very thin layer of glucose or inert material to mask their taste. If crushed or opened, the bitter taste is experienced. Other drugs stain the teeth or cause an anesthetic-like effect on the tongue if crushed and exposed to the oral cavity. In addition, some drugs irritate the oral mucosa.

Selected drugs that should not be crushed are shown in Table 5. The student should refer to a current drug guide for a more comprehensive list.

TABLE 4 General Drug Administration Guidelines
Verify the medication order for accuracy.
Check the allergy history on the chart.
Identify any conditions that may result in a change in dosage, such as cardiac, renal, or hepatic impairment or potential drug–drug interactions. Notify the prescriber of any discrepancies.
Wash hands and apply gloves, if indicated (e.g., parenteral, rectal, vaginal routes).
Use aseptic technique when preparing and administering parenteral medications.
Identify the patient by asking the person to state his or her full name (or by asking the parent or guardian), checking the identification band, and comparing this information with the MAR.
Ask the patient about known allergies.
Inform the patient of the name of the drug, the expected actions and adverse effects, and how it will be administered.
Position the patient for the appropriate route of administration.
For enteral drugs, assist the patient to a sitting position.
If the drug is prepackaged (unit dose), remove it from the packaging at the bedside when possible.
Unless specifically instructed to do so in the orders, do not leave drugs at the bedside.
Document the medication administration and any pertinent patient responses on the MAR.
Evaluate the patient's response to the drug, reporting any adverse effects.

TABLE 5 Selected Drugs That Should Not Be Crushed or Opened

Trade Name	Generic Name	Dosage Form	Comments
Accutane	isotretinoin	Capsule	Mucous membrane irritant
Adalat CC	nifedipine	Tablet	Sustained release
Adderall XR	amphetamine	Capsule	Sustained release
Ambien CR	zolpidem	Tablet	Controlled release
Augmentin XR	amoxicillin	Tablet	Sustained release
Bayer Caplet	aspirin, enteric coated	Caplet	Enteric coated
Calan SR	verapamil	Tablet	Sustained release
Cardizem LA, Cardizem CD, Cardizem SR	diltiazem	Tablet Capsule Tablet	Sustained release; capsules may be opened and contents taken without chewing or crushing
Cipro XR	ciprofloxacin	Tablet	Sustained release
Compazine Spansule	prochlorperazine	Capsule	Sustained release; capsules may be opened and contents taken without chewing or crushing
Cotazym S	pancrelipase	Capsule	Enteric coated; capsules may be opened and contents taken without chewing or crushing
Covera-HS	verapamil	Tablet	Sustained release
Cymbalta	duloxetine	Capsule	Sustained release
Depakene	valproic acid	Capsule	Sustained release; mucous membrane irritant
Depakote ER	valproate	Tablet	Sustained release
Dilacor XR	diltiazem	Capsule	Sustained release
Dilatate SR	isosorbide dinitrate	Capsule	Sustained release
Eskalith CR	lithium	Tablet	Sustained release
Feosol	ferrous sulfate	Tablet	Enteric coated
Glucotrol XL	glyburide	Tablet	Sustained release
Inderal LA	propranolol	Capsule	Sustained release
Indocin SR	indomethacin	Capsule	Sustained release; capsules may be opened and contents taken without chewing or crushing
Isoptin SR	verapamil	Tablet	Sustained release
Isosorbide dinitrate SR	isosorbide dinitrate	Tablet	Sustained release
Kaon CL, Klor-Con, Klotrix, K-Tab, Slow-K	potassium chloride	Tablet	Sustained release
Morphine sulfate extended release	morphine	Tablet	Sustained release
Nexium	esomeprazole	Capsule	Sustained release
Nicotinic acid	niacin	Tablet, capsule	Sustained release
Nitrostat	nitroglycerin	Tablet	Sublingual
OxyContin	oxycodone	Tablet	Sustained release
Plendil	felodipine	Tablet	Sustained release
Prevacid	lansoprazole	Capsule	Sustained release; capsules may be opened and contents taken without chewing or crushing
Prilosec	omeprazole	Capsule	Sustained release
Procardia XL	nifedipine	Tablet	Sustained release
Ritalin SR	methylphenidate	Tablet	Sustained release
Sinemet SR	levodopa, carbidopa	Tablet	Sustained release; tablet is scored and may be broken in half
Tessalon Perles	benzonatate	Capsule	Will anesthetize tongue and mouth if chewed
Toprol XL	metoprolol	Tablet	Sustained release
Trental	pentoxifylline	Tablet	Sustained release
Wellbutrin SR, XL	bupropion	Tablet	Sustained release

As an alternative to crushing, some drugs are available in liquid form for patients who have difficulty swallowing tablets or capsules. Liquid forms include elixirs, syrups, and suspensions. Liquid drugs are usually heavily flavored and sweetened to mask their bitter taste.

Another more recent alternative to crushing is the orally disintegrating tablet (ODT). Most ODTs are soft and designed to dissolve on the tongue in less than 30 seconds, without the need to drink water. ODTs are convenient and are appropriate for certain patient populations, such as those who have difficulty chewing or swallowing and patients who are mentally retarded, nauseated, or uncooperative. Because of their widespread acceptance, ODTs are now available for dozens of medications.

A few drugs are formulated as lozenges, or **troches**, which are allowed to slowly dissolve in the mouth. Most patients are familiar with OTC throat lozenges, which are used to dampen a cough or ease a sore throat. One of the most common prescription troches is clotrimazole (Mycelex Troche), a drug for treating fungal infections of the oral cavity. The nurse should teach patients to allow the troche to slowly dissolve and not to swallow it whole.

Tablets (other than ODTs), liquids, and capsules have certain disadvantages. The patient must be conscious and able to swallow properly. Certain types of drugs, including proteins such as insulin, are inactivated by the digestive enzymes in the stomach and small intestine. Furthermore, drugs absorbed from the stomach and small intestine first travel to the liver, where they may be inactivated before they ever reach their target organs—a process called first-pass metabolism. There is also significant variation among patients in the motility of the GI tract and in its ability to absorb medications. In addition, children and some adults have an aversion to swallowing large tablets and capsules or to taking oral medications that taste bad.

PharmFACT

Although both are given by mouth, the same drug administered by the oral and ODT routes may have different doses. This is because the oral cavity mucosa absorbs some drugs at a different rate than the gastric mucosa (Hirani, Rathod, & Vadalia, 2009).

Sublingual and Buccal Drug Administration

Sublingual and buccal administrations are enteral routes in which the tablets are not swallowed but instead are kept in the mouth. Unlike troches, which are slowly dissolved in the mouth to treat a local condition (sore throat or oral infections), sublingual and buccal drugs are intended to be absorbed. The mucosa of the oral cavity contains extensive capillaries that provide an excellent absorptive surface for certain drugs. Medications given by this route are not subjected to destructive stomach acid, and they do not undergo hepatic first-pass metabolism.

For the sublingual route, the medication is placed under the tongue and allowed to slowly dissolve. Because of the rich blood supply to this region, the sublingual route results in a rapid onset of drug action. Sublingual dosage forms are most often formulated as rapidly disintegrating tablets or as soft gelatin capsules filled with liquid drug.

When multiple medications are ordered, the sublingual preparations should be administered after oral medications have been swallowed. The patient should be instructed not to move the drug with the tongue or to eat or drink anything until the medication has completely dissolved. The sublingual mucosa is not suitable for extended release formulations because it is a relatively small area and is constantly being bathed by a substantial amount of saliva that will remove these drugs from the region. Figure 2a illustrates sublingual drug administration.

To administer drugs by the buccal route, the tablet is placed in the oral cavity between the gum and cheek. The patient must be instructed not to manipulate the drug with the tongue; otherwise it could get displaced to the sublingual area, where it will be more rapidly absorbed, or to the back of the throat, where it could be swallowed. The buccal mucosa is thicker and less permeable to medications than the sublingual area, providing for slower absorption. The buccal route is preferred over the sublingual route for sustained release delivery because of its greater mucosal surface area. For example, testosterone, a drug normally given by injection, is available in a buccal form (Striant). Buccal testosterone releases the drug over 12 hours and gives a more consistent, sustained drug level than does the transdermal patch delivery system for testosterone. Drugs formulated for buccal administration generally do not cause irritation and are small enough to not cause discomfort to the patient. Like the sublingual route, drugs administered by the buccal route avoid first-pass metabolism by the liver and the enzymatic processes of the stomach and small intestine. Figure 2b illustrates buccal drug administration.

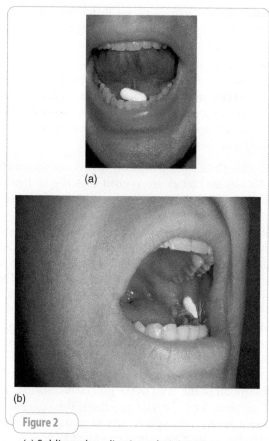

(a)

(b)

Figure 2

(a) Sublingual medication administration;
(b) buccal medication administration.

35

Nasogastric and Gastrostomy Drug Administration

Patients with a nasogastric (NG) tube or an enteral feeding mechanism, such as a gastrostomy (G) tube, may have their medications administered through these devices. An NG tube is a soft, flexible tube inserted by way of the nasopharynx with the tip lying in the stomach. A G tube is surgically placed directly into the patient's stomach. Generally, an NG tube is used for short-term treatment, whereas the G tube is inserted for patients requiring long-term care. Drugs administered through these tubes are usually in liquid form. Although solid drugs can be crushed or dissolved, they tend to clog the tubes. Sustained release medications should not be crushed and administered through NG or G tubes. Drugs administered by these routes are exposed to the same physiological processes as those given orally. NG and G tubes should be flushed according to agency policy to maintain patency before and after administration of medications.

8 Topical medications are applied to the skin or mucous membranes.

The **topical route** of drug administration includes medications applied to the skin or the membranous linings of the eye, ear, nose, respiratory tract, urinary tract, vagina, and rectum. Types of topical applications include the following:

- Dermatologic preparations are drugs applied to the skin. Skin is the topical route most commonly used. Formulations include creams, lotions, ointments, gels, powders, and sprays.

- Instillations and irrigations are drugs applied into body cavities or orifices. These include the eyes, ears, nose, urinary bladder, rectum, and vagina.

- Inhalations are drugs applied to the respiratory tract by inhalers, nebulizers, or positive pressure breathing machines. The most common indication for inhaled drugs is bronchoconstriction caused by asthma. However, a number of illegal, abused drugs are taken by this route because it provides a very rapid onset of drug action.

Many drugs are applied topically to produce a local effect. For example, antibiotics are applied topically to treat skin infections. Antineoplastic agents may be instilled into the urinary bladder via catheter to treat localized tumors of the bladder mucosa. Corticosteroids are sprayed into the nostrils to reduce inflammation of the nasal mucosa due to allergic rhinitis. Topical delivery produces fewer adverse effects compared to the same drug given orally or parenterally. This is because, when given topically, drugs are absorbed more slowly and the amount of the drug reaching the general circulation is minimal. The most common adverse events resulting from topical administration are transient burning, stinging, or redness of the area where they are applied.

Some drugs are given topically to provide for slow release and absorption of the drug to the general circulation. These agents are given for their systemic effects. For example, a nitroglycerin patch is not applied to the skin to treat a local skin condition but to treat a systemic condition such as coronary artery disease. Likewise, prochlorperazine (Compazine) suppositories are inserted rectally not to treat a disease of the rectum but to alleviate nausea.

The distinction between topical drugs given for local effects and those administered for systemic effects is an important one for the nurse. In the case of local drugs, absorption is undesirable and may result in adverse effects if the drug reaches the systemic circulation. For systemic drugs, absorption across the skin or mucous membrane is essential for the therapeutic action of the drug. With either type of topical agent, medication should not be applied to abraded or denuded skin because this could affect drug absorption.

Transdermal Delivery System

The use of **transdermal patches** provides an effective means of delivering certain medications. Examples include nitroglycerin to treat angina pectoris, testosterone for hypogonadism, and scopolamine (Transderm Scop) for motion sickness. Transdermal patches contain a specified amount of medication, although the rate of delivery and the actual dose received can vary. Patches are changed on a regularly scheduled basis using a site rotation routine, which should be documented in the MAR. Before applying a transdermal patch, the nurse should verify that the previous patch has been removed and disposed of appropriately. For optimum dosing, patches should not be applied to hairy areas of the skin, and they should never be applied to skin that is abraded or denuded. Medications administered by this route avoid the first-pass effect in the liver and bypass digestive enzymes. Figure 3 illustrates the application of a transdermal drug.

Ophthalmic Administration

The ophthalmic route is used to treat local conditions of the eye and surrounding structures. Common indications include excessive dryness, eye infections, glaucoma, and dilation of the pupil during eye examinations. Ophthalmic medications are available in the form of eye irrigations, drops, ointments, and medicated disks. Ophthalmic drugs are absorbed into the systemic circulation via drainage of the drug into the nasolacrimal ducts and subsequently to the nasopharynx and the GI tract. Generally this is a slow process and only small amounts reach the general circulation; thus ophthalmic drugs cause few systemic adverse effects. Infants are an exception. The concentration of drugs reaching the systemic circulation is higher than in an adult, giving a greater chance for adverse drug events. With a child, it is advisable to enlist the help of an adult caregiver to better immobilize the patient to prevent accidental injury to the eye during administration. Ophthalmic administration is shown in Figure 4a.

Otic Administration

The otic route is used to treat local conditions of the ear, including infections and accumulations of earwax in the auditory canal. Otic medications include eardrops and irrigations, which are usually ordered for cleaning purposes, as shown in Figure 4b. Administration to infants and young children must be performed carefully to avoid injury to the tympanic membrane. Otic medications should always be brought to

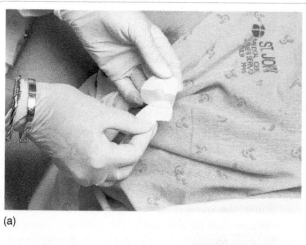

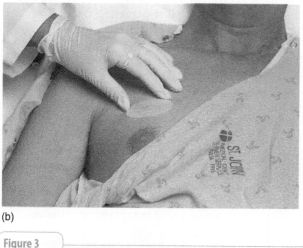

Figure 3

Transdermal patch administration: (a) Protective coating is removed from the patch. (b) The patch is immediately applied to clean, dry, and hairless skin and labeled with the date, time, and initials.

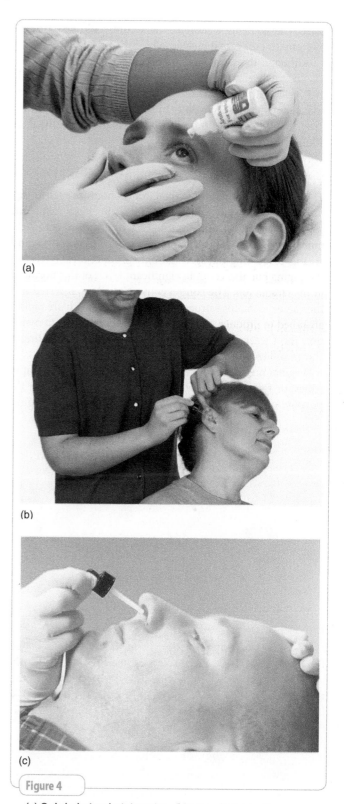

Figure 4

(a) Ophthalmic administration; (b) otic administration; (c) intranasal administration.
Source: (b) DK Images

room temperature before administration because cold medications may cause dizziness or nausea. Systemic adverse effects from otic preparations are not observed unless the drug is applied to areas of open abrasions or injury, such as a ruptured tympanic membrane.

Intranasal Administration

Drugs are applied by the intranasal route for their local effects on the nasal mucosa or for systemic absorption. Advantages of this route include convenience and rapid onset of action. Local indications include the application of drops or sprays for shrinking swollen nasal mucous membranes or for loosening secretions and facilitating drainage. For example, decongestant nasal sprays bring immediate relief from the nasal congestion caused by the common cold. Intranasal formulations of corticosteroids have revolutionized the treatment of allergic rhinitis due to their effectiveness and high safety margin when administered by this route.

The nasal mucosa also provides an excellent absorptive surface for certain medications to produce systemic actions.

Advantages of this route include avoidance of the first-pass effect and digestive enzymes. For example, an intranasal form of vitamin B_{12} is available that is used for patients lacking intrinsic factor, a substance required for the absorption of this vitamin in the GI tract. Intranasal calcitonin is available to treat osteoporosis. Being a protein, calcitonin would be destroyed by stomach enzymes if given orally.

Although the nasal mucosa provides an excellent surface for drug delivery, there is a potential for damage to the ciliated cells within the nasal cavity, and mucosal irritation is common. Mucus secretion is unpredictable and may inhibit drug absorption from this site. Figure 4c illustrates the nasal administration of drugs.

Vaginal Administration

The **vaginal route** is used to treat local conditions such as vaginal infections, pain, and itching. The vagina has a rich blood supply, and drugs inserted into it may be absorbed across the mucosa and produce systemic effects. For example, vaginal creams containing estrogen not only produce local effects on the vagina but also result in significant levels of this hormone in the circulation. The contraceptive NuvaRing, inserted into the vagina, contains estrogen and progestin, which are rapidly absorbed to produce serum levels sufficient to prevent ovulation for a week. Intravaginal administration of NuvaRing is shown in Figure 5.

Vaginal medications are inserted as suppositories, creams, jellies, or foams. It is important for the nurse to explain the purpose of treatment and provide for privacy during vaginal administration. Before inserting vaginal medications, the patient should be instructed to empty the bladder so there will be less discomfort during treatment and less possibility of irritating or injuring the vaginal lining.

Rectal Administration

The **rectal route** may be used for either local or systemic drug delivery. It is a safe and effective means of delivering medications to comatose patients or to those who are experiencing nausea and vomiting. Rectal medications are normally in suppository form, although a few laxatives and diagnostic agents are given via enema. Although absorption is slower than by other routes, the rectal route is steady and reliable provided the medication can be retained by the patient. Venous blood from the lower rectum is not transported to the circulation by way of the liver; thus the first-pass effect is avoided as are the digestive enzymes of the upper GI tract.

CONNECTION Checkpoint 3.2

Pharmaceutical companies are always exploring novel methods of drug delivery so they may be granted exclusivity. Why is exclusivity important to the pharmaceutical company? *See Answer to Connection Checkpoint 3.2 on student resource website.*

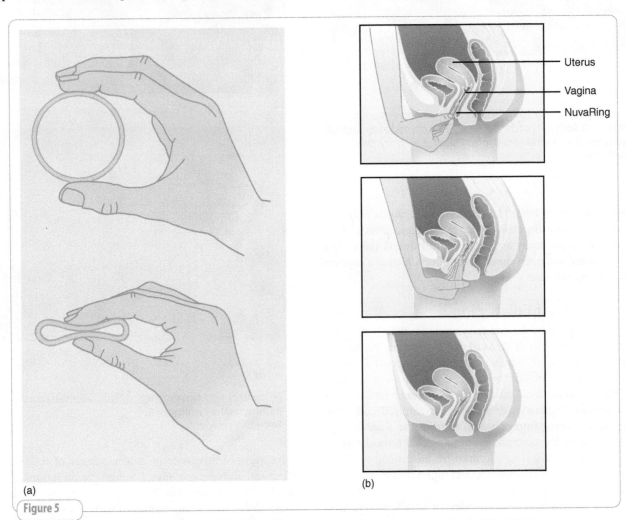

(a)　(b)

Figure 5

Vaginal medication administration: (a) The NuvaRing® contraceptive; (b) proper insertion of the NuvaRing.

9 Parenteral administration is the dispensing of medications via a needle, usually into the skin layers, subcutaneous tissue, muscles, or veins.

The parenteral route refers to the administration of drugs by routes other than enteral or topical. A needle is used to deliver drugs into the skin layers, subcutaneous tissue, muscles, or veins. Less common parenteral delivery methods include administration into arteries (intra-arterial), bone (intraosseous), body cavities (intrathecal), or organs (intracardiac). Parenteral drug administration is more invasive than topical or enteral because of the potential for introducing pathogenic microbes directly into the blood or body tissues. Specialized equipment and techniques are employed in the preparation and administration of injectable products. The nurse must know the correct anatomic locations for parenteral administration, proper administration technique, and safety procedures regarding disposal of hazardous equipment. Injectable medications are frequently supplied in prefilled unit dose systems from the pharmacy.

Intradermal and Subcutaneous Administration

Injection into the skin delivers drugs to the blood vessels that supply the various layers of the skin. Medications may be injected either intradermally or subcutaneously. The major difference between these methods is the depth of injection. An advantage of both methods is that they offer a means of administering drugs to patients who are unable to take medications orally. Drugs administered by these routes avoid digestive enzymes and the hepatic first-pass effect. However, only small volumes can be administered by these routes, and injections can result in pain and swelling at the injection site.

The intradermal (ID) route administers drugs into the dermis layer of the skin. Because the dermis contains more blood vessels than the deeper subcutaneous layer, drugs are more readily absorbed. This route is usually employed for allergy and disease screening or for local anesthetic delivery prior to venous cannulation. ID injections are limited to very small volumes of medication, usually only 0.1 to 0.2 mL. The usual sites for ID injections are the nonhairy skin surfaces of the upper back, over the scapulae, the high upper chest, and the inner forearm. An ID injection is illustrated in Figure 6.

The subcutaneous route delivers drugs to the deepest layers of the skin. Insulin, heparin, vitamins, some vaccines, and other medications are given in this area because the sites are easily accessible and provide for rapid absorption. Body sites that are ideal for subcutaneous injections include the following:

- Outer aspect of the upper arm, above the triceps muscle
- Anterior thigh
- Subscapular area of the upper back
- Upper dorsogluteal and ventrogluteal areas
- Abdomen, above the iliac crest and below the diaphragm, 1½ to 2 inches out from the umbilicus

Subcutaneous doses are small in volume, usually ranging from 0.5 to 1 mL. The needle size varies with the patient's quantity of body fat. The length is usually one half the size of a pinched/bunched skinfold that can be grasped between the thumb and forefinger. It is important to rotate injection sites in an orderly and documented manner to promote absorption, lessen tissue damage, and minimize discomfort. For insulin, rotation should be within an anatomical area to promote reliable absorption and to maintain consistent blood glucose levels. When performing subcutaneous injections, it is not necessary to aspirate prior to the injection. Figure 7 illustrates subcutaneous drug administration.

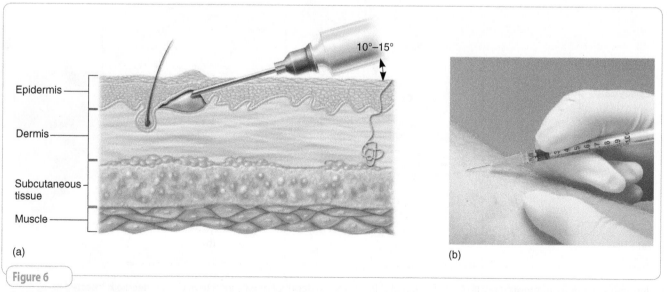

Epidermis

Dermis

Subcutaneous tissue

Muscle

10°–15°

(a)

(b)

Figure 6

Intradermal drug administration: (a) Cross section of skin showing the depth of needle insertion. (b) The needle is inserted with the bevel up at 10–15°.

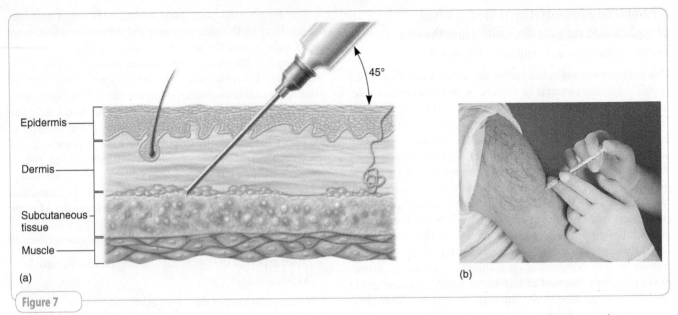

Epidermis

Dermis

Subcutaneous tissue

Muscle

45°

(a)

(b)

Subcutaneous drug administration: (a) Cross section of skin shows the depth of needle insertion. (b) The needle is inserted at a 45° angle.

Intramuscular Administration

The intramuscular (IM) route delivers drugs directly into large muscles. Because muscle tissue has a rich blood supply, drug molecules quickly move into blood vessels to produce a more rapid onset of action than with oral, ID, or subcutaneous administration. In a few cases, the drug is formulated in an oily, viscous base that promotes slow and continuous absorption from the muscle.

The anatomic structure of muscle permits this tissue to receive a larger volume of drug than the subcutaneous region. Adults with well-developed muscles can tolerate up to 3 mL in the gluteus maximus and gluteus medius muscles. In the deltoid muscle, volumes of 0.5 to 1 mL are recommended.

A major consideration for the nurse regarding IM drug administration is the selection of an appropriate injection site. Injection sites must be located away from bone, large blood vessels, and nerves. The size and length of the needle are determined by body size and muscle mass, the specific drug to be administered, the amount of adipose tissue overlying the muscle, and the age of the patient. Figure 8 illustrates IM injections. The four common sites for IM injections are listed in Table 6.

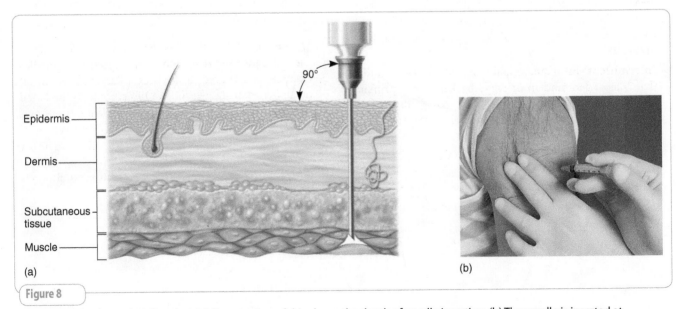

Epidermis

Dermis

Subcutaneous tissue

Muscle

90°

(a)

(b)

Intramuscular drug administration: (a) Cross section of skin shows the depth of needle insertion. (b) The needle is inserted at a 90° angle.

TABLE 6	Sites for Intramuscular Injections
Site	**Description**
Deltoid	Used in well-developed teens and adults for volumes of medication not to exceed 1 mL. Because the radial nerve lies in proximity, the deltoid is not generally used except for small-volume vaccines, such as for hepatitis B in adults.
Dorsogluteal	Used for adults and for children who have been walking for at least 6 months. The site is rarely used due to the potential for damage to the sciatic nerve.
Vastus lateralis	Usually thick and well developed in both adults and children, the middle third of the muscle is the site for IM injections. Sometimes this is considered the site of choice for infants 12 months and younger.
Ventrogluteal	A common site for IM injections. This area provides the greatest thickness of gluteal muscles, contains no large blood vessels or nerves, is sealed off by bone, and contains less fat than the buttock area, thus eliminating the need to determine the depth of subcutaneous fat. It is a suitable site for children and infants older than 7 months of age.

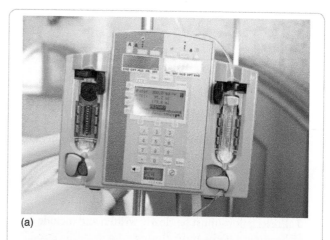

(a)

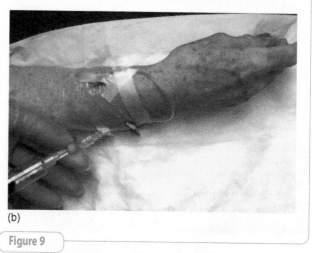

(b)

Figure 9

Intravenous drug administration: (a) syringe pump for IV infusion; (b) injecting a medication by IV push.
Source: (a) © Paul Velgos/istockphoto.com; (b) Carol Urban

Intravenous Administration

The intravenous (IV) route delivers drugs and fluids directly into the bloodstream, which immediately distributes them throughout the body. The IV route is used when a very rapid onset of action is desired. Unlike other routes in which absorption may be unpredictable, an exact level of drug in the bloodstream can be attained by fine adjustments to the IV flow rate. Like other parenteral routes, IV drugs bypass the enzymatic processes of the alimentary canal and avoid the first-pass effect of the liver. The IV route is useful for patients who are comatose or otherwise unable to take oral medications. The three basic types of IV administration include the following:

- **Large-volume infusion.** For fluid maintenance, replacement, or supplementation. Compatible medications may be mixed into a large-volume IV container with fluids such as normal saline or Ringer's lactate, as shown in Figure 9a.

- **Intermittent infusion.** Small amount of IV solution that is arranged tandem or piggy-backed to the primary large-volume infusion. This is used to instill adjunct medications, such as antibiotics or analgesics over a short period.

- **IV bolus (push) administration.** Concentrated dose delivered directly to the circulation via syringe to administer single-dose medications. Bolus injections may be given

through an intermittent injection port or by direct IV push for treating emergencies. The bolus method of administration is illustrated in Figure 9b.

Although the IV route offers the fastest onset of drug action, it is also the most dangerous. Once injected, the medication cannot be retrieved. If the drug solution or the needle is contaminated, pathogens have a direct route to the bloodstream and body tissues. Patients receiving IV injections must be closely monitored for adverse reactions. Although some adverse reactions occur immediately after injection, others may take hours or days to appear. Antidotes for drugs that can cause potentially dangerous or fatal reactions must always be readily available.

UNDERSTANDING THE CHAPTER

Key Concepts Summary

1 Achieving patient adherence with pharmacotherapy can be a major challenge for the nurse.

2 Drugs should be stored properly and never used past their expiration date.

3 Prescriptions must be clearly written and include a heading, a body, and a closing.

4 For maximum effectiveness, drugs must be administered at the proper dosing intervals.

5 The primary system of measurement used in pharmacology is the metric system.

6 Medication administration should be properly recorded as soon as possible after the drug is administered.

7 Enteral drugs are administered by the oral route or through gastrostomy or nasogastric tubes.

8 Topical medications are applied to the skin or mucous membranes.

9 Parenteral administration is the dispensing of medications via a needle, usually into the skin layers, subcutaneous tissue, muscles, or veins.

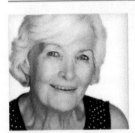

Making the PATIENT Connection

Remember the patient "Lavenia Deberry" at the beginning of the chapter? Now read the remainder of the case study. Based on the information presented within this chapter, respond to the critical thinking questions that follow.

Eighty-seven-year-old Lavenia Deberry lives in an assisted living facility. She is quite capable of caring for herself and is strongly independent. Today, she has come to her health care provider's office with fever and a productive cough that she has had for the past 10 days. She admits to self-medicating with various "leftover" antibiotics. She had hoped that one of the antibiotics would cure her infection.

Lavenia is also on a medication for high blood pressure and diabetes. However, she has been known to take her medications inconsistently. She says she does not like taking pills and most of the time she feels pretty good without them. She has difficulty remembering to take medications. Ms. Deberry states that sometimes "I forget whether I've taken the medication or not. Besides, I don't want to become dependent on any medications."

Critical Thinking Questions

1. What factors contribute to nonadherence with medication regimens?
2. Identify ways to promote patient adherence with medication regimens.
3. Prepare a list of concepts to teach the patient about taking medications.
4. What factors influence effective patient teaching related to drug therapy?

See Answers to Critical Thinking Questions on student resource website.

NCLEX-RN® Review

1 The client who received a prescription for an antibiotic 2 weeks ago now presents with the same symptoms of bacterial infection. Which should the nurse suspect?

1. Faulty and low-quality medication
2. Toxic adverse effects of the drug
3. Excessive dosage of the prescription
4. Nonadherence to the prescribed therapy

2 Prior to administering a liquid medication to a client, the nurse notices that the medication color looks different than usual. Based on this observation the nurse should:

1. Administer the medication.
2. Consult the hospital pharmacist.
3. Notify the health care provider.
4. Call the poison control center.

3 The client is to receive a vaginal suppository. Which should the nurse include in the instructions to the client concerning the drug's administration?

1. Remove the suppository 5 minutes after insertion.
2. Cleanse the perineal area with soap and water before insertion.
3. Insert the suppository only in the morning.
4. Urinate before insertion of the suppository.

4 Cipro XR has been prescribed for a client with a gastrostomy tube. Which is the appropriate nursing action for this medication?

1. Crush the medication and dilute it in tepid tap water.
2. Instruct the client to take the medication with only sips of water.

3. Request the hospital pharmacist to send a substitute drug.

4. Notify the health care provider and request that another form of the drug be prescribed.

5. The prescriber orders Lasix 40 mg intravenous stat to a client with heart failure. Which of the following describes the correct response of the nurse to this medication order?

1. Give the medication at the next meal.

2. Administer the medication immediately.

3. Dispense the medication when the client requests it.

4. Oversee the self-administration of the medication.

6. The older adult client has a new prescription for cyanocobalamin (Vitamin B$_{12}$). Which of the following activities should the nurse perform before giving this drug? Select all that apply.

1. Identify the client by checking identification band and asking the client to state full name.

2. Position the client in the proper position for medication administration.

3. Evaluate the client's response to the drug.

4. Document the medication administration on the chart.

5. Check the chart for drug allergies and verify these with the client.

6. Verify the medication for accuracy.

Additional Case Study

Albert Lewis, a 52-year-old hospitalized patient, is receiving multiple medications. While in the hospital, Albert receives the following drugs:

- Nitroglycerin tablet sublingual prn for chest pain
- Nifedipine Extended Release (ER) orally every 6 hours
- Mycelex Troche twice a day
- Clorafan 500 mg intravenously (IV)
- Insulin subcutaneous injections every morning
- Garamycin optic solution, 2 drops to each eye, 3 times per day
- Fentanyl transdermal patch every 12 hours.

1. How would you respond when the patient asks you, "Why can't I take all my medications orally?"

2. Discuss the advantages and disadvantages of each route for each of the medications listed above.

3. What special precautions should you take with drugs with an enteric coating and those that are extended release?

See Answers to Additional Case Study on student resource website.

Pearson Nursing Student Resources

Find additional review materials at nursing.pearsonhighered.com

Prepare for success with additional NCLEX®-style practice questions, interactive assignments and activities, web links, animations, videos, and more!

References

Henry J. Kaiser Family Foundation. (2008). *Prescription drug trends*. Retrieved from http://www.kff.org/rxdrugs/upload/3057_07.pdf

Hirani, J. J., Rathod, D. A., & Vadalia, K. R. (2009). Orally disintegrating tablets: A review. *Tropical Journal of Pharmaceutical Research, 8*(2), 161–172.

U.S. Food and Drug Administration. (2011). *For Consumers: How to dispose of unused medications*. Retrieved from http://www.fda.gov/ForConsumers/ConsumerUpdates/ucm101653.htm

Selected Bibliography

Berman, A., & Snyder, S. (2012). *Kozier & Erb's Fundamentals of Nursing* (9th ed.). Upper Saddle River, NJ: Pearson Education.

Briesacher, M., Andrade, S. Fouayzi, H., & Chan, K. (2008). Comparison of drug adherence rates among patients with seven different medical conditions. *Pharmacotherapy, 28*(4), 437–443. doi:10.1592/phco.28.4.437

Christensen, J. M. (2009). *Dosage forms and drug delivery systems*. New York, NY: McGraw-Hill.

Cramer, J. A. (2011). Doctors diagnose and prescribe: Patients decide what to do. *Medical Care, 49*(5), 425–426. doi:10.1097/MLR.0b013e318217479e

Doggrell, S. A. (2010). Adherence to medicines in the older-aged with chronic conditions: Does intervention by an allied health professional help? *Drugs & Aging, 27*(3), 239–254. doi:10.2165/11532870-000000000-00000

Elganzouri, E. S., Standish, C. A., & Androwich, I. (2009). Medication administration time study (MATS): Nursing staff performance of medication administration. *Journal of Nursing Administration, 39*(5), 204–210. doi:10.1097/NNA.0b013e3181a23d6d

Gould, E., & Mitty, E. (2010). Medication adherence is a partnership, medication compliance is not. *Geriatric Nursing, 31*(4), 290–298. doi:10.1016/j.gerinurse.2010.05.004

Institute for Safe Medication Practices. (2010). *ISMP's list of error-prone abbreviations, symbols, and dose designations*. Retrieved from http://www.ismp.org/Tools/errorproneabbreviations.pdf

Mansur, N., Weiss, A., & Beloosesky, Y. (2009). Is there an association between inappropriate prescription drug use and adherence in discharged elderly patients? *Annals of Pharmacotherapy, 43*(2), 177–184.

Answers to NCLEX-RN® Review

1 Answer: 4   Rationale: Nonadherence to drug therapy, especially antibiotics, is a major problem. Many people will discontinue a medication when their symptoms disappear. It is critical that the client be instructed to take the medication as prescribed and for the entire specified time. Options 1, 2, and 3 are incorrect. Strict standards for the manufacture of prescription medications is set by governmental regulation and medications must meet approved quality and safety measures. Toxic adverse effects do not produce the same symptoms of the condition for which the drug is prescribed. Excessive dosage also produces toxicity-related adverse effects. Cognitive Level: Applying; Client Need: Physiological Integrity; Nursing Process: Evaluation

2 Answer: 2   Rationale: The rule—when in doubt, throw it out—is most often a good one to follow. However, hospitals and pharmacies sometimes change brands. Before wasting a medication, it is often wise to consult the pharmacist about any concerns related to the appearance of the medication. Options 1, 3, and 4 are incorrect. The nurse must never administer a medication that has a questionable appearance. Physicians do not usually administer medications and in some cases are less likely to be capable of identifying what a drug should look like. Poison control centers are a valuable part of the health care team when there is a question of an accidental ingestion or overdose. Cognitive Level: Applying; Client Need: Safe and Effective Care Environment; Nursing Process: Evaluation

3 Answer: 4   Rationale: Vaginal suppositories can be very uncomfortable when the client's bladder is full and emptying the bladder may make insertion more comfortable. Options 1, 2, and 3 are incorrect. Vaginal suppositories dissolve once in place and should not be removed. Cleansing the perineal area is not necessarily required before the insertion of a vaginal suppository. Vaginal suppositories can be used any time during the day and are not restricted to the morning. Cognitive Level: Applying; Client Need: Safe and Effective Care Environment; Nursing Process: Implementation

4 Answer: 4   Rationale: The nurse should contact the prescriber to clarify the order and request that another form of the drug be prescribed. The letters "XR" in Cipro XR indicate that this drug is released over a prolonged time frame. Sustained or extended release drugs should never be crushed or tampered with in any way. Options 1, 2, and 3 are incorrect. Altering the form of these medications may greatly influence the absorption rate of the drug. When clients have gastrostomy or any gastric tubes, the nurse should suspect that there is a reason why the oral route cannot be used to administer medication. Pharmacists are prohibited from changing a drug order without consulting the original prescriber. Cognitive Level: Applying; Client Need: Safe and Effective Care Environment; Nursing Process: Implementation

5 Answer: 2   Rationale: Stat is the abbreviation for *statim*, the Latin word for "immediately." Options 1, 3, and 4 are incorrect. The order for Lasix has no reference to mealtimes. The "stat" order suggests that there is an immediate client need. The nurse is responsible for administering the drug intravenously. Cognitive Level: Applying; Client Need: Safe and Effective Care Environment; Nursing Process: Implementation

6 Answer: 1, 2, 5, 6   Rationale: Prior to giving any medication, the nurse should verify the order for accuracy. The allergy history should be assessed by checking the chart and verifying listed allergies with the client. The client should be identified using the identification badge and by asking the client to state his or her full name. Other methods of identification such as asking for a birth date or asking a family member these questions may be necessary if the client appears confused or disoriented. The client should be placed in the proper position for medication administration. Options 3 and 4 are incorrect answers. Evaluating a client's response to medication and documenting the administration are activities that the nurse performs after the medication is given. Cognitive Level: Applying; Client Need: Safe and Effective Care Environment; Nursing Process: Implementation

Pharmacokinetics

From Chapter 4 of *Pharmacology: Connections to Nursing Practice*, Second Edition. Michael Patrick Adams, Carol Quam Urban. Copyright © 2013 by Pearson Education, Inc. All rights reserved.

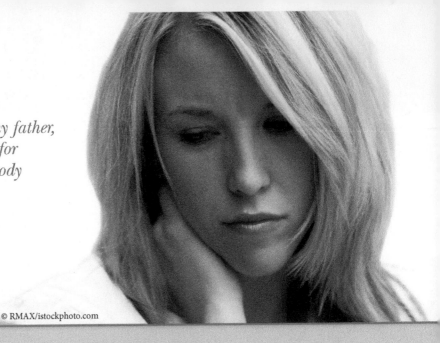

"I'm terribly worried about my father, John Kessler. He's been so ill for so long. I don't know if his body can take much more."

Patient's daughter, "Emily Kessler Myers"

© RMAX/istockphoto.com

Pharmacokinetics

Learning Outcomes

After reading this chapter, the student should be able to:

1. Identify the four primary processes of pharmacokinetics.
2. Explain mechanisms by which drugs cross plasma membranes.
3. Discuss factors affecting drug absorption.
4. Discuss how drugs are distributed throughout the body.
5. Describe how plasma proteins affect drug distribution.
6. Explain the metabolism of drugs and its applications to pharmacotherapy.
7. Identify major processes by which drugs are excreted.
8. Explain how enterohepatic recirculation affects drug activity.
9. Explain how a drug reaches and maintains its therapeutic range in the plasma.
10. Explain the applications of a drug's plasma half-life ($t_{1/2}$) to pharmacotherapy.
11. Differentiate between loading and maintenance doses.

Chapter Outline

Introduction to Pharmacokinetics

Primary Processes of Pharmacokinetics

Absorption

Distribution

Metabolism

Excretion

Time–Response Relationships

Drug Plasma Levels

Drug Half-Life

Loading and Maintenance Doses

To produce a therapeutic effect, a drug must reach its target cells in sufficient quantities. For many medications, such as topical agents used to treat superficial skin conditions, this is an easy task. For most medications, however, the process of reaching target cells to cause a physiological change is challenging. Drugs are exposed to a myriad of different barriers and destructive processes after they enter the body. The purpose of this chapter is to examine factors that act on the drug as it attempts to reach its target cells.

Introduction to Pharmacokinetics

1 Pharmacokinetics focuses on what the body does to drugs after they are administered.

The term **pharmacokinetics** is derived from the root words *pharmaco,* which refers to medicines, and *kinetics,* which means "movement" or "motion." Pharmacokinetics is thus the study of drug movement throughout the body. In practical terms, it describes what the body does to the medication after it is administered. Pharmacokinetics is a core subject in pharmacology, and a firm grasp of this topic allows nurses to better understand and predict the actions and adverse effects of medications in their patients.

Drugs face numerous obstacles in reaching their target cells. For most medications, the greatest barrier is crossing the many membranes that separate the drug from its target cells. A drug taken by mouth, for example, must cross the plasma membranes of the mucosal cells of the gastrointestinal (GI) tract and the endothelial cells of the capillaries to enter the bloodstream. To leave the bloodstream, it must again cross capillary cells, travel through interstitial fluid, and perhaps enter target cells by passing through their plasma membranes. Depending on the mechanism of action, the drug may also need to enter cellular organelles such as nuclei, which are surrounded by additional membranes. Some of the membranes and barriers that many drugs must successfully penetrate before they can elicit a response are illustrated in Figure 1.

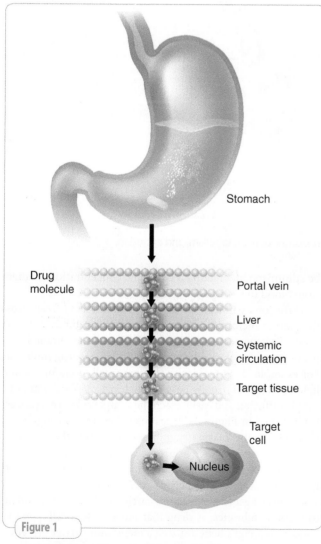

Stomach

Drug molecule

Portal vein

Liver

Systemic circulation

Target tissue

Target cell

Nucleus

Figure 1

Barriers that a drug administered by the oral route must cross before interacting with a target cell.

While seeking their target cells and attempting to pass through the various membranes, drugs are subjected to numerous physiological processes. For medications given by the enteral route, stomach acid and digestive enzymes often break down the drug molecules. Enzymes in the liver and other organs may chemically change the drug molecule, making it less active. If seen as foreign by the body, phagocytes may attempt to remove the drug, or an immune response may be triggered. The kidneys, large intestine, and other organs attempt to excrete the drug from the body.

The preceding examples all illustrate pharmacokinetic processes: how the body handles drugs. The many processes of pharmacokinetics are grouped into four categories: absorption, distribution, metabolism, and excretion, which are illustrated in Figure 2. All four of these processes have drug movement in common. Whether it involves movement to its target site or movement out of the body, kinetics is certainly an appropriate name for this important branch of pharmacology.

Key Terms

absorption

affinity

blood–brain barrier

diffusion

distribution

drug-protein complexes

enterohepatic recirculation

enzyme induction

excretion

fetal–placental barrier

first-pass effect

hepatic microsomal enzyme system

isozymes

loading dose

maintenance doses

metabolism

minimum effective concentration

pharmacokinetics

plasma half-life ($t_{1/2}$)

prodrugs

substrate

therapeutic drug monitoring

therapeutic range

toxic concentration

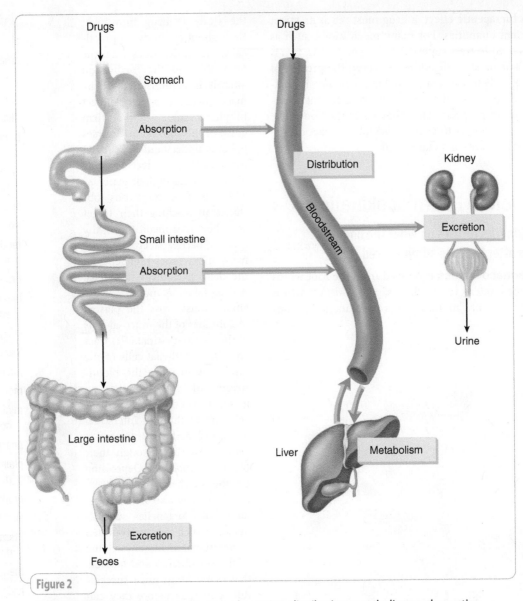

Figure 2

The four processes of pharmacokinetics: absorption, distribution, metabolism, and excretion.

2 Drugs use diffusion and active transport to cross plasma membranes to reach their target cells.

With few exceptions, drugs must cross plasma membranes and enter cells to produce their effects. Plasma membranes are composed of a lipid bilayer, with proteins and other molecules interspersed in the membrane. Like other chemicals, drugs use two primary processes to cross membranes: diffusion and active transport.

Simple **diffusion** or passive transport is the movement of a chemical from an area of higher concentration to an area of lower concentration. This is best explained by the use of an example. When first administered, a drug given by the intravenous (IV) route is in high concentration in the blood but has not yet entered the tissues. The drug will move quickly by passive diffusion from its region of high concentration (blood) to a region of low concentration (tissues) to produce its action. With time the drug will be inactivated (metabolized) by the tissue and more doses of the drug may

be administered, creating a continual concentration gradient from blood to tissue.

Diffusion assumes that the chemical is able to freely cross the plasma membrane. This, however, is not the case for all drugs. Passage across the lipid-rich plasma membrane is dependent on the physical characteristics of the drug molecule. For example, drug molecules that are small, nonionized, and lipid soluble will usually pass through plasma membranes by simple diffusion and easily reach their target cells. This process is illustrated in Figure 3. Drugs may also enter through open channels in the plasma membrane; however, the molecule must be very small, such as urea, alcohol, and water.

Large molecules, ionized drugs, and water-soluble agents have difficulty crossing plasma membranes by simple diffusion. These agents may require carrier, or transport, proteins to cross membranes. A drug that moves into a cell along its concentration gradient utilizing a membrane carrier protein is using the process of facilitated diffusion. This process does not require energy expenditure from the cell, but it does require

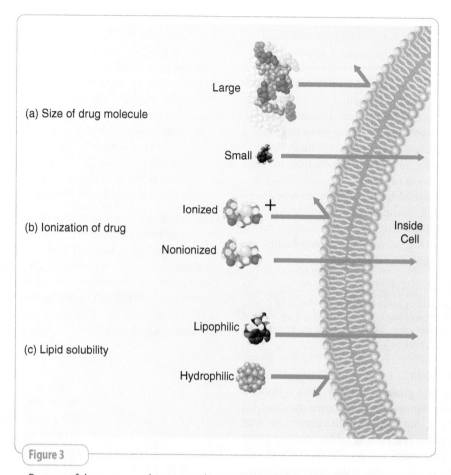

(a) Size of drug molecule

Large

Small

(b) Ionization of drug

Ionized

Nonionized

Inside Cell

(c) Lipid solubility

Lipophilic

Hydrophilic

Figure 3

Passage of drugs across plasma membranes: (a) small drugs; (b) nonionized drugs; and (c) lipophilic drugs are more likely to cross membranes.

that a specific carrier protein be present on the plasma membrane. Transport proteins are selective and only carry molecules that have specific structures.

Some drugs cross membranes against their gradient, from low concentration to high concentration, through the process of active transport. This requires expenditure of energy on the part of the cell and a carrier protein. Carrier proteins that assist in active transport are sometimes called pumps.

Primary Processes of Pharmacokinetics

3 Absorption is the process of moving a drug from the site of administration to the bloodstream.

For most medications the first step toward reaching target cells is **absorption**, the process by which drug molecules move from their site of administration to the blood. Oral medications enter the bloodstream by being absorbed across epithelial cells lining the GI tract. Drugs administered by the intradermal (ID) or subcutaneous routes are absorbed by blood vessels in the skin; intramuscular (IM) drugs cross membranes to enter the rich blood supply serving skeletal muscle. Topical drugs may be absorbed across the skin or associated mucous membranes lining the vagina, the respiratory tract, or the nasal passages. With the exception of a few topical medications, GI anti-infectives, and some radiologic contrast agents, the majority of drugs must be absorbed in order to produce an effect. Of course, drugs administered directly into blood vessels by IV or intra-arterial routes are not absorbed because they are already in the bloodstream.

Absorption is the primary pharmacokinetic factor determining the onset of drug action—the length of time it takes a drug to produce its effect. In general, the more rapid the absorption, the faster the onset of drug action. Drugs used in critical care are designed to be absorbed within seconds or minutes, or they are given intravenously. At the other extreme are drugs such as the contraceptive Mirena, which is a polyethylene tube placed in the uterus. The drug inside Mirena, levonorgestrel, is absorbed slowly from the tube and provides contraceptive protection for up to 5 years.

In addition to onset time, absorption determines the intensity of drug action. For any given drug, a specific percentage of the drug is absorbed, ranging from 0% to 100%. Everything else being equal, drugs with higher absorption rates produce a more effective response than those with lower absorption rates. The degree of absorption is conditional on many factors.

Route of administration: Because drugs administered by the IV route bypass absorption entirely, they have the most rapid onset of action. Inhalation also produces a very rapid response because the membrane separating the inhaled drug from the bloodstream is very thin, making absorption easier. Subcutaneous and IM formulations are absorbed rapidly, though they have a slower onset of action than IV or inhalation.

Tablets and capsules must dissolve before the drug is available for absorption, thus their onset time is relatively slow. The dissolution rate of a tablet or capsule is often the slowest part of the absorption process of an oral medication. Because oral liquid formulations do not undergo dissolution, they are absorbed faster than tablets or capsules.

Topical medications applied to the skin are absorbed very slowly because it is difficult for the drug to penetrate the thick, keratin layer. However, topical drugs applied to mucous membranes are absorbed quickly because these membranes are relatively thin and have a rich blood supply.

CONNECTION Checkpoint 4.1

Crushing a tablet enhances a drug's rate of absorption because it does not have to dissolve. What type of medications should not be crushed or opened? *See Answer to Connection Checkpoint 4.1 on student resource website.*

Drug concentration and dose: For almost all drugs, higher doses produce a faster and greater response. This is because a higher dose produces a greater concentration gradient for diffusion. As an example, consider the antihypertensive drug diltiazem (Cardizem) given as a 100-mg tablet, which is about 50% absorbed. Half of the drug (50 mg) will reach the bloodstream for distribution to target cells. If the dose of diltiazem is doubled to 200 mg, greater amounts of the drug (100 mg) will be absorbed in the bloodstream. Although the percentage absorbed remains the same (50%), the higher dose results in a greater quantity of drug in the blood and, subsequently, more drug is available to produce an action at its target cells.

GI tract environment: For drugs given by mouth, the physical and chemical conditions within the GI tract play a significant role in drug absorption. Most absorption occurs in the small intestine, because this portion of the GI tract is longer, and the absorptive surfaces of the microvilli are much more extensive as compared to the stomach. Furthermore the time spent by food and drugs in the stomach is brief, and the thick mucous layer in the organ discourages absorption.

Digestive motility is variable among patients; very rapid motility may speed the drug through the GI tract before complete absorption occurs. Abnormally slow motility may cause the drug to be retained in the stomach, where it is exposed for a longer time to destructive enzymes and high acidity. Fatty foods in the stomach nearly always slow drug absorption. With few exceptions, absorption is most complete when the drug is taken between meals; the presence of food in the stomach may lessen the incidence of nausea and vomiting, but it also slows absorption. All these factors contribute to wide patient variability with regard to absorption, as well as to drug action when drugs are administered orally.

Blood flow to the absorption site: For a drug to be absorbed, there must be adequate blood flow to the site of administration;

thus drugs are absorbed faster from areas of the body where blood flow is high. IM injections are placed into large muscles because they have a high blood flow that maximizes absorption. During heart failure or shock, the amount of blood flow to certain tissues is reduced and absorption from the GI tract or IM sites may be diminished. Topical drugs placed on the skin have slow absorption due to the poor blood supply to the upper layers of the skin.

In some circumstances blood flow can be manipulated to purposely slow absorption. For example, local anesthetics can be toxic if absorbed too quickly. To purposely slow absorption, a vasoconstrictor (epinephrine) is sometimes added to local anesthetics to reduce blood flow to the treated region.

Drug ionization: Ionized molecules are those that carry a positive or a negative charge. Most drugs can exist in either a charged or uncharged state, depending on the pH of the surrounding fluid. The ionization of a drug affects its ability to cross plasma membranes and to be excreted by the body (see Section 6). Aspirin, or acetylsalicylic acid, provides an example of the effects of ionization on absorption, as depicted in Figure 4. In the highly acidic environment of the stomach, aspirin is in its

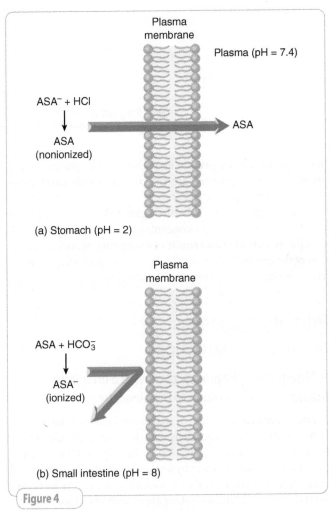

(a) Stomach (pH = 2)

(b) Small intestine (pH = 8)

Figure 4

Effect of pH on drug absorption: (a) A weak acid such as aspirin (ASA) is in a nonionized form in an acidic environment and absorption occurs. (b) In a basic environment, aspirin is mostly in an ionized form and absorption is prevented.

nonionized form and is thus readily absorbed and distributed in the bloodstream. As aspirin enters the alkaline environment of the small intestine, however, it becomes ionized. In its ionized form, the aspirin molecule is less likely to be absorbed and distributed to target cells. Unlike acidic drugs such as aspirin, medications that are weakly basic are in their nonionized form in an alkaline environment; therefore, basic drugs are much more likely to be absorbed in alkaline environments such as the small intestine. In simplest terms, it may help the student to remember the following:

- Acids are absorbed in acids because they are nonionized.
- Bases are absorbed in bases because they are nonionized.

Drug interactions: Drug–drug and food–drug interactions have the capability of affecting absorption. For example, administering oral tetracyclines with food or drugs containing calcium, iron, or magnesium can significantly delay absorption of the antibiotic. High-fat meals can slow stomach motility significantly and delay the absorption of oral medications taken with the meal.

Surface area: Other factors being equal, drugs will be absorbed faster when applied to regions of the body having a larger surface area. This is one reason why the small intestine is such an important organ for drug absorption. Relative to the oral cavity and stomach, the microvilli of the small intestine provide a vast surface area that is richly supplied with blood vessels. Another region with an enormous surface area is the lung. Inhaled substances such as bronchodilators or crack cocaine act almost instantaneously due the large absorptive surface provided by terminal bronchioles and alveoli.

CONNECTION Checkpoint 4.2

Classify the following routes of administration as topical, enteral, or parenteral: buccal, subcutaneous, intravaginal, sublingual, and rectal. *See Answer to Connection Checkpoint 4.2 on student resource website.*

4 Distribution describes how drugs are transported throughout the body.

Distribution is the phase of pharmacokinetics describing the *movement* of pharmacologic agents throughout the body after they are absorbed. Drugs are not simply passive agents, being swept along an inert path to their target tissues. Rather, drugs may interact with blood components and may be chemically and physically changed before they reach their targets. Like absorption, several key factors influence drug distribution.

Blood flow to tissues: The simplest factor determining drug distribution is the amount of blood flow to body tissues. Because the heart, liver, and kidneys receive a great percentage of the blood supply, these organs receive the highest exposure to absorbed drugs. Skin, bone, and adipose tissue receive a meager blood flow; therefore, it is more difficult to deliver high concentrations of drugs to these areas.

Blood flow should also be considered at the local level. For example, after traumatic injury, the blood supply to a fractured bone may be reduced due to damaged blood vessels, or blocked by cellular debris from the inflammatory process. Antibiotics may have difficulty reaching the injured area until blood flow can be restored. The delivery of high concentrations of drugs to injured, necrotic, or abscessed areas that have inadequate perfusion is always challenging.

Drug solubility: The physical properties of a drug greatly influence how it moves throughout the body after administration. Lipid solubility is an important characteristic because it determines how quickly a drug is absorbed, mixes within the bloodstream, crosses membranes, and becomes localized in body tissues. Lipid-soluble agents are not limited by the barriers that normally stop water-soluble drugs; thus they are more completely distributed to body tissues.

Tissue storage: Some tissues have the ability to accumulate and store drugs in high concentrations relative to other tissues. The bone marrow, teeth, eyes, and adipose tissue have an especially high **affinity**, or attraction, for certain medications. Examples of agents that are stored in adipose tissue are diazepam (Valium), lipid-soluble vitamins, and tetracycline, which binds to calcium salts and accumulates in bones and teeth. Once stored in tissues, drugs may remain in the body for many months and be released very slowly back to the circulation. For example, the therapeutic effects of alendronate (Fosamax), a drug for osteoporosis, will continue for 4–7 months after the drug is discontinued.

Drug-protein binding: Many drugs bind reversibly to plasma proteins, particularly albumin, to form **drug-protein complexes**. Drug-protein complexes are too large to cross capillary membranes; the drugs continue circulating in the bloodstream and are unavailable for distribution to their site of action. Drugs will remain trapped in the bloodstream bound to plasma proteins until they are released or displaced from the drug-protein complex. Only unbound, or free, drugs can reach their target cells or be excreted by the kidneys. This concept is illustrated in Figure 5. Some drugs, such as the anticoagulant warfarin (Coumadin), are highly bound; 99% of the drug in the plasma exists in drug-protein complexes, and only 1% exists as a free drug available to reach target cells.

Drugs and other chemicals compete with one another for plasma protein binding sites, and some agents have a greater affinity for these binding sites than other agents. Drug–drug and drug–food interactions may occur when one agent displaces another from plasma proteins. The displaced medication can quickly reach high levels in the blood and produce adverse effects. For example, drugs such as aspirin or cimetidine (Tagamet) will displace warfarin from its protein binding sites and raise blood levels of free warfarin, dramatically increasing the risk of hemorrhage. Most drug guides give the percentage of the drug bound to plasma proteins; when giving multiple medications that are highly bound, the nurse should carefully monitor for adverse effects.

Special barriers to drug distribution: Most capillaries in the body are relatively porous due to spaces between the endothelial cells. Many drugs can exit the bloodstream by traveling through the spaces and enter the interstitial fluid with relative ease. The brain and placenta, however, possess

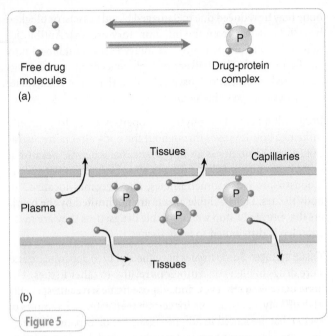

Figure 5

Plasma protein binding and drug availability: (a) The drug exists in a free state or is bound to plasma protein. (b) Drug-protein complexes are too large to cross membranes.

special anatomic barriers that inhibit many chemicals and drugs from exiting the blood. These barriers are referred to as the **blood–brain barrier** and **fetal–placental barrier.**

Unlike other capillaries, those in the brain have endothelial cells that are sealed by tight junctions and a thick basement membrane. Brain cells known as astrocytes press firmly against the basement membrane, secreting chemicals that adjust the capillary permeability. The purpose of the blood–brain barrier is obvious: to protect the brain from pathogens and toxic substances. Some highly lipid-soluble agents such as general anesthetics, sedatives, antianxiety agents, and anticonvulsant drugs readily cross the blood–brain barrier to produce their actions on the central nervous system (CNS). In contrast, most antitumor medications and antibiotics do not easily cross this barrier, making brain cancers and infections difficult to treat. The blood–brain barrier becomes more permeable when it is inflamed due to infections such as meningitis. In neonates, the blood–brain barrier is not fully developed, allowing drugs to cross the barrier more readily.

The series of membranes that separate the maternal blood from the fetal blood serves as a fetal–placental barrier that prevents potentially harmful substances from passing from the mother's bloodstream to the fetus. In reality, the placenta is an ineffective barrier because substances such as alcohol, cocaine, caffeine, and certain prescription medications can easily cross the placental barrier and cause potential harm to the fetus. Consequently, no prescription medication, over-the-counter (OTC) drug, or herbal therapy should be taken by a pregnant woman without first consulting a health care provider. The nurse should always question women of child-bearing age regarding their pregnancy status before a drug is prescribed.

5 Metabolism is a process that changes the activity of a drug and makes it more likely to be excreted.

Drug **metabolism**, also called biotransformation, is the process used by the body to chemically change a drug molecule. Metabolism involves hundreds of complex biochemical pathways and reactions that alter the structure and function of drugs, nutrients, vitamins, and minerals. The liver is the primary site of drug metabolism, although the kidneys and cells of the intestinal tract also have high metabolic rates. To survive, all cells must undergo metabolism to some extent. The types of metabolic reactions, however, are specific to each type of cell: Reactions occurring in liver cells are very different from those in skin cells or brain cells.

In most cases, metabolic reactions change the structure of a drug so that it can be more easily excreted by the body. This often changes the drug from lipid soluble (easily absorbed and distributed) to water soluble, which is more easily excreted by the kidneys. In addition, once the molecule has been changed to water soluble, it is less able to enter tissues. This serves as a detoxifying effect for drugs and other substances entering the body.

Chemical changes to drugs always result in functional changes. The products of drug metabolism, or metabolites, usually have less pharmacologic activity than the original molecule. On rare occasions a metabolite may have greater activity than the original drug. This is the case for codeine. Although 90% of codeine is changed to inactive metabolites by the liver, 10% is converted to morphine, which has significantly greater ability to relieve severe pain. In a few cases, the metabolite has greater toxicity than the original drug. Probably the most common example of this is acetaminophen (Tylenol), which is converted to a metabolite that is highly toxic to the liver.

In a few cases, the drug administered to the patient has no pharmacologic activity until it undergoes metabolism. Agents that require metabolism to produce their action are called **prodrugs.** For example, the antihypertensive enalapril (Vasotec) is converted in the liver to enaliprat, which has considerably more ability to lower blood pressure than the original drug. Examples of other prodrugs include benazepril (Lotensin) and losartan (Cozaar).

Hepatic microsomal enzymes: Most metabolism in the liver is accomplished by the **hepatic microsomal enzyme system.** This enzyme complex is known as the P450 system, named after cytochrome P450 (CYP), which is a key component of the system. Although this system is complex, a key point to remember is that CYP is simply an enzyme that metabolizes drugs as well as nutrients and other endogenous substances. Although the liver is the major site for CYP activity, nearly every tissue in the body has some CYP enzymes.

It was once thought that a single CYP enzyme was responsible for all drug metabolism, but scientists have since identified more than 50 CYPs. These different forms are called **isozymes** of cytochrome P450. Although very similar, each isozyme performs slightly different metabolic functions. CYPs

TABLE 1 Isozymes of Cytochrome P450: Selected Substrates, Inducers, and Inhibitors

Isozyme	Substrates	Inducers	Inhibitors
CYP1A2	acetaminophen, amitriptyline, caffeine, dantrolene, diazepam, estradiol, haloperidol, imipramine, lidocaine, methadone, ondansetron, ritonavir, tacrine, tamoxifen, verapamil, warfarin	omeprazole, phenobarbital, phenytoin, rifampin, ritonavir	cimetidine, ciprofloxacin, erythromycin, grapefruit juice, isoniazid, ketoconazole, levofloxacin, paroxetine
CYP2C9	amiodarone, amitriptyline, dapsone, ethosuximide, ibuprofen, imipramine, naproxen, nifedipine, omeprazole, phenytoin, progesterone, propranolol, ritonavir, sulfonamides, tamoxifen, testosterone, tricyclic antidepressants, valproic acid, warfarin	barbiturates, carbamazepine, ethanol, phenobarbital	cimetidine, disulfiram, fluconazole, fluoxetine, fluvastatin, ketoconazole, omeprazole, ritonavir, sertraline
CYP2C19	diazepam, omeprazole	none	
CYP2D6	amitriptyline, captopril, chlorpromazine, citalopram, codeine, fluoxetine, haloperidol, imipramine, lidocaine, loratadine, meperidine, methamphetamine, metoprolol, mexiletine, odansetron, oxycodone, paroxetine, propranolol, ritonavir, tamoxifen, tramadol, trazodone, venlafaxine	carbamazepine, phenobarbital, phenytoin, rifampin, ritonavir	amiodarone, cimetidine, citalopram, fluoxetine, haloperidol, methadone, paroxetine, ritonavir, sertraline
CYP3A4	alprazolam, amiodarone, carbamazepine, chlorpromazine, cocaine, cortisol, cyclosporine, diltiazem, erythromycin, ketoconazole, lidocaine, lovastatin, nifedipine, omeprazole, prednisone, ritonavir, sertraline, tamoxifen, venlafaxine, verapamil	dexamethasone, ethosuximide, nevirapine, phenobarbital, phenytoin, prednisone	clotrimazole, diltiazem, erythromycin, fluconazole, fluoxetine, ketoconazole, metronidazole, nifedipine, norfloxacin, omeprazole, fluoxetine, ritonavir, sertraline, verapamil, zafirlukast

are named by assigning numbers to indicate their subfamily, such as CYP1, CYP2, CYP3, and so on. Additional letters and numbers are added to further identify the specific gene, such as CYP1A1, CYP3A4, and CYP26C1. Fortunately for nursing students, only a handful of the 50-plus isozymes are responsible for the majority of drug metabolism, as shown in Table 1. Indeed, a single isozyme, CYP3A4, is responsible for about 50% of all drug metabolism in the liver.

The CYPs are important to pharmacotherapy because they determine the speed at which most drugs are metabolized and they contribute significantly to drug–drug interactions. Changes in hepatic microsomal enzymes can significantly affect drug action. There are three major consequences of the CYP system that have importance to pharmacotherapy:

- **Drugs as substrates.** When a drug is metabolized by a CYP, it is said to be a **substrate** for the enzyme. For example, naproxen and warfarin are substrates for CYP2C9. Codeine and amphetamine are substrates for a different isozyme, CYP2D6. Each isozyme of CYP can metabolize many different drugs, and a drug may be metabolized by multiple CYPs. Because of this overlap, two drugs that are administered concurrently may compete for binding sites on the same CYP isozyme, resulting in a drug–drug interaction.

- **Drugs as enzyme inhibitors.** Some drugs are able to inhibit the action of CYP isozymes. The inhibition may affect all hepatic microsomal enzymes or it may be specific to a single isozyme. Because most drugs are inactivated by metabolism, inhibiting a CYP enzyme could affect the amount of active drug available. For example, ciprofloxacin (Cipro) inhibits CYP1A2. Administering Cipro concurrently with naproxen (a substrate for CYP1A2) could result in less metabolism of naproxen, higher amounts of naproxen in the blood, and a prolonged drug effect. Because naproxen is a relatively safe drug, this higher level may not produce noticeable toxicity. However, giving Cipro with a more toxic drug such as warfarin (also a substrate for CYP1A2) has the potential

to cause a serious drug interaction. The dose of warfarin would need to be adjusted downward to avoid toxicity. It is important to note that CYP enzyme inhibition can occur after a single dose of an inhibitor.

- **Drugs as enzyme inducers.** A few drugs have the ability to increase metabolic activity in the liver, a process called **enzyme induction**. For example, phenobarbital causes the liver to synthesize greater amounts of microsomal enzymes, including CYP3A4, CYP2C19, and CYP2C9. By doing so, phenobarbital accelerates the metabolism (inactivation) of most drugs metabolized in the liver. In fact, with continued therapy phenobarbital increases the rate of its own destruction. In these patients, because drugs will be inactivated at a much faster rate, higher doses may be required to achieve an optimum therapeutic effect. Unlike CYP inhibition, which can occur after a single dose, enzyme induction generally takes from days to weeks.

Metabolism has a number of additional therapeutic consequences. As illustrated in Pharmacotherapy Illustrated 1, drugs absorbed after oral administration cross directly into the hepatic-portal circulation, which carries blood to the liver before it is distributed to other body tissues. Some drugs can be completely metabolized to an inactive form on their first trip through the liver *before they even reach the general circulation*. This **first-pass effect** is important to pharmacology, because a large number of oral drugs are rendered inactive by hepatic metabolic reactions. Alternate routes of delivery that bypass the first-pass effect, such as the sublingual, rectal, or parenteral routes, may need to be considered for these drugs. Remember, however, that even drugs administered by parenteral routes may be rapidly inactivated when passing through the liver.

Patient variation in metabolism: Certain patients have diminished hepatic metabolic activity, which may result in altered drug action. Infants do not develop a mature microsomal enzyme system until at least 1 year of age. Hepatic enzyme

PHARMACOTHERAPY ILLUSTRATED

First-Pass Effect: Oral Drug Is Metabolized to an Inactive Form Before It Has an Opportunity to Reach Target Cells

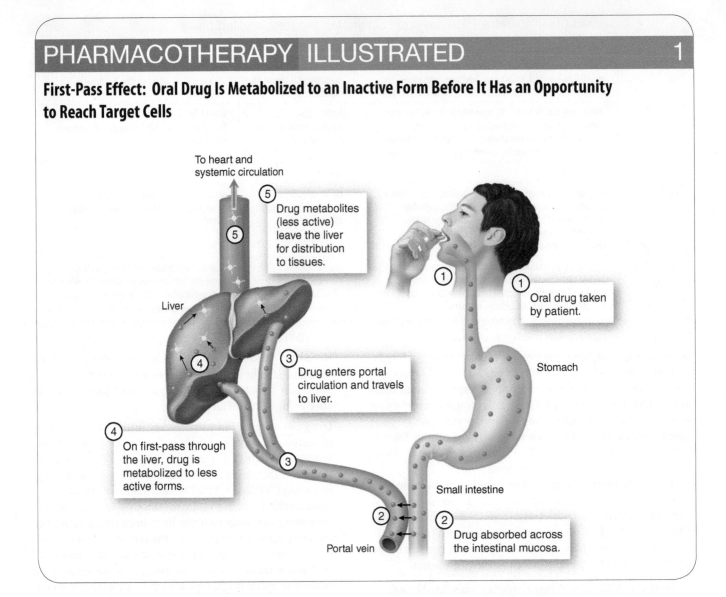

To heart and systemic circulation

5 Drug metabolites (less active) leave the liver for distribution to tissues.

Liver

4 On first-pass through the liver, drug is metabolized to less active forms.

3 Drug enters portal circulation and travels to liver.

1 Oral drug taken by patient.

Stomach

Small intestine

2 Drug absorbed across the intestinal mucosa.

Portal vein

activity is generally reduced in older adults; thus these patients may require lower doses. Patients with liver impairment will require reductions in drug dosage because of the decreased metabolic activity. The nurse should pay careful attention to laboratory values that may indicate liver disease so that drug doses may be adjusted accordingly.

The baseline functions of hepatic microsomal enzyme systems are genetically determined. Genetic differences in the function of CYP enzymes may cause people to metabolize drugs at widely different rates. Some patients metabolize at a faster rate, others at a slower rate. Certain genetic disorders have been recognized in which patients lack specific metabolic enzymes. In these "slow metabolizers" normal drug doses may cause toxicity. Genetic differences are not always predictable, although some occur at a higher rate in certain ethnic populations.

Certain lifestyle factors also affect CYP enzyme activity and thus may influence response to medications. Chronic alcohol consumption and tobacco use induce certain CYP enzymes. St. John's wort, a popular herbal remedy for depression, is an enzyme inducer and can affect the therapeutic response to certain medications. On the other hand, grapefruit juice is an

inhibitor of CYP3A4 activity. These examples underscore the importance of obtaining a thorough patient history prior to initiating drug therapy.

6 Excretion processes remove drugs from the body.

Drugs will continue to act on the body until they are either metabolized to an inactive form or removed from the body by **excretion**. The rate at which a drug is excreted determines its concentration in the blood and, ultimately, its duration of action. Pathologic states, especially liver or kidney disease, often increase the duration and intensity of drug action in the body because they interfere with natural excretion mechanisms.

Renal excretion: Although drugs are removed from the body by numerous organs and tissues, the primary site of excretion is the kidney. In an average size person, the kidneys filter approximately 180 L of blood each day. Unbound (free) drugs, water-soluble agents, electrolytes, and small molecules easily pass through the pores of Bowman's capsule and enter the filtrate. Proteins, blood cells, and drug-protein complexes are not filtered because of their large size.

Treating the Diverse Patient   One Size Does Not Fit All

One of the difficult challenges of modern pharmacology is to develop medications that produce an optimal result with minimal adverse effects for all users. Although humans vary in their individual response to medications, drugs have traditionally been designed to target the "average" person, a one-size-fits-all approach, when the "average" person does not exist. A solution to this dilemma may come in the near future with pharmacogenomics, the science that predicts when a patient will have a positive or an adverse response to a drug based on inherited genes.

Scientists have determined that the way a person responds to a medication depends on certain traits found in the genes: small variations in the sequence of their nucleotide bases. Without knowing the specific genes involved in the drug response, one cannot predict the individual response to a medication.

Gene variation diagnostic tools called SNPs (pronounced snips) are expensive to access. However, DNA microarrays (DNA chips) are part of an evolving technology that will open the door to a targeted drug response for a group of patients. Review of gene susceptibility prior to prescribing the drug may be a possibility in the future.

This technology would also be beneficial in clinical trials. By predetermining patients' responses, those with known adverse reaction to a drug would be excluded. Clinical trials would be conducted with smaller groups, resulting in less expense and, ultimately, in reduced cost of drugs to the consumer. The health care provider could prescribe in confidence, unlike the current method in which the prescriber gives the patient a medication that may or may not be effective or have adverse effects based on the individual response.

After filtration at the renal corpuscle, drugs may undergo reabsorption in the renal tubule. Mechanisms of reabsorption are the same as absorption elsewhere in the body. Nonionized and lipid-soluble drugs cross renal tubular membranes more easily and return to the circulation; ionized and water-soluble drugs generally remain in the filtrate.

Drug-protein complexes and other substances too large to be filtered in Bowman's capsule are sometimes secreted into the distal tubule of the nephron. For example, only 10% of a dose of penicillin G is filtered in Bowman's capsule; 90% is secreted into the renal tubule. As with metabolic enzyme activity, secretion mechanisms are less active in infants and in older adults.

The renal excretion of drugs is dependent on the pH of the filtrate in the renal tubule. Weak acids like aspirin are excreted more efficiently when the filtrate is slightly alkaline. This is because aspirin is ionized in an alkaline environment, and the ionized drug will remain in the filtrate to be excreted in the urine. Weakly basic drugs such as diazepam (Valium) are excreted more quickly if the filtrate is slightly acidic because they are ionized in that environment. The pH of the filtrate may be intentionally manipulated to speed up renal excretion. For example, following an overdose of an acidic drug such as aspirin, nurses may administer sodium bicarbonate. Sodium bicarbonate makes the urine more basic, which ionizes the aspirin molecule, facilitating its urinary excretion. The excretion of diazepam, on the other hand, can be enhanced by giving ammonium chloride, which acidifies the filtrate and ionizes the diazepam molecule.

Impairment of kidney function can dramatically affect pharmacokinetics. Patients with renal failure will have diminished ability to excrete medications and may retain drugs for extended periods. Doses for these patients must be reduced to prevent drug toxicity. Because small to moderate changes in renal function can cause rapid increases in serum drug levels, kidney function must be constantly monitored in patients receiving nephrotoxic drugs or medications that have a narrow margin of safety.

Pulmonary excretion: Drugs delivered by gaseous or volatile liquid forms are especially suited for excretion by the respiratory system. The rate of respiratory excretion is dependent on factors that affect gas exchange, including diffusion, gas solubility, and blood flow to the lungs. The elimination of gaseous and volatile anesthetics following surgery is primarily dependent on respiratory activity: The faster the breathing rate, the greater the excretion. On the other hand, the respiratory removal of water-soluble agents such as alcohol is more dependent on blood flow to the lungs. The greater the blood flow through lung capillaries, the greater the pulmonary excretion. In contrast with other methods of excretion, the lungs excrete most drugs in their original unmetabolized form.

Glandular secretion: Glandular activity is another elimination mechanism. Water-soluble drugs may be secreted into the saliva, sweat, or breast milk. The "funny taste" that patients experience when given certain drugs is an example of the secretion of medications into saliva. Another example is the garlic smell that can be detected when standing next to a perspiring person who has recently eaten garlic. Excretion into breast milk is of considerable importance for basic drugs such as morphine or codeine, because these can achieve high concentrations and potentially affect the nursing infant. Lactating women should always check with their health care provider before taking any prescription medication, OTC drug, or herbal supplement.

Fecal and biliary excretion: Certain oral drugs travel through the GI tract without being absorbed and are excreted in the feces. Examples include mebendazole (Vermox), a drug used to kill intestinal worms, and barium sulfate, a radiologic contrast agent.

Some drugs are secreted in bile, a process known as biliary excretion. Drugs secreted into bile will enter the duodenum via the common bile duct and eventually leave the body in the feces. However, most bile is circulated back to the liver by **enterohepatic recirculation**, as illustrated in Figure 6. Drugs may be recirculated numerous times with the bile, thus extending their stay in the body; biliary excretion is influential in prolonging the activity of digoxin (Lanoxin), certain antibiotics, and phenothiazines. Recirculated drugs are eventually metabolized by the liver and may be excreted by the kidneys.

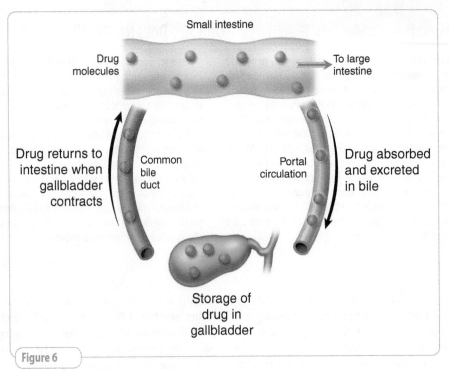

Small intestine

Drug molecules

To large intestine

Drug returns to intestine when gallbladder contracts

Common bile duct

Portal circulation

Drug absorbed and excreted in bile

Storage of drug in gallbladder

Figure 6

Enterohepatic recirculation of a drug can increase its half-life in the body and prolong its duration of action.

Recirculation and elimination of drugs through biliary excretion may continue for several weeks after therapy has been discontinued.

Time–Response Relationships

7 The therapeutic response of most drugs depends on their concentration in the plasma.

The therapeutic response from most drugs is directly related to their concentration in the plasma. Although the concentration of the drug at its target tissue is more predictive of drug action, this quantity is impossible to measure. For example, although it is possible to conduct a laboratory test that measures the serum level of lithium carbonate (Eskalith) by taking a blood sample, it is a far different matter to measure the quantity of this drug in neurons within the brain.

It is common practice to monitor the plasma levels of drugs that have a low safety margin and to use these data to predict drug action or toxicity. Results of **therapeutic drug monitoring** are used by the health care provider to keep the drug dose within a predetermined therapeutic range. For example, the therapeutic range for the antibiotic vancomycin (Vancocin) is 20 to 40 mcg/mL and the toxic level is considered to be greater than 80 mcg/mL. For patients with severe infections, the nurse would carefully monitor the laboratory results for vancomycin to be certain that serum levels fall within the therapeutic range. Dosages would be adjusted upward or downward based on therapeutic drug monitoring and the patient responses. The nurse should always remember, however, that individual responses to drugs are highly variable and patients may experience toxic

effects (or no effects) even if the serum concentration of the drug lies in the normal range.

A number of important pharmacokinetic principles can be illustrated by measuring the drug plasma level following a single dose administered by the oral route. These pharmacokinetic values are shown graphically in Figure 7. In this example, the plasma drug level slowly increased and took about 2 hours before the **minimum effective concentration** was reached. The minimum effective drug plasma concentration, that amount of drug required to produce a therapeutic effect, is 6 mcg/mL. The level of drug then entered the **therapeutic range** of the drug, which in this case lies between 6 and 12 mcg/mL. In this range, the drug produced its desired therapeutic action. After peaking, the drug plasma level slowly began to fall out of the therapeutic range due to excretion processes. A higher dose might have caused the drug plasma level to reach a **toxic concentration**, that level of drug that results in serious adverse effects. The goal of pharmacotherapy is to reach and maintain a plasma drug level in the therapeutic range while avoiding the toxic concentration.

These values have great clinical significance. For example, if the patient has a severe headache and is given half of an aspirin tablet, the plasma drug level will remain below the minimum effective concentration, and the patient will not experience pain relief. Two or three tablets will increase the plasma level of aspirin into the therapeutic range, and the pain will subside. Taking six or more tablets may result in adverse effects, such as GI bleeding or tinnitus. For each drug administered, the nurse's goal is to keep its plasma concentration in the therapeutic range. For some drugs, this therapeutic range is quite wide.

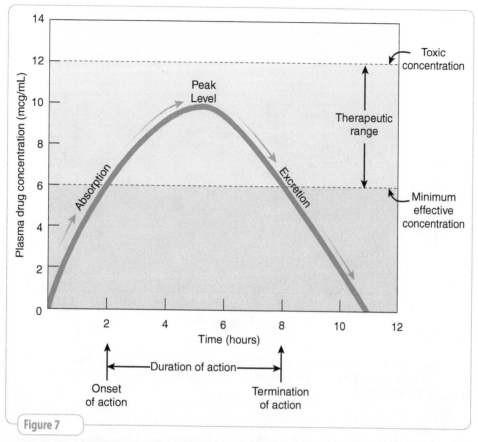

Figure 7

Single-dose drug administration. Pharmacokinetic values for this drug are as follows: onset of action = 2 hours; duration of action = 6 hours; termination of action = 8 hours after administration; peak plasma concentration = 10 mcg/mL; time to peak drug effect = 5 hours; $t_{1/2}$ = 4 hours.

For other medications, the difference between a minimum effective dose and a toxic dose can be extremely narrow.

8 The drug half-life estimates the duration of action for most medications.

In the example illustrated in Figure 7, the serum concentration of the drug reached a peak and then fell back below the therapeutic range. The length of time a drug concentration remains in the therapeutic range is its *duration of action*. In this example, the duration of action was 6 hours. The duration of action is an important pharmacokinetic variable that is determined by how rapidly the drug is metabolized and excreted.

The most common description of a drug's duration of action is its **plasma half-life ($t_{1/2}$)**: the length of time required for the plasma concentration of a drug to decrease by one half after administration. Some drugs have a half-life of only a few minutes, whereas others have a half-life of several hours or days. A few drugs have exceptionally long half-lives; for example, amiodarone (Cordarone) has a $t_{1/2}$ of 40 to 55 days.

Is it better to administer a drug with a short or long half-life? The answer depends on the patient's condition and the treatment goal. Drugs with short half-lives are ideal for conditions and procedures having a brief duration. For example, during a dental procedure, local anesthesia may only be needed for 15 to 20 minutes; thus procaine (Novocain), with a half-life of 8 minutes, may be sufficient. Giving a drug with a long duration of action could cause adverse effects after the patient leaves the office. As another example, a simple headache can be relieved with a short-acting drug such as aspirin ($t_{1/2}$ = 15 to 20 minutes), rather than a drug with a 10- or 12-hour duration. Because short-acting drugs are rapidly excreted, the risk of long-term adverse effects is reduced.

Long-duration drugs also have certain advantages. In the preceding example, procaine would not be suitable for a dental procedure that lasts 2 hours because multiple injections would be necessary. Long-duration drugs are beneficial in treating chronic conditions such as heart failure or hypertension and for the prevention of conditions such as migraine headaches, seizures, or pregnancy. Short-acting drugs such as aspirin must be given every 3 to 4 hours, whereas medications with longer half-lives, such as felodipine ($t_{1/2}$ = 10 hours), need to be given only once a day. As drugs stay in the body for prolonged periods, however, the risk for long-term adverse effects increases. This can become particularly serious for patients with significant renal or hepatic impairment; diminished metabolism and excretion will cause the plasma half-life of a drug to increase, and the concentration may reach toxic levels. In these patients, medications must be given less frequently, or the dosages must be reduced.

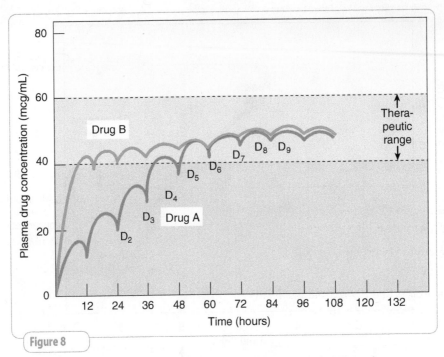

Figure 8

Multiple-dose drug administration. Drug A and drug B are administered every 12 hours. Drug B reaches the therapeutic range faster, because the first dose is a loading dose.

As a rule of thumb, when a drug is discontinued it takes approximately four half-lives before the agent is considered "functionally" eliminated. After four half-lives, 94% of the drug has been eliminated. In the case of procaine with a half-life of only 8 minutes, the drug is considered eliminated in 32 minutes. Although some drug remains, the amount is too small to produce any beneficial or toxic effect. In the example of felodipine ($t_{1/2}$ = 10 hours), the drug would take 40 hours to be eliminated. Note, however, that this "rule of thumb" does not apply to all drugs; it certainly does not apply to medications administered to patients with renal or hepatic impairment.

9 Repeated dosing allows a plateau drug plasma level to be reached.

Few drugs are administered as a single dose. When multiple doses are administered over an extended period, the goal is to keep the drug plasma level continuously within the therapeutic range. In other words, the next dose should be administered before the drug plasma level falls below the minimum effective concentration.

Multiple doses result in an accumulation of drug in the bloodstream, as shown in Figure 8. If doses are timed correctly, a plateau drug plasma level will be reached and maintained within the therapeutic range. From a pharmacokinetic perspective, at the plateau level the amount of drug absorbed equals the amount of drug being excreted, resulting in a steady therapeutic level of drug being distributed to body tissues. Theoretically, it takes approximately four half-lives to reach this equilibrium. If the medication is given as a continuous infusion, the plateau can be reached very quickly

and maintained with little or no fluctuation in drug plasma levels.

Note that in Figure 8, plasma drug levels are not necessarily smooth and continuous: There are peaks as well as troughs. When giving oral drugs, there is always some degree of fluctuation in peak concentration and trough concentration levels. A key point is that the peak should not rise into the toxic range, nor should the trough fall below the therapeutic range. Sustained or extended release formulations are designed to slowly release the drug so peak and trough fluctuations are minimized. Changing the dosing schedule can also reduce fluctuations. For example, rather than giving 60 mg of codeine once daily, it may be given 30 mg bid or 20 mg tid to reduce wide variation in the peak and trough levels.

The plateau may be reached faster by administration of loading doses followed by regular maintenance doses. A **loading dose** is a higher amount of drug, often given only once or twice, that is administered to "prime" the bloodstream with a level sufficient to quickly induce a therapeutic response. Before plasma levels drop back toward zero, intermittent **maintenance doses** are given to keep the plasma drug concentration in the therapeutic range. Although blood levels of the drug fluctuate with this approach, the equilibrium state can be reached almost as rapidly as with a continuous infusion. Loading doses are particularly important for drugs with prolonged half-lives and for situations in which it is critical to raise drug plasma levels quickly, as might be the case when administering an antibiotic for a severe infection. In Figure 8, it took almost five doses (48 hours) before a therapeutic level was reached using a routine dosing schedule. With a loading dose, a therapeutic level was reached within 12 hours.

UNDERSTANDING THE CHAPTER

Key Concepts Summary

1 Pharmacokinetics focuses on what the body does to drugs after they are administered.

2 Drugs use diffusion and active transport to cross plasma membranes to reach their target cells.

3 Absorption is the process of moving a drug from the site of administration to the bloodstream.

4 Distribution describes how drugs are transported throughout the body.

5 Metabolism is a process that changes the activity of a drug and makes it more likely to be excreted.

6 Excretion processes remove drugs from the body.

7 The therapeutic response of most drugs depends on their concentration in the plasma.

8 The drug half-life estimates the duration of action for most medications.

9 Repeated dosing allows a plateau drug plasma level to be reached.

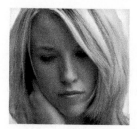

Making the PATIENT Connection

Remember the patient "John Kessler" at the beginning of the chapter? Now read the remainder of the case study. Based on the information presented within this chapter, respond to the critical thinking questions that follow.

John Kessler has been ill for a long time and his prognosis is poor. He is 84 years old with multiple debilitating and chronic conditions. He has had uncontrolled diabetes for more than 20 years, and has experienced many complications due to this condition. Three years ago, he developed chronic renal failure and requires dialysis three times a week. To further complicate his condition, John has continued to consume alcohol every day, and smokes one pack of cigarettes per day. He has a long history of both alcohol and tobacco use.

Five days ago, his daughter noticed that he was becoming increasingly weak and lethargic. Last night when his temperature reached 38.8°C (102°F) and he became confused, his daughter took him to the emergency department, and he was admitted to the medical unit. A chest x-ray this morning revealed bilateral pneumonia. John is receiving multiple medications through both the intravenous and inhalation routes.

Critical Thinking Questions

1. What factors may influence drug metabolism or excretion in this patient?

2. Discuss why drug elimination for this patient may complicate the pharmacotherapy.

3. How will the IV or inhalation drug therapy affect the absorption of his medications?

4. John will receive a loading dose of IV antibiotic and then be placed on maintenance doses every 6 hours. What is the purpose of this regimen? Why would this patient be a candidate for a loading dose?

See Answers to Critical Thinking Questions on student resource website.

NCLEX-RN® Review

1 The nurse is teaching the client about a newly prescribed medication. Which statement made by the client would indicate the need for further medication education?

1. "The liquid form of the drug will be absorbed faster than the tablets."

2. "If I take more, I'll have a better response."

3. "Taking this drug with food will decrease how much drug gets into my system."

4. "I can consult my health care provider if I experience unexpected adverse effects."

2 The nurse is caring for several clients. Which client will the nurse anticipate is most likely to experience an alteration in drug metabolism?

1. A 3-day-old premature infant

2. A 22-year-old pregnant female

3. A 32-year-old man with kidney stones

4. A 50-year-old executive with hypertension

3 The client is receiving multiple medications, including one drug specifically used to stimulate gastric peristalsis. The nurse knows that this drug could have what influence on additional oral medications?

1. Increased absorption
2. Reduced excretion
3. Decreased absorption
4. Enhanced distribution

4 A client is being discharged from the hospital with a nebulizer for self-administration of inhalation medication. Which statement made by the client indicates to the nurse that client education has been successful?

1. "Inhaled medications should only be taken in the morning."
2. "Doses for inhaled medication are larger than those taken orally."
3. "Medicines taken by inhalation produce a very rapid response."
4. "Inhaled drugs are often rendered inactive by hepatic metabolic reactions."

5 The nurse is caring for a client with hepatitis and resulting hepatic impairment. The nurse would expect the duration of action for most medications to:

1. Decrease.
2. Improve.
3. Be unaffected.
4. Increase.

6 The nurse is monitoring the therapeutic drug level for a client on vancomycin (Vancocin) and notes that the level is within the accepted range. What does this indicate to the nurse? Select all that apply.

1. The drug should cause no toxicities or adverse effects.
2. The drug level is appropriate to exert therapeutic effects.
3. The dose will not need to be changed for the duration of treatment.
4. The nurse will need to continue monitoring because each client response to a drug is unique.
5. This drug will effectively treat the client's condition.

Additional Case Study

Janice Albertson is a student nurse caring for a patient on the unit in which you are the RN. She has researched every drug her patient will be receiving and is familiar with the dose, mechanism of action, and possible adverse effects. Now she comes to you and asks, "Why is the drug's plasma half-life listed in the drug reference book? What is the value of this information?"

1. How would you respond to Janice's questions?
2. When is the use of drugs with short half-lives indicated?
3. List the indications for the use of a drug with a long half-life.

See Answers to Additional Case Study on student resource website.

Pearson Nursing Student Resources

Find additional review materials at nursing.pearsonhighered.com

Prepare for success with additional NCLEX®-style practice questions, interactive assignments and activities, web links, animations, videos, and more!

Selected Bibliography

Amur, S., Zineh, I., Abernethy, D. R., Huang, S. & Lesko, L. J. (2010). Pharmacogenomics and adverse drug reactions. *Personalized Medicine, 7*(6), 633-642. doi:10.2217/pme.10.63

Bauer, L. A. (2011). Clinical pharmacokinetics and pharmacodynamics. In J. T. DiPiro, R. L. Talbert, G. C. Yee, G. R. Matzke, B. G. Wells, & L. M. Posey (Eds.), *Pharmacotherapy: A Pathophysiology Approach* (8th ed., pp. 12–35). New York, NY: McGraw-Hill.

Buxton, I. L., & Benet, L. Z. (2011). Pharmacokinetics: The dynamics of drug absorption, distribution, action and elimination. In L. L. Brunton, B. A. Chabner, & B. C. Knollman (Eds.), *The pharmacological basis of therapeutics* (12th ed., pp. 17–40). New York, NY: McGraw-Hill.

Custodio, J. M., & Benet, L. Z. (2008). Predicting drug disposition, absorption/elimination/transporter interplay and the role of food on drug absorption. *Advanced Drug Delivery Systems, 60*(6), 717–733. doi:10.1016/j.addr.2007.08.043

Delafuente, J. C. (2008). Pharmacokinetic and pharmacodynamic alterations in the geriatric patient. *The Consultant Pharmacist, 23*(4), 564. doi:10.4140/TCP.n.2008.324

Klotz, U. (2009). Pharmacokinetics and drug metabolism in the elderly. *Drug Metabolism Reviews, 41*(2), 67–76. doi:10.1080/03602530902722679

Papadopoulos, J., & Smithburger, P. L. (2010). Common drug interactions leading to adverse drug events in the intensive care unit: Management and pharmacokinetic considerations. *Critical Care Medicine, 38*, S126-S135. doi:10.1097/CCM.0b013e3181de0acf

Rosenbaum, S. E. (2011). *Basic pharmacokinetics and pharmacodynamics: An integrated textbook and computer simulations.* Hoboken, NJ: John Wiley & Sons.

Yengi, L. G., Leung, L., & Kao, J. (2007). The evolving role of drug metabolism in drug discovery and development. *Pharmaceutical Research, 24*(5), 842–858. doi:10.1007/s11095-006-9217-9

Answers to NCLEX-RN® Review

1 Answer: 2 Rationale: Although taking a larger dose of a medication usually results in a greater therapeutic response, the response also depends on the drug's plasma concentration. If a toxic level is reached from too large a dose, the drug will have adverse effects instead of a better therapeutic response. Options 1, 3, and 4 are incorrect because they are true statements. The liquid form of a drug will be absorbed faster than its tablet form. Food decreases the absorption rate of most drugs. Clients should always consult a health care provider if unexpected adverse effects develop. Cognitive Level: Applying; Client Need: Health Promotion and Maintenance; Nursing Process: Evaluation

2 Answer: 1 Rationale: Infants do not develop a mature microsomal enzyme system until they are a year old and therefore do not metabolize drugs very efficiently. Options 2, 3, and 4 are incorrect. Pregnancy does not significantly affect drug metabolism. The concern with pregnant clients is primarily focused on alterations in distribution due to the fetal–placental barrier. The presence of kidney stones would not influence drug metabolism. Hypertension is not a factor that directly results in abnormal metabolism. Cognitive Level: Applying; Client Need: Physiological Integrity; Nursing Process: Implementation

3 Answer: 3 Rationale: Peristalsis is the wavelike muscular contraction that pushes food into the stomach and helps to mix stomach contents. An increase in this activity would decrease the time that drugs would remain in the GI system, and therefore decrease absorption. Options 1, 2, and 4 are incorrect. Excretion for most drugs occurs mostly through the kidneys, lungs, and glands. Peristalsis would not reduce excretions of medications. A delay in peristalsis would prolong absorption time, and peristalsis is not involved in the distribution of drugs to their target sites. Cognitive Level: Applying; Patient Need: Physiological Integrity; Nursing Process: Evaluation

4 Answer: 3 Rationale: Inhaled drugs produce an immediate therapeutic response. Options 1, 2, and 4 are incorrect. Inhaled medication can be used at any time during the day and is not restricted to the morning. Doses for inhaled drugs are small compared to orally ingested medications, and because these drugs go directly to the lung surface area and are readily absorbed, very little of the substance is lost due to metabolism. Cognitive Level: Applying; Client Need: Health Promotion and Maintenance; Nursing Process: Evaluation

5 Answer: 4 Rationale: The length of time a drug concentration remains in the therapeutic range is its duration of action. Clients with hepatic impairment do not effectively metabolize drugs, which increases the duration of action. Options 1, 2, and 3 are incorrect. In clients with hepatic disease, the duration of action most likely will increase since drug metabolism is impaired. Although the duration of action is extended, the effects of the drug are not improved. Cognitive Level: Applying; Client Need: Safe and Effective Care Environment; Nursing Process: Evaluation

6 Answer: 2, 4 Rationale: A therapeutic drug level that is in the accepted range indicates that the drug is at a minimally effective concentration but not at a toxic level. Because each client response to a drug is unique, the nurse should continue monitoring the client throughout the drug's use. Options 1, 3, and 5 are incorrect. Because individual client responses to drugs can be highly variable, adverse effects, toxicities, or even no effect may occur at levels within the therapeutic range. For that reason, the drug dose may need to be adjusted throughout therapy. Therapeutic effectiveness of a drug depends on many factors and the therapeutic range of a drug is the level between minimally effective and toxic levels. It is not an indicator of how effective a drug will be in treating an individual condition. Cognitive Level: Applying; Client Need: Physiological Integrity; Nursing Process: Evaluation

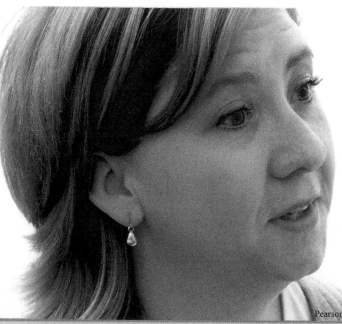

"I am totally confused by all the antacid commercials on television. Some say their medication is the most efficient and others claim their brand is the most potent. What does it all mean?"

Patient "Katherine Hunter"

Pearson Education/PH College

Pharmacodynamics

Chapter Outline

Interpatient Variability

Therapeutic Index

Dose–Response Relationship

Potency and Efficacy

Receptor Theory

Agonists and Antagonists

Pharmacogenetics

Learning Outcomes

After reading this chapter, the student should be able to:

1. Employ principles of pharmacodynamics to explain variations in drug response in a population.

2. Apply frequency distribution curves to explain interpatient variability in medication response.

3. Explain the importance of the median effective dose (ED_{50}) to clinical practice.

4. Compare and contrast median lethal dose (LD_{50}) and median toxicity dose (TD_{50}).

5. Relate a drug's therapeutic index to its margin of safety.

6. Identify the significance of the dose–response relationship to clinical practice.

7. Compare and contrast the terms *potency* and *efficacy*.

8. Describe the relationship between receptors and drug action.

9. Distinguish between an agonist, partial agonist, and antagonist.

10. Explain possible future developments in the field of pharmacogenetics.

From Chapter 5 of *Pharmacology: Connections to Nursing Practice*, Second Edition. Michael Patrick Adams, Carol Quam Urban. Copyright © 2013 by Pearson Education, Inc. All rights reserved.

Key Terms

The term *pharmacodynamics* is comprised of the root words *pharmaco*, which refers to medicines, and *dynamics*, which means "change." In simplest terms, pharmacodynamics refers to how a drug changes the body. A more complete definition explains **pharmacodynamics** as the branch of pharmacology concerned with the mechanisms of drug action and the relationships between drug concentration and responses in the body. This chapter examines the mechanisms by which drugs affect patients, and how the nurse can apply these principles to clinical practice.

Interpatient Variability

1 Patients have widely different responses to drugs, which can be depicted on a frequency distribution curve.

The principles of pharmacodynamics have important clinical applications. Health care providers must be able to predict whether a given dose of medication will produce a therapeutic change in their patients. Why does the "average" dose obtained from a drug guide sometimes produce a hyperresponse and at other times no response at all? Knowledge of dose–response relationships, therapeutic indexes, and drug–receptor interactions—all topics of pharmacodynamics—can help nurses provide safer and more effective treatment.

The interpatient variability observed during drug therapy can best be illustrated by examining a frequency distribution curve. Shown in Figure 1, a **frequency distribution curve** is a graphic representation of the actual number of patients responding with a particular drug action at different doses. On the horizontal axis, notice the wide range in doses that produced the patient responses shown on the curve. A few patients responded to the drug at very low doses (10 to 20 mg). As the dose was increased, more and more patients responded. The peak of the curve (50 mg) indicates the largest number of patients responding to the drug. Some patients required very high doses (80 to 90 mg) to elicit the desired response. The curve does not show the magnitude of the response, only whether or not a measurable response occurred among the patients. As an example, think of the given response to an antihypertensive drug as defined by a reduction of 20 mm in systolic blood pressure. A few patients experienced the desired 20-mm reduction at a drug dose of only 10 mg; a 50-mg dose gave the largest number of patients the 20-mm reduction in blood pressure. However, a few patients needed as much as 90 mg of the drug to produce the same 20-mm reduction.

The dose in the middle of the frequency distribution curve represents the drug's **median effective dose (ED$_{50}$)**. The ED$_{50}$ is the dose required to produce a specific therapeutic response in 50% of a group of patients. Drug guides usually use the ED$_{50}$ as the "average" or standard dose for a drug.

The interpatient variability shown in Figure 1 has important clinical implications. First, the nurse should realize that the standard or average dose predicts a satisfactory therapeutic response for only half the population. But what about responses in the rest of the patients? Many patients will require more or less than the average dose for optimum pharmacotherapy. Using the systolic blood pressure example, assume that a large group of patients is given the average dose of 50 mg. Some of these patients will experience toxicity at this level because they only need 10 mg to achieve blood pressure reduction. Other patients in this group will probably have no reduction in blood pressure at all. By monitoring the patient, taking vital signs, and interpreting any associated laboratory data, the nurse is key in determining whether the average dose is effective for the patient. *It is not enough to simply memorize an average dose for a drug; the nurse must have the skills to know when and how to adjust this dose to obtain the optimum therapeutic response.*

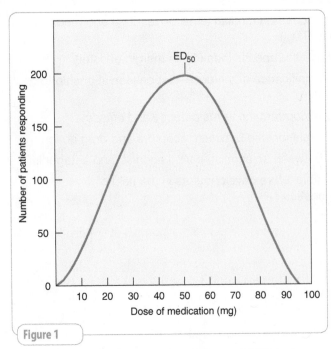

Figure 1

Frequency distribution curve: interpatient variability in drug response.

Therapeutic Index

2 The therapeutic index describes a drug's margin of safety.

Selecting a dose that produces an optimum therapeutic response for each individual patient is certainly important, but the nurse must also be able to predict whether that dose is safe for that patient. Frequency distribution curves can also be used to illustrate the safety of a drug.

The **median lethal dose (LD$_{50}$)** is a value often determined in laboratory animals in preclinical experiments during the drug development process. The LD$_{50}$ is the dose of drug that will kill 50% of a group of animals. Just as with ED$_{50}$, a population of animals will exhibit considerable variability in lethal dosage; what may be a nontoxic dose for one animal may kill another.

To examine the safety of a particular drug, the LD$_{50}$ is compared to ED$_{50}$, as shown in Figure 2a. In this example, 10 mg of drug is the average effective dose, and 40 mg is the average lethal dose. The ED$_{50}$ and LD$_{50}$ are used to calculate one of the most important values in pharmacology, a drug's therapeutic index. The **therapeutic index (TI)** is defined as the ratio of a drug's LD$_{50}$ to its ED$_{50}$.

$$\text{Therapeutic index} = \frac{\text{median lethal dose (LD}_{50})}{\text{median effective dose (ED}_{50})}$$

The larger the difference between the two doses, the greater the TI. In Figure 2a, the TI is 4 (40 mg ÷ 10 mg). Essentially, this means that it would take an error in magnitude of approximately four times the average dose to be lethal to a patient. In terms of dosage, this is a relatively safe drug, and small to moderate medication errors or changes in the drug's bioavailability would likely not be fatal. Thus, the TI is a measure of a drug's safety margin: the higher the value, the safer the medication. Drugs exhibit a wide range of TIs, from 1 to 2 to greater than 100.

As another example, the TI of a second drug is shown in Figure 2b. Drug Z has the same ED$_{50}$ as drug X but shows a different LD$_{50}$. The TI for drug Z is only 2 (20 mg ÷ 10 mg). The difference between an effective dose and a lethal dose is very small for drug Z; thus the drug has a narrow safety margin. Small medication errors or changes in the drug's metabolism or excretion could have lethal consequences. The TI offers the nurse practical information on the safety of a drug and a means to compare one drug to another.

In Figure 2b, notice that the two curves overlapped. Some patients required a dose of 15 to 20 mg to produce the desired effect, yet this same dose was lethal in other patients. This type of drug would require careful assessment of hepatic and renal function prior to the initiation of therapy. With drugs exhibiting a low TI, it is prudent to begin with the lowest dose possible, then increase the amount of drug with careful monitoring.

Because the LD$_{50}$ cannot be experimentally determined in humans, other estimates of drug safety are available. The **median toxicity dose (TD$_{50}$)** is the dose that will produce a

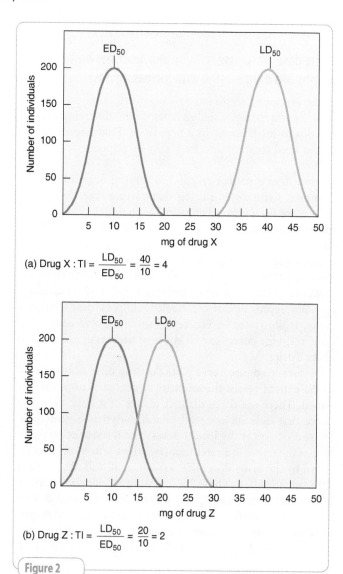

(a) Drug X : TI = $\dfrac{\text{LD}_{50}}{\text{ED}_{50}} = \dfrac{40}{10} = 4$

(b) Drug Z : TI = $\dfrac{\text{LD}_{50}}{\text{ED}_{50}} = \dfrac{20}{10} = 2$

Figure 2

Therapeutic index: (a) Drug X has a therapeutic index of 4. (b) Drug Z has a therapeutic index of 2.

given toxicity in 50% of a group of patients. The TD$_{50}$ value may be extrapolated from animal data or based on adverse effects recorded in patient clinical trials.

The **margin of safety (MOS)** is another index of a drug's effectiveness and safety. The MOS is calculated as the amount of drug that is lethal to 1% of animals (LD$_1$) divided by the amount of drug that produces a therapeutic effect in 99% of the animals (ED$_{99}$). In general, the higher the MOS value, the safer the medication. Of course this considers only the lethality of the drug and does not account for nonlethal, though serious, adverse effects that may occur at lower doses.

CONNECTION Checkpoint 5.1

Before a pharmaceutical company tests a drug in patients after preclinical trials have been completed, what document must be submitted to the FDA? *See Answer to Connection Checkpoint 5.1 on student resource website.*

Dose–Response Relationship

3 The dose–response relationship describes how the actions of a drug change with increasing dose.

In the preceding section, frequency distribution curves were used to graphically visualize interpatient differences in responses to medications in a *population*. Pharmacodynamics is also used to study the variability in responses in a *single patient*.

How does a patient respond to varying doses of a drug? Common sense would suggest that a larger dose would produce more drug effect. For example, an antibiotic would kill more bacteria if the dose was increased from 10 to 20 mg. An antihypertensive drug would cause a greater reduction in blood pressure if the dose was increased from 50 to 100 mg. These simple examples describe the **dose–response relationship**, one of the most fundamental concepts in pharmacology. A graphic representation of this relationship, the dose–response curve, is illustrated in Figure 3. Examining and comparing dose–response curves can yield a large amount of information about a drug.

A dose–response curve plots the drug dose administered to the patient versus the intensity or degree of response obtained. There are three distinct phases of a dose–response curve that indicate essential pharmacodynamic principles. Phase 1 occurs at the lowest doses. The flatness of this portion of the curve indicates that few target cells have been affected by the drug; doses that are too small will not produce a therapeutic effect. Phase 2 is the rising, straight line portion of the curve. In this portion, there is a linear relationship between the amount of drug administered and the degree of response obtained from the patient. For example, if the dose is doubled, twice as much response may be obtained.

This is the most desirable range of doses for pharmacotherapeutics, because giving more drug results in proportionately more effect; a lower drug dose gives less effect. In phase 3 increasing the drug dose produces no additional therapeutic response—a plateau has been reached. This may occur for a number of reasons. One possible explanation is that all the target receptors for the drug are occupied. It could also mean that the drug has brought 100% relief, such as when a migraine headache has been terminated; giving higher doses produces no additional relief. Although increasing the dose during phase 3 does not result in additional therapeutic effects, the nurse should be mindful that increasing the dose may produce more adverse effects.

The dose–response curve in Figure 3 is smooth and continuous; thus it is sometimes called a graded dose–response curve. This is important to pharmacotherapeutics because, by adjusting the dose in small increments, the prescriber is able to attain virtually any degree of therapeutic response (0% to 100%) within the linear range of drug doses. This is especially true when using the intravenous (IV) route, during which the nurse can adjust the infusion rate in very small increments.

Many types of adverse effects also follow a graded dose–response relationship: the higher the dose, the more intense the adverse effect. By adjusting the dose lower, while still keeping it within the therapeutic range, adverse effects may be lessened. Some adverse effects, such as anaphylaxis, are independent of dose in that even the smallest amount of drug may trigger a serious adverse response.

Potency and Efficacy

4 Potency and efficacy are fundamental concepts of pharmacodynamics that describe a drug's activity.

Within a pharmacologic class, not all drugs are equally effective at treating a disorder. For example, some antineoplastic drugs kill more cancer cells than others; some antihypertensive agents lower blood pressure to a greater extent than others; and some analgesics are more effective at relieving severe pain than others in the same class. Furthermore, drugs in the same class are effective at different doses: One antibiotic may be effective at a dose of 1 mg/kg, whereas another is most effective at 100 mg/kg. Nurses need a method to compare one drug to another so that they can administer treatment effectively.

There are two fundamental ways to compare medications within therapeutic and pharmacologic classes. First is the concept of **potency**, which is the strength of a drug at a specified concentration or dose. A drug that is more potent will produce its therapeutic effect at a lower dose, compared to another drug in the same class. As an example, consider two calcium channel blockers used for hypertension: amlodipine (Norvasc) and nifedipine (Procardia). Amlodipine produces its decrease in blood pressure at 10 mg (maximum dose) and nifedipine at 180 mg. Amlodipine is clearly more potent than nifedipine because it took a lower dose (18 times less) to produce its antihypertensive effect.

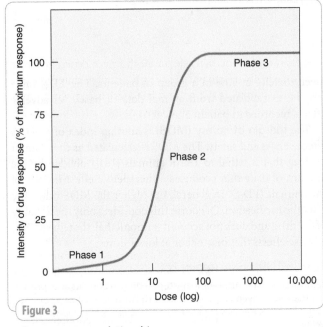

Figure 3

Dose–response relationship.

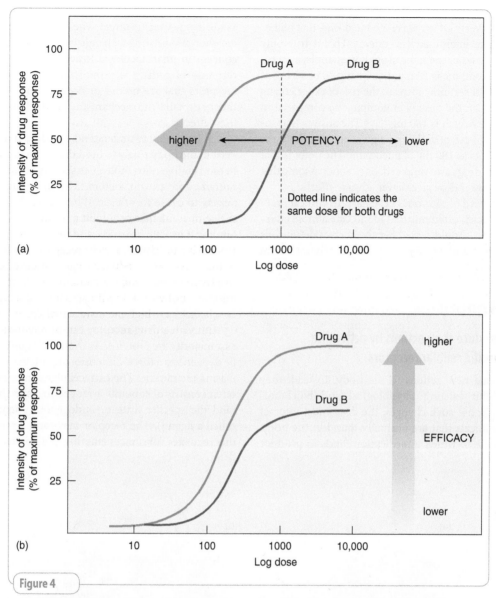

Figure 4

Potency and efficacy: (a) Drug A has a higher potency than drug B. (b) Drug A has a higher efficacy than drug B.

Thus, potency is a way to compare the doses of two independently administered drugs in terms of how much is needed to produce a particular response. A useful way to visualize the concept of potency is by examining dose–response curves. When comparing the two drugs shown in Figure 4a, drug A is more potent because it requires a lower dose to produce the same response.

A second method used to compare drugs is called **efficacy**, which is defined as the greatest maximal response that can be produced from a particular drug. In the example in Figure 4b, drug A is more efficacious because it produces a higher maximal response.

Which is more important to the outcomes of pharmacotherapy: potency or efficacy? Perhaps the best way to understand these important concepts is to use the specific example of headache pain. Two common over-the-counter (OTC) analgesic therapies are ibuprofen, 200 mg, and aspirin, 650 mg. The fact that ibuprofen relieves pain at a lower dose indicates that this agent is more potent than aspirin. At the given doses, however, both are equally effective at relieving headaches; thus they have the same efficacy. If the patient is experiencing severe pain, however, neither aspirin nor ibuprofen has sufficient efficacy to bring relief. Narcotic analgesics, such as morphine, have a greater efficacy than aspirin or ibuprofen and could effectively treat this type of pain. From a pharmacotherapeutic perspective, efficacy is almost always more important than potency. In the preceding example, the average dose is unimportant to the patient, but headache relief is essential. As another comparison, the patient with cancer is much more concerned with how many cancer cells have been killed (efficacy) than with the dose the nurse administered (potency). In the comparison of Norvasc to Procardia, although Norvasc is clearly more potent, both drugs reduce blood pressure to the same degree; thus they have the same efficacy. Although the nurse will often hear claims that one drug is more potent than another, a more compelling concern is which drug is more efficacious.

A word of caution is necessary at this point. In Section 3, it is stated that many adverse effects are related to dose—that higher doses produce more intense adverse effects. This is true only when comparing doses of the same drug. For example, a therapeutic dose for amlodipine is 10 mg/day. Giving 20 or 30 mg of amlodipine will most certainly increase the risk of experiencing an adverse effect. Can the dose of amlodipine be compared to a dose of nifedipine, which is 180 mg/day? The answer is absolutely not. In fact, 10 mg of amlodipine gives roughly the same risk of adverse effects as 180 mg of nifedipine. The point is that when two different drugs are compared, one cannot assume that the drug with the lower dose gives fewer adverse effects.

An additional word of caution is necessary. In clinical practice the term *potency* is often misused to indicate a more effective drug. The nurse should remember the correct definitions of the words *potency* and *efficacy* and try to incorporate them into clinical practice.

Receptor Theory

5 Most drugs produce their actions by activating or inhibiting specific cellular receptors.

Drugs rarely create new actions in the body; instead, they enhance or inhibit existing physiological and biochemical processes. To cause such changes, the drug must interact with specific chemicals that are normally found in the body. A cellular molecule to which a medication binds to produce its effects is called a **receptor**. A receptor may be thought of as the drug's specific target. The concept of a drug binding to a receptor and causing a change in physiology is a fundamental concept in pharmacology. Receptor theory predicts that the response of a drug is proportional to the concentration of receptors that are bound or occupied by the drug. Receptor theory explains the mechanisms by which most drugs produce their effects.

It is important to understand, however, that receptors do not exist in the body solely to bind drugs; their normal function is to bind endogenous molecules such as hormones, neurotransmitters, and growth factors. The drug simply uses existing targets to cause its effects. When drugs bind to the receptor they either enhance or inhibit a normal cellular function. The binding is usually reversible and the action of the drug is terminated once the drug leaves its receptor. In a few cases, binding of the drug is irreversible. Drugs that have the ability to bind to a receptor and produce a strong action are said to have high **intrinsic activity**. Intrinsic activity and efficacy are related. Drugs that have high intrinsic activity have high efficacy.

Although a drug receptor can be any type of molecule, the vast majority are proteins. As shown in Figure 5, a receptor may be depicted as a three-dimensional protein spanning across the plasma membrane. The extracellular component of a receptor often consists of subunits arranged in a specific shape that will bind the specific drug or endogenous chemical (sometimes called a ligand). The receptor may form a membrane channel that regulates substances entering and leaving the cell.

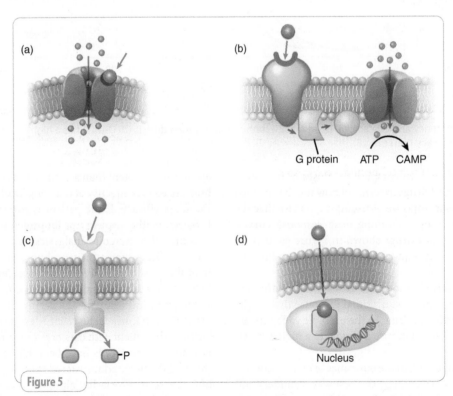

(a)

(b)

G protein   ATP   CAMP

(c)

P

(d)

Nucleus

Figure 5

Types of cellular receptors: (a) Drug binds to the receptor opening channel. (b) Drug binds to the receptor, causing a G protein–mediated reaction in the cell. (c) Drug binds to the transmembrane receptor to signal a change inside the cell. (d) Drug enters the cell nucleus to increase synthesis of specific proteins.

A drug binds to its receptor in a very selective manner, much like a lock and key. Once the receptor is occupied, a series of **second messenger** events is triggered within the cell such as the conversion of adenosine triphosphate (ATP) to cyclic adenosine monophosphate (cyclic AMP), the release of intracellular calcium, or the activation of specific G proteins and associated enzymes. These cascades of biochemical events initiate the drug's action by either stimulating or inhibiting the normal activity of the cell. Small changes to the structure of a drug, or its receptor, may weaken or even eliminate binding between the two molecules, rendering the drug ineffective.

Not all receptors are proteins bound to the plasma membrane: Some are intracellular molecules such as DNA or enzymes in the cytoplasm. By interacting with these types of receptors, medications are able to inhibit protein synthesis or regulate events such as cell division and metabolism. Examples of agents that bind intracellular components include steroid hormones and certain vitamins.

Receptor subtypes have been discovered that permit the "fine-tuning" of pharmacotherapy. For example, the first drugs affecting the autonomic nervous system affected all types of autonomic receptors. These agents were not very useful because they produced such a broad range of therapeutic and adverse effects. Later, it was discovered that two basic receptor types existed in the body, alpha and beta, and drugs were then developed that were selective for only one type. This permitted more specific drug therapy (and fewer adverse effects). Still later, several subtypes of alpha and beta receptors, including alpha-1, alpha-2, beta-1, and beta-2, were discovered that allowed even more specificity in pharmacotherapy. In recent years, researchers have further divided and refined various drug receptor subtypes. It is likely that research will continue to result in the development of new medications that activate very specific receptors to cause therapeutic responses while avoiding some adverse effects.

Some drugs act independently of cellular receptors. These agents are associated with other mechanisms, such as changing the permeability of cellular membranes, depressing membrane excitability, or altering the activity of cellular pumps. Actions such as these are often described as nonspecific cellular responses. Ethyl alcohol, general anesthetics, and osmotic diuretics are examples of agents that act by nonspecific mechanisms.

Agonists and Antagonists

6 Agonists, partial agonists, and antagonists compete for cellular receptors and can modify drug action.

When a drug binds to a receptor, several possible consequences can result. In simplest terms, some specific activity of the cell is either enhanced or inhibited. The actual biochemical mechanism underlying the therapeutic effect, however, may be extremely complex. In some cases, the mechanism of action is not known.

When a drug binds to its receptor, it may produce a response that mimics the effect of the endogenous regulatory molecule. For example, when the drug bethanechol is administered, it binds to acetylcholine receptors in the autonomic nervous system and produces the same actions as acetylcholine.

A drug that activates a receptor and produces the same type of response as the endogenous substance is called an **agonist**. Agonists sometimes produce a greater maximal response than the endogenous chemical. The term **partial agonist** is used to describe a medication that produces a weaker, or less efficacious, response than an agonist.

A second possibility is that a drug will occupy a receptor and prevent the endogenous chemical from binding to produce its action. This type of drug, an **antagonist**, often competes with agonists for receptor binding sites. For example, the drug atropine competes with acetylcholine for certain receptors in the autonomic nervous system. If the dose is high enough, atropine may completely block the effects of acetylcholine because acetylcholine cannot reach its receptors. Antagonists may be used as medications when the body is producing too much of a response from an endogenous chemical or from a drug overdose, such as high blood pressure, fast heart rate, secretion of excess stomach acid, or sedation. Giving an antagonist in these situations may reverse the adverse effects. An antagonist has no intrinsic activity; the actions observed after administering an antagonist are caused by lack of agonist action.

Not all antagonism is associated with receptors, as in the previous example. Functional antagonists inhibit the effects of an agonist, not by competing for a receptor but by changing pharmacokinetic factors. For example, antagonists may slow the absorption of an agonist, resulting in less pharmacologic effect. An antagonist may change the pH of the surrounding fluid and neutralize the agonist before it is even absorbed. By speeding up metabolism or excretion, an antagonist can enhance the removal of an agonist from the body. The relationships that occur between agonists and antagonists explain many of the drug–drug and drug–food interactions that occur in the body. Figure 6 illustrates the concept of agonist and antagonist drug action.

CONNECTION Checkpoint 5.2

Phenytoin is an inducer of CYP1A2, the enzyme that metabolizes acetaminophen. Would phenytoin be considered a functional agonist or an antagonist to acetaminophen? *See Answer to Connection Checkpoint 5.2 on student resource website.*

Pharmacogenetics

7 In the future, pharmacogenetics may allow customization of drug therapy.

Until quite recently, it was thought that drugs provided safe and effective treatment to every patient in the same manner. Unfortunately, a significant portion of the population either develops unacceptable adverse effects to certain drugs or is unresponsive to them. Some scientists and clinicians are now discarding the "one size fits all" approach to drug therapy, which was designed to treat the entire population without addressing important interpatient variation.

With the advent of the Human Genome Project and other advances in medicine, pharmacologists are hopeful that future drugs can be customized for patients with specific genetic similarities. In the past, any unpredictable and unexplained

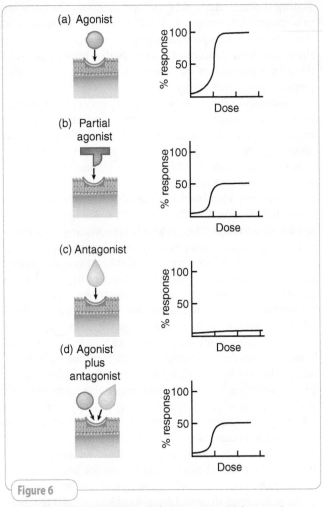

Figure 6

Agonists, partial agonists, and antagonists: (a) An agonist results in maximum response. (b) A partial agonist results in less than maximum response. (c) An antagonist results in little or no response. (d) An agonist plus antagonist results in diminished response.

drug reaction has been labeled **idiosyncratic response**. It is hoped that, by analyzing a DNA test before prescribing a drug, these idiosyncratic adverse effects can someday be avoided.

Pharmacogenetics is the branch of pharmacology that examines the role of genetics in drug response. The most important advances in pharmacogenetics so far have been the identification of subtle genetic differences in drug-metabolizing enzymes. Genetic differences in these enzymes are responsible for a significant portion of drug-induced toxicity. It is hoped that the use of pharmacogenetic information may someday allow for drug therapy that is customized to a patient's individual molecules. Although therapies based on a patient's genetically based response may not be cost effective at this time, pharmacogenetics may radically change the way pharmacotherapy will be practiced in the future.

CONNECTIONS

Treating the Diverse Patient
Enzyme Deficiencies in Ethnic Populations

Pharmacogenetics has identified ethnic populations of people, such as males of Mediterranean and African descent, who are deficient in glucose-6-phosphate dehydrogenase (G6PD), an enzyme that is essential in carbohydrate metabolism. As reviewed by Carter (2009), G6PD deficiency is the most common enzyme deficiency, with about 400 million people affected worldwide. Over 60 different mutations that encode for G6PD have been identified. When certain oxidative drugs are given, such as primaquine, sulfonamides, or nitrofurantoin (Macrobid), an acute hemolysis of red blood cells (RBCs) occurs due to the breaking of chemical bonds in the hemoglobin molecule, with large numbers of circulating RBCs being destroyed. Genetic typing does not always predict toxicity. Patients may report a history of severe allergy to fava beans, which induce the hemolytic symptoms. The role of the nurse is critical in observing patients carefully for 24 to 72 hours following administration of these medications. Prevention is the best treatment.

UNDERSTANDING THE CHAPTER

Key Concepts Summary

1 Patients have widely different responses to drugs, which can be depicted on a frequency distribution curve.

2 The therapeutic index describes a drug's margin of safety.

3 The dose–response relationship describes how the actions of a drug change with increasing dose.

4 Potency and efficacy are fundamental concepts of pharmacodynamics that describe a drug's activity.

5 Most drugs produce their actions by activating or inhibiting specific cellular receptors.

6 Agonists, partial agonists, and antagonists compete for cellular receptors and can modify drug action.

7 In the future, pharmacogenetics may allow customization of drug therapy.

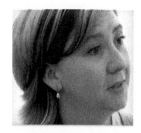

Making the PATIENT Connection

Remember the patient "Katherine Hunter" at the beginning of the chapter? Now read the remainder of the case study. Based on the information presented within this chapter, respond to the critical thinking questions that follow.

Katherine Hunter prides herself on being a wise consumer and cautiously examines the claims by manufacturers for all her purchases. She researches everything she buys, such as automobiles, household appliances, and medications. Recently, she has begun to seriously consider assertions made by the advertisements for various types of antacids. Most brands claim to be the most efficient in relieving the symptoms of indigestion. Others say that their brand is the most potent antacid available without a prescription. Some products claim that they not only relieve heartburn, but also supply the body with needed vitamins and minerals. When purchasing an OTC medication, all Katherine wants is something that will work quickly with few adverse effects.

Critical Thinking Questions

1. How would you teach Katherine the difference between potency and efficacy?

2. Which of the two concepts (potency and efficacy) would be most important for selecting a drug? Why?

3. What are the drawbacks of comparing two different medications?

See Answers to Critical Thinking Questions on student resource website.

NCLEX-RN® Review

1 What parameters would the nurse use to determine whether the average dose of a medication is effective for a client? Select all that apply.

1. Physical examination
2. Vital signs
3. Laboratory values
4. Dosage time
5. Efficacy

2 The nurse knows that a drug with a high therapeutic index is:

1. Probably safe.
2. Often dangerous.
3. Frequently risky.
4. Most likely effective.

3 While reviewing a drug manufacturer's package insert, the nurse reads about the dose–response curve. The purpose of the dose–response curve is to illustrate the relationship between:

1. The amount of a drug administered and the degree of response it produces.
2. The prevalence of toxic effects in a given population.
3. The degree of response and the total duration of action of the drug.
4. The peak serum drug level when half the dose is administered.

4 A research nurse is discussing the TD_{50} of a drug with the other members of the investigation team. On which of the following would the discussion focus?

1. Effectiveness
2. Dose response
3. Receptor subtypes
4. Toxicity

5 A client with myasthenia gravis has been receiving neostigmine, a cholinergic agonist, for the past 2 years. The nurse is ready to administer benztropine, a cholinergic antagonist. Which result will likely occur when these drugs are combined?

1. Neostigmine will exhibit a greater effect.
2. Neostigmine will exhibit a lesser effect.
3. Neostigmine will not be affected by the administration of benztropine.
4. Neostigmine will first exhibit a greater effect, followed by a lesser effect.

6 When considering pharmacodynamic principles for a client's drug therapy, the nurse is aware that affinity for a receptor is most closely associated with a drug's:

1. Potency.
2. Efficacy.
3. Metabolism.
4. First-pass effect.

Additional Case Study

As the nurse practicing in a middle school, you have been asked to speak to the eighth-grade pre-health professionals' class. The topic for today's discussion is "how drugs work in the body." The teacher has provided you with an outline of concepts that you will need to address.

1. Describe the link between a drug's action and drug receptors.
2. Why do people respond differently to medication?
3. What are drug agonists and drug antagonists?

See Answers to Additional Case Study on student resource website.

Pearson Nursing Student Resources

Find additional review materials at nursing.pearsonhighered.com

Prepare for success with additional NCLEX®-style practice questions, interactive assignments and activities, web links, animations, videos, and more!

Reference

Carter, S. M. (2009). *Glucose-6-phosphate dehydrogenase deficiency*. Retrieved from http://emedicine.medscape.com/article/200390-overview

Selected Bibliography

Bauer, L. A. (2011). Clinical pharmacokinetics and pharmacodynamics. In J. T. DiPiro, R. L. Talbert, G. C. Yee, G. R. Matzke, B. G. Wells, & L. M. Posey (Eds.), *Pharmacotherapy: A pathophysiology approach* (8th ed., pp. 15–37). New York, NY: McGraw-Hill.

Blumenthal, D. K., & Garrison, J. C. (2011). Pharmacodynamics: Molecular mechanisms of drug action. In L. L. Brunton, B. A. Chabner, & B. C. Knollman (Eds.), *The pharmacological basis of therapeutics* (12th ed., pp. 41–72). New York, NY: McGraw-Hill.

Bowie, M. W., & Slattum, P. W. (2007). Pharmacodynamics in older adults: A review. *The American Journal of Geriatric Pharmacotherapy, 5*(3), 263–303. doi:10.1016/j.amjopharm.2007.10.001

Howland, R. H. (2009). Psychopharmacology: Effects of aging on pharmacokinetic and pharmacodynamic drug processes. *Journal of Psychosocial Nursing and Mental Health Services, 47*(10), 15–18. doi:10.3928/02793695-20090902-06

Kudzma, E. C., & Carey, E. T. (2009). Pharmacogenomics: Personalizing drug therapy. *American Journal of Nursing, 109*(10), 50–57.

Soldin, O. P., & Mattison, D. R. (2009). Sex differences in pharmacokinetics and pharmacodynamics. *Clinical Pharmacokinetics, 48*(3), 143–157. doi:10.2165/00003088-200948030-00001

Whitley, H., & Lindsey, W. (2009). Sex-based differences in drug activity. *American Family Physician, 80*(11), 1254–1258.

Zineh, I., Pebanco, G. D., Aquilante, C. L., Gerhard, T., Beitelshees, A. L., Beasley, B. N., & Hartzema, A. G. (2006). Discordance between availability of pharmacogenetics studies and pharmacogenetics-based prescribing information for the top 200 drugs. *Annals of Pharmacotherapy, 40*(4), 639–644. doi:10.1345/aph.1G4

Zopf, Y., Rabe, C., Neubert, A., Hanson, C., Brune, K., Hahn, E. G., & Dormann, H. (2009). Gender-based differences in drug prescription: relation to adverse drug reactions. *Pharmacology, 84*(6), 333–339. doi:10.1159/000248311

Answers to NCLEX-RN® Review

1 Answer: 1, 2, 3, 5   Rationale: One of the critical determinants of the effectiveness of drug therapy is a physical examination. Nurses will utilize assessment skills to ascertain whether the drug is being effective. In many cases, a client's vital signs such as a decrease in body temperature, a change in blood pressure and pulse, or improved respiratory status may indicate the effectiveness of a drug. The effects of many drugs are monitored by diagnostic laboratory values such as white blood cell counts, cultures, and electrolyte levels. Efficacy is the term that describes the ability of a drug to produce the desired therapeutic effect. Option 4 is incorrect. The dosage time does not directly evaluate the effectiveness of drug therapy. Cognitive Level: Applying; Client Need: Physiological Integrity; Nursing Process: Evaluation

2 Answer: 1   Rationale: Therapeutic index is the ratio between the therapeutic dose and the toxic dose of a drug, and is used as a measure of the relative safety of the drug. The higher the therapeutic index is, the greater the safety of the drug. Options 2, 3, and 4 are incorrect. A drug may be labeled "dangerous" for many reasons other than the therapeutic index, including the potential for abuse. The higher the therapeutic index is, the lower the risk of drug toxicity. A high degree of safety does not signify the effectiveness of the drug. Cognitive Level: Applying; Client Need: Physiological Integrity; Nursing Process: Implementation

3 Answer: 1   Rationale: A dose response curve is a graphic representation that shows the relationship between the amount of a drug administered and the extent of the response it produces. Options 2, 3, and 4 are incorrect. A dose response curve does not illustrate the toxic effects of a drug or any specific population, or graphically present the duration of action of a drug. Serum drug levels must be measured to determine the peak level. It is unique to each client and the dose response curve only represents a maximum (toxic) dose level. Cognitive Level: Applying; Client Need: Safe and Effective Care Environment; Nursing Process: Assessment

4 Answer: 4　Rationale: The TD_{50} measures the median toxicity dose. This information indicates the dose that will produce a given toxicity in 50% of a group of clients. Options 1, 2, and 3 are incorrect. Effectiveness, dose response, and receptor subtypes are not represented by the TD_{50} level. Cognitive Level: Applying; Client Need: Physiological Integrity; Nursing Process: Implementation

5 Answer: 2　Rationale: Antagonists bind to receptors and block the effects of an endogenous chemical or another drug by competing with receptor binding sites or inhibiting the drug effect. As an antagonist, benztropine would block the effects of neostigmine and the neostigmine would exhibit a lesser effect. Options 1, 3, and 4 are incorrect. A drug that produces an effect after binding with a receptor is an agonist. Cognitive Level: Analyzing; Client Need: Physiological Integrity; Nursing Process: Implementation

6 Answer: 1　Rationale: Potency is a reflection of a drug's ability to bind to a receptor. Options 2, 3, and 4 are incorrect. Efficacy and the affinity of a drug to bind to a receptor are separate variables from potency. Metabolism is a function of pharmacokinetics not pharmacodynamics. First-pass effect is a phenomenon that occurs during enteral absorption and does not affect drug affinity. Cognitive Level: Applying; Client Need: Safe and Effective Care Environment; Nursing Process: Implementation

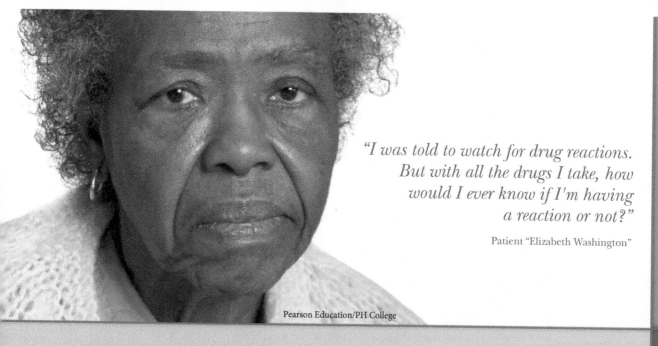

"I was told to watch for drug reactions. But with all the drugs I take, how would I ever know if I'm having a reaction or not?"

Patient "Elizabeth Washington"

Pearson Education/PH College

Adverse Drug Effects and Drug Interactions

Chapter Outline

Adverse Drug Effects

The Role of the Nurse in Managing Adverse Effects

Allergic Reactions

Idiosyncratic Responses

Carcinogenicity and Teratogenicity

Organ-Specific Drug Toxicity

Drug Interactions

Pharmacokinetic Drug Interactions

Pharmacodynamic Drug Interactions

Drug Interactions with Food and Dietary Supplements

Learning Outcomes

After reading this chapter, the student should be able to:

1. Differentiate between adverse effects and side effects.

2. Create a plan to minimize or prevent adverse drug events in patients.

3. Explain the advantages and disadvantages of the Adverse Event Reporting System.

4. Describe the incidence and characteristics of drug allergies.

5. Explain how idiosyncratic reactions differ from other types of adverse effects.

6. Explain why certain drugs with carcinogenic or teratogenic potential are used in pharmacotherapy.

7. Report the characteristic signs, symptoms, and treatment for each of the following organ-specific adverse events: nephrotoxicity, neurotoxicity, hepatotoxicity, dermatologic toxicity, bone marrow toxicity, cardiotoxicity, and skeletal muscle toxicity.

8. Use examples to explain the importance of drug interactions to pharmacotherapy.

9. Describe the mechanisms of drug interactions that alter absorption, distribution, metabolism, or excretion.

10. Differentiate among additive, synergistic, and antagonistic drug interactions.

11. Identify examples of drug–food interactions that may impact pharmacotherapeutic outcomes.

From Chapter 6 of *Pharmacology: Connections to Nursing Practice*, Second Edition. Michael Patrick Adams, Carol Quam Urban. Copyright © 2013 by Pearson Education, Inc. All rights reserved.

Key Terms

Drugs are administered with the goal of producing a therapeutic effect. All drugs, however, produce both intended therapeutic effects as well as unintended effects. An **adverse drug effect** is an undesirable and potentially harmful action caused by the administration of medication. Adverse effects, also called adverse events, are a significant component of pharmacotherapy and, when severe, may cause treatment to be discontinued or result in permanent harm to the patient. The purpose of this chapter is to examine the different types of adverse effects and drug interactions, so that the nurse can minimize their impact on treatment outcomes.

Adverse Drug Effects

1 The nurse plays a key role in preventing and managing adverse drug effects.

Although every drug has the *potential* to produce adverse events, most pharmacotherapy can be conducted without significant undesirable effects. Indeed, drugs that produce serious adverse effects are screened and removed from consideration during the drug development and approval process, or are restricted for treating serious health conditions such as cancer. Patients expect that their drugs, including over-the-counter (OTC) agents, herbal products, and dietary supplements, will be free from serious adverse effects when taken as directed. Although the majority of drugs are very safe, adverse effects cannot be entirely avoided.

Side effects are types of drug effects that are predictable and which may occur even at therapeutic doses. Side effects are less serious than adverse effects. Patients are often willing to tolerate annoying side effects if they believe the drug will improve their condition or prevent a disease. The distinction between an adverse effect and a side effect, however, is often unclear. For example, is headache a side effect or an adverse effect? What about nausea? The answer lies in the severity of the symptoms. Headache or nausea may be minor (side effects), or they may become intense and disabling (adverse effects). The U.S. Food and Drug Administration (FDA) defines serious drug effects as those that:

- Result in a patient's death, hospitalization, or disability.
- Cause a congenital abnormality.
- Cause a life-threatening event.
- Require an intervention to prevent permanent damage.

Adverse drug events may be specific to a single type of tissue or affect multiple organ systems. The most common adverse events are nausea and vomiting, which may occur when drugs are administered by any route. Headache and changes in blood pressure are also very common. Some adverse effects, though rare, are serious enough to warrant regular or continuous monitoring. Examples of serious events include impairment or failure of entire organs, such as cardiac, hepatic, or renal failure or loss of vision or hearing. Anaphylaxis, Stevens–Johnson syndrome (SJS), cancer, and birth defects are additional rare, adverse drug events that occur with certain drugs.

Many adverse effects are extensions of a drug's pharmacologic actions. These types of events are considered dose dependent: As the drug dose increases, the risk for adverse effects also increases. For example, antihypertensive drugs are given to lower blood pressure, but high doses cause hypotension, which may manifest as dizziness or fainting. Drugs for treating insomnia or anxiety may depress brain activity too much at higher doses, resulting in drowsiness or daytime sedation. Knowing the therapeutic actions of the drug enables the nurse to predict the signs and symptoms of many of the adverse effects that occur during treatment. It is important for nurses and their patients to understand that the difference between a substance being a beneficial drug or a poison is often simply a matter of dose.

Can adverse effects be prevented? Although nurses play a key role in minimizing the number and severity of adverse events in their patients, some adverse effects simply cannot be predicted or prevented. Skilled health care providers and nurses, however, have multiple ways to minimize or prevent adverse effects, from having expert knowledge of how a drug acts to obtaining a comprehensive medical history from their patients. The following are means that health care providers use to minimize or prevent adverse drug events in their patients:

- **Take a thorough medical history.** The medical history of the patient may reveal drug allergies or conditions that contraindicate the use of certain drugs. The history may also identify other drugs taken by the patient that could negatively interact with the prescribed medication.

- **Thoroughly assess the patient and all diagnostic data.** Assessment may reveal underlying hepatic or renal impairment that will affect the way the drug is handled by the body. The very young and the elderly are most susceptible to drug reactions because metabolism and excretion of drugs in these populations are less predictable. To prevent adverse effects, average drug doses should be adjusted based on careful patient assessment.

- **Prevent medication errors.** Administering the incorrect dose or giving the drug to the wrong patient may cause unnecessary adverse effects.

- **Monitor pharmacotherapy carefully.** Monitor patient signs and symptoms regularly after initial drug doses or when doses are increased, especially when giving parenteral agents and for very ill patients. Patients receiving drugs that have frequent or potentially severe adverse effects should be monitored continuously until the baseline effects of the drug have been established.

- **Know the drugs.** It is essential for nurses to know the most frequent and most serious adverse effects for every drug administered. A comprehensive knowledge of the drugs, herbal products, and supplements taken by their patients helps nurses to monitor for and identify adverse effects and provide the necessary interventions before they become serious.

- **Be prepared for the unusual.** Anaphylaxis may occur immediately and unpredictably (see Section 3). Other adverse effects may be delayed, occurring days, weeks, or months after therapy is initiated. Some drugs produce actions opposite to those expected (see Section 4). Patients may be reluctant to report certain adverse effects (such as impotence) without prompting by the nurse.

- **Question unusual orders.** If the nurse suspects that the wrong dose has been ordered or the pharmacy has filled the order incorrectly, the drug should not be administered until the prescriber or the pharmacy has been contacted.

- **Teach patients about adverse effects.** The patient is the nurse's ally in identifying and preventing adverse effects. Teaching patients what therapeutic and adverse effects to expect from the drug and which types of symptoms to report to their health care provider are important in preventing serious adverse effects. In addition, inadequate teaching may result in poor patient adherence to the drug regimen and suboptimal treatment outcomes.

PharmFACT

According to Davies et al. (2009), approximately one in seven hospitalized patients experiences an adverse drug reaction. The drugs most frequently associated with these adverse events were diuretics, opioid analgesics, and anticoagulants.

2 The FDA continues to monitor for new adverse events after a drug is approved and marketed.

Before approving a drug, the FDA carefully examines all clinical information supplied by the manufacturer regarding drug effectiveness and safety. Although extensive premarketing testing may be conducted, clinical research has certain limitations and the FDA's decision is based on a relatively small number of clinical trials. Once marketed, the drug is disseminated to a larger and more diverse patient population, at which point adverse effects that were not discovered during clinical trials may begin to surface. For this reason, the FDA continues to monitor the safety of drugs after they are approved.

Established in 1993, the FDA's MedWatch Safety Information and **Adverse Event Reporting System (AERS)** is a voluntary program that encourages health care providers and consumers to report suspected adverse effects directly to the FDA or the product manufacturer. By law, reports received by the manufacturers are forwarded to the FDA to be added to the computerized information database.

The number of adverse events reported to the FDA has steadily grown every year. In 2000, the FDA received 266,866 adverse event reports. More than 500,000 events are now reported annually; approximately 60% by health care providers and 40% by consumers.

Data from the AERS are analyzed by clinical reviewers, usually a physician, pharmacist, or nurse, at the Center for Drug Evaluation and Research of the FDA. If a potential safety concern is identified, the FDA may take one of the following actions:

- Conduct additional epidemiologic studies to determine the validity or extent of the safety concern.
- Require changes to a product's labeling information.
- Require a **Black Box Warning** in the drug insert that warns prescribers that the drug carries a risk for a serious or even fatal adverse effect.
- Restrict the use of the drug in specific populations.
- Communicate safety information to health care providers and consumers.
- Recall a product that may have quality or performance concerns.
- Remove the product from the market.

The FDA disseminates changes in safety information through its MedWatch website. Interested parties may subscribe to podcasts, electronic newsletters, and even cell phone text message alerts giving them the latest drug safety information.

The AERS provides a national database for making safety decisions about drugs, but it does have limitations. Health care providers are not required by law to report suspected adverse events to MedWatch. Because the system relies on voluntary reports, not all adverse events are reported. The FDA does not attempt to prove causation, that is, whether the adverse event was caused by the drug or by some other factor involved in treatment. Reports sometimes do contain insufficient or vague details regarding the incident.

A word of caution is necessary regarding the reporting of adverse drug events. The placebo effect predicts that a certain percentage of patients will respond with positive therapeutic outcomes to a treatment, even if the substance is inert and has no pharmacologic properties (essentially a "sugar pill"). The same holds true for side and adverse effects. A certain percentage of patients will experience headache, nausea and vomiting, rash, changes in blood pressure, or pain following the administration of a placebo. Thus when examining drug information, the nurse should always examine the incidence of adverse effects that occur over and above that caused by a placebo. It is important to understand that the patient is not faking symptoms that result from placebo administration; they truly believe, and may be visibly experiencing, side effects. However, the drug itself may not be responsible for the effects.

3 Allergic reactions are caused by a hyperresponse of the immune system.

Drug allergies are common events, comprising 6% to 10% of all adverse drug effects. Although drug allergies may elicit a diverse range of patient symptoms, all are caused by a hyperresponse of body defenses. Depending on the type of allergic response, basophils, mast cells, eosinophils, or lymphocytes secrete chemical mediators that trigger the allergic response. Specific chemical mediators of allergy include histamine, serotonin, leukotrienes, prostaglandins, and complement.

Several characteristics define a drug allergy. Allergies typically occur with very small amounts of drug; the severity of allergy symptoms is usually not proportional to the dose. The symptoms of allergy are unrelated to the pharmacologic actions of the drug; anaphylaxis has the same symptoms regardless of the drug that induces it. Patients often exhibit cross-allergy, an allergic reaction to drugs with a similar structure, such as those from the same pharmacologic class. Drug allergies require a previous exposure to the drug (or a very similar drug). This sensitizes the patient to subsequent exposures, during which a hyperresponse of body defenses is rapidly mounted upon reexposure to the drug.

The signs and symptoms of drug allergy are variable and range from minor to life threatening. Symptoms may appear within minutes after the drug is administered or they may develop after prolonged pharmacotherapy. Because the signs and symptoms of drug allergy are nonspecific, it is sometimes difficult to attribute an allergy symptom to any given drug, especially in patients receiving multiple drugs. Complicating an accurate diagnosis is that symptoms of drug allergy are the same as those of allergy to other substances, such as certain foods, or environmental triggers, such as animal dander or dust mites. It is important to determine the source of allergy, especially in patients with severe reactions, so that the offending drug or environmental substance can be avoided in the future.

Although allergic reactions are possible with most drugs, some agents exhibit a relatively higher incidence. The drugs or drug classes most likely to cause allergic reactions include penicillins and related antibiotics (monobactams and cephalosporins), radiologic contrast media containing iodine, insulin, nonsteroidal anti-inflammatory drugs (NSAIDs, including aspirin), sulfonamides, cancer chemotherapy agents, preservatives (sulfites and paraben), and certain antiseizure agents.

Patients are usually unaware of the true definition of allergy and often report any adverse effect they experience as a drug allergy. For example, many patients experience acute nausea and vomiting with narcotic analgesics such as codeine and will report that they have an allergy to codeine during a drug history. In fact, these symptoms are not caused by an overactive immune response and are thus not a true allergy. Inaccurate reporting of allergies may lead to the health care provider avoiding the use of entire drug classes and prescribing less effective or more expensive "second-choice" agents.

4 Idiosyncratic reactions are unusual drug responses often caused by genetic differences among patients.

An **idiosyncratic response** is an adverse drug effect that produces an unusual and unexpected response that is not related to the pharmacologic action of the drug. Idiosyncratic

reactions are not classified as allergies because they are not immune related. They are rare, unpredictable, and vary from patient to patient.

Many, though not all, idiosyncratic reactions are due to unique, individual genetic differences among patients. For example, mutations involving specific metabolic enzymes may cause certain patients to be extremely sensitive to the effects of a drug or to be resistant. The drug may be handled by a different metabolic pathway, resulting in the accumulation of a metabolite that gives a different and unexpected response from the original drug.

Historically, the term *idiosyncratic* has been used to denote any drug effect that could not be explained. With advances in the understanding of drug mechanisms, fewer and fewer drug responses are not understood, at least to some extent. With improved reporting of adverse drug events, rare "unexpected" events are now documented and may be "expected." Thus use of the term *idiosyncratic*, although still common in clinical practice, will likely continue to diminish with time.

PharmFACT

Between 3% and 11% of hospital admissions are caused by adverse drug effects.

5 Some drugs have the ability to induce cancer or cause birth defects.

Most adverse effects occur within minutes or hours after a drug is administered; some develop after several days or weeks of pharmacotherapy. In a few instances, the adverse effect may occur years or even decades after the drug was administered. Such is the case with drug-induced cancer.

Why would a drug be approved by the FDA if it was known to cause cancer in humans? In most cases, drugs that produce cancer in laboratory animals during preclinical trials are not submitted for approval to the FDA. However, there are a few conditions that may warrant the approval of a drug with carcinogenic potential. The answer lies in the **risk–benefit ratio**. If a patient has a condition that is likely to cause premature death if left untreated, the benefits of taking a drug with carcinogenic potential may outweigh the long-term risks. This assumes, of course, that effective, safer alternatives are not available.

Of the thousands of drugs and drug combinations approved for pharmacotherapy, only a few increase the risk of acquiring cancer. These drugs, shown in Table 1, fall into three primary classes: antineoplastics, immunosuppressants, and hormonal agents.

Some of the antineoplastics used to treat cancer are known chemical carcinogens. Molecular damage from these drugs results from mutations in deoxyribonucleic acid (DNA). Although much of the DNA damage is repaired by cellular enzymes, some mutations persist and accumulate in cells as a person ages, increasing cancer risk. The initial damage done by the drug may take decades to manifest as cancer. Leukemia is the type of cancer with the greatest cancer risk from antineoplastic therapy. However, the patient may never develop cancer; indeed, the majority of patients receiving antineoplastic drugs do not develop the disease. Furthermore, the patient

TABLE 1 Selected Drugs Suspected of Causing Cancer in Humans

Class	Drug	Type of Cancer
Antineoplastic	chlorambucil	Leukemia, urinary bladder
	cyclophosphamide	
	dacarbazine	
	doxorubicin	
	etoposide	
	nitrosoureas	
	teniposide	
Hormones and hormone antagonists	anabolic steroids	Uterus, breast, hepatic
	estrogen replacement therapy and oral contraceptives	
	tamoxifen	
Immunosuppressants	azathioprine	Lymphoma, skin
	cyclosporine	

TABLE 2 Organ-Specific Toxicity

Toxicity	Example Drugs and Classes
Bone marrow	ACE inhibitors, antimalarials, antineoplastics, antiseizure agents (phenytoin, carbamazepine), antithyroid drugs, cephalosporins, chloramphenicol, chlorpropamide, chlorpromazine, cimetidine, furosemide, methyldopa, NSAIDs, phenylbutazone, sulfonamides
Cardiotoxicity	anthracycline antineoplastics (doxorubicin, daunorubicin, epirubicin, idarubicin, mitoxantrone)
Dermatologic	antiseizure agents (phenobarbital, phenytoin, carbamazepine), cephalosporins, erythromycin, NSAIDs, penicillin, radiologic contrast media, sulfonamides, tetracyclines
Hepatotoxicity	carbamazepine, chlorpromazine, halothane
Nephrotoxicity	ACE inhibitors, acyclovir, aminoglycosides, amphotericin B, cisplatin and other platinum-based antineoplastics, cocaine, cyclosporine, NSAIDs, radiologic contrast media, sulfonamides, tacrolimus
Neurotoxicity	aminoglycosides, cisplatin, ethanol, loop diuretics, methyldopa, salicylates, vincristine
Skeletal muscle toxicity	statins (HMG CoA reductase inhibitors)

may have benefited from additional decades of life he or she would never have experienced had it not been for treatment with these drugs. Because pharmacotherapy combined with surgery and radiation therapy can result in a total cure for some patients, the benefit of drug therapy outweighs the small risk of developing cancer later in life.

The second class of drugs that can induce cancer are the immunosuppressive agents. These agents are administered to dampen the immune system for patients receiving transplanted tissues or who have serious inflammatory disorders. Because the immune system is responsible for removing cancer cells after they form in the body, any drug that inhibits this system would be expected to have some degree of cancer risk. Lymphoma is the greatest type of cancer risk from immunosuppressants.

The third group of drugs that may cause cancer consists of hormones or hormone antagonists. Little is known about the mechanisms by which hormone imbalances lead to cancer, and the topic is a subject of ongoing research. In some cases, hormones protect the patient from cancer, or they may reduce the incidence of one type of cancer but increase the risk of another type. Cancers from hormones or hormone antagonists tend to affect reproductive organs, such as the vagina, uterus, or breast.

A similar question might be asked regarding drugs that cause birth defects, or **teratogens**. Why would a drug be approved by the FDA if it was shown to produce birth defects in laboratory animals during the preclinical stage of drug testing? The answer to this question is very different from that for cancer-inducing drugs.

Teratogens affect a smaller percentage of the population: those who are pregnant. In most cases these drugs do not affect males, and they are also safe to use in older adults. Thus, known teratogens may be approved for indications in patients who do not have the potential to become pregnant. When approved for females with reproductive potential, however, these drugs have increased risks. Although a pregnancy test may be performed prior to pharmacotherapy and the nurse may warn the patient to discontinue the drug if pregnancy is suspected, the potential still remains for exposing an embryo or fetus to a toxic agent. In females with reproductive potential, teratogenic drugs are not used unless they have clear benefits that outweigh the possible risk of birth defects. All health care providers must carefully assess patient compliance with instructions against this potential risk.

The nurse should remember that drugs are not tested in pregnant humans before FDA approval, and that animal testing cannot predict with great accuracy the effects on the human fetus. In some cases, the risks to a human embryo or fetus have been determined after a drug has been approved. The FDA has established pregnancy categories, which gauge the risk of a drug causing birth defects. All drug use should be assumed dangerous during pregnancy, unless data have otherwise demonstrated the drug to be safe. No woman should take a drug, herbal product, or dietary supplement during pregnancy unless approved by the patient's health care practitioner.

6 Drug toxicity may be specific to particular organs.

Very few drugs produce adverse effects in every organ system; these agents would be too toxic for safe pharmacotherapy. Instead, adverse effects are often organ specific, targeting one or a few organs. It is important for the nurse to learn these specific toxicities so that appropriate signs, symptoms, and diagnostic tests can be carefully monitored. Selected organ-specific toxicities are summarized in Table 2.

Nephrotoxicity: The kidneys are one of the most common organ systems affected by drugs. This is because these organs filter large volumes of blood, and most drugs are excreted by the renal route. Some drugs are reabsorbed or secreted by the kidney, exposing renal tubule cells to high concentrations of these agents. A few obstruct the urinary system by causing crystalluria in the urinary tract. Drug nephrotoxicity may manifest as acute symptoms that appear after one or several doses, or as chronic symptoms that appear after several months of pharmacotherapy.

It is critical for the health care provider to identify at-risk patients and attempt to prevent drug-induced nephrotoxicity. Means for prevention include providing proper hydration, monitoring urinary lab values, and adjusting doses appropriately for patients with renal impairment. Patients with serious renal impairment should not receive nephrotoxic drugs unless other therapeutic options have been exhausted.

Neurotoxicity: Although the blood–brain barrier prevents many drugs from reaching the brain, neurotoxicity is a relatively common adverse effect of certain drug classes. This is because the brain receives a large percentage of the blood supply and is especially sensitive to small amounts of toxic substances. For sedatives, antidepressants, antianxiety agents, antiseizure agents, and antipsychotic drugs, the difference between a therapeutic dose and one that produces adverse effects may be very small. Indeed, drowsiness is seen in a majority of patients receiving these drugs when therapy is initiated. Signs and symptoms of toxicity in the central nervous system (CNS) include depression, mania, sedation, behavioral changes, hallucinations, and seizures. The special senses may be affected, including visual changes, loss of balance, and hearing impairment.

Effective teaching is essential when patients are beginning therapy with potentially neurotoxic drugs. The nurse should warn patients not to drive vehicles or perform other hazardous tasks until they are certain of the effects of these drugs. Caregivers should be taught to report changes in patient behavior, because the person receiving the medication may have difficulty recognizing these signs. The nurse should be aware that neurotoxic drugs can significantly worsen preexisting CNS disease. Serious symptoms such as seizures, delirium, suicidal ideation, or significant visual or hearing impairment should be immediately reported to the prescriber.

Hepatotoxicity: A major function of the liver is to detoxify foreign chemicals that enter the body; thus it should not be surprising that hepatotoxicity is one of the most common adverse drug effects. Effects of hepatotoxic drugs range from minor, reversible symptoms to fatal hepatitis.

The nurse should regularly monitor liver enzyme tests when administering hepatotoxic drugs, because changes in these laboratory values are early signs of liver toxicity. Symptoms of liver impairment are vague and nonspecific and include right upper quadrant pain, anorexia, bloating, fatigue, and nausea or vomiting. During chronic hepatotoxicity, jaundice, itching, and easy bruising are evident. In serious cases, the liver will be unable to metabolize other drugs, resulting in high serum drug levels. Extreme care must be taken when administering potentially hepatotoxic drugs to patients with preexisting liver disease.

Dermatologic toxicity: Drug reactions affecting the skin are some of the most common types of adverse effects. These reactions may be caused by a hypersensitivity response or by nonimmune-type responses. Rash, the most common cutaneous drug reaction, usually occurs within 1 to 2 weeks of initiation of drug therapy and resolves without serious complications. Drug-induced rash is sometimes accompanied by itching (pruritus). Although almost any drug can cause rash, antibiotics are the most frequent drug class causing this condition. Urticaria (hives) are raised welts that are often accompanied by intense pruritus and, although less common than rash, are a symptom of a potential allergic reaction that could lead to anaphylaxis.

Drug-induced dermatologic toxicity may be serious. In angioedema, swelling occurs in the dermis, periorbital region, and around the mouth and throat. Angioedema is considered a severe drug reaction because the swelling may impair breathing and may be fatal. SJS is another drug-induced condition that can be fatal. This syndrome causes severe blistering of the skin, usually accompanied by mucous membrane involvement and fever.

Phototoxicity is a type of drug-induced dermatologic toxicity in which certain drugs cause the skin to absorb excess ultraviolet radiation from the sun or heat lamps. Symptoms resemble sunburn and are best prevented by advising patients to avoid direct sunlight. Phototoxicity resolves when the drug is discontinued.

Most types of drug-induced dermatologic toxicity do not require pharmacologic treatment. If pruritus is prominent, an antihistamine or corticosteroid may be administered. In all cases of serious drug-induced hypersensitivity, the nurse should discontinue the drug until the cause of the skin condition can be diagnosed.

Bone marrow toxicity: Drugs affecting the bone marrow are of great concern due to the possibility of serious and perhaps fatal outcomes. The bone marrow serves as a nursery for the production of red blood cells, white blood cells, and platelets. Drugs may affect only one of these types of cells or all three. When all three groups are affected, drug-induced pancytopenia or aplastic anemia occurs, and the patient is at great risk for serious illness. Loss of white blood cells may cause agranulocytosis or neutropenia, which places the patient at risk for serious infections. The drug class most likely to cause bone marrow toxicity is the antineoplastics class. Bone marrow toxicity is the dose-limiting factor with these drugs.

The role of the nurse in preventing bone marrow toxicity is to carefully monitor laboratory data and recognize changes that suggest impending toxicity, such as decreases in red cells, white cells, or platelets. In many cases, bone marrow toxicity can be quickly reversed if the condition is recognized early and the drug is discontinued. Furthermore, the nurse should carefully monitor the therapeutic regimen of patients who have preexisting blood cell disorders because adding a drug with bone marrow toxicity may worsen these conditions.

Cardiotoxicity: Some drugs damage cardiac muscle cells, affecting the ability of the heart to effectively pump blood to the tissues. The most common cardiotoxic drugs belong to a chemical class called the anthracyclines, which include daunorubicin (Cerubidine, DaunoXome), doxorubicin (Adriamycin), epirubicin (Ellence), idarubicin (Idamycin), and mitoxantrone (Novantrone). These are all antineoplastic medications. The cardiotoxicity of these drugs can be severe and lead to bradycardia, tachycardia, heart failure, and acute left ventricular failure. The nurse administering cardiotoxic drugs must be vigilant in observing for signs of cardiotoxicity such as excessive fatigue, cough, shortness of breath (especially when recumbent), weight gain, or peripheral edema.

A second type of cardiotoxicity is manifested as prolongation of the QT interval on the electrocardiogram (ECG). The QT interval is the duration for activation and recovery of the ventricular myocardium. Extending the QT interval is associated with a rare type of ventricular tachycardia known as torsade de pointes, which can cause sudden cardiac death. More than a hundred drugs have been shown to cause QT prolongation and several have been removed from the market because of this adverse effect. Since 2005, the FDA has required all new drugs to be tested for QT prolongation prior to approval. Patients with preexisting cardiac disease must be monitored carefully when being administered drugs that prolong the QT interval.

Skeletal muscle toxicity: Skeletal muscle is relatively resistant to the effects of drugs, despite its extensive blood supply. In skeletal muscle the incidence of drug-induced myopathy is low but may be serious when it does occur. The most severe myopathy is rhabdomyolysis, a syndrome characterized by extensive muscle necrosis with the release of muscle enzymes and other constituents into the circulation. Rhabdomyolysis is a rare, though serious adverse effect of statins, common medications used to treat excessive lipid levels in the blood.

To prevent skeletal muscle toxicity, the nurse should assess for unexplained muscle soreness or pain during therapy. Laboratory tests such as creatine kinase (CK) should be evaluated regularly during therapy with drugs that have muscle toxicity.

Drug Interactions

7 Drug interactions may significantly affect pharmacotherapeutic outcomes.

A **drug interaction** occurs when a substance increases or decreases a drug's actions. The substance causing the drug interaction may be another drug, a dietary supplement, an herbal product, or a food. The substance participating in the drug interaction must be external to the body and is usually taken concurrently with the medication. Although substances that are naturally found in the body (endogenous substances) routinely interact with drugs, these are not considered drug interactions because they are part of the body's "normal" response to the drug.

Because patients often take multiple drugs concurrently, drug interactions occur continually. Even if only one drug is taken, the potential for a drug–food interaction still exists. Drug interactions are impossible to totally eliminate and

should be considered an important component of pharmacotherapy. In the large majority of cases, the drug interaction goes unnoticed and treatment outcomes are unaffected. Indeed, it is likely that most drug interactions have yet to be documented or researched because they do not cause clinically noticeable effects or harm to the patient.

Some drug interactions are important to pharmacology because they are known to cause adverse effects or otherwise affect treatment outcomes. By studying the mechanisms of potential drug interactions, the nurse can prevent certain adverse effects and optimize treatment outcomes. For example, if the patient is receiving gentamicin, the nurse should use caution when administering acyclovir, because the drug combination can cause higher than normal levels of acyclovir in the blood. The nurse may suggest that the prescriber reduce the dose or substitute a different drug. *Understanding drug interactions can directly affect the success of pharmacotherapy.*

Drug interactions occur by dozens of different mechanisms. To simplify their study, it may be helpful to remember that drug interactions can have three basic effects on the action of a drug:

- The actions of the drug can be inhibited, resulting in less therapeutic action. For example, milk interferes with the absorption of tetracycline, causing a lower serum level of antibiotic, thus diminishing its therapeutic effects.

- The actions of the drug may be enhanced, causing a greater therapeutic response. For example, coadministration of the two antiviral drugs lopinavir and ritonavir causes a greater reduction in levels of HIV than occurs when either drug is used alone.

- The drug interaction may produce a totally new and different response. For example, when used alone disulfiram (Antabuse) has no pharmacologic effects. When taken with alcohol, however, the combination produces dramatic, new actions such as severe headache, flushing, dyspnea, palpitations, and blurred vision.

8 Pharmacokinetic drug interactions include changes in the absorption, distribution, metabolism, or excretion of medications.

Pharmacokinetics is the branch of pharmacology dealing with how the body acts on a drug after it is administered. Many drug interactions involve some aspect of the pharmacokinetics of the medication. When studying drug interactions, it is convenient to use the same categories for pharmacokinetics. The general types of pharmacokinetic interactions are illustrated in Figure 1.

Absorption: Most drugs need to be absorbed to produce their actions. Any substance that affects absorption has the potential to influence drug response. In fact, this is one of the most common mechanisms of drug interactions. By interfering with normal absorption, drug action may be inhibited or enhanced. Increasing absorption will raise drug serum levels and produce an enhanced effect; substances inhibiting absorption have the opposite effect.

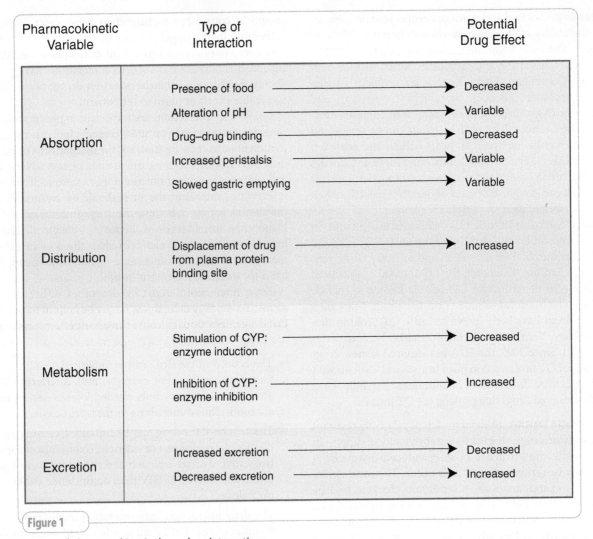

Pharmacokinetic Variable	Type of Interaction	Potential Drug Effect
Absorption	Presence of food	Decreased
	Alteration of pH	Variable
	Drug–drug binding	Decreased
	Increased peristalsis	Variable
	Slowed gastric emptying	Variable
Distribution	Displacement of drug from plasma protein binding site	Increased
Metabolism	Stimulation of CYP: enzyme induction	Decreased
	Inhibition of CYP: enzyme inhibition	Increased
Excretion	Increased excretion	Decreased
	Decreased excretion	Increased

Figure 1

Types of pharmacokinetic drug–drug interactions.

The simplest way to affect absorption is to change the speed of substances moving through the gastrointestinal (GI) tract. Opioids such as morphine or heroin will slow peristalsis, giving drugs additional time for absorption. Laxatives and drugs that stimulate the parasympathetic nervous system will speed substances through the GI tract, diminishing the absorption time of drugs concurrently administered. The bile acid resins such as cholestyramine (Questran) bind other drugs and prevent their absorption.

Many drug–drug interactions caused by changes in absorption may be prevented by taking the two drugs at least 2 to 3 hours apart. In the case of drug–food interactions, the interacting food should be avoided, or the drug may be taken on an empty stomach. Taking drugs on an empty stomach, however, may increase the incidence of nausea or vomiting, which could result in loss of the drug before complete absorption occurs. The nurse must teach patients with drug-induced nausea not to take drugs with antacids or milk unless approved by the prescriber. Antacids are alkaline (basic) substances that raise the pH of the GI contents and have the potential to change the percentage of ionized drug. Ionized forms of drugs are less able to cross the intestinal mucosa than nonionized forms.

Distribution: Distribution is the movement of a drug from its site of absorption to its site of action. Many drugs travel through the blood bound to plasma proteins and, when bound, the drug is unable to leave the blood to reach its target. Drugs may compete for available binding sites on plasma proteins; one drug may prevent another from binding to plasma proteins or may displace a drug from its binding sites. If this occurs, the amount of unbound or free drug increases, potentially raising the drug serum concentration to toxic levels. For example, diazepam displaces phenytoin from plasma proteins, causing a rapid increase in the plasma concentration of free phenytoin and an increased risk of adverse effects. Drugs that have a high potential for displacing other drugs from protein binding sites include aspirin and other NSAIDs, phenylbutazone, and sulfonamides.

A second potential drug–drug interaction involving distribution can occur if the pH of the plasma is altered by a drug. For example, when an alkaline substance such as sodium bicarbonate is infused, the pH of plasma increases, causing acidic drugs to become ionized. The ionized acidic drugs are less able to cross membranes and they accumulate in the extracellular spaces, creating an ionization (pH) gradient. The pH gradient moves acidic drugs from inside cells to the extracellular spaces, thus altering distribution.

Metabolism: A large number of drugs are metabolized by hepatic enzymes. Drug metabolites generally have less activity than the original drug and are more readily excreted by the kidneys. Any drug-induced change in the activity of hepatic enzymes has the potential to cause drug–drug interactions.

Certain drugs have the ability to increase (induce) or decrease (inhibit) hepatic enzyme activity. Inducers such as phenobarbital will increase drug metabolism, thus promoting the inactivation and excretion of drugs administered concurrently. Clinically, this will be observed as diminished drug effectiveness. For example, if phenobarbital is administered concurrently with the antihypertensive drug nifedipine, less blood pressure reduction will result. The dose of nifedipine will need to be increased to produce an optimal therapeutic effect. However, care must be taken if the inducer is discontinued because hepatic enzymes will return back to baseline levels in a few days or weeks. Once hepatic enzymes return to normal, the dose of nifedipine will have to be adjusted downward to avoid toxicity. Also, remember that a few drugs (prodrugs) are *activated* by metabolism. Increasing the metabolism of prodrugs will cause an increase, rather than a decrease, in therapeutic response.

Inhibitors of hepatic metabolism will cause drug interactions that are opposite to those of inducers. For example, ritonavir inhibits the hepatic enzyme CYP3A4 and will decrease the metabolism of other drugs that are substrates for this enzyme. Giving ritonavir concurrently with nifedipine causes an increased blood pressure reduction due to the diminished metabolism of the antihypertensive. The nifedipine dose must be lowered to avoid toxicity. After ritonavir is discontinued, hepatic enzyme levels return to baseline and the nifedipine dose must be adjusted once again to maintain blood pressure control.

Drug interactions involving hepatic metabolism are some of the most complex in pharmacology. Although many of these interactions are not clinically significant, others clearly have the potential to affect therapeutic outcomes. The nurse will need to remember which drugs are inducers, inhibitors, and substrates of CYP enzymes to optimize pharmacotherapeutic outcomes and minimize adverse effects.

CONNECTION Checkpoint 6.1

Explain the significance of the first-pass effect on pharmacotherapy. *See Answer to Connection Checkpoint 6.1 on student resource website.*

Excretion: Most drugs are eliminated from the body through renal excretion. A drug interaction may occur if a substance changes the glomerular filtration rate (GFR), the amount of fluid filtered (mL) by the kidney per minute. The GFR is directly related to cardiac output; drugs that increase cardiac output will affect the GFR and hasten the excretion of other drugs.

A second type of excretion-related interaction may occur if one drug changes the secretion or reabsorption of another drug in the renal tubule. For example, methotrexate competes with NSAIDs for the same secretion mechanism. Taken concurrently, NSAIDs block the secretion of methotrexate, raising drug serum levels and increasing the risk of methotrexate toxicity.

Renal elimination may also be affected by drugs that change the pH of the filtrate in the renal tubules. Changing the pH causes drugs to become more (or less) ionized. The excretion of weak acids can be significantly increased by alkalinizing the urine through the administration of sodium bicarbonate. This drug interaction may be used therapeutically to promote more rapid excretion of acidic drugs such as aspirin during overdose situations. Similarly, excretion of weak bases can be increased by acidifying the urine through the administration of ammonium chloride.

Not all excretion-related drug interactions involve the kidneys. Some drugs are extensively excreted by the biliary system and two drugs may interact through this mechanism. For example, pravastatin and cyclosporine use the same carrier protein to move drug molecules from the liver to bile. Giving the two drugs concurrently will slow the biliary excretion of pravastatin and raise its serum concentration to potentially toxic levels. Because biliary excretion is not the dominant form of elimination for most drugs, this type of drug–drug excretion interaction is far less common than those involving the kidneys.

PharmFACT

Polycyclic aromatic hydrocarbons (PAHs) found in tobacco smoke are potent inducers of several hepatic microsomal enzymes. Smoking may reduce the effectiveness of drugs such as oral contraceptives, corticosteroids, clozapine, tacrine, and olanzapine (Kroon, 2007).

9 Pharmacodynamic drug interactions include additive, synergistic, or antagonistic effects.

Pharmacodynamics is the branch of pharmacology examining the mechanisms of drug action, meaning how a drug changes the body. Many drugs produce their actions by binding to specific receptors. When two drugs compete for the same receptor, or activate receptors that produce opposite effects, drug interactions are possible. Many common interactions encountered in clinical practice are pharmacodynamic in nature.

Two possible events can occur during a pharmacodynamic drug interaction: Drug action may be enhanced or inhibited. "Drug action" in the context of a drug interaction may be a therapeutic effect or an adverse effect. Thus, the drug interaction may be desirable (increased therapeutic response/decreased adverse effect) or undesirable (decreased therapeutic response/increased adverse effect). The basic pharmacodynamic drug–drug interactions are illustrated in Figure 2.

The pharmacodynamic drug interaction that is easiest to visualize is the **additive effect**. In this interaction, two drugs from a similar therapeutic class produce a combined summation response. This is used extensively in treating hypertension. For example, a diuretic may be used to lower systolic blood pressure by 10 mmHg, and a beta blocker may be added to the regimen to produce another 15-mmHg reduction. Combined, the two drugs produce a 25-mmHg reduction.

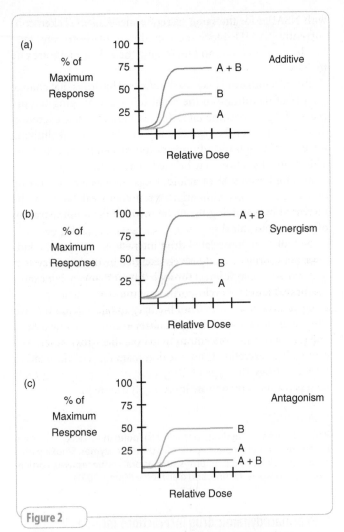

Figure 2

Additive, synergistic, and antagonistic drug interactions: (a) additive response; (b) synergistic response; (c) antagonistic response.

Why would two drugs be prescribed (with more expense to the patient), rather than a single drug? There are two rationales. First, to produce a 25-mmHg reduction using only the diuretic, the dose would have to be increased. Keeping the doses of both the diuretic and beta blocker low and taking advantage of their additive effect reduces the potential for adverse drug events. Second, some drugs have low efficacy and it may not be possible to achieve a 25-mmHg reduction with a single drug. The maximum effect from the diuretic may have been a 10-mmHg reduction, and another drug would need to be added to the regimen to achieve a greater response. In this example, the two drugs act at very different types of receptors to produce the additive therapeutic response: beta blockers in cardiac muscle and diuretics in the renal tubules.

Another pharmacodynamic drug interaction that produces an enhanced response is a **synergistic effect**. In this interaction, the effect of the two drugs is greater than would be expected from simply adding the two individual drugs' responses. This type of interaction is used extensively in treating infections. For example, Synercid is a combination drug

that contains quinupristin and dalfopristin, two antibiotics that are effective against resistant *Staphylococcus* infections. Both drugs bind to the bacterial ribosome and produce greater killing than would be predicted from adding the two individual drugs' effects. Another example is the combination antibiotic Bactrim, which combines trimethoprim and sulfamethoxazole to produce a synergistic effect on bacterial cell killing.

A third type of pharmacodynamic interaction occurs when adding a second drug results in a diminished pharmacologic response. This **antagonistic effect** can result in drug actions being "cancelled." For example, drugs activating the sympathetic nervous system such as epinephrine, will increase the heart rate and dilate the bronchi. A drug such as carvedilol (Coreg) will have the opposite effects: slowed heart rate and bronchoconstriction. Thus, carvedilol is considered an antagonist to epinephrine and may cancel its actions, depending on the doses of the two drugs. Why would a nurse administer drugs with opposite actions? This is generally done to reduce the adverse effects of a drug. For example, if a drug given to treat hypertension has an expected adverse effect of increasing heart rate, an antagonist may be given to slow the heart rate and keep it within normal limits. When given intentionally, an antagonist does not necessarily reverse all actions of the first drug: It may selectively inhibit an undesirable action.

In some cases, antagonists are used to treat symptoms of drug overdose. For example, patients taking an overdose of narcotics such as morphine or heroin, experience coma and life-threatening CNS depression. The administration of naloxone (Narcan), a specific narcotic antagonist, can quickly reverse some of the serious adverse effects of morphine.

Pharmacodynamic interactions can be indirect and complex. The well-documented drug interaction between digoxin (Lanoxin) and diuretics such as furosemide (Lasix), is an excellent example of an indirect effect. Furosemide enhances the excretion of potassium ion (hypokalemia), which increases the cardiotoxicity of digoxin. This can be a life-threatening interaction. Another example is the inhibition of vitamin K production in the intestine caused by antibiotics. If the patient is also taking warfarin (Coumadin), bleeding may occur because the liver is prevented from producing certain clotting factors. Again, the antibiotic did not directly interact with warfarin, yet the combination produced a serious adverse effect.

CONNECTION Checkpoint 6.2

The types of curves shown in Figure 2 are called dose–response curves. Explain the three phases of these curves. *See Answer to Connection Checkpoint 6.2 on student resource website.*

10 Food, nutrients, and dietary supplements may interact with medications and affect their actions.

Historically, interactions between drugs and food, dietary supplements, and herbal products have been largely dismissed as clinically unimportant. Although a few interactions, such as tetracyclines with calcium products, have been documented for decades, only since the late 1980s have drug–food interactions been recognized as important to maximizing pharmacotherapeutic outcomes. The interaction that prompted the increased interest in this topic was that of a benign and healthy substance: grapefruit juice. The interaction was discovered by chance in a research study designed to examine the effects of alcohol on felodipine, a calcium channel blocker. The researchers used grapefruit juice incidentally to disguise the taste of the alcohol.

Patients often take medications with juice because it covers up the bitter taste of many drugs and provides a plentiful source of vitamins and minerals. Unfortunately, grapefruit juice also contains substances that increase the absorption of certain oral drugs. This occurs because grapefruit juice inhibits the enzyme CYP3A4 in the wall of the intestinal tract. As drugs are absorbed, they are not inactivated by CYP3A4, and higher amounts reach the circulation. Surprisingly, the inhibition from grapefruit juice may last up to 3 days after drinking the juice. The substances in the juice inhibiting CYP3A4 enzymes are called furanocoumarins. Fortunately, only a few drug classes interact with grapefruit juice. These include benzodiazepines, certain calcium channel blockers, and statins (HMG CoA reductase inhibitors).

Most of the drug–food interactions discovered thus far act by either increasing or decreasing the absorption or bioavailability of the drug. Some of these interactions are shown in Table 3. Drug–food interactions are easily avoided by timing the drug dose appropriately with the food or supplement. In most cases, there should be a 2-hour time gap between ingestion of the food and drug. In a few cases, the drug should be administered with food to increase its absorption.

Interactions of drugs with herbal products have also largely been undocumented. As more patients take these products, research is demonstrating that certain drug–herb

TABLE 3 Selected Drug–Food and Drug–Herbal Interactions

Drug	Interaction
antiplatelet and anticoagulant drugs	Feverfew can increase the risk of bleeding.
atovaquone (Malarone)	Fatty food enhances absorption.
azithromycin (Zithromax)	Food reduces absorption.
calcium channel blockers and cyclosporine	Grapefruit juice enhances absorption.
cholestyramine (Questran)	Drug binds iron, folic acid, and vitamin A to decrease their absorption.
CNS depressants	Kava can increase drowsiness and sedation.
etidronate (Didronel)	Milk, calcium, and iron bind the drug and decrease absorption.
fluoroquinolones	Calcium, iron, and other metal ions bind the drug and decrease absorption.
lovastatin (Mevacor)	Food increases absorption.
MAO inhibitors	Foods containing tyramine can cause hypertensive crisis.
NSAIDs	Food reduces the incidence of side effects.
penicillin G	Food (milk) and metal ions reduce absorption.
selective serotonin reuptake inhibitors (SSRIs)	St. John's wort and grapefruit juice increase risk of adverse effects (serotonin syndrome).
sucralfate (Carafate)	Food protein binds the drug to decrease absorption.
tetracyclines	Dairy products and iron reduce absorption.
warfarin (Coumadin)	Vitamin K antagonizes the action of warfarin; ginkgo, garlic, and St. John's wort may increase risk of bleeding.
zidovudine (AZT)	Food reduces bioavailability.

To the Community   Food–Drug Interactions

CONNECTIONS

The nurse has a critical role in patient education related to food–drug interactions. One of the common questions a patient will ask is "Do I take this drug with food?" Most medications can be administered with food, so of greater importance is what foods the patient should avoid when taking the drug.

Foods may contain naturally occurring substances or be fortified with vitamins that do not mix well with medications. The drug ingredients may not work as well as they should when certain foods are taken concurrently. Food nutrients can affect absorption, metabolism, or elimination of the drug by binding with ingredients in the medication. One common food–drug interaction is taking grapefruit juice with selected statins, calcium channel blockers, estrogen-containing birth control pills, tricyclic antidepressants, the antidysrhythmic drug amiodarone, or the immunosuppressant tacrolimus (Prograf).

The stimulation effects of caffeine may be increased when taken with ciprofloxacin or other fluoroquinolones. Other food–drug interactions can occur with dairy and other calcium products, antacids, protein-rich foods, high-fat meals, fiber, vitamin C, cranberry and other fruit juices, tyramine-containing foods, alcohol, leafy green vegetables, soy milk, and dietary supplements. Fad diets may include foods that interact with medications. In short, the safest way to take a medication is with a glass of water.

Here is what to teach the patient:

- Always read the prescription label because the pharmacist will indicate if the medication must be taken with food. If not, take with just a glass of water.
- Read drug handouts carefully because these give more details about possible food–drug interactions. The same is true for OTC medications. Read all inserts for warnings. If anything is unclear, ask the pharmacist or the health care provider who prescribed the medication.
- Drink a full 8-ounce glass of water with the medication.
- Avoid taking herbal supplements and vitamins at the same time as prescription medications to avoid interactions.
- Avoid taking a drug with a hot drink or opening or crushing the pill to stir in liquid. Both can affect the effectiveness of the drug.
- Avoid drinking alcohol when taking medication.
- Provide a list of current prescription and nonprescription medications to the pharmacist. Filling all prescriptions at the same store will assist the pharmacist in comparing your current and new medications for possible interactions.
- Seek information from the pharmacist or health care provider if uncertain about medications. A phone call can clear up any questions and support an improved therapeutic outcome.

combinations have a significant impact on pharmacotherapy. Because patients view herbal products as "natural," they do not usually mention them when recording their drug history; thus the health care provider must ask specific questions about their use.

Perhaps the most widely studied herb is St. John's wort, which is taken by patients as a complementary or alternative therapy for depression. The herb induces hepatic metabolic enzymes, which can reduce the effectiveness of certain prescription medications, including antidepressants, warfarin, and benzodiazepines. A second herb that has been extensively studied is ginkgo biloba, which is taken by patients to improve circulation and memory. Ginkgo may produce additive anticoagulant effects when taken with warfarin or antiplatelet drugs. It can also antagonize the effects of antiseizure drugs, thus increasing the risk for seizures.

UNDERSTANDING THE CHAPTER

Key Concepts Summary

1 The nurse plays a key role in preventing and managing adverse drug effects.

2 The FDA continues to monitor for new adverse events after a drug is approved and marketed.

3 Allergic reactions are caused by a hyperresponse of the immune system.

4 Idiosyncratic reactions are unusual drug responses often caused by genetic differences among patients.

5 Some drugs have the ability to induce cancer or cause birth defects.

6 Drug toxicity may be specific to particular organs.

7 Drug interactions may significantly affect pharmacotherapeutic outcomes.

8 Pharmacokinetic drug interactions include changes in the absorption, distribution, metabolism, or excretion of medications.

9 Pharmacodynamic drug interactions include additive, synergistic, or antagonistic effects.

10 Food, nutrients, and dietary supplements may interact with medications and affect their actions.

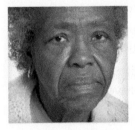

Making the PATIENT Connection

Remember the patient "Elizabeth Washington" at the beginning of the chapter? Now read the remainder of the case study. Based on the information presented within this chapter, respond to the critical thinking questions that follow.

The more medication an individual takes, the more likely it is that an adverse reaction may occur. For Elizabeth Washington this is a real possibility because she takes multiple medications for various physical problems. Elizabeth is a 77-year-old African American woman with several chronic conditions that require pharmacotherapy, including diabetes, heart failure, arthritis, and depression. She has been wheelchair bound since her stroke 2 years ago and has lost functional ability of her left side.

Unfortunately, she does not have a regular health care provider. Elizabeth obtains all her health care from a clinic operated for lower income individuals. The primary health care providers in the clinic are medical residents and interns who rotate every month as part of their medical training. Therefore, it is unlikely that she will see the same prescriber more than a couple of times. Her medical record is quite extensive and spans her health history for the last 15 years. Because her medical history record is so lengthy, Elizabeth fears that the new doctors will not take the time to read the entire chart before prescribing the newest treatment or therapy.

Critical Thinking Questions

1. Identify ways that you can minimize or prevent adverse drug events in this patient.

2. What existing conditions make Elizabeth more susceptible to a drug reaction?

3. Discuss how drug reactions can affect pharmacokinetics.

4. Differentiate among additive, synergistic, and antagonist drug effects.

See Answers to Critical Thinking Questions on student resource website.

NCLEX-RN® Review

1 Prior to the administration of an antibiotic, the client informs the nurse that 4 years ago the client experienced an allergic reaction. Based on this information what should the nurse do first?

1. Ask the client to describe the reaction further.
2. Notify the health care provider on call about the client's statements.
3. Administer the dose and observe the client for a reaction.
4. Check the medical administration record for documented allergies.

2 The nurse is researching a new drug prior to administration. The drug handbook states that the adverse effects are "dose related" which means that:

1. As the dose increases, the risk of adverse effects also increases.
2. The adverse effects should be expected after the first dose.
3. Oral preparations will produce the most adverse effects.
4. The timing of each dose should be correlated with the presence of adverse effects.

3 The client is receiving a medication that may cause nephrotoxicity. To prevent this adverse reaction the nurse should encourage the client to:

1. Avoid sunbathing and exposure to direct sunlight.
2. Increase the intake of potassium-enriched foods.
3. Abstain from alcoholic beverages.
4. Increase fluid intake to promote adequate hydration.

4 On physical examination, the nurse observes raised hive-like welts covering the client's trunk and arms. The client also reports intense itching after receiving a new medication. The nurse will suspect what dermatologic adverse effect?

1. Angioedema
2. Stevens–Johnson syndrome
3. Urticaria
4. Phototoxicity

5 When observing a client for bone marrow toxicity, the nurse would monitor for:

1. Increased complaints of muscle and bone pain in the lower extremities.
2. Decrease in red blood cells, white blood cells, and platelets.
3. Decrease in the range of motion of the upper and lower extremities.
4. Increase in hepatic enzymes.

6 The client is receiving a medication that causes hepatotoxicity. What symptoms would alert the nurse that this drug-related toxicity has occurred?

1. Black furry tongue and vaginal yeast infection
2. A sudden reduction in blood pressure on rising
3. Right upper quadrant pain and anorexia
4. Uncontrollable movements in the face, arms, and legs

Additional Case Study

As the triage nurse in the emergency department, you determine the patient's chief complaint, obtain vital signs, collect past medical history information, and ask about drug and food allergies. While assessing a patient with a suspected ankle fracture, she tells you that she is allergic to codeine because it makes her nauseated and sleepy.

1. What further questions would you ask the patient about drug allergies?
2. Differentiate among an adverse effect, side effect, and drug allergy.
3. Is this patient experiencing an idiosyncratic reaction? Explain.

See Answers to Additional Case Study on student resource website.

Pearson Nursing Student Resources

Find additional review materials at nursing.pearsonhighered.com

Prepare for success with additional NCLEX®-style practice questions, interactive assignments and activities, web links, animations, videos, and more!

References

Davies, E. C., Green, C. F., Taylor, S., Williamson, P. R., Mottram, D. R. & Pirmohamed, M. (2009). Adverse drug reactions in hospital in-patients: A prospective analysis of 3695 patient-episodes. *PLoS ONE, 4*(2), e4439. doi:10.1371/journal.pone.0004439

Kroon, L. A. (2007). Drug interactions with smoking. *American Journal of Health-System Pharmacy, 64*(18), 1917–1921. doi:10.2146/ajhp060414

Selected Bibliography

Akamine, D., Filho, M. K., & Peres, C. M. (2007). Drug–nutrient interactions in elderly people. *Current Opinion in Clinical Nutrition and Metabolic Care, 10*(3), 304–310. doi:10.1097/MCO.0b013e3280d646ce

Bilyeu, K. M., Gumm, C. J., Fitzgerald, J. M., Fox, S. W., & Selig, P. (2011). Cultivating quality: Reducing the use of potentially inappropriate medications in older adults. *American Journal of Nursing, 111*(1), 47–52. doi:10.1097/01.NAJ.0000393060.94063.15

Boullata, J. I., & Armenti, V. T. (Eds). (2010). *Handbook of drug-nutrient interactions* (2nd ed.) New York, NY: Humana Press.

George, E. L., Henneman, E. A., & Tasota, F. J. (2010). Nursing implications for prevention of adverse drug events in the intensive care unit. *Critical Care Medicine, 38*(6 suppl), S136–S144. doi:10.1097/CCM.0b013e3181de0b23

Izzo, A. A., & Edzard, E. (2009). Interactions between herbal medicines and prescribed drugs: An updated systematic review, *Drugs, 69*(13), 1777–1798. doi:10.2165/11317010-000000000-00000

Jordan, S. (2011). Adverse events: Expecting too much of nurses and too little of nursing research. *Journal of Nursing Management, 19*(3), 287-292. doi:10.1111/j.1365-2834.2011.01265.x

Lund, B. C., Carnahan, R. M., Chrischilles, E. A., & Kaboli, P. J. (2010). Inappropriate prescribing predicts adverse drug events in older adults. *Annals of Pharmacotherapy, 44*(6), 957–963. doi:10.1345/aph.1P182

Pronsky, Z. (2010). *Food–medication interactions handbook* (16th ed.). Pottstown, PA: Food Medication Interactions.

Reimche, L., Forster, A. J. & van Walraven, C. (2010, October 6). Incidence and contributors to potential drug–drug interactions in hospitalized patients. Advance online publication. *Journal of Clinical Pharmacology.* doi:10.1177/0091270010378858

Valente, S., & Murray, L. P. (2011). Creative strategies to improve patient safety: Allergies and adverse drug reactions. *Nurses in Staff Development, 27*(1), E1–E5. doi:10.1097/NND.0b013e31819b5f0b

Wilmer, A., Louie, K., Dodek, P., Wong, H., & Ayas, N. (2010). Incidence of medication errors and adverse drug events in the ICU: A systematic review. *Quality and Safety in Health Care, 19*(5), 1–9. doi:10.1136/qshc.2008.030783

Answers to NCLEX-RN® Review

1 Answer: 1   Rationale: Collecting additional information will provide the prescriber with knowledge about the type and severity of the reaction to that specific drug and will assist in determining the appropriateness of the order. Options 2, 3, and 4 are incorrect. The nurse should gather additional information from the client or family member before notifying the prescriber. A medication is never administered to a client when allergic sensitivity is suspected until further investigation into the type and severity of the reaction has been completed. Although documentation of the event may be in the client's medical record, the reaction may not have been documented or may have happened after the last health care visit. Cognitive Level: Applying; Client Need: Physiological Integrity; Nursing Process: Implementation

2 Answer: 1   Rationale: The nurse knows to closely monitor the client for the onset of adverse effects whenever the dose of the drug is increased. Options 2, 3, and 4 are incorrect. Although adverse effects are sometimes noted after the first dose, they may occur at any time during drug administration. Although some adverse effects are common when a drug is given PO, others are more common when given by other routes, such as IV or IM. The timing of medication is not a factor associated with dose-related adverse effects. Cognitive Level: Applying; Client Need: Physiological Integrity; Nursing Process: Implementation

3 Answer: 4   Rationale: Promoting hydration may dramatically reduce the risk of renal damage produced by drug therapies. Options 1, 2, and 3 are incorrect. Avoiding direct sunlight is teaching given to clients receiving drugs that cause phototoxicity. The consumption of potassium-enriched foods will not reduce the risk of drug-induced nephrotoxicity, nor will avoiding alcohol consumption. Cognitive Level: Applying; Client Need: Physiological Integrity; Nursing Process: Implementation

4 Answer: 3   Rationale: Urticaria or hives, with raised, itchy areas of skin, is usually a sign of an allergic reaction. Options 1, 2, and 4 are incorrect. Angioedema is a notable swelling around the eyes and lips and sometimes of the hands and feet that occurs beneath the skin instead of on the surface. SJS is characterized by a flulike period of fever, sore throat, and headache followed by the sudden development of circular lesions that cover the majority of the skin. Phototoxicity occurs when a drug renders the skin susceptible to damage by sunlight. Cognitive Level: Applying; Client Need: Physiological Integrity; Nursing Process: Evaluation

5 Answer: 2   Rationale: The function of the bone marrow is to produce blood cells. When drugs cause bone marrow toxicity, the condition manifests as a decrease in all blood cell types. Options 1, 3, and 4 are incorrect. Muscle and bone pain are most often associated with muscle toxicity. Bone marrow toxicity is not related to a decline in an individual's range of motion. Liver enzymes are not typically affected by bone marrow toxicity. Cognitive Level: Applying; Client Need: Physiological Integrity; Nursing Process: Evaluation

6 Answer: 3   Rationale: The presence of right upper quadrant pain and anorexia are the vague symptoms often associated with drug-induced liver damage. Options 1, 2 and 4 are incorrect. Black, "furry" tongue or infections elsewhere are not related to liver damage. A sudden drop in BP is orthostatic hypotension. Unusual and uncontrolled movements are neurologic-related effects. Cognitive Level: Analyzing; Client Need: Physiological Integrity; Nursing Process: Evaluation

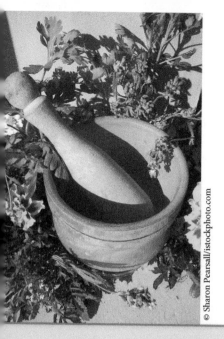

© Sharon Pearsall/istockphoto.com

"My daughter is getting so frustrated with me. It seems that I can't remember anything. Just last week I forgot to take my medications twice and failed to pick up my grandson at his weekly tae kwon do lesson."

Patient "Larry Bunch"

The Role of Complementary and Alternative Therapies in Pharmacotherapy

Chapter Outline

Types of Complementary and Alternative Therapies

History of Herbal Therapies

Standardization of Herbal Products

Dietary Supplement Regulation

Herb–Drug Interactions

Specialty Supplements

Learning Outcomes

After reading this chapter, the student should be able to:

1. Explain the role of complementary and alternative therapies in promoting patient wellness.

2. Analyze why herbal and dietary supplements have increased in popularity.

3. Identify the parts of an herb that contain active ingredients and the types of formulations made from these parts.

4. Compare the strengths and weaknesses of the Dietary Supplement Health and Education Act of 1994 with the Dietary Supplement and Nonprescription Drug Consumer Protection Act of 2006.

5. Describe specific adverse effects that may be caused by herbal preparations.

6. Discuss the role of the nurse in teaching patients about complementary and alternative therapies.

7. Identify common herb–drug interactions.

8. Explain why it is important to standardize herbal products based on specific active ingredients.

From Chapter 15 of *Pharmacology: Connections to Nursing Practice*, Second Edition. Michael Patrick Adams, Carol Quam Urban. Copyright © 2013 by Pearson Education, Inc. All rights reserved.

Complementary and alternative medicine represents a multibillion dollar industry. Sales of dietary supplements alone now exceed $26 billion annually, with an estimated 200 million consumers using them. Despite the fact that these therapies have not been subjected to the same scientific scrutiny as prescription medications, consumers have turned to these treatments for a wide variety of reasons. Many people have the impression that natural substances have more healing power than synthetic medications. The availability of herbal supplements at a reasonable cost has convinced many consumers to try them. This chapter focuses on the role of complementary and alternative therapies in the prevention and treatment of disease.

TABLE 1 Complementary and Alternative Therapies

Healing Method	Examples
Biologic-based therapies	Herbal therapies
	Nutritional supplements
	Special diets
Alternative health care systems	Naturopathy
	Homeopathy
	Chiropractic
	Native American medicine (e.g., sweat lodges, medicine wheel)
	Chinese traditional medicine (e.g., acupuncture, Chinese herbs)
Manual healing	Massage
	Pressure-point therapies
	Hand-mediated biofield therapies
Mind–body interventions	Yoga, Pilates
	Meditation
	Hypnotherapy
	Guided imagery
	Biofeedback
	Movement-oriented therapies (e.g., music, dance)
Spiritual	Shamans
	Faith and prayer
Others	Bioelectromagnetics
	Detoxifying therapies
	Animal-assisted therapy

Types of Complementary and Alternative Therapies

1 Complementary and alternative therapies are used by a large number of people to prevent and treat disease.

Complementary and alternative medicine (CAM) comprises an extremely diverse set of therapies and healing systems that are considered to be outside of mainstream health care. Although diverse, the major CAM systems have certain common characteristics:

- Focus on treating the individual person
- Consideration of the health of the whole person
- Integration of mind and body
- Emphasis on disease prevention, self-care, and self-healing
- Recognition of the role of spirituality in health and healing.

Because of its popularity, the scientific community has begun to examine the effectiveness, or lack of effectiveness, of CAM therapies. Although research into these alternative systems has begun to appear worldwide, few CAM therapies have been subjected to rigorous, controlled clinical and scientific studies. It is likely that some of these therapies will be found ineffective, whereas others will become mainstream treatments. The definition of a complementary therapy as being "outside the mainstream" is somewhat ambiguous because the line between an alternative therapy and a conventional therapy is constantly changing. Increasing numbers of health care providers are now recommending CAM therapies to their patients. Table 1 lists the most common CAM therapies.

Nurses have long known the value of CAM in preventing and treating disease. Prayer, meditation, massage, and yoga have been used to treat both body and spirit for centuries. From a pharmacologic perspective the value of CAM therapies lies in their ability to reduce the need for medications. For example, if a patient can find anxiety relief through massage or biofeedback therapy, the use of antianxiety drugs may be reduced or eliminated. Reduction of drug dose leads to fewer adverse effects.

The nurse should be sensitive to the patient's beliefs about and need for alternative treatment and not be judgmental. Both the advantages and the limitations must be presented to patients so they may make rational and informed decisions about their treatment. Both pharmacotherapy and alternative therapies can play complementary roles in healing.

History of Herbal Therapies

2 Natural products from plants have been used as medicines for thousands of years.

An **herb** is technically a **botanical** (plant-based substance) that does not have any woody tissue such as stems or bark. In common usage, however, consumers tend to use "herb" to refer to a wide variety of products including substances such as ginkgo biloba (which is a tree) and chondroitin (which is derived from animals). Over time, the term *herb* has come to refer to any plant product with some useful application either as a food enhancer, such as flavoring, or as a medicine.

The use of herbs has been recorded for thousands of years. One of the earliest recorded uses of plant products was a prescription for garlic written in 3000 BC. Eastern and Western medicine have recorded thousands of herbs and herb combinations reputed to have therapeutic value. Over time, the popularity of specific herbs and remedies has varied, depending on the availability of the botanical (i.e., geographical region) and perceived effectiveness. The most popular herbals in the United States and their primary uses are shown in Table 2.

With the birth of the pharmaceutical industry in the late 1800s, the interest in herbal medicine began to wane. Synthetic drugs could be standardized and produced more cheaply than natural herbal products. Regulatory agencies required that products be safe and effective. The focus of health care was on diagnosing and treating specific diseases, rather than promoting wellness and holistic care. Most alternative therapies were no longer taught in medical or nursing schools. These healing techniques were criticized as being unscientific relics of the past.

Beginning in the 1970s and continuing to current times, however, alternative therapies and herbal medicine have experienced a remarkable resurgence, such that the majority of adult Americans are either currently taking herbal therapies on a regular basis or have taken them in the past. Why would people turn to folk remedies and products with uncertain effectiveness when effective prescription medications

TABLE 2 Top-Selling Herbal Supplements

Rank	Herb	Medicinal Part	Primary Use(s)	Herb Feature (Chapter)
1	Cranberry	Berries/juice	Prevent urinary tract infection	53
2	Flaxseed (ground) and/or oil	Seeds and oil	Lower cholesterol levels, reduce the risk of heart disease, laxative	—
3	Saw palmetto	Berries	Treatment of benign prostatic hyperplasia	74
4	Soy	Beans	Source of protein, vitamins, and minerals; relief of menopausal symptoms, prevent cardiovascular disease, anticancer	72
5	Garlic	Bulbs	Reduce blood cholesterol, reduce blood pressure, anticoagulation	41
6	Ginkgo	Leaves and seeds	Improve memory, reduce dizziness	25
7	Wheat or barley grass	Leaves	Improve digestion, vitamin and mineral supplement	—
8	Echinacea	Entire plant	Enhance immune system, treat the common cold	45
9	Aloe vera	Leaves	Topical application for minor skin irritations and burns	76
10	Tumeric	Roots and bulbs	Indigestion, dyspepsia, reduce inflammation	—
11	Milk thistle	Seeds	Antitoxin, protection against liver disease	
12	Stevia	Leaves	Natural sweetener	—
13	Black cohosh	Roots	Relief of menopausal symptoms	73
14	St. John's wort	Flowers, leaves, stems	Reduce depression, reduce anxiety, anti-inflammatory	23
15	Ginseng	Root	Relieve stress, enhance immune system, decrease fatigue	38
16	Elderberry	Berries and flowers	Congestion in respiratory system due to colds and flu	
17	Green tea	Leaves	Antioxidant; lower LDL cholesterol; prevent cancer; relieve stomach problems, nausea, vomiting	66
18	Acai	Berries	Vitamin and mineral supplement, antioxidant, possible weight loss	—
19	Evening primrose	Seeds/oil	Source of essential fatty acids, relief of premenstrual or menopausal symptoms, relief of rheumatoid arthritis and other inflammatory symptoms	—
20	Valerian	Roots	Relieve stress, promote sleep	—
21	Chlorophyll/chlorella	Leaves	Improve digestion, vitamin and mineral supplement	
22	Horny goat weed	Leaves and roots	Enhance sexual function	—
23	Bilberry	Berries and leaves	Terminate diarrhea, improve and protect vision, antioxidant	77
24	Grape seed	Seeds/oil	Source of essential fatty acids, antioxidant, restore microcirculation to tissues	37
25	Ginger	Root	Antiemetic, antithrombotic, diuretic, promote gastric secretions, anti-inflammatory, increase blood glucose, stimulation of peripheral circulation	62

are available? This increase in popularity has been due to a number of factors:

- Herbal products and dietary supplements were once available only in specialty health food stores but can now be purchased in virtually all supermarkets and pharmacies.
- Complementary therapies are aggressively marketed by the supplement industry as viable and natural alternatives to conventional medicine. The increased availability of the Internet as a marketing tool has led to sites with misleading information about the effectiveness of herbal and dietary supplements.
- The baby-boom generation has demonstrated a renewed interest in natural alternatives and preventive medicine.
- The gradual aging of the population has led people to seek therapeutic alternatives for chronic conditions such as pain, arthritis, anxiety, depression, hormone-replacement therapy, and prostate difficulties.
- Several high-profile drugs such as Vioxx have been removed from the market or their use severely restricted due to "un-expected" adverse effects. People have the impression that natural substances are safer than synthetic pharmaceuticals.
- The high cost of prescription medicines has driven people to seek less expensive alternatives.
- Nurses and other health care providers have been more proactive in promoting self-care and recommending alternative therapies for their patients

Numerous surveys have been conducted to determine the extent of alternative therapy use in the United States. Results of these studies agree that there is widespread and progressively increasing use of these therapies. One of the largest studies of Americans' use of complementary therapies conducted by the National Center for Complementary and Alternative Medicine (NCCAM) surveyed over 23,000 people (Barnes, Bloom, & Nahin, 2008). Findings of this study included the following:

- Thirty-eight percent of adults and about 12% of children are currently using CAM.
- Women and those with higher educational levels are most likely to use CAM.
- Of those who take natural products, the most commonly used are fish oil (37%), glucosamine (20%), echinacea (20%), flaxseed (16%), ginseng (14%), ginkgo biloba (11%), chondroitin (11%), garlic (11%), and coenzyme Q (9%).
- The most frequent conditions treated with CAM are back pain (17%), head or chest cold (10%), joint pain/arthritis (5%), neck pain (5%), and anxiety or depression (5%).
- People are more likely to use CAM when they are unable to afford conventional health care.

This pharmacology text emphasizes CAM by the use of features. The inclusion of these therapies is not an endorsement, nor does it imply their effectiveness. They are included because the nurse will frequently need to teach specific natural therapies, and because some of them have the potential to impact pharmacotherapy (see Section 5). The student should

refer to the current medical literature for complete dosing and safety information. Several excellent sources of reliable information are available. The National Center for Complementary and Alternative Medicine (NCCAM) is a branch of the National Institutes of Health (NIH). It offers current information on research involving these products. Although somewhat dated, another extensive source of reliable information is *The Complete German Commission E Monographs: Therapeutic Guide to Herbal Medicines*, which evaluates the safety and effectiveness of over 380 herbs licensed for medical prescribing in Germany.

PharmFACT

According to Broussard, Louik, Honein, and Mitchell (2010), 9.4% of women take herbal products during pregnancy, with ginger and ephedra being the most frequently consumed. Potentially, this results in as many as 395,000 births in the United States in which the fetus received prenatal exposure to herbal products.

Standardization of Herbal Products

3 Herbal products are available in a variety of formulations, some containing standardized extracts and others containing whole herbs.

The pharmacologically active chemicals in an herbal product may be present in only one specific part or in all parts of the plant. For example, the active chemicals in chamomile are in the aboveground portion such as the leaves, stems, or flowers. For other herbs, such as ginger, the underground rhizomes and roots are used for their healing properties. It is, therefore, essential to know which portion of the plant contains the active chemicals if growing or collecting herbs for home use.

Most prescription drugs contain only one active chemical. This chemical can be standardized and measured, so that the amount of drug received by the patient is precisely known. Herbs, however, may contain dozens of active chemicals, many of which have not yet been isolated, studied, or even identified. It is possible that some of these substances work together synergistically and may not have the same activity if isolated. Furthermore, the strength of an herbal preparation can vary from batch to batch, depending on where it was grown and how it was collected, stored, and preserved.

Some attempts have been made to standardize herbal extracts, using a marker substance such as the percent flavone glycosides in ginkgo or the percent hypericins in St. John's wort. Some of these standardizations are shown in Table 3. In some cases, manufacturers have isolated this component and market only one active chemical in the herb. Until science can better characterize these substances, however, it is best to conceptualize the active ingredient of an herb as being the entire herb. Taking one single component in high doses can increase the risk for adverse effects from an herb. An example of the ingredients and standardization of ginkgo biloba using a marker substance is shown in Figure 1. It should not be

TABLE 3 Standardization of Selected Herb Extracts

Herb	Standardization	Percent
Black cohosh rhizome	Triterpene glycosides	2.5
Cascara sagrada bark	Hydroxyanthracenic heterosides	20
Echinacea purpurea, whole herb	Echinacosides Phenolics	4
Ginger rhizome	Pungent compounds (gingerols)	>10
Ginkgo leaf	Flavone glycosides	24–25
	Lactones	6
Ginseng root	Ginseosides	20–30
Kava kava rhizome	Kavalactones	40–45
Milk thistle root	Silymarin	80
St. John's wort, whole herb	Hypericins	0.3–0.5
	Hyperforin	3–5
Saw palmetto berries	Fatty acids and sterols	80–90

TABLE 4 Liquid Formulations of Herbal Products

Product	Description
Tea	Fresh or dried herbs are soaked in hot water for 5–10 min before ingestion; convenient
Infusion	Fresh or dried herbs are soaked in hot water for long periods, at least 15 min; stronger than teas
Decoction	Fresh or dried herbs are boiled in water for 30–60 min until much of the liquid has boiled off; very concentrated
Tincture	Active ingredients are extracted using alcohol by soaking the herb; alcohol remains as part of the liquid
Extract	Active ingredients are extracted using organic solvents to form a highly concentrated liquid or solid form; solvent may be removed or be part of the final product

Figure 1

Two ginkgo biloba labels. Note the lack of standardization: (a) 60 mg of extract, 24% Ginkgo Flavone Glycosides, and 6% Terpene Lactones; (b) 50:1 Ginkgo Biloba Leaf Extract, 24% Ginkgo Flavinoglycosides.

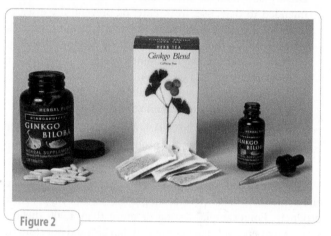

Figure 2

Three different ginkgo formulations: tablets, tea bags, and liquid extract.

assumed that an herb is safe or effective simply because it contains the standard amount of marker substance.

The two basic formulations of herbal products are solid and liquid. Solid products include pills, tablets, and capsules made from the dried herbs. Other solid products are salves and ointments that are administered topically. Liquid formulations are made by extracting the active chemicals from the plant using solvents such as water, alcohol, or glycerol. The liquids are then concentrated in various strengths and ingested. The types of liquid herbal formulations are described in Table 4. Figure 2 illustrates some of the formulations of ginkgo biloba, one of the most popular herbals.

Dietary Supplement Regulation

4 Herbal products and dietary supplements are regulated by the Dietary Supplement Health and Education Act of 1994.

Since the passage of the Food, Drug, and Cosmetic Act in 1936, Americans have come to expect that all approved prescription and over-the-counter (OTC) drugs have passed rigid standards of safety prior to being marketed. Furthermore, it is expected that these drugs have been tested for effectiveness and that they truly provide the medical benefits claimed by the manufacturer. For herbal products, however, Americans cannot and should not expect the same quality standards. These products are regulated by a far less rigorous law, the **Dietary Supplement Health and Education Act of 1994 (DSHEA)**.

According to the DSHEA, dietary supplements are exempted from the Food, Drug, and Cosmetic Act that regulates prescription drugs. **Dietary supplements** are defined as products intended to enhance or supplement the diet such as botanicals, vitamins, minerals, or any other extract or metabolite that is not already approved as a drug by the FDA (as of 1994). A major strength of the legislation is that it gives the FDA the authority to remove from the market any product that poses a "significant or unreasonable" risk to the public. It also requires these products to be clearly labeled as "dietary supplements." An example of an herbal label for black cohosh is shown in Figure 3.

Unfortunately, the DSHEA has several significant flaws that lead to a lack of standardization in the dietary supplement industry and, ultimately, to less protection for the consumer. These flaws include:

- The manufacturer does not have to test the safety of the dietary supplement prior to marketing. If it is to be removed from the market, the FDA has the burden of proving that the dietary supplement is harmful.

- Effectiveness does not have to be demonstrated by the manufacturer.

- Dietary supplements must state that the product is not intended to diagnose, treat, cure, or prevent any disease; however, the label may make claims about the product's effect on body structure and function, such as the following:
  - Helps promote healthy immune systems
  - Reduces anxiety and stress
  - Helps to maintain cardiovascular function
  - May reduce pain and inflammation

- The accuracy of the label is not regulated; the product may or may not contain the product listed in the amounts claimed.

Lax government oversight has resulted in a lack of quality and sometimes blatant mislabeling of herbal and supplement products. For example, testing of more than 1,200 dietary supplement products has determined that 25% did not contain the correct amount of labeled ingredients. In some cases, the products contained none of the ingredients claimed on the label, and others were contaminated with potentially dangerous heavy metals such as cadmium and lead.

Several steps have been taken to address the lack of purity and mislabeling of herbal and dietary supplements. The United States Pharmacopoeia (USP) is a nonprofit public health organization that has attempted to raise the standards and quality of pharmaceuticals and dietary supplements. The USP has developed a voluntary process by which a manufacturer may submit a product for the **USP Verification Program**. Using a multistep approach, the USP examines the manufacturing processes used to create a supplement and tests the product to see if it contains the ingredients specified on the label and whether the product will break down and release its ingredients in the body (bioavailability). If the product meets the stringent standards of the USP, it may then carry the USP verified dietary supplement mark on the label. The verification mark, shown in Figure 4, indicates to consumers that the product has been manufactured under acceptable standards of purity, has been tested for active ingredients stated on the label, and is free of harmful contaminants. However, it does not indicate that the product is safe or effective.

In another attempt to protect consumers, Congress passed the **Dietary Supplement and Nonprescription Drug Consumer Protection Act**, which took effect in 2007. Companies that market herbal and dietary supplements are now required to include their contact information (address and phone number) on the product labels so consumers can report adverse events. Companies must notify the FDA of any serious adverse event reports within 15 days of receiving such reports. Under this act, a "serious adverse event" is defined as any adverse reaction resulting in death, a life-threatening experience, inpatient hospitalization, a persistent or significant disability or incapacity, or a congenital anomaly or birth defect, as well as any event requiring a medical or surgical intervention to prevent one of these conditions based on reasonable medical judgment. Companies must keep records of such events for at least 6 years, and the records are subject to inspection by the FDA.

Also in 2007, the FDA announced a final rule that requires the manufacturers of dietary supplements to evaluate the

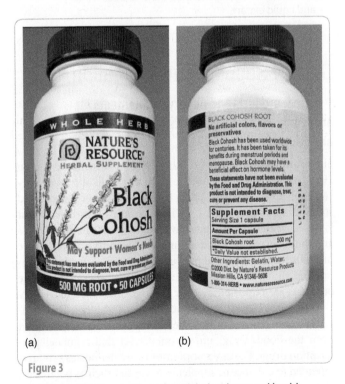

Labeling of black cohosh: (a) front label with general health claim; (b) back label with more health claims and FDA disclaimer.

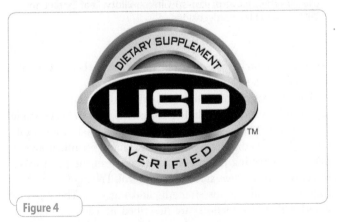

USP verified dietary supplement mark.
Source: U.S. Pharmacopeia

identity, purity, potency, and composition of their products. The labels must accurately reflect the content of the products, which must be free of contaminants such as pesticides, toxins, glass, or heavy metals. The rule was phased in over a 3-year period.

CONNECTION Checkpoint 15.1

What is a pharmacopeia? What function does it serve in the United States? *See Answer to Connection Checkpoint 15.1 on student resource website.*

Herb–Drug Interactions

5 Natural products may have pharmacologic actions and can interact with conventional drugs.

A key concept to remember when learning about alternative therapies is that "natural" is not synonymous with "better" or "safe." It is likely that some botanicals do indeed contain active chemicals that are as powerful as, and perhaps more effective than, some currently approved medications. Thousands of years of experience, combined with current scientific research, have shown that some of these herbal remedies have therapeutic actions. Just because a substance comes from a natural product, however, does not make it safe or effective. For example, poison ivy is natural but it certainly is not safe or therapeutic. The dried seed pods of the poppy plant yield opium, which has therapeutic effects but can also kill if taken inappropriately. Some natural products may not offer an improvement over conventional therapy in treating certain disorders and, indeed, may be of no value whatsoever. Furthermore, a patient who substitutes an unproven alternative therapy for an established, effective medical treatment may delay healing and cause irreparable harmful effects.

Some herbal products contain ingredients that may cause additive, synergistic, or antagonistic interactions with prescription or OTC drugs. For example, ginkgo biloba and ginger have the ability to increase bleeding time. If used concurrently with anticoagulants, these herbs may increase the potential for adverse bleeding events. St. John's wort, kava, and valerian cause relaxation and may result in excessive sedation if taken concurrently with central nervous system (CNS) depressants. A few herbals have organ-specific toxicity. The herb comfrey given concurrently with large doses of acetaminophen may increase the patient's risk of hepatotoxicity. Herbals such as psyllium, aloe, and flaxseed may bind to drugs in the gastrointestinal (GI) tract, thus slowing their absorption.

The true extent of herb–drug interactions is unknown. Most reports in the medical literature are anecdotal, often given as a case report on a single patient. It is often impossible to know the exact amount of herb taken because there is such a wide variation in the quality of products on the market or even to know what chemical within the herb (either active ingredients or contaminants) may have caused the reported interaction. Relatively few controlled scientific studies of herb–drug or dietary supplement–drug interactions have been conducted. The majority of the information regarding these interactions is theoretical, rather than clinically based.

CONNECTIONS

Lifespan Considerations
Older Adults at Risk for Polyherbacy

One of the most important health issues affecting older adults is the excessive or inappropriate use of medications. Although health care providers assess for polypharmacy, elderly patients may not divulge the use of herbs and supplements when talking to health care providers. With the increased use of herbs and supplements by older adults, a new health care dilemma— **polyherbacy**, the use of multiple herbs or other supplements.

There are many issues related to the use of herbals and nutritional supplements that should be considered with older adults. For example, there may be:

- Inadequate data that examine the effects and impact that supplements have on the natural physiological changes that occur during the aging process. Because older adults experience diminished kidney and liver function, they may be at greater risk for toxicity.
- Altered pharmacokinetic processes that would increase the older adult's incidence of serious adverse effects.
- Unknown chemicals in the preparation that could interact with other medications.

Health care providers should always inquire about herbal use and should also be aware of the adverse effects that may result from such products.

When obtaining medical histories nurses should include questions on the use of herbal and dietary supplements because these products are contraindicated for certain patients. Patients taking medications with potentially serious adverse effects such as insulin, warfarin (Coumadin), antiepileptic drugs, antineoplastic agents, or digoxin (Lanoxin) should be warned to never take any herbal product or dietary supplement without first discussing their needs with a health care provider. Pregnant or lactating women should not take these products without approval of their health care provider. The nurse should also remember that the potential for any drug interaction increases in older adults, especially those with hepatic or renal impairment. Potential drug interactions with selected herbs are shown in Table 5.

Another warning that must be heeded with natural products is to beware of allergic reactions. It is not unusual to find dozens of different chemicals in teas and infusions made from the flowers, leaves, or roots of a plant. Patients who have known allergies to food products or medicines should seek medical advice before taking a new herbal product. It is always wise to take the smallest amount possible when starting herbal therapy, even less than the recommended dose, to see if allergies or other adverse effects occur.

Nurses have an obligation to seek the latest medical information on herbal products, because there is a good possibility that their patients are using them to supplement traditional medicines. Each patient who takes an herbal product does so for a reason. The nurse needs to listen, assess, and understand the patient's goals for taking the supplement. Does the patient have an accurate understanding of the actions of the herb? Are

TABLE 5 Documented Herb–Drug Interactions

Common and (Scientific) Name	Interacts with	Effects of Interaction
Echinacea (*Echinacea purpurea*)	amiodarone, anabolic steroids, ketoconazole, methotrexate	May increase hepatotoxicity
Feverfew (*Tanacetum parthenium*)	aspirin and other NSAIDs; heparin; warfarin	Increases bleeding risk
Flaxseed (*Linum usitatissimum*)	most drugs	Binds to drugs; decreases absorption
Garlic (*Allium sativum*)	aspirin and other NSAIDs; warfarin	Increases bleeding risk
	insulin; oral antidiabetic agents	Has additive hypoglycemic effects
	saquinavir	Induces CYP3A4 enzymes; decreases drug effectiveness
Ginger (*Zingiber officinale*)	aspirin and other NSAIDs; heparin; warfarin	Increases bleeding risk
Ginkgo (*Ginkgo biloba*)	anticonvulsants	Decreases drug effectiveness
	tricyclic antidepressants	May decrease seizure threshold
	omeprazole	Induces CYP2C19 enzymes; decreases drug effectiveness
	trazodone	Increases drug effects
Ginseng (*Panax quinquefolius/ Eleutherococcus senticosus*)	CNS depressants	Potentiates sedation
	digoxin	Increases toxicity
	diuretics	May attenuate diuretic effects
	insulin; oral antidiabetic agents	Increases hypoglycemic effects
	MAO inhibitors	May cause hypertension, manic symptoms, headaches, nervousness
	warfarin	Decreases anticoagulant effects
Goldenseal (*Hydrastis canadensis/ Eleutherococcus senticosus*)	diuretics	May attenuate diuretic effects
Green tea	warfarin	Decreases anticoagulant effects
Kava kava (*Piper methysticum*)	barbiturates; benzodiazepines; alcohol and other CNS depressants	Potentiates sedation
	levodopa/carbidopa	Worsens Parkinson's symptoms
	phenothiazines	Increases risk and severity of dystonic reactions
St. John's wort (*Hypericum perforatum*)	opioids, alcohol, and other CNS depressants	Potentiates sedation
	cyclosporine	May decrease cyclosporine levels
	efavirenz, indinavir	Decreases antiretroviral activity
	MAO inhibitors	May cause hypertensive crisis
	oral contraceptives	Decreases drug effectiveness
	selective serotonin reuptake inhibitors; tricyclic antidepressants	Increases risk of serotonin syndrome
	warfarin	Decreases anticoagulant effects
Soy	warfarin	Decreases anticoagulant effects
Valerian (*Valeriana officinalis*)	barbiturates; benzodiazepines and other CNS depressants	Potentiates sedation

there more effective therapies, either pharmacologic or non-pharmacologic, for the patient's condition? Is there a potential for harmful effects from the product due to high doses or herb–drug interactions? Establishing a supportive attitude toward the use of CAM is important. Nurses often need to educate their patients on the role of alternative therapies in the treatment of their disorder and discuss which treatment or combination of treatments will best meet their patients' health goals. Patients should be advised to be skeptical of marketing claims for herbal products and to seek health information from reputable sources.

CONNECTION Checkpoint 15.2

St. John's wort induces hepatic CYP metabolic enzymes. How could this herb affect therapy with antidepressants or benzodiazepines that are substrates for CYP enzymes? *See Answer to Connection Checkpoint 15.2 on student resource website.*

Specialty Supplements

6 Specialty supplements are nonherbal dietary products that are widely used to promote wellness.

Specialty supplements are nonherbal dietary products used to enhance a wide variety of body functions. These supplements form a diverse group of products obtained from plant and animal sources. They are more specific in their action than herbal products and are generally targeted for one condition or a smaller group of related conditions. The most popular specialty supplements are listed in Table 6.

In general, specialty supplements have a legitimate rationale for their use. For example, chondroitin and glucosamine are natural substances in the body necessary for cartilage growth and maintenance. Amino acids are natural building blocks of muscle protein. Flaxseed and fish oils contain omega fatty acids that have been shown to reduce the risk of heart disease in certain patients.

As with herbal products, the link between most specialty supplements and their claimed benefits is unclear. In most cases, the body already has sufficient quantities of the substance; thus taking additional amounts may be of no benefit. In other cases, the supplement is marketed for conditions for which the supplement has no proven effect. The good news is that these substances are generally not harmful unless taken in large amounts. The bad news, however, is that they can give patients false hopes of an easy cure for chronic conditions such as heart disease or the pain of arthritis. As with herbal products, the health care provider should advise patients to be skeptical about any health claims regarding the use of these supplements.

TABLE 6 Selected Specialty Supplements

Name	Primary Uses	Supplement Feature (Chapter)
Amino acids	Build protein, muscle strength, and endurance	—
Carnitine	Enhance energy and sports performance, heart health, memory, immune function, and male fertility	39
Chromium	Treatment of diabetes; hyperglycemia	69
Coenzyme Q10	Prevent heart disease, provide antioxidant therapy	32
DHEA	Boost immune and memory functions	—
Fish oil	Reduce cholesterol levels, enhance brain function, increase visual acuity owing to the presence of the omega-3 fatty acids	71
Glucosamine and chondroitin	Alleviate arthritis and other joint problems	75
Lactobacillus acidophilus	Maintain intestinal health	63
Melatonin	Reduce sleeplessness and jet-lag during travel	22
Methyl sulfonyl methane (MSM)	Reduce allergic reactions to pollen and foods, relieve pain and inflammation of arthritis and similar conditions	—
Selenium	Reduce the risk of certain types of cancer	—
Vitamin C	Prevent colds	48

UNDERSTANDING THE CHAPTER

Key Concepts Summary

1 Complementary and alternative therapies are used by a large number of people to prevent and treat disease.

2 Natural products from plants have been used as medicines for thousands of years.

3 Herbal products are available in a variety of formulations, some containing standardized extracts and others containing whole herbs.

4 Herbal products and dietary supplements are regulated by the Dietary Supplement Health and Education Act of 1994.

5 Natural products may have pharmacologic actions and can interact with conventional drugs.

6 Specialty supplements are nonherbal dietary products that are widely used to promote wellness.

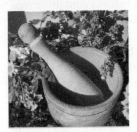

Making the PATIENT Connection

Remember the patient "Larry Bunch" at the beginning of the chapter? Now read the remainder of the case study. Based on the information presented within this chapter, respond to the critical thinking questions that follow.

Sixty-nine-year old Larry Bunch was not only frustrating his daughter, but his forgetfulness was annoying him as well. Since the death of his wife 2 years ago, his forgetfulness seemed to be worsening. To remedy the situation, he purchased a bottle of ginkgo biloba at the health food store and began taking the supplement about 6 months ago.

Larry was hospitalized 3 years ago for a cardiac condition (atrial fibrillation). When he was discharged from the hospital, he was placed on an anticoagulant therapy to prevent blood clots from forming in his heart. Today, Larry comes to his health care provider's office for a scheduled blood test to determine the effectiveness of his anticoagulant.

When the results from the blood test return, it is noted that Larry's coagulation time is abnormally high. Based on the test, Larry is at high risk of hemorrhaging. As the nurse, you note that his vital signs are within normal limits, and he states he feels well. However, you also observe some large bruises on Larry's arms, which he cannot explain.

Critical Thinking Questions

1. What is the relationship between this patient's use of ginkgo and the laboratory results?

2. What instructions should this patient receive about taking the supplement?

3. Discuss the hazards that patients face when using complementary and alternative therapies.

4. What should the health care provider do concerning Larry's forgetfulness?

See Answers to Critical Thinking Questions on student resource website.

NCLEX-RN® Review

1 A client asks why all health care providers do not rely on complementary and alternative medicine. When talking to this client the nurse knows that many complementary and alternative therapies:

1. Have not been subjected to rigorous clinical studies.
2. Consist only of old wives' tales and fables.
3. Only provide a placebo effect.
4. Are costly and not worth the risk.

2 Which health teaching concept should be included in the instructions for a client taking echinacea?

1. Dosage can be doubled if symptoms fail to resolve in 48 hours.
2. Limit fluid intake while taking this supplement.
3. Take the smallest amount possible when starting herbal therapy.
4. Allergic reactions are not possible with natural supplements.

3 Which client is most likely to experience drug toxicity while taking herbal supplements?

1. An 80-year-old female with cirrhosis
2. A 58-year-old male with cardiac irregularities
3. A 30-year-old female with pneumonia
4. An 18-year-old male with chronic acne

4 The client asks the nurse, "Why are herbal supplements so popular?" The nurse's answer is based on which factors? (Select all that apply.) Herbal supplements:

1. Can now be purchased in virtually all supermarkets.
2. Are aggressively marketed by the herbal and supplement industry.
3. Cost less than prescription medicines.
4. Are safer than synthetic pharmaceuticals.
5. Appeal to the aging population.

5 The nurse is teaching at a community wellness seminar when one participant asks, "How can I be sure that my herbal supplement is pure?" Which of the following labeling marks indicates that the product meets acceptable standards of purity?

1. USP verified dietary supplement mark
2. DEA prescriber number
3. FDA identification and regulation code
4. U.S. Customs Service integers

6 Polyherbacy may be of concern in the older adult population. A pharmacokinetic factor for this concern is that the older adult:

1. Is more likely to have difficulty using herbal products correctly.
2. May spend too much on herbal products rather than prescriptions.
3. May hold unrealistic expectations for the outcomes of herbal therapy.
4. May have age-related changes in liver or kidney function.

Additional Case Study

"It must be safe, after all, it is sold in the grocery store!" exclaimed Linda. As you, the nurse, talk with the patient, Linda Thomas, she explains to you that she takes multiple OTC dietary supplements. Because the bottle states that the ingredients are "all natural," she knows it must be good for her.

1. What are the hazards associated with believing that all medication-type substances sold in the supermarket are safe?

2. Discuss how the words "all natural ingredients" can be confusing.

3. Identify the nurse's role in working with patients who participate in complementary and alternative therapies.

See Answers to Additional Case Study on student resource website.

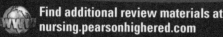

Pearson Nursing Student Resources

Find additional review materials at nursing.pearsonhighered.com

Prepare for success with additional NCLEX®-style practice questions, interactive assignments and activities, web links, animations, videos, and more!

References

Barnes, P. M., Bloom, B., & Nahin, R. L. (2008). Complementary and alternative medicine use among adults and children: United States, 2007 (National Health Statistics Reports No 12). Hyattsville, MD: National Center for Health Statistics.

Broussard, C. S., Louik, C., Honein, M. A., & Mitchell, A. A. (2010). Herbal use before and during pregnancy. *American Journal of Obstetrics & Gynecology, 202*(5), 443.e1–443.e6.

Selected Bibliography

Anastasi, J. K., Chang, M., & Capilli, B. (2011). Herbal supplements: Talking with your patients. *The Journal for Nurse Practitioners, 7*(1), 29–35. doi:10.1016/j.nurpra.2010.06.004

Anderson, E. (2009). Complementary therapies and older adults. *Topics in Geriatric Rehabilitation, 25*(4), 320–328.

Bent, S. (2007). Herbal medicine in the United States: Review of efficacy, safety, and regulation. *Journal of General Internal Medicine, 23*(6):854–859. doi:10.1007/s11606-008-0632-y

Blumenthal, M. (Ed.). (2000). *Herbal medicine: Expanded Commission E monographs.* Austin, TX: American Botanical Council.

Blumenthal, M., Lindstrom, A., & Lynch, M. E. (2011). Herbal sales continue growth–up 3.3% in 2010. *HerbalGram: The Journal of the American Botanical Council,*

90, 64-67. Retrieved from http://cms.herbalgram.org/herbalgram/issue90/MarketReport.html

Booth-LaForce, C., Scott, C. S., Heitkemper, M. M., Cornman, B. J., Lan, M. C., Bond, E. F., & Swanson, K. M. (2010). Complementary and alternative medicine (CAM) attitudes and competencies of nursing students and faculty: Results of integrating CAM into the nursing curriculum. *Journal of Professional Nursing, 26*(5), 293–300. doi:10.1016/j.profnurs.2010.03.003

Cassileth, B. R., Heitzer, M., & Wesa, K. (2009). The public health impact of herbs and nutritional supplements. *Pharmaceutical Biology, 47*(8), 761–767. doi:10.1080/13880200902991581

Chavez, M. L. (2005). Herbal–drug interactions. *InetCE, 9*(10), 2–30.

DerMarderosian, A., Liberti, L., Beutler, J. A., Grauds, C., Tatro, D. S., Cirigliano, M., & DeSilva, D. (2010). *The review of natural products* (6th ed.). St. Louis, MO: Wolters Kluwer Health.

Fontaine, K. L. (2009). *Complementary and alternative therapies for nursing practice* (3rd ed.). Upper Saddle River, NJ: Prentice Hall.

Gagnier, J. J., van Tulder, M., Berman, B., & Bombardier, C. (2007). Herbal medicine for low back pain: A Cochrane review. *Spine, 32*(1), 82–92. doi:10.1097/01.brs.0000249525.70011.fe

Gardiner, P., Graham, R., Legedza, A. T., Ahn, A. C., Eisenberg, D. M., & Phillips, R. S. (2007). Factors associated with herbal therapy use by adults in the United States. *Alternative Therapies Health Medicine, 13*(2), 22–29.

Hung, S. K., & Ernst, E. (2010). Herbal medicine: An overview of the literature from three decades. *Journal of Dietary Supplements, 7*(3), 217–226. doi:10.3109/19390211.2010.487818

Izzo, A., & Edzard, E. (2009). Interactions between herbal medicines and prescribed drugs: An updated systematic review. *Drugs, 69*(13), 1777–1798. doi:10.2165/11317010-000000000-00000

Myles, D. (2007). Saving wild ginseng, goldenseal, and other native plants from mountain top removal. *HerbalGram, 73*(50).

Picciano, M. F., & McGuire, M. K. (2009). Use of dietary supplements by pregnant and lactating women in North America. *The American Journal of Clinical Nutrition, 89*(2), 6635–6675. doi:10.3945/ajcn.2008.26811B

White House Commission on Complementary and Alternative Medicine Policy. (2002). *Final report.* Retrieved from http://govinfo.library.unt.edu/whccamp

Answers to NCLEX-RN® Review

1 Answer: 1 Rationale: Although CAM medications have been used for thousands of years, many of these substances lack adequate scientific clinical studies to verify their effectiveness. Most health care providers are hesitant to recommend a substance that has questionable effectiveness. Options 2, 3, and 4 are incorrect. CAM has a rich history of use over thousands of years in treating certain diseases and conditions. To imply that all alternative therapies are nothing more than fable is incorrect. There is no evidence that response to CAM therapies is related to the placebo effect. In many cases the CAM therapy may be less expensive than prescription medications. Cognitive Level: Applying; Client Need: Safe and Effective Care Environment; Nursing Process: Implementation

2 Answer: 3 Rationale: It is best to advise the client to take small amounts of a new supplement to determine any initial intolerance. Options 1, 2, and 4 are incorrect. Doubling dosages can be extremely dangerous and is seldom, if ever, advisable. There is no indication that fluid intake should be reduced with echinacea. Allergic reactions are possible with natural supplements. Clients should be taught to read the label carefully and avoid any supplement that contains any known allergy-provoking substances. Cognitive Level: Applying; Client Need: Physiological Integrity; Nursing Process: Implementation

3 Answer: 1 Rationale: Older adults with hepatic disease are at higher risk of developing serious drug reactions when taking herbal supplements. Options 2, 3, and 4 are incorrect. Clients with cardiac irregularities, pneumonia, or acne may require traditional medications and should be encouraged to consult their health care provider. If the client prefers to use CAM, this can also be discussed with the provider at the time of the health care visit. Cognitive Level: Applying; Client Need: Physiological Integrity; Nursing Process: Evaluation

4 Answer: 1, 2, 3, 5 Rationale: Herbal supplements can be found in almost every supermarket, pharmacy, and health food store. Due to aggressive marketing, herbal supplements are also extremely popular. Most herbal supplements are less expensive than prescribed medications and are therefore more appealing to individuals for whom cost is a critical issue. Older clients may also seek therapeutic alternatives for chronic health conditions. Option 4 is incorrect. Natural substances are not necessarily safer than synthetic products and do not undergo the same rigorous testing as synthetic products. Cognitive Level: Applying; Client Need: Safe and Effective Care Environment; Nursing Process: Implementation

5 Answer: 1 Rationale: The USP verified dietary supplement mark is awarded to dietary supplements that pass verification processes. The mark represents that USP has tested the supplement to verify that the label accurately reflects the product in the bottle and that the supplement does not contain harmful levels of contaminants. Options 2, 3, and 4 are incorrect. A DEA number is assigned to a health care provider and allows them to write prescriptions for controlled substances such as a narcotic. The FDA does not control herbal supplements and this code does not exist. U.S. Customs is not responsible for ensuring that herbal supplements are pure. Cognitive Level: Applying; Client Need: Safe and Effective Care Environment; Nursing Process: Implementation

6 Answer: 4 Rationale: Changes in liver or kidney function in the older adult may lead to changes in metabolism or excretion for herbal as well as synthetic medications. Options 1, 2, and 3 are incorrect. Older adults are no more likely to have difficulty taking herbal medications or to spend more money on these products than the younger adult population. These difficulties are client specific at any age. Due to aggressive marketing campaigns by the herbal and dietary supplement industry, all age groups are as likely to hold unrealistic expectations for herbal products. Cognitive Level: Applying; Client Need: Physiological Integrity; Nursing Process: Evaluation

Pharmacotherapy of Severe Pain and Migraines

From Chapter 29 of *Pharmacology: Connections to Nursing Practice*, Second Edition. Michael Patrick Adams, Carol Quam Urban. Copyright © 2013 by Pearson Education, Inc. All rights reserved.

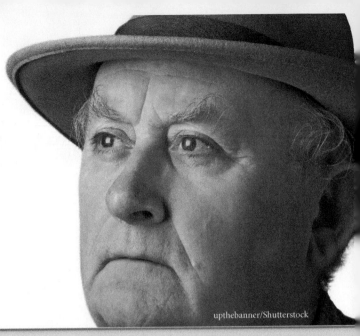

"I'm having urological surgery tomorrow and I am worried about pain. I've taken pain medicine daily for years because of chronic pain from back problems and numerous back surgeries. Will I experience severe pain after this procedure?"

Patient "Larry Smith"

Pharmacotherapy of Severe Pain and Migraines

Learning Outcomes

After reading this chapter, the student should be able to:

1. Identify changes that have occurred in pain management during the past two decades.
2. Differentiate the types and classifications of pain.
3. Refute the common pain myths, using objective evidence.
4. Explain the phases of pain physiology: transduction, transmission, perception, and modulation.
5. Describe the role of nonpharmacologic therapies in pain management.
6. Describe the nursing assessment of pain.
7. Identify the classes of drugs used for minor, moderate, and severe pain.
8. Compare and contrast the actions of opioid agonists, mixed opioid agonists-antagonists, and opioid antagonists.
9. Describe the advantages of combining opioid, nonopioid, and adjuvant analgesics in the treatment of pain.
10. Compare and contrast the actions and adverse effects of the opioids and nonopioids for analgesia.
11. For each of the classes shown in the chapter outline, identify the prototype and representative drugs and explain the mechanism(s) of drug action, primary indications, contraindications, significant drug interactions, pregnancy category, and important adverse effects.
12. Explain the role of opioid antagonists in the diagnosis and treatment of acute opioid toxicity.
13. Compare the types of drugs used for preventing migraines to those for terminating migraines.
14. Apply the nursing process to care for patients receiving pharmacotherapy for pain.

Chapter Outline

General Principles
of Pain Management

Pharmacotherapy of Acute
and Chronic Pain

Opioid Analgesics

PROTOTYPE **Morphine Sulfate (Astramorph PF, Duramorph RF, Roxanol, Others)**

Mixed Agonist-Antagonist Opioids

Nonopioid Analgesics

Nonsteroidal Anti-Inflammatory Drugs (NSAIDs) and Acetaminophen

Centrally Acting Analgesics

PROTOTYPE **Tramadol (Ultram)**

Adjuvant Analgesics

Pharmacotherapy
with Opioid Antagonists

PROTOTYPE **Naloxone (Narcan)**

Pharmacotherapy of Migraines

PROTOTYPE **Sumatriptan (Imitrex)**

Pain is a subjective experience that has both physiological and emotional components. Usually associated with trauma or disease, pain may be viewed as a natural defense mechanism that helps people avoid potentially damaging situations and encourages them to seek medical help. Pain medications are some of the most frequently prescribed drugs in medicine. This chapter examines the drug classes used in pain management and for the pharmacotherapy of migraines.

General Principles of Pain Management

1 Strategies for pain management have changed during the past two decades.

In recent years health care professionals have come to realize that accurate pain assessment and treatment are essential for quality patient care. To this end, the American Pain Society coined the phrase "Pain: The Fifth Vital Sign" to elevate the awareness of pain treatment among health care providers. Many health care agencies now include assessment of pain as part of the process of monitoring vital signs.

The perception of pain can clearly be influenced by comorbid conditions such as anxiety, fatigue, and depression. For example, knowing that health care providers and caregivers are attentive and actively engaged in pain management may lower patients' anxiety, thus reducing pain perception and increasing pain tolerance. Furthermore, culture and ethnicity can also influence pain perception and expression. Listening, showing respect, and allowing patients to help develop and choose treatment options consistent with their beliefs and customs are the most culturally sensitive approaches to attain optimum pain relief.

Beginning in the early 1990s, groups such as the American Pain Society established guidelines for the management of pain in different populations. The Agency for Healthcare Research and Quality of the United States Department of Health and Human Services maintains the *Clinical Guideline Clearinghouse*, that serves as a database of evidence-based practice guidelines. The *Clearinghouse* contains many guidelines for pain management established by different professional groups. These guidelines are updated regularly as research determines optimum strategies for pain management.

An important and effective advance in pain management was the adoption of the guidelines on pain published by The Joint Commission (formerly the Joint Commission on Accreditation of Healthcare Organizations [JCAHO] in 2001). Its standards required appropriate assessment and management of pain as an integral component of health care, essentially "guaranteeing" every patient the right to effective pain management. As a result of the guidelines, most institutions have implemented the practice of assessing every patient's pain from the time of admission, ensuring staff competency regarding pain management, and educating patients and their families about pain.

2 Pain is classified by its duration and its source.

The purpose of classifying pain is to guide appropriate treatment rationales based on the type of pain reported by the patient. A simple classification is to group types of pain as either acute or chronic. Acute pain has an abrupt onset but brief duration; it subsides as healing takes place or the pain stimulus ceases. Examples of acute pain include that associated with surgical incisions, labor and delivery, sprained joints, or myocardial infarction (MI). Although it may be severe, acute pain is often self-limiting; high doses of pain medication may be necessary, but therapy is usually of short duration. There is little risk of chronic drug adverse effects or dependence because of the relatively limited length of the treatment period.

Chronic pain persists longer than 6 months, can interfere with daily activities, and is sometimes associated with feelings of helplessness or hopelessness. Chronic pain can be further classified as either nonmalignant or malignant (cancer) pain. Chronic nonmalignant pain is not life threatening and usually responds favorably to a consistent, stable dose of pain medication as part of a treatment regimen. The most common example is low back pain. Cancer pain ends with control of the disease or death. Although the majority of patients with cancer experience pain during the advanced stages of the disease, 90% of the cancer pain can be controlled with oral (PO) drugs, using around-the-clock dosing, with prn doses or augmentation as needed for breakthrough pain.

PharmFACT

Low Back Pain in America

- Low back pain (LBP) is the second most common cause of disability in adults.
- More than 80% of the population will experience LBP during their lifetime. Of those who experience LBP, 85% will have recurring episodes.
- LBP costs an estimated $100 billion to $200 billion each year, two-thirds of which is due to lost wages and productivity (Freburger et al., 2009).

Pain can also be classified as to its source: nociceptors or neuropathic. **Nociceptors** are the sensory nerve receptors strategically located throughout the body that initiate pain transmission when stimulated. For example, a needlestick will activate pain receptors in the finger, producing **nociceptor pain**. This type of pain may be further subdivided into somatic pain, which produces sharp, localized sensations usually experienced in muscles and joints, or visceral pain, which is described as a generalized dull, throbbing, or aching pain usually located in internal organs. Nociceptor pain

addiction

adjuvant analgesics

analgesics

auras

endorphins

gate control theory

kappa receptors

migraine

mu receptors

narcotic

neuropathic pain

nociceptor pain

nociceptors

nonopioid analgesics

opiates

opioid

opium

tension headache

CONNECTIONS

Evidence-Based Practice   Opioids for Chronic Noncancer Pain Management

Clinical Question

Are opioids appropriate for the management of chronic noncancer pain?

Evidence

Opioids for acute pain and pain associated with cancer are accepted treatments but the use of chronic opioid therapy (COT) for chronic noncancer pain (CNCP) is controversial. Many diseases lead to chronic pain including osteoarthritis, fibromyalgia, and back pain. In addition, current drug therapy and other nondrug treatments result in large health care costs. Any decisions to use COT must be balanced against the very real concerns of abuse, diversion (use for recreational purposes, especially by persons not prescribed the drug), and addiction. The American Pain Society and American Academy of Pain Management sought to develop recommendations for the use of opioids for pain management in chronic noncancer pain.

After systematic review of over 8,000 studies by Chou et al. (2009), recommendations were established for the use of COT for CNCP, including:

- A thorough health history should be conducted including assessment of risk for substance abuse or addiction. The impact of pain on the patient's quality of life should be considered, and benefits and risks of COT should be evaluated.
- Patients should discuss benefits and risks of COT with their provider, sign an informed consent document, and a written plan of care should be established with the patient.
- A trial of opioids over several weeks to months should be tried to determine whether COT is appropriate. Drug type and dosing

(short versus long-acting opioids, around-the-clock versus as-needed dosing) may be evaluated during this period. Adverse effects or substance abuse or diversion during this period should be evaluated before continuing the COT plan of care.

- Patients on COT require frequent ongoing assessments, including for therapeutic and adverse effects as well as substance abuse, addiction, or diversion. Escalating doses and high-dose opioid use may suggest the need to consider options such as opioid rotation to different drugs.
- Any patient exhibiting substance abuse behaviors or intolerable adverse effects should be tapered off COT.
- Nondrug therapies such as cognitive–behavioral therapy should be considered along with COT.

Implications

Opioid therapy for chronic noncancer pain is an effective method for pain relief for select patients, but a thorough health history, continuous monitoring, and a consideration of nondrug therapies to supplement the opioid therapy should be part of the drug regimen.

Critical Thinking Question

Select two of the preceding recommendations and develop strategies that the nurse can incorporate in the care of a patient with chronic noncancer pain.

See Answers to Critical Thinking Questions on student resource website.

---

responds quite well to **analgesics**, which are medications that relieve pain.

In contrast, **neuropathic pain** is caused by injury or irritation to nerve tissue and typically is described as burning, shooting, or numbing pain. The cause of neuropathic pain may be difficult to determine. Analgesic treatment of neuropathic pain is often unsuccessful or high doses may be required. Neuropathic pain responds best to adjuvant analgesics such as antiseizure drugs and antidepressants (see Section 12).

3 Health care providers and patients sometimes hold myths about pain that impede optimum pain management.

Commonly held but untrue beliefs by both patients and health care providers may interfere with effective pain management. For example, health care providers may undertreat pain because of common misconceptions about pain. Furthermore, patients may not report their pain accurately or may refuse pain medications because of similar misconceptions.

A pervasive myth is that health care professionals can successfully recognize pain, independent of the patient's report. The nurse must understand that patients are the authorities on their own pain. Pain is whatever the patient says it is, existing whenever the patient says it does. Patient self-report of pain is sufficient for a nursing diagnosis of pain.

A closely related myth is that a person in pain must look and act like he or she is in pain. Some patients do not show or report pain accurately because they feel it is a sign of weakness. In addition, vital signs are sometimes unreliable indicators of

pain. Although they may be elevated during the initial experience of acute pain owing to sympathetic arousal, vital signs return to normal as the body adapts. A related misconception is the belief that if a person is able to sleep, he or she must not be experiencing much pain. Although it is certainly true that pain can interfere with sleep quality and quantity, social withdrawal and excessive sleep may be indicators of coping mechanisms for some people with severe or chronic pain.

Both patients and health care providers may share the myth that the use of potent analgesics inevitably leads to addiction. **Addiction** is the continued use of a substance despite serious health and social consequences. The incidence of addiction to opioids, which are used in the treatment of severe pain, is less than 1% in patients with no previous history of drug abuse. Related to this myth is the belief that patients experiencing chronic pain overreport pain because they are addicted to opioids.

Another contradictory myth is the belief that the more pain a person experiences, the more he or she is likely to tolerate it. In fact, the opposite is more likely to occur. Unrelieved pain creates anxiety and fatigue, both of which increase pain perception and decrease tolerance. A related myth is that there is no physiological basis for the moderating effects of emotions of pain perception.

4 Pain transmission processes allow multiple targets for pharmacologic intervention.

Pain physiology has four phases: transduction, transmission, perception, and modulation. These phases are illustrated in Figure 1.

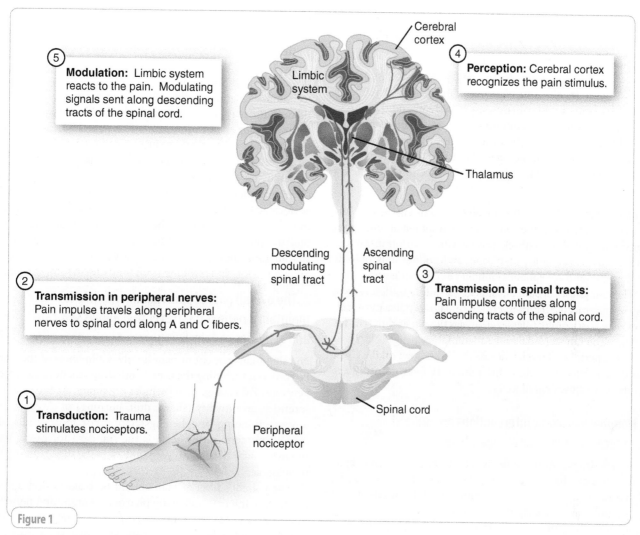

Figure 1

Phases of pain physiology.

Pain transduction: Pain transduction begins when nociceptor nerve endings in the peripheral nervous system are stimulated. This occurs when local tissue injury causes the release of chemical mediators of inflammation, including prostaglandins, leukotrienes, histamine, bradykinin, and substance P. These substances sensitize peripheral nociceptors, making them easier to activate.

Pain transmission: The nerve impulse signaling the pain travels from the nociceptor to the spinal cord along two types of sensory neurons called A and C fibers. A fibers are wrapped in myelin, a lipid substance that speeds nerve transmission, and carry signals for intense, well-defined pain. On the other hand, C fibers are unmyelinated and thus carry information more slowly and conduct poorly localized pain, which is often perceived as burning or a dull ache.

A fibers have three subtypes: alpha (α), beta (β), and delta (Δ). Aα fibers have the fastest transmission and respond to touch and pressure on muscle; Aβ fibers are slower and respond to touch and pressure on skin. Finally, AΔ fibers are the slowest of the A fibers and respond to tissue injury, producing the sensation of sharp pain.

The sensory nerve fibers enter the dorsal horn of the spinal cord and have adjacent synapses in an area called the substantia gelatinosa. The **gate control theory** proposes a gating mechanism for the transmission of pain in the spinal cord. Signals from faster Aα or Aβ fibers reach the spinal cord and close the gate before those of C fibers reach the region (or gate), in effect blocking the transmission of these types of pain impulses. The gate control theory, proposed in 1965, has withstood the test of time and has been found to be more complex than originally proposed. The "gates" can also be closed when flooded with nonnociceptor impulses. Gate control explains the effectiveness of massage, transcutaneous electrical nerve stimulation, and possibly acupuncture in reducing pain.

Once a pain impulse reaches the spinal cord, neurotransmitters are responsible for passing the message along to the next neuron. At the spinal cord, glutamate is the neurotransmitter for A fibers, whereas both glutamate and substance P are neurotransmitters for C fibers. Impulse transmission from the spinal cord to the brain is moderated by both excitatory and inhibitory neurotransmitters. The activity of substance P may be affected by other neurotransmitters released from neurons in the central nervous system (CNS). One group of neurotransmitters functions as endogenous opioids, or natural pain modifiers; these include **endorphins** and enkephalins.

Pain perception: Perception, the conscious experience of pain, occurs in the brain. Numerous cortical structures and pathways are involved in perception, including the reticular activating system, the somatosensory system, and the limbic system. When the pain impulse reaches the brain, it may respond to the sensation with a wide variety of possible actions, ranging from signaling the skeletal muscles to jerk away from a sharp object to mental depression in those experiencing chronic pain.

Pain modulation: Modulation involves descending nervous impulses traveling down the spinal cord that inhibit afferent pain transmission via a feedback mechanism. Neurotransmitters such as serotonin, norepinephrine, and endogenous opioids (endorphins and enkephalins) inhibit pain transmission.

The four phases of pain physiology allow for multiple targets for the pharmacologic intervention of pain impulse transmission. The two primary classes of analgesics act at different locations: The nonsteroidal anti-inflammatory drugs (NSAIDs) act at the peripheral level, whereas the opioids act on the CNS. Drugs that affect or mimic the inhibitory neurotransmitters are used as adjuvant analgesics.

5 Nonpharmacologic interventions are utilized to reduce and augment analgesic use.

Although drugs are quite effective at relieving pain in most patients, they can have significant adverse effects. For example, high doses of aspirin cause gastrointestinal (GI) bleeding, and the opioids can cause significant drowsiness and respiratory depression. Nonpharmacologic techniques may be used to attain adequate pain relief in place of drugs, or they may serve as adjuncts to analgesics. When used concurrently with medication, nonpharmacologic techniques may allow for improved comfort, lower doses, and the potential for fewer drug-related adverse events. Nondrug interventions should routinely be considered in the nursing plan of care for patients with pain. Some complementary and alternative therapies (CATs) used for reducing pain include the following:

- Acupressure and acupuncture
- Application of cold or heat
- Biofeedback therapy
- Distraction, including art or music therapy, or laughter
- Electrical nerve stimulation
- Hypnosis
- Massage
- Meditation
- Physical therapy
- Yoga.

Some of these interventions are part of standard nursing practice and can be performed by nurses; for example, massage, and application of heat and cold packs. Other CATs such as therapeutic touch, Reiki, acupressure or acupuncture require additional training. Some of these techniques appear to act by increasing endogenous endorphin release. Others use gate control as the probable physiological mechanism to reduce the perception of pain.

Patients with intractable cancer pain require more invasive techniques because rapidly growing tumors often press on vital tissues and nerves. Furthermore, chemotherapy and surgical treatments for cancer can cause severe pain. Radiation therapy may provide pain relief by shrinking solid tumors that may be pressing on nerves. Surgery may be used to reduce pain by removing part of or the entire tumor. Injection of alcohol or another neurotoxic substance into neurons is occasionally performed to cause nerve blocks. Nerve blocks irreversibly stop impulse transmission along the treated nerves and have the potential to provide total pain relief. Injection of local anesthetics or steroid hormones as nerve blocks can provide relief for months and is used for pain resulting from pressure on spinal nerves.

6 The overall goal of pain management is to maintain a patient pain level that allows self-care and activities of daily living.

Nursing management of pain involves all phases of the nursing process, including the use of both drug and nondrug interventions. Pain assessment includes documenting the location, intensity, and quality (sharp, dull, burning) of the pain and any precipitating or relieving factors. For most adults, the 0-to-10 numeric rating scale is the standard for rating pain intensity, with 0 being no pain and 10 being the greatest pain imaginable.

The patient's level of pain should be reassessed at appropriate time intervals following pharmacotherapy and nondrug interventions. The pain rating is used as a reference point, initially as a baseline level of pain and later as an indicator of effectiveness as to how well the treatment is achieving the patient's goals. Assessment needs to include the patient's ability to perform activities of daily living (ADLs) such as eating, sleeping, self-care, and ambulation—especially for chronic pain.

CONNECTIONS

Lifespan Considerations
Pain Assessment in the Very Young

According to Voepel-Lewis, Zanotti, Danmeyer, and Merkel (2010), behavioral rating scales such as the FLACC scale have been used with children as young as 3 months to 7 years of age. Developed by the University of Michigan Health System, FLACC stands for the five categories assessed: face, legs, activity, cry, and consolability. Each category is scored 0 to 2 and then added to get a 0-to-10 rating. For example, an infant with a pain rating of 0 would have no particular facial expression (F), legs relaxed (L), be lying quietly (A), without crying (C), and relaxed (C). On the other extreme, a rating of 10 would be seen as an infant crying steadily, with a rigid body and drawn up or kicking legs, clenched jaw or quivering chin, and who is difficult to console or comfort. The scale has undergone extensive testing for construct validity and reliability over the years since it was developed, and is now used for assessing pain in nonverbal patients of all ages.

Goals and principles of pain management:

The immediate goal of pain management is to reduce pain to a level that allows the patient to perform reasonable ADLs. An acceptable level of pain is one that enables the patient to sleep, eat, and perform other required or desired physical activities. For acute pain the primary goal is to reduce pain during the healing process until the source of the pain is eliminated. For chronic pain the long-term goal is to reduce pain to a level that allows for self-care and ADLs. The patient should understand that the total elimination of chronic pain may not be a realistic goal, or that it may require a long period of treatment. Several key principles underlie the nursing management of pain:

- The patient should be considered the expert on his or her own pain; the nurse should always believe the patient's self-assessment of pain.

- Pain management is a patient right and should be based on the patient's goals. The patient should be screened for pain during an initial assessment and periodically thereafter. If pain cannot be effectively managed, then a pain management specialist should be consulted.

- Nondrug interventions should routinely be utilized in pain management. A combination of therapies is optimum because different modalities work by different mechanisms, thus improving the effectiveness of pain management.

- Dosing should be individualized and titrated to produce the desired effect.

- Adverse effects should be actively and proactively managed.

- Preventive around-the-clock dosing for moderate to severe pain should be implemented. It is much easier to maintain a comfort level than to eliminate existing or escalating pain. A fixed dosing schedule avoids the unnecessary discomfort and anxiety sometimes associated with prn dosing.

Pharmacologic therapies:

Dozens of over-the-counter (OTC) and prescription pain medications are available, and the selection of a specific medication depends on many factors. Foremost is the severity of the pain. The drug selected must be capable of providing adequate pain relief. Secondarily, the choice of analgesic depends on potential adverse events and drug interactions and contraindications. A key point is that every analgesic, even an OTC pain reliever, has the potential to cause serious adverse effects in susceptible patients. This reinforces the need to utilize nonpharmacologic therapies for pain relief whenever possible.

The two broad categories of analgesics are the opioids and nonopioids. A third category of drugs for the management of pain is the adjuvant analgesics. The adjuvant analgesics have no pain relief activity when used alone but they are able to enhance the analgesic action of opioids and nonopioids.

The drug class of choice for severe pain is the opioids. Minor to moderate pain is treated with nonopioids such as NSAIDs, centrally acting agents, or acetaminophen. There are dozens of opioids and NSAIDs to choose from and it is difficult for beginning students, and even experienced health care providers, to learn the subtle differences of drugs within each class. Although the large number of analgesics appears overwhelming, many of them are quite similar and prescribers most often use only a few drugs in each class. The various drugs used for analgesia and the levels at which they act are shown in Pharmacotherapy Illustrated 1.

The pharmacologic management of acute and chronic pain is based on the analgesic ladder proposed by the World Health Organization and shown in Figure 2. Pain ratings of less than 4 are treated with nonopioid analgesics, CATs, or a combination of the two. When pain ratings become moderate (4 to 6), PO opioids are added to the baseline treatment. When pain is severe (7 to 10), parenteral opioids are used. If chronic pain has neuropathic qualities, adjuvant analgesics are added.

Opioid and nonopioid combinations:

It is common practice to use opioid and nonopioid analgesics concurrently in the pharmacotherapy of pain. For convenience, these combinations are available as fixed-dose tablets or capsules. The two classes of analgesics work synergistically to relieve pain, and the dose of opioid can be kept small to avoid dependence and opioid-related adverse effects. Use of these combinations in chronic pain management has a dose ceiling due to the toxicities of the nonopioid analgesic. For example, patients taking a combination product containing acetaminophen need to have their liver enzyme levels monitored regularly and take care not to exceed the maximum daily dosages for acetaminophen. Common combination analgesics include:

- Endocet (oxycodone HCl, 5–10 mg; acetaminophen, 325–650 mg)
- Norco (hydrocodone, 5–10 mg; acetaminophen, 325 mg)
- Percocet (oxycodone HCl, 2.5–10 mg; acetaminophen, 325–650 mg)
- Percodan (oxycodone HCl, 4.8355 mg; aspirin, 325 mg)
- Vicodin or Lortab (hydrocodone, 5 mg; acetaminophen, 500 mg)
- Vicodin HP (hydrocodone, 10 mg; acetaminophen, 660 mg)

Patient-controlled analgesia:

Patient-controlled analgesia (PCA) is a method of drug delivery that uses an infusion pump to deliver a prescribed amount of opioid by patient self-administration. By pressing a button, the patient can self-administer the opioid, thus relieving the anxiety of waiting for a prn drug administration.

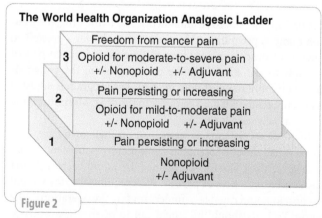

The World Health Organization Analgesic Ladder

Figure 2

The World Health Organization analgesic ladder.
Source: From *Cancer Pain Relief*, 2nd ed., by World Health Organization, 1996, Geneva: Author. Copyright © World Health Organization (WHO), 2006. All rights reserved.

PHARMACOTHERAPY ILLUSTRATED

Sites of Analgesic Action

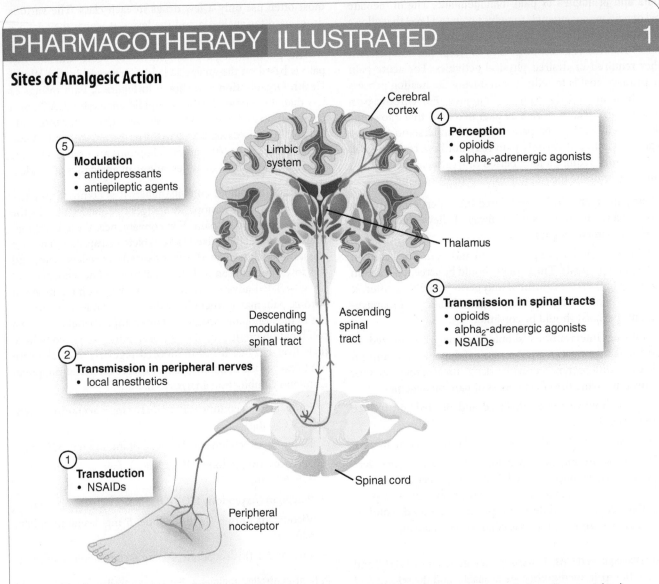

⑤ Modulation
- antidepressants
- antiepileptic agents

④ Perception
- opioids
- alpha$_2$-adrenergic agonists

Cerebral cortex

Limbic system

Thalamus

③ Transmission in spinal tracts
- opioids
- alpha$_2$-adrenergic agonists
- NSAIDs

Descending modulating spinal tract

Ascending spinal tract

② Transmission in peripheral nerves
- local anesthetics

① Transduction
- NSAIDs

Spinal cord

Peripheral nociceptor

(1) Trauma stimulates nociceptors, which generate a pain signal that is blocked by NSAIDs. (2) The pain impulse travels along afferent peripheral nerves to the spinal cord and is blocked by local anesthetics. (3) The pain impulse continues along ascending tracts of the spinal cord and is blocked by NSAIDs, opioids, and alpha$_2$ agonists. (4) The cerebral cortex perceives pain that is blocked by opioids and alpha$_2$ agonists. (5) The limbic system sends modulating impulses along descending tracts of the spinal cord that are blocked by antiepileptic and antidepressant drugs.

The patient does not have unlimited access to the drug; the infusion pump is programmed by the nurse to deliver a prescribed amount of drug over a designated time period. If the patient attempts to self-administer the drug too often, the patient is locked out until the next dose interval. The program is adjusted depending on the patient's response to the drug. Morphine is the opioid usually used for PCA.

PCA allows patients to participate in their own care. Frequent, small doses of analgesics give a more consistent serum drug level than would be obtained by administering larger doses three to four times per day. PCA requires that the patient be conscious and capable of understanding the operation of the pump. Patients should be taught not to be overly concerned about activating the pump because the program is set to prevent the possibility of overdose. Family members or visitors should not use the device to give the patient more medication,

but should consult with the nurse or health care provider if they feel that the patient's pain is not relieved.

Pharmacotherapy of Acute and Chronic Pain

7 Opioid analgesics exert their effects by interacting with specific receptors in the central nervous system.

Opium is one of the oldest known natural remedies; it has been used to relieve pain for thousands of years. Extracted from the unripe seeds of the poppy plant, *Papaver somniferum*, **opium** is a milky substance that contains over 20 different chemicals having pharmacologic activity. Opium contains 9% to 14% morphine and 0.8% to 2.5% codeine. Natural substances obtained from opium (such as morphine and codeine) are called **opiates**.

In the late 1800s, scientists began to create synthetic and semisynthetic substances with morphine-like properties. There are now over a dozen different synthetic drugs with morphine-like activity. **Opioid** is a general term referring to any of these substances, natural or synthetic, and is often used interchangeably with the term *opiate*.

Pharmacotherapy with opioids is predominantly used to relieve moderate to severe pain. With proper dosing, opioids can relieve any degree of pain; they are most effective in treating constant, dull types of pain. In large quantities opioids produce euphoria and severe CNS depression that can lead to stupor, coma, or death. When used for prolonged periods at high doses, opioids cause physical and psychological dependence.

Narcotic is another term commonly used to describe morphine-like drugs that produce analgesia and CNS depression. In clinical practice, a narcotic analgesic is the same as an opioid, and the terms may be used interchangeably. In the context of law enforcement, however, the term *narcotic* is often used to describe a much broader range of abused illegal drugs such as hallucinogens, cocaine, amphetamines, and marijuana.

Opioids exert their actions by interacting with at least six types of receptors in the CNS; mu, kappa, and delta are the three major receptor types. From the perspective of pain management, the **mu** and **kappa receptors** are the most important, as shown in Figure 3. Activation of the mu receptor is responsible for the analgesic properties of the opioids as well as some of the adverse effects such as respiratory depression and physical dependence. Drugs that activate opioid receptors are called opioid agonists; those that block these receptors are called opioid antagonists. Because there are multiple opioid receptors, three general types of drug–receptor interactions are possible:

- **Opioid agonist.** Drugs that activate both mu and kappa receptors; for example, morphine and codeine (see Section 8)
- **Mixed opioid agonist-antagonist.** Drugs that occupy one receptor and block (or have no effect) on the other; for example, pentazocine (Talwin), butorphanol (Stadol), and buprenorphine (Buprenex) (see Section 9)
- **Opioid antagonist.** Drugs that block both mu and kappa receptors; for example, naloxone (Narcan) (see Section 13)

The types of agonist actions produced by activating the mu and kappa receptors are shown in Table 1. Analgesia is obviously the desired response in pain management. The other responses constitute adverse effects of opioid therapy and must be assessed, prevented, or managed as part of the plan of care for a patient receiving opioid therapy (see Nursing Practice Application for Patients Receiving Opioid Analgesic Therapy.

Opioids do not lower the threshold for pain at the nociceptors and they do not slow or block the transmission of the pain impulse. It is the perception and emotional response to pain that is altered. Essentially the patient knows that the pain still exists, but it does not cause concern or anxiety.

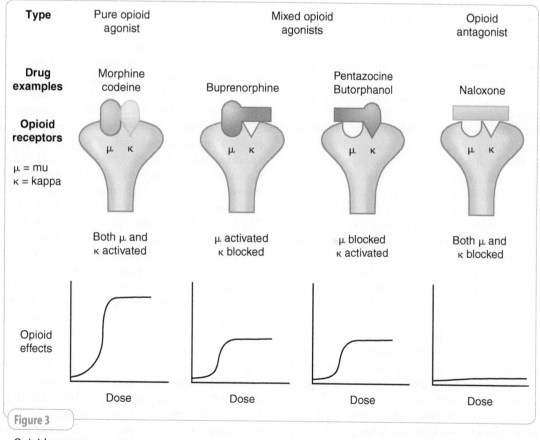

Figure 3

Opioid receptors.

TABLE 1 Responses Produced by Activation of Specific Opioid Receptors

Response	Mu Receptor	Kappa Receptor
Analgesia	Yes	Yes
Decreased GI motility	Yes	Yes
Euphoria	Yes	No
Miosis	No	Yes
Physical dependence	Yes	No
Respiratory depression	Yes	No
Sedation	Yes	Yes

8 Opioids are the drugs of choice for moderate to severe pain that cannot be controlled with other classes of analgesics.

Over 20 different opioids are available as medications. This large group is split into subclasses by similarities in their chemical structures, mechanisms of action, and effectiveness. Each classification is useful in explaining some of the similarities and differences among the opioids. The most basic classification is by effectiveness, which places opioids into the two basic categories of strong or moderate analgesic activity. The opioids are listed in Table 2. Some opioids that have very short durations of action are used primarily as anesthesia adjuncts.

Opioids produce many important physiological actions in addition to analgesia. They are effective at suppressing the cough reflex and at slowing the motility of the GI tract in patients with severe diarrhea. Opioids are powerful CNS depressants and can cause sedation, which may be considered a therapeutic effect or an adverse effect, depending on the patient's disease state. Some patients experience euphoria and intense relaxation, which are reasons why these drugs are frequently abused.

Opioids have the potential to produce many serious adverse effects, including respiratory depression, sedation, nausea, vomiting, and constipation. Table 2 compares the major adverse effect potentials of the individual opioids.

Management of opioid adverse effects is summarized in Table 3. Through activation of primarily the mu receptors, opioids can cause profound respiratory depression, which is the most serious adverse effect of drugs in this class. Respiratory depression is most problematic during the initial period of drug administration and with patients who have not previously taken these drugs (opiate naïve). Patients at greatest risk include those with preexisting respiratory impairment or those concurrently taking other respiratory depressant drugs. A current medication history is very important, especially alcohol use and other CNS depressants, because these drugs will cause additive respiratory depression and sedation. Tolerance to respiratory depression usually occurs within 48 to 72 hours of initiation of therapy.

Respirations should be monitored before initiating therapy and regularly throughout opioid pharmacotherapy. The drugs should be withheld if respirations fall below 12 per minute. Narcotic antagonists such as naloxone (Narcan) should be readily available if respirations fall below 10 per minute (see Section 13). If opioids are administered by continuous epidural or intravenous (IV) routes, interventions should be taken to reduce the risk of respiratory depression. These include frequent monitoring of vital signs, level of consciousness (LOC), and pain rating as well as proper body positioning. Airway equipment and narcotic antagonists are usually kept at the bedside.

Opioids can cause orthostatic hypotension by inhibiting the baroreceptor reflex and by causing peripheral vasodilation. Dizziness and fainting are possible; assistance may therefore be needed with ambulation. Hydromorphone and meperidine are especially prone to causing hypotension. Patients with hypovolemia are more sensitive to this hypotensive effect; therefore, volume deficiencies should be corrected before initiating opioid therapy.

Increased intracranial pressure (ICP) is a severe adverse reaction that can occur as an indirect result of respiratory depression. When respiration is suppressed, the CO_2 content of the blood increases. The result is vasodilation of cerebral blood vessels and rising ICP. This is of particular concern in patients with conditions that might cause elevated ICP, such as those with head injury, intracranial bleeding, or brain tumors. Narcotic analgesics are usually contraindicated in these patients.

Opioids promote urinary retention by increasing the tone in the bladder sphincter and through suppression of stimuli that normally signal bladder fullness. If the patient has not voided within 6 hours, especially after surgery, insertion of a urinary catheter may be necessary. Patients prone to urinary hesitancy, such as those with benign prostatic hyperplasia, must be carefully monitored.

Constipation, nausea, and vomiting frequently occur during opioid administration. Constipation occurs because the drugs suppress intestinal peristalsis, increase the tone of the anal sphincter, and inhibit secretion of fluids into the intestine. Bowel function should be closely monitored, especially after surgery or with long-term use. The plan of care for these patients should include a bowel program to prevent or manage constipation. A baseline program would include increased dietary fiber, adequate fluid intake, and a stool softener such as docusate. More active interventions are implemented if the patient does not resume or maintain normal bowel elimination. The constipation-promoting effect of the opioids is used to advantage in the treatment of severe diarrhea (see Chapter 63).

Opioids directly stimulate the chemoreceptor trigger zone in the medulla to cause intense nausea and vomiting in certain patients. An antiemetic such as promethazine (Phenergan) or ondansetron (Zofran) may be indicated. Orders for prn antiemetics should be made available whenever parenteral opioids are used.

Prolonged use of opioids results in tolerance. Typically, tolerance is noted when patients report that the duration of analgesia is decreasing or admit to taking the drug more frequently as therapy progresses. Increasingly higher doses will be needed to produce the same degree of analgesia. Tolerance does not develop equally for all opioid actions. Whereas

TABLE 2 Selected Opioid Analgesic Comparison

Drug	Route and Dose (maximum dose where indicated)	Equianalgesic Dose*	Analgesic Duration	Respiratory Depression	Emesis	Constipation	Dependence Potential
Opioid Agonists with High Effectiveness							
fentanyl (Sublimaze)	IM: 0.05–0.1 mg Transdermal: 25–100 mcg every 72 h	0.1–0.2 mg 25 mcg/h	1–2 h 3 days	Y	Y	?	Y
hydromorphone (Dilaudid)	PO: 1–4 mg every 4–6 h Subcutaneous/IM/IV: 1–4 mg every 4–6 h	7.5 mg 1.5 mg	4–5 h	YY	Y	Y	YYY
levorphanol (Levo-Dromoran)	PO: 2–3 mg tid/qid Subcutaneous/IV: 1–2 mg every 6–8 h	4 mg 2 mg	4–8 h	YY	Y	YY	YY
meperidine (Demerol)	PO: 50–150 mg every 3–4 h IM: 50–100 mg every 3–4 h IV: 1–1.5 mg/kg every 3–4 h	300 mg 75 mg 50 mg	2–4 h	YY		Y	YYY
methadone (Dolophine)	PO: 20 mg every 6–8 h	20 mg	4–8 h	YY	Y	YY	Y
morphine	PO: 30 mg every 4 h Sustained release IM: 10 mg every 4 h IV: 2–10 mg every 2–4 h; 0.1–1 mg/mL continuous	30 mg 30 mg SR 10 mg 10 mg	4–5 h 8–12 h 4–5 h 4–5 h	YY	YY	YY	YYYY
oxymorphone (Opana)	Subcutaneous: 1.0–1.5 mg every 4–6 h Rectal: 1 suppository (5 mg) every 4–6 h PO (extended release): 5–20 mg bid	1 mg 10 1	3–6 h 36 h 12 h	YY	YY	YY	YYY
Opioids with Moderate Effectiveness							
codeine	PO: 15–60 mg qid IM: 15–30 mg every 4–6 h	200 mg 120 mg	4–6 h				
hydrocodone (Hycodan)	PO: 5–10 every 4–6 h	30 mg	4–6 h	Y		Y	Y
oxycodone (OxyContin)	PO: 5–10 mg qid Controlled release: 10–20 mg every 12 h	20 mg 20 mg	4–6 h 8–12 h	YY	YY	YY	YY
Opioids with Mixed Agonist-Antagonist Effects							
buprenorphine (Buprenex)	IM/IV: 0.3 mg every 6 h	0.3 mg	6 h	YY	Y		YY
butorphanol (Stadol)	IM: 1–4 mg every 3–4 h IV: 0.5–2 mg IV every 3–4 h	2 mg 1 mg	3–4 h	YYY	Y		YY
nalbuphine (Nubain)	Subcutaneous/IM/IV: 10–20 mg every 3–6 h	10 mg	3–6 h	Y	Y		YY
pentazocine (Talwin)	PO: 50–100 every 3–4 h Subcutaneous/IM: 30 mg every 3–4 h	25 mg 30 mg	4–6 h	Y	YY		YY

* Dose in milligrams that produces the same degree of analgesia as that produced by 10 mg of morphine.
Y = low incidence, YY = moderate incidence, YYY = high incidence, YYYY = highest incidence.

TABLE 3 Management of Opioid Adverse Effects

Adverse Effect	Management
Constipation	Assume it will occur and initiate preventive measures: Increase dietary fiber and fluid intake; use stool softeners and mild laxatives if needed.
Nausea	Usually transient. Antiemetics are administered, as needed.
Orthostatic hypotension	Assess blood pressure before ambulation; change positions slowly; assist with ambulation if needed.
Respiratory depression	Monitor respiratory status frequently—especially initially and with dosage increases. Avoid other CNS depressants that could have additive effects such as alcohol, antidepressants, and barbiturates. Use coughing, deep breathing, and incentive spirometry. If the patient is unresponsive and the respiratory rate is less than 12 breaths/min, administer naloxone per protocol.
Sedation	Common with initiation of therapy or during dosage increase. Tolerance develops in several days. Use safety precautions, especially with ambulation.
Urinary retention	Monitor for bladder distention. More common in elderly men. Tolerance usually develops with long-term dosing. Monitor; if receiving epidural administration, use an indwelling catheter.

tolerance to respiratory depression, sedation, and euphoria develop rapidly, tolerance never develops to the constipation or miosis effects. It should be remembered that as doses of opioids are increased to more effectively manage pain, the incidence of adverse effects will also increase.

All of the narcotic analgesics have the potential to cause physical and psychological dependence. Dependence is most likely to occur when high doses are taken for extended periods. Many health care providers and nurses are hesitant to administer the proper amount of opioid analgesics for fear of causing patient dependence or of producing serious adverse effects such as sedation or respiratory depression. Undermedication, however, results in patients not receiving adequate pain relief. When used according to accepted medical practice, patients can, and indeed should, receive the pain relief they need without fear of dependence or serious adverse effects.

Opioids are frequently abused for nonmedical purposes. The risk of abuse is especially high in patients with a history of substance abuse. Opioids are frequently diverted from medical sources (e.g., patients, pharmacies, hospitals), either stolen or sold for criminal intent. Opioids are even stolen from family members, especially the elderly. Illicit users may "doctor shop" and obtain opioids from different prescribers then sell the pills for profit.

Many patients who experience an adverse reaction to an opioid will report that they are allergic to these drugs. For example, patients who experience nausea, vomiting, or severe dizziness will often state they are allergic to narcotics. True allergic (Type I hypersensitivity) reactions to opioids, however, are actually rare. Although some of the opioids do indeed cause direct histamine release from mast cells, these types of idiosyncratic reactions do not result in the classic signs of anaphylaxis, thus they are not true allergic reactions. Morphine, codeine, and meperidine have the highest potential for nonimmune histamine release. When a real immune hypersensitivity reaction does occur, it may extend to other drugs in the opioid class.

Equianalgesic use in pain management: Table 2 includes a column labeled "Equianalgesic Dose." It is often necessary to change the route of a patient's pain medication or even the drug itself. One of the most frequently occurring examples that a nurse may encounter is the transition a patient makes from IV medications after surgery to PO analgesics prior to discharge. Using relative potency information (equivalent dose), the primary health care provider can determine the appropriate new dose. Following surgery, it is not unusual to have orders for a parenteral opioid for severe pain, an oral opioid for moderate pain, and a combination opioid and nonopioid for mild pain. The nurse can use these same equivalencies in choosing the drug and dose when a range of analgesic options is ordered.

CONNECTION Checkpoint 29.1

A common abbreviation for morphine sulfate is MS or MSO₄. Why should this abbreviation be avoided and what can you do to prevent this type of medication error? *See Answer to Connection Checkpoint 29.1 on student resource website.*

PROTOTYPE DRUG	Morphine Sulfate (Astramorph PF, Duramorph RF, Roxanol, Others)

Classification: **Therapeutic:** Narcotic analgesic
Pharmacologic: Opioid agonist

Therapeutic Effects and Uses: Morphine sulfate is the narcotic analgesic of choice for the management of most types of acute and severe chronic pain. Morphine is a drug of choice for relieving acute chest pain associated with MI. The drug was in use for thousands of years prior to its approval by the U.S. Food and Drug Administration (FDA) in 1939 and is still obtained from unripe seeds of the poppy plant.

In addition to relieving severe pain, morphine is used off-label to treat several other conditions. Its CNS depressant action may be used to provide preanesthetic sedation and to calm severely agitated patients. In patients who are terminally ill, its respiratory depressant action may be used to relieve the shortness of breath associated with end-stage cancer, heart failure, or pulmonary edema.

The advantages of morphine therapy, especially in the treatment of chronic cancer pain where dosing increases over time, are that morphine has no upper end dose limit, and that patients develop tolerance to all the adverse effects except constipation. Extended release tablets (MS Contin, Oramorph SR) or capsules (Avinza, Kadian) are available. Initiation of therapy is usually begun with shorter acting agents. Once the correct dose has been titrated, the patient may be switched to extended release formulations. In 2004, the FDA approved an extended release liposome injection (DepoDur), which is given by a single epidural injection for postsurgical pain.

Mechanism of Action: Morphine occupies mu and kappa receptor sites in the brain and dorsal horn of the spinal cord that alter the release of afferent neurotransmitters. The dominant effect alters the perception of and emotional response to pain, producing analgesia and euphoria. The drug mimics the actions of endogenous endorphins.

Pharmacokinetics:

Routes(s)	PO, IV, subcutaneous, intramuscular (IM), rectal, epidural, intrathecal
Absorption	PO variable, 30%; subcutaneous or IM may be erratic or delayed
Distribution	Widely distributed; crosses the placenta; is secreted in breast milk
Primary metabolism	Hepatic; significant first-pass metabolism
Primary excretion	Renal; 7–10% in bile and feces
Onset of action	PO: 30–60 min; IV: rapid; epidural: 15–30 min
Duration of action	PO: 4–7 h; IV: 4–5 h; epidural: 4–24 h

Adverse Effects: Morphine depresses the CNS, causing sedation, dizziness, anxiety, and a feeling of floating or disorientation. Tolerance often develops to these CNS effects after a few days of therapy. Hallucinations and seizures may occur at high doses. Morphine reduces the sensitivity of the respiratory center to CO_2, thus decreasing tidal volume and rate and producing respiratory depression. The resulting increase in CO_2 produces cerebral vasodilation and increases cerebrospinal fluid (CSF) pressure. Morphine stimulates the chemoreceptor trigger zone in the medulla, producing nausea and vomiting, which may require the administration of an antiemetic drug during the first few days of therapy. The drug delays digestion, increases smooth muscle tone in the intestinal tract, and slows peristalsis in the colon, leading to constipation. Morphine also causes spasm of the sphincter of Oddi, which can result in intense pain (biliary colic) and potential obstruction of bile flow. Urinary retention may occur due to increasing bladder sphincter tone. Peripheral vasodilation may cause orthostatic hypotension. Pruritus is more common when morphine is given by the IV and epidural routes and is not considered a sign of hypersensitivity in the absence of skin rash. **Black Box Warnings:** Morphine is a Schedule II controlled substance with a high potential for physical and psychological dependence. The extended release forms are prescribed for opioid-tolerant patients only and are not intended for prn use. The extended release forms should never be opened, chewed, dissolved, or crushed because this can lead to fatal overdose. Alcohol and products containing alcohol should never be consumed when taking Avinza.

Contraindications/Precautions: Morphine is contraindicated in patients with hypersensitivity to opioids. Premature infants are especially sensitive to the effects of morphine; thus the drug should not be used during pregnancy or during the delivery of premature infants. It should be used with caution in the elderly and in those with undiagnosed abdominal pain, hepatic or renal impairment, shock, CNS depression, head injury or increased ICP, chronic obstructive pulmonary disease (COPD), or other conditions with decreased respiratory reserve, including severe obesity. Mothers should wait 4 to 6 hours after a dose of morphine before breast-feeding; withdrawal symptoms have been noted in nursing infants whose mothers abruptly discontinue opioid use. Morphine should never be withdrawn abruptly because this will precipitate symptoms of acute opioid withdrawal. Discontinuation should be conducted gradually over several days.

Drug Interactions: When used with other CNS depressants, including alcohol, skeletal muscle relaxants, and monoamine oxidase inhibitors (MAOIs), increased sedation will result. Administration of an opioid antagonist such as naloxone will reverse the effects of morphine and may produce immediate withdrawal symptoms. Concurrent use with antidiarrheal drugs such as loperamide will cause additive constipation. **Herbal/Food:** Use of kava, valerian, or chamomile can increase CNS depression. St. John's wort may decrease the analgesic action of morphine.

Pregnancy: Category C.

Treatment of Overdose: Morphine overdose can cause coma and life-threatening respiratory depression and requires immediate treatment. Naloxone is a specific antidote for morphine intoxication (see Section 13).

Nursing Responsibilities: Key nursing implications for patients receiving morphine are included in the Nursing Practice Application for Patients Receiving Opioid Analgesic Therapy.

Lifespan and Diversity Considerations:

- Use special caution when administering morphine to the older adult who is at greater risk for hypotension, dizziness, drowsiness, and falls. Provide assistance with ambulation as needed.

- Monitor for constipation in the older adult and increase fluids and fiber in the diet. Stool softeners or other drugs may be required.

- Assess the older adult patient frequently for urinary retention, and report if difficulty with urination occurs.

Patient and Family Education:

- Inform the health care provider if pain increases above the selected goal rating or larger doses are required to maintain pain relief.

- Maintain adequate fluid intake to prevent constipation and to reduce the likelihood of hypotension related to fluid volume deficit.

Drugs Similar to Morphine Sulfate (Astramorph PF, Duramorph RF, Roxanol, Others)

Other opioids used for pain management are shown in Table 2. Propoxyphene (Darvon, Darvocet), a widely used opioid with weak analgesic activity, was removed from the U.S. market in 2010 due to an unacceptable risk of cardiac rhythm abnormalities. The following are descriptions of opioids with pure agonist activity. All these agents have the same actions and adverse effects as morphine. All are controlled substances.

Codeine: Approved by the FDA in 1939, codeine can be administered by the PO, subcutaneous, or IM routes. Because it has stronger antitussive action than morphine, it is often used for suppression of severe cough. At the low doses needed for cough suppression, codeine does not produce the serious adverse effects characteristic of morphine. When used to treat cough and other severe cold symptoms, low doses are usually combined with guaifenesin (a nonnarcotic antitussive), promethazine (a phenothiazine with antihistamine action), phenylephrine (a decongestant), or brompheniramine (an antihistamine). Doses required to produce analgesia are much higher than those needed for cough suppression. When prescribed for analgesia, it is usually in combination with acetaminophen and its use is often limited by nausea and vomiting. During the metabolism of codeine in the CNS, about 10% is converted to morphine, which is responsible for its analgesic effects. Codeine may also be used off-label to treat serious diarrhea. This drug is pregnancy category C; the category changes to D if used in high doses or close to term.

Fentanyl (Abstral, Actiq, Duragesic, Fentora, Onsolis, Sublimaze): Originally approved in 1968 as an IV anesthetic (Sublimaze) for short-term surgical procedures, fentanyl has since been introduced in multiple formulations. These include oral tablets (Fentora), buccal film (Onsolis), sublingual tablets (Abstral), oral transmucosal lozenges (Actiq), and transdermal patches (Duragesic).

All the nonanesthetic formulations of fentanyl are restricted to the management of breakthrough pain in patients who are already receiving and who are tolerant to around-the-clock opioid therapy for their chronic, persistent pain. This includes intractable cancer pain. Giving these formulations to patients who are opioid naïve can result in serious or fatal respiratory depression. Generally, the initial dose depends on how much morphine the patient has been receiving, that is, how tolerant the patient has become to the effects of opioids. Doses are gradually increased until the breakthrough pain is relieved. The buccal, transdermal, and transmucosal forms of fentanyl have black box warnings regarding the dependence potential for this drug and the serious adverse effects that can occur if the drug is misused.

Several other opioids, for example, remifentanil (Ultiva), alfentanil (Alfenta), and sufentanil (Sufenta), are closely related to fentanyl and are used as IV anesthetics.

Hydrocodone (Hycodan, others): Approved in 1957, hydrocodone is used for analgesia, most often combined with acetaminophen, aspirin, or ibuprofen in fixed dose combinations such as Vicodin, Lortab, and Norco. Acetaminophen has a dose ceiling that limits the use of such combinations in chronic pain management. Hydrocodone is an effective antitussive and is combined with decongestants or antihistamines for severe cold and flu symptoms. Although it is slightly more effective than codeine as an antitussive, it causes more sedation. This drug is pregnancy category C; the category changes to D if used in high doses or close to term.

Hydromorphone (Dilaudid, Exalgo): Approved in 1984, hydromorphone is available by the PO, rectal, and parenteral routes. Its primary application is analgesia, including PCA. Hydromorphone produces less nausea but more orthostatic hypotension than morphine. It has a more rapid onset of action and a shorter duration of activity than morphine, requiring PO dosing every 3 to 6 hours. An extended duration formulation of the drug (Exalgo) was approved in 2010. Hydromorphone has black box warnings regarding the dependence potential for this drug and the serious adverse effects that can occur if the drug is misused. This drug is pregnancy category C.

Levorphanol (Levo-Dromoran): Approved in 1953, levorphanol is a pure opioid agonist available by the PO and parenteral routes for severe pain. At equianalgesic doses, levorphanol exhibits the same actions and adverse effects as morphine. It offers no advantages over the use of other drugs in this class. This drug is pregnancy category B; the category changes to D if used in high doses or close to term.

Meperidine (Demerol): Approved in 1942, meperidine is available by both the PO and parenteral routes for the treatment of severe pain. Toxicity can occur due to its active metabolite, called normeperidine, which is a CNS stimulant with a half-life of 15 to 30 hours. Accumulation of this metabolite can result from doses greater than 400 to 600 mg per day or administration longer than 48 hours. Normeperidine can cause tremors and seizures, which are not reversed with narcotic antagonists (naloxone). For this reason, meperidine is not recommended for use longer than 48 hours, for chronic pain, or for use in PCA. When meperidine is used in high doses or longer than 48 hours, the nurse needs to consult with the prescriber and report any incidences of tremors and irritability before giving the next dose. Because of these adverse effects, meperidine is considered a second-line agent that is used when other opioids are contraindicated. An off-label use for meperidine is for the management of shivering, a common complication in the postoperative period. The drug has a short half-life that requires dosing every 3 to 4 hours. This drug is pregnancy category C; the category changes to D if used in high doses or close to term.

Methadone (Dolophine): Approved in 1947, methadone is an oral preparation with pharmacologic effects similar to those of morphine; adverse effects are similar with lower incidence. Methadone is the most frequently prescribed agent in the management of opiate dependency and is increasingly used for management of chronic pain. Methadone has a very long duration of action and can be dosed once daily. Oral liquid (Methadose) and dispersible tablets (Diskets) are available in treating opiate withdrawal symptoms because they offer less risk for abuse than regular tablets. IV methadone is used for the short-term therapy of hospitalized patients. A black box warning indicates that when converting from other analgesics to methadone particular diligence is necessary because deaths have been reported during the conversion period. The deaths were likely due to titrating the dose of methadone too quickly, resulting in cardiac and respiratory failure. This drug is pregnancy category C.

Oxycodone (OxyContin, Others): Approved in 1976, oxycodone is an oral opioid that is often combined with acetaminophen (Endocet, Percocet) or with aspirin (Percodan) for the management of moderate to severe pain. The drug is used when around-the-clock analgesia in needed for an extended period of time. It is not indicated for short-term or prn use. Oxycodone causes less nausea, vomiting, and hallucinations than morphine. The immediate release forms of this drug have a short duration of action, requiring dosing every 3 to 4 hours. The extended release form (OxyContin) can be dosed twice a day. OxyContin has become a popular drug of abuse. A black box warning states that all patients receiving oxycodone should be routinely monitored for signs of misuse, abuse, and addiction. Breaking, cutting, chewing, crushing, or dissolving the extended release tablets may result in a potentially fatal overdose. This drug is pregnancy category B; the category changes to D if used in high doses or close to term.

9 Mixed agonist and antagonist opioids exhibit moderate analgesia with less risk of dependence than morphine.

The mixed agonist-antagonist opioids are narcotic analgesics that were developed with the intention of producing drugs with strong analgesia that have fewer adverse effects than morphine and other pure opioid agonists. The four drugs in this class are used to treat moderate pain but are not as effective as morphine in treating severe pain. Their advantage is that they cause less respiratory depression and have a lower potential for dependence. These drugs have some abuse potential but less so than the pure opioid agonists. The types of adverse effects, contraindications, and nursing responsibilities are similar to those of the pure opioid agonists (see Section 8).

With both agonist and antagonist actions, what would happen if a person addicted to morphine or heroin took one of the drugs in this class? Blocking opioid receptors would cause the patient to experience opioid withdrawal symptoms. In fact, some of the mixed agonist-antagonist drugs are indicated for the induction of opioid withdrawal and the maintenance of opioid dependence.

Buprenorphine (Buprenex, Butrans, Suboxone, Subutex): Originally approved in 1981, buprenorphine is a partial agonist at the mu receptors and an antagonist at the kappa receptors. It is indicated for the relief of moderate to severe pain when given by the parenteral route (Buprenex). The sublingual form (Suboxone, Subutex) is reserved for the management of opioid withdrawal and dependence. Suboxone is a combination drug that also contains the narcotic antagonist naloxone. In 2010, a transdermal patch system (Butrans) was approved that provides 7 days of analgesia. Abuse of buprenorphine has been reported but is less common because the drug is unable to produce the degree of euphoria observed with the pure opioid agonists. Furthermore, withdrawal symptoms from this drug are generally mild and its onset may be delayed 1 to 2 weeks. Buprenorphine is a Schedule III drug. Respiratory depression can be a serious adverse effect at high doses. A black box warning states that when using the transdermal form of the drug, do not exceed a dose of 20 mcg/h (the highest dose patch, worn for 7 days) due to a risk of QT interval prolongation. Do not expose the patch application site to high external temperatures because this increases drug release and can cause overdose or death. This drug is pregnancy category C.

Butorphanol (Stadol): Approved in 1978, butorphanol is an agonist at the kappa receptors and is a weak antagonist at the mu receptors. Delivered by the IV or IM route, it is approved for moderate to severe pain and as a preanesthetic medication that supplements general anesthesia. A nasal spray form of the drug (Stadol NS) has a fast onset of 20 to 40 minutes but it must be repeated every 4 to 6 hours for continuous pain control. Drowsiness and dizziness are experienced by a large number of patients, and the intranasal form can cause nasal congestion. Like buprenorphine, the drug is not commonly abused and withdrawal symptoms are mild. Butorphanol is a Schedule III drug. This drug is pregnancy category C.

Nalbuphine (Nubain): Approved in 1979, nalbuphine is an agonist at the kappa receptors and a weak antagonist at the mu receptors. Given by the IV, IM, or subcutaneous route, it is approved for moderate to severe pain and as a preanesthesia or general anesthesia adjunct. Drowsiness is the most common adverse effect. The risk for dependence is low, and nalbuphine is not a scheduled drug. Abrupt discontinuation, however, can precipitate mild opioid withdrawal symptoms. This drug is pregnancy category B (category D with prolonged use or high doses at term).

Pentazocine (Talwin): Approved in 1967, pentazocine was the first of the agonist-antagonist opioids marketed. Available by both the PO and parenteral routes, it is approved to treat moderate to severe pain an as a supplement to general anesthesia. The drug is available in combination tablets with acetaminophen and naloxone. The drug acts as an agonist at the kappa receptors and a weak antagonist at the mu receptors. Pentazocine causes less nausea, vomiting, and respiratory depression than morphine. Like other drugs in this class, drowsiness and dizziness are common adverse effects. Also like other mixed agonists-antagonists, pentazocine does not produce euphoria and has a low potential for abuse (Schedule IV). Withdrawal symptoms are similar to those of other opioids but milder. A major advantage is that overdose with pentazocine does not result in the high mortality observed with morphine. This drug is pregnancy category C.

Patients Receiving Opioid Analgesic Therapy

Assessment	Potential Nursing Diagnoses
Baseline assessment prior to administration: • Understand the reason the drug has been prescribed in order to assess for therapeutic effects. • Obtain a complete health history including cardiovascular, neurologic, respiratory, hepatic, renal, cancer, gallbladder or urologic disease, pregnancy, or breast-feeding. Note recent surgeries or injuries. Obtain a drug history including allergies, current prescription and OTC drugs, and herbal preparations. Be alert to possible drug interactions. • Assess the level of pain. Use objective screening tools when possible (e.g., FLACC [face, limbs, arms, cry, consolability] for infants or very young children, Wong-Baker FACES scale for children, numerical rating scale for adults). Assess pain history and what has worked successfully or not for the patient in the past. • Obtain baseline vital signs and weight. • Evaluate appropriate laboratory findings (e.g., CBC, hepatic, and renal function studies). • Assess the patient's ability to receive and understand instructions. Include family and caregivers as needed. **Assessment throughout administration:** • Assess for desired therapeutic effects (e.g., absent or greatly diminished pain, ability to move more easily without pain or carry out postoperative treatment care). Continue to use pain rating scale to quantify level of improvement. • Continue periodic monitoring of CBC, hepatic, and renal function studies. • Assess vital signs, especially blood pressure, pulse, and respiratory rate. • Assess for and report adverse effects: excessive dizziness, drowsiness, confusion, agitation, hypotension, tachycardia, bradypnea, pinpoint pupils.	• *Acute Pain* • *Chronic Pain* • *Ineffective Breathing Pattern* • *Constipation*, related to adverse drug effects • *Deficient Knowledge*, (Drug Therapy) • *Risk for Injury*, related to adverse drug effects • *Risk for Falls*, related to adverse drug effects

Planning: Patient Goals and Expected Outcomes

The patient will:

• Experience therapeutic effects dependent on the reason the drug is being given (e.g., absent or decreased pain, ease in movement and postoperative care).
• Be free from or experience minimal adverse effects.
• Verbalize an understanding of the drug's use, adverse effects, and required precautions.
• Demonstrate proper self-administration of the medication (e.g., dose, timing, and when to notify the provider).

Implementation

Interventions and (Rationales)	Patient-Centered Care
Ensuring therapeutic effects: • Continue assessments as above for therapeutic effects. Give the drug before the start of acute pain and encourage regularly scheduled doses for the first 24 to 48 hours postoperatively for adequate postoperative pain relief. Provide additional comfort measures to supplement drug therapy. (Consistent use of a pain rating scale by all providers will help quantify level of pain relief and leads to better pain control. Watch for subtle signs of pain: hesitancy to move, shallow breaths to avoid increasing pain, grimacing on movement. Encouraging the patient to maintain regular doses around-the-clock during the acute postoperative or pain period may provide better relief than giving prn doses on-request when pain has increased to the point medication is needed.)	• Teach the patient that pain relief, rather than merely control, is the goal of therapy. • Encourage the patient to take the drug consistently during the acute postoperative or procedure period rather than requesting only when pain is severe. • Explain the rationale behind the pain rating scale (i.e., it allows consistency among all providers). • Encourage the patient, family, or caregiver to use additional, nonmedicinal pain relief techniques (e.g., distraction with television or music, massage, or guided imagery).
Minimizing adverse effects: • Continue to monitor vital signs, especially respirations and pulse oximetry as ordered, postoperatively and in patients with acute pain. For terminal cancer pain, obtain instructions from the oncologist or hospice provider on any dose restrictions. (Respiratory depression is most common with the first dose of an opioid and when given in the presence of other CNS depressants, e.g., postoperatively when the patient may still be experiencing the effects of general anesthesia agents. Count respirations before giving the opioid drug, and contact the provider before giving if the respirations are below 12 per minute in the adult patient, or as ordered in the child. Continue to assess the respiratory rate every 15 to 30 minutes for the first 4 hours. For terminal cancer pain, the drug might not be withheld regardless of respiratory rate, dependent on the provider.)	• Encourage the patient to take deep breaths in the postoperative period. • Encourage consistent pain medication usage to increase activity tolerance. • Encourage patients with terminal cancer to take the dose consistently around the clock with prn doses as required. Advise the family or caregiver of the provider's instructions for adequate pain relief, and to contact the provider if any pain remains.
• Monitor blood pressure and pulse periodically or if symptoms warrant. Ensure patient safety; monitor ambulation until the effects of the drug are known. Be particularly cautious with older adults who are at increased risk for falls. (Opioids may cause hypotension as an adverse effect and increase the risk of falls.)	• Teach the patient to rise from lying or sitting to standing slowly to avoid dizziness or falls. • Instruct the patient to call for assistance prior to getting out of bed or attempting to walk alone, and to avoid driving or other activities requiring mental alertness or physical coordination until the effects of the drug are known.

• Continue to assess bowel sounds. Increase fluid intake and dietary fiber intake. (Decreased peristalsis is an adverse effect of opioid drugs. Significantly diminished or absent bowels sounds should be reported to the health care provider immediately. Additional fluids and fiber may ease constipation but additional medications such as MiraLAX or Colace may be required.)	• Teach the patient to increase fluids to 2 L per day and increase intake of dietary fiber such as fruits, vegetables, and whole grains. • Instruct the patient to report severe constipation to the health care provider for additional advice on laxatives or stool softeners.
• Monitor for itching or reports of itching. (Opioids may cause histamine release with itching or a sensation of itching. In severe cases, antihistamines may be required. Assess for itching as an expected side effect versus signs and symptoms of true allergy or anaphylaxis: changes in vital signs especially hypotension, tachycardia, dyspnea, or urticaria.)	• Teach the patient to report itching to the health care provider, especially if severe or increasing. • Instruct the patient to immediately report any itching associated with dizziness or lightheadedness, difficulty breathing, palpitations, or significant hives.
• Assess for changes in level of consciousness, disorientation or confusion, agitation, headache, sluggish or pinpoint pupils, or seizures immediately. (Neurologic changes may indicate overmedication, increased intracranial pressure, or adverse drug effects. Older adults may be at risk for confusion and falls.)	• Instruct the patient, family, or caregiver to immediately report increasing lethargy, disorientation, confusion, changes in behavior or mood, agitation or aggression, slurred speech, ataxia or seizures. • Ensure patient safety if disorientation is present.
• Assess for urinary retention, especially in the postoperative period. (Opioids may cause urinary retention as an adverse effect.)	• Encourage the patient to move about in bed and to start early ambulation as soon as allowed postoperatively. Assist to normal voiding position if unable to use the bathroom or commode. • Instruct the patient to immediately report the inability to void, increasing bladder pressure, or pain.
• Administer antiemetics 30 to 60 minutes before opioid dose if nausea and vomiting occur. (Nausea and vomiting are common adverse effects.)	• Encourage the patient to report nausea if it occurs. Small amounts of food intake (e.g., dry crackers) and sips of carbonated beverages (e.g., ginger ale) may help if the patient is not NPO.
• Monitor pain relief in patients on PCA pumps. If a basal dose is not given continuously, assess that pain relief is adequate and contact the provider if pain remains present. Teach and encourage the patient to use the self-medication control button whenever pain is present or increasing, or before activities. (PCA-administered pain control has greatly improved pain relief for patients with regular dosing, but is only effective when taken as needed. Review dosage history and patient symptoms to ensure adequate pain relief. Contact the provider if dose, frequency, or basal dose seems inadequate for relief.)	• Instruct the patient, family, or caregiver on the use of the PCA pump. Encourage use on an as-often-as-needed basis, and emphasize the limitations present to protect the patient (i.e., overdose is not possible).
• For IV push administration, dilute the drug with 4 to 5 mL of sterile normal saline and administer over 4 to 5 min unless otherwise ordered. The patient should remain supine to prevent dizziness or hypotension. Monitor blood pressure, pulse rate, and respiratory rate before and after the dose. (Opioids may cause hypotension and significant dizziness. Keeping the patient supine will limit these effects.)	• Explain the rationale to the patient for the need to remain flat during the drug administration and for 15 to 30 minutes after the dose, and to call for assistance before getting out of bed.
• Assess the home environment for medication safety and need for appropriate interventions. Advise the family on restrictions of prescription renewal. (Opioids are Scheduled drugs and may not be used by any person other than the patient. Safeguard medication in the home to prevent overdose.)	• Instruct the patient, family, or caregiver in proper medication storage and need for the drug to be used by the patient only. • Teach the family or caregiver about prescription renewal restrictions (i.e., new prescription each time, no refills, prescription may not be called in) as appropriate for the Schedule of the drug.
Patient understanding of drug therapy: • Use opportunities during administration of medications and during assessments to discuss the rationale for drug therapy, desired therapeutic outcomes, commonly observed adverse effects, parameters for when to call the health care provider, and any necessary monitoring or precautions. (Using time during nursing care helps to optimize and reinforce key teaching areas.)	• The patient should be able to state the reason for the drug, appropriate dose and scheduling, what adverse effects to observe for, and when to report them.
Patient self-administration of drug therapy: • When administering the medication, instruct the patient, family, or caregiver in the proper self-administration of drug (e.g., take the drug as prescribed when needed). (Utilizing time during nurse-administration of these drugs helps to reinforce teaching.)	Teach the patient to take the medication: • Before the pain becomes severe and for cancer pain, as consistently as possible. • If using a PCA pump, use the self-dosage button whenever pain begins to increase or before activities such as sitting at the bedside. • Take with food to decrease GI upset. • Because opioids are Scheduled drugs (most often C-II through IV), federal law restricts the sale and use of the drug to the person receiving the prescription only. Additional prescriptions may be necessary if the drug is continued beyond the first prescription (e.g., phone-in refills are not allowed for C-II drugs). Do not share with any other person and do not discard unused drug down drains or in the garbage or flush it down the toilet. Return the drug to the pharmacy or health care provider for proper disposal.

Evaluation of Outcome Criteria

Evaluate effectiveness of drug therapy by confirming that patient goals and expected outcomes have been met (see "Planning").

TABLE 4 Nonopioid Centrally Acting Analgesics

Drug	Route and Adult Dose for Pain (maximum dose where indicated)	Adverse Effects
clonidine (Duraclon)	Epidural: 30–40 mcg/h by continuous infusion or 100–900 mcg bolus	*Drowsiness, orthostatic hypotension, dry mouth, anxiety, constipation* <u>Severe hypotension, dysrhythmias</u>
tramadol (Ultram)	PO (immediate release): 25–100 mg every 4–6 h prn (max: 400 mg/day) PO (extended release): 100 mg once daily (max: 300 mg/day)	*Dizziness, nausea, vomiting, constipation, lethargy* <u>Hallucinations, emotional lability, respiratory depression</u>
ziconotide (Prialt)	Intrathecal: 0.1 mcg/h via infusion; may increase as needed up to 0.1 mcg/h no more than every 2–3 days (max: 0.8 mcg/h)	*Dizziness, nausea, diarrhea, somnolence, asthenia* <u>Confusion, memory impairment, hallucinations</u>

Note: Italics indicate common adverse effects. <u>Underline</u> indicates serious adverse effects.

10 Nonsteroidal anti-inflammatory drugs are the medications of choice for mild to moderate pain.

The **nonopioid analgesics** include NSAIDs, acetaminophen, and a few centrally acting agents. NSAIDs, such as aspirin and ibuprofen, are the drugs of choice for mild to moderate pain, especially for pain associated with inflammation. Nonopioids have many advantages over the opioids. Acetaminophen, aspirin, and many NSAIDs are available OTC and are inexpensive. They are available in many different formulations, including those designed for children. For most patients, they are safe and produce adverse effects only at high doses. NSAIDs have antipyretic and anti-inflammatory actions as well as analgesic properties. Indeed, some NSAIDs are used primarily for their anti-inflammatory effects. Nursing practice applications for the nonopioid analgesics are similar to those for the opioid analgesics and are presented in the Nursing Practice Application for Patients Receiving Opioid Analgesic Therapy.

NSAIDs act at peripheral sites by inhibiting pain mediators at the nociceptor level. When tissue is damaged, chemical mediators, including histamine, potassium ion, hydrogen ion, and bradykinin, are released locally. Also released during tissue damage is arachidonic acid, which is metabolized into chemical mediators of inflammation and pain such as prostaglandins. Prostaglandins can induce pain through the formation of free radicals.

NSAIDs inhibit cyclooxygenase, an enzyme responsible for the formation of prostaglandins. Because they act by a different mechanism than opioids, NSAIDs do not produce the severe adverse effects of NSAIDs observed with the narcotic analgesics. The most prominent effects are GI related and include nausea, vomiting, anorexia, dyspepsia, and ulceration of the GI mucosa. At high doses, the ulceration can be severe, resulting in bleeding and even perforation. In 2010 a fixed combination of naproxen and omeprazole (Vimovo) was approved to

reduce the risk of developing NSAID-induced gastric ulcers. Other common adverse events include dizziness, headache, and rash. These drugs do not cause physical or psychological dependence. When combined with opioids in fixed dose combinations, NSAIDs produce a synergistic analgesic effect that allows the dose of opioid to be lowered.

It is important to note that several important nonopioid analgesics are not classified as NSAIDs. Acetaminophen is a nonopioid analgesic whose effectiveness in relieving pain and reducing fever is equal to aspirin and ibuprofen. Clonidine (Catapres) and tramadol (Ultram) are nonopioid analgesics that act centrally, rather than at the nociceptors. These agents are presented in the following section.

11 A few miscellaneous analgesics reduce pain by acting on the central nervous system.

Three analgesics suppress pain by acting on the CNS but are not classified as opioids. Clonidine (Catapres), tramadol (Ultram), and ziconotide (Prialt) act by unique mechanisms but only tramadol is widely prescribed. The doses of the three centrally acting agents are listed in Table 4.

PROTOTYPE DRUG | Tramadol (Ultram)

Classification: **Therapeutic:** Analgesic
Pharmacologic: Centrally acting nonopioid analgesic

Therapeutic Effects and Uses: Tramadol was approved for the treatment of moderate pain in 1995. It is available as an immediate release formulation for acute pain and as an extended release form (Ryzolt, Tramadol ER) for chronic pain that requires long-term, continuous analgesia. An orally disintegrating tablet (Rybix, Ultram ODT) was marketed in 2005 for patients who have difficulty swallowing tablets. Ultracet is a fixed dose combination of tramadol and acetaminophen. Off-label uses of tramadol include treatment of neuropathic pain and restless leg syndrome.

Tramadol has gained in popularity as an alternative to NSAIDs and opioids. It does not exhibit the GI ulceration typical of high-dose NSAID therapy, and it does not cause the severe respiratory depression characteristic of opioids.

Mechanism of Action: Tramadol has a unique mechanism that involves both opioid and nonopioid actions. The drug and one of its metabolites bind to the opioid mu receptor. This opioid agonist activity is weak: approximately 10 times less than that of codeine. In addition to its central opioid action, tramadol inhibits norepinephrine and serotonin reuptake in spinal neurons, which inhibits the transmission of pain impulses.

Pharmacokinetics:

Routes(s)	PO
Absorption	75% absorbed
Distribution	Widely distributed; crosses the placenta; small amounts secreted in breast milk; 20% bound to protein
Primary metabolism	Hepatic; significant first-pass metabolism
Primary excretion	Renal
Onset of action	30–60 min
Duration of action	3–7 h

Adverse Effects: Tramadol is well tolerated, and its most common adverse effects are vertigo, dizziness, headache, nausea, vomiting, constipation, and lethargy. Because it acts centrally, symptoms of CNS stimulation such as nervousness, tremor, anxiety, agitation, confusion, visual impairment, and hallucinations are possible. Some patients experience drowsiness or depression rather than CNS excitation. Seizures have been reported, especially in patients who are concurrently taking antidepressants. Although respiratory depression can occur, it is not as severe as that caused by opioids. Physical dependence is possible although at much less risk than morphine; tramadol is not a controlled substance. Symptoms of opioid withdrawal, such as anxiety, sweating, tremors, panic attacks, and paresthesias, may occur if the drug is abruptly discontinued.

Contraindications/Precautions: Patients with a hypersensitivity to tramadol should not be given the drug. Caution should be exercised in patients allergic to codeine and other opioid agonists because cross-hypersensitivity has been reported. Although the risk for dependence is low, the drug should be used with caution in patients with a history of substance abuse.

Tramadol should not be administered to patients with a history of depression or suicidal ideation because the drug can be fatal in overdose situations, especially if combined with alcohol or other CNS depressants. Because tramadol causes some degree of respiratory depression, it should be used cautiously in patients with COPD. The drug should be used with caution in patients with renal or hepatic impairment or in those with increased ICP. Because tramadol lowers the seizure threshold, it should be used with caution in patients with a history of seizures. Tramadol should be avoided during pregnancy and lactation because its chronic use can cause physical dependence and postpartum withdrawal symptoms in the newborn.

Drug Interactions: Use of tramadol concurrently with carbamazepine or certain antidepressants increases the risk of seizures. Carbamazepine also has additive CNS depressant effects and may reduce the analgesic activity of tramadol. Ethanol combined with tramadol may result in death. When used with other CNS depressants, the dose of tramadol should be reduced. Concurrent use of tramadol with MAOIs can result in seizures or serotonin syndrome. Tramadol is changed to an active metabolite by the hepatic CYP2D6 enzyme. If inhibitors of this enzyme (e.g., amiodarone, chloroquine, haloperidol, ritonavir, quinidine) are given concurrently with tramadol, a reduced analgesic effect may result. **Herbal/Food:** Food significantly affects the absorption of the extended release form of tramadol. St. John's wort is contraindicated due to the possibility of serotonin syndrome. Caution should be observed when using herbs such as valerian or kava that may have an additive CNS depressant effect.

Pregnancy: Category C.

Treatment of Overdose: Overdose with tramadol will result in serious CNS depression, respiratory depression, and perhaps death. Administration of naloxone will reduce some, but not all, of the symptoms of tramadol overdose and may precipitate convulsions.

Nursing Responsibilities: Key nursing implications for patients receiving tramadol are similar to those for opioid agents and are included in the Nursing Practice Application for Patients Receiving Opioid Analgesic Therapy.

CONNECTIONS

Lifespan Considerations
Influence of Increasing Age on Pain Expression and Perception

Pain control in the older adult can be challenging. Knowledge of the aging process, behavioral cues, subtle signs of discomfort, and verbal and nonverbal responses to pain are a must when it comes to effective pain management. Older patients may have a decreased perception of pain or simply ignore pain as a natural consequence of aging. Because these patients frequently go undermedicated, a thorough assessment is a necessity. Older adults may have difficulty with numerical rating scales and may respond more appropriately to the Wong-Baker Faces scale. When administering opioids for pain relief, the nurse should always monitor older adult patients closely. Aging decreases both hepatic metabolism and renal excretion; smaller doses are usually indicated and adverse effects may be heightened. Initial doses should be 25% to 50% lower with frequent reassessment. The nurse should closely monitor decreased respirations, LOC, and dizziness. Body weight should be taken prior to the start of opioid administration and doses calculated accordingly. Bed rails should be kept raised and the bed in a low position at all times to prevent injury from falls. Some opioids, such as meperidine (Demerol) or hydromorphone (Dilaudid), should be used cautiously due to orthostatic hypotension. Many older adults take multiple drugs (polypharmacy); therefore, it is important to obtain a complete list of all medications taken and to check for interactions.

Drugs Similar to Tramadol (Ultram)

The two other centrally acting, nonopioid analgesics are clonidine and ziconotide. These drugs act by very different mechanisms than tramadol and are much less frequently prescribed.

Clonidine (Catapres, Duraclon): Originally approved as an oral drug for hypertension (Catapres) in 1974, clonidine has been used off-label for a large number of other indications, including hot flashes, Tourette's syndrome, attention deficit/hyperactivity disorder (ADHD), and withdrawal from ethanol, nicotine, and opioids. It has a very limited role in treating severe, intractable cancer pain that is refractory to other drugs, including opioids. For this indication, it is administered as an epidural infusion, usually in combination with opioids. Clonidine activates alpha₂-adrenergic receptors in the spinal cord, resulting in decreased pain signals reaching the brain. Because this drug is absorbed into the circulation, the most serious adverse effects from the epidural use of clonidine are the same as those from PO administration: severe hypotension and bradycardia. Clonidine is also available as a transdermal therapeutic system (clonidine TTS), which consists of a patch that releases the drug over 7 days. Clonidine (Kapvay) was approved by the FDA to treat ADHD in 2010. Clonidine is pregnancy category C.

Ziconotide (Prialt): Ziconotide, approved in 2004, is unusual in that it was originally obtained from a species of saltwater snail. Like clonidine, its use is limited to patients whose pain is refractory to all other analgesics, including morphine. It is only administered by intrathecal infusion. An off-label use is for severe muscle spasticity due to spinal cord injury. The drug provides analgesia by blocking N-type calcium channels at the presynaptic nerve terminals in the spinal cord. This prevents neurotransmitter release, thus blocking pain transmission. Ziconotide has the potential for frequent and serious adverse effects. The drug carries a black box warning regarding the potential for severe psychiatric symptoms and neurologic impairment, including impaired cognition, decreased consciousness, and hallucinations. Dizziness, nausea, and vomiting occur in about half the patients receiving the drug. Although these adverse effects are serious, the student should remember that cancer patients receiving this agent are terminally ill and pain relief is often the primary therapeutic goal. This drug is pregnancy category C.

12 Adjuvant analgesics have primary indications other than pain but can enhance analgesia.

Some types of pain are not adequately relieved by analgesics alone. **Adjuvant analgesics** are a diverse group of drugs that are used to enhance analgesia for specific indications. All of these drugs have other primary classifications, such as antidepressant, antiseizure, tranquilizer, or anti-inflammatory. The use of adjuvant analgesics includes two primary indications:

- Pain that is refractory to opioids, such as intractable cancer pain
- Neuropathic pain, which is caused by damage to the nerve itself, and pain caused by swelling in the CNS, which puts pressure on nerves.

In patients with intractable cancer pain, adjuvant analgesics are used in combination with analgesics to enhance the level of pain relief. It is important to understand that these agents supplement pain relief; they do not substitute for proper dosing of opioid analgesics in patients with severe pain. Adjuvant analgesics are generally not used if the pain is well managed with opioids, because these drugs have additional adverse effects and drug interactions that can complicate therapy.

Neuropathic pain is difficult to control with analgesics. The most common cause of neuropathic pain is diabetes, but herpes zoster infections, acute trauma, cancer, and certain autoimmune conditions can also cause this type of pain. Neuropathic pain is commonly described as steady burning, electric shock, or "pins and needles" sensations. Rather than treat with high doses of opioids, several adjuvant analgesics have been found to be effective at relieving neuropathic pain. These drugs may be used alone or in combination with opioids.

Adjuvant analgesics can be added at any step in the pain management ladder; they are usually dosed on a regular schedule as opposed to prn. The use of specific adjuvant analgesics and their doses are often guided by experience, rather than controlled clinical trials, and the majority of these drugs are prescribed off-label for their analgesic effects. Table 5 summarizes the effects and uses of selected adjuvant analgesics.

Antidepressants: Some of the most commonly prescribed adjuvant analgesics come from the antidepressant drug class. Both of the common classes of antidepressants, tricyclics and selective serotonin reuptake inhibitors (SSRIs), are used as adjuncts in the management of neuropathic pain. Although the tricyclics seem to be more effective, the SSRIs cause fewer serious adverse effects. These drugs increase the levels of the inhibitory neurotransmitters serotonin and norepinephrine in the CNS, resulting in increased pain modulation and decreased pain perception. Patients experiencing neuropathic pain may need trials with different antidepressants until the right combination of effectiveness and tolerable adverse effects is found. Doses of these drugs are generally lower than those used to treat depression, and the drugs act to relieve pain within 5 to 7 days. If improvement in pain relief is not noted within 1 week, the drug is discontinued. Duloxetine (Cymbalta) was the first of the antidepressants to receive approval for the treatment of diabetic peripheral neuropathic pain, chronic musculoskeletal pain, and fibromyalgia pain. Other drugs used for this purpose include amitriptyline (Elavil), imipramine (Tofranil), doxepin (Sinequan), paroxetine (Paxil), and venlafaxine (Effexor).

CONNECTION Checkpoint 29.2

Use of tricyclic antidepressants has declined in recent decades due to a higher incidence of adverse effects compared to drugs in the SSRI class, but they are useful in the treatment of neuropathic pain. What type of adverse effects would likely be observed in patients taking tricyclics for migraines? *See Answer to Connection Checkpoint 29.2 on student resource website.*

Antiseizure drugs: Antiseizure drugs commonly prescribed for neuropathic pain include gabapentin (Neurontin), valproic acid (Depakene), phenytoin (Dilantin), and carbamazepine (Tegretol). The antiseizure drugs act by suppressing neuronal

TABLE 5 Adjuvant Analgesics

Drug Class	Examples	Effect	Use
Antiseizure agent	carbamazepine (Tegretol) clonazepam (Klonopin) gabapentin (Gralise, Neurontin)	Decrease nerve impulse transmission and spontaneous neuron firing. (Phantom pain is theorized as a type of sensory seizure.)	Reduce peripheral nerve pain in neuropathy and phantom pain after amputation.
Benzodiazepine	diazepam (Valium) lorazepam (Ativan)	Potentiate effects of gamma aminobutyric acid (GABA) and other inhibitory neurotransmitters.	Relax skeletal muscle in muscle spasm; reduce anxiety in terminal dyspnea.
Bisphosphonate	pamidronate (Aredia) zoledronate (Reclast, Zometa)	Inhibit bone resorption.	Reduce cancer-related bone pain.
Corticosteroid	dexamethasone (Decadron) prednisone (various)	Reduce cerebral and spinal edema via various mechanisms in prostaglandin cascade.	Reduce swelling and pain in CNS cancer, spinal cord compression, postspinal surgery.
Selective serotonin reuptake inhibitor (SSRI)	citalopram (Celexa) fluoxetine (Prozac) fluvoxamine (Luvox) sertraline (Zoloft)	Increase concentrations of inhibitory neurotransmitters (serotonin and norepinephrine) in the CNS.	Reduce neuropathic pain.
Tricyclic antidepressant	amitriptyline (Elavil) amoxapine desipramine (Norpramin) doxepin (Sinequan) imipramine (Tofranil) nortriptyline (Aventyl) protriptyline (Vivactil)	Increase concentrations of inhibitory neurotransmitters (serotonin and norepinephrine) in the CNS.	Reduce neuropathic pain.

discharges and reducing the hyperexcitability that occurs after nerve injury. These drugs may cause nausea, vomiting, sedation, confusion, or dizziness. Gabapentin is considered a first-line drug for treating neuropathic pain, and an extended release tablet form of the drug (Gralise) was approved to treat postherpetic neuralgia in 2011.

Corticosteroids: Corticosteroids are used as adjuvants in pain management because they reduce inflammatory swelling and pressure on the brain, spinal cord, and spinal nerves. Dexamethasone (Decadron) is a drug of choice when given parenterally to reduce either cerebral or spinal cord edema; oral prednisone (Deltasone) may follow for a period of time. Steroids can also be injected directly into joints in refractory arthritis, or epidural/spinal tracts for chronic musculoskeletal pain.

Local anesthetics: Mexiletine (Mexitil) is a Class IB antidysrhythmic drug with anesthetic properties that is given PO for neuropathic pain refractory to other analgesics. Caution must be used when giving this drug to patients with heart disease or dysrhythmias. Short IV infusions of lidocaine (Xylocaine) may also provide temporary relief for some patients. A 5% lidocaine patch is approved for postherpetic neuralgia.

Muscle relaxants: Muscle relaxants such as the benzodiazepines may be used effectively as adjuvant analgesics when muscle spasm is a component of the pain. Muscle spasm can be present following orthopedic injury or with musculoskeletal disease or degenerative nervous system conditions. Benzodiazepines can also be used to reduce anxiety in the terminal dyspnea of heart failure or end-stage respiratory disease. Examples include diazepam (Valium), lorazepam (Ativan), and oxazepam (Serax).

Bone-specific agents: Patients with bone cancer or metastases may experience severe pain. For palliative care, the administration of calcitonin, either subcutaneously or intranasally, may provide some relief for bone pain. The adjuvant analgesic activity of the bisphosphonates such as pamidronate (Aredia) and zolendronate (Reclast, Zometa) has been well established.

Miscellaneous agents: Capsaicin is a product obtained from chili peppers that is available as a cream to treat minor musculoskeletal pin. A prescription patch containing 8% capsaicin (Qutenza) was approved in 2010 for the relief of pain associated with postherpetic neuralgia. Milnacipran (Savella) was approved in 2009 for the treatment of fibromyalgia. The exact mechanism by which these drugs inhibit pain pathways is unknown.

Pharmacotherapy with Opioid Antagonists

13 The primary indication for an opioid antagonist is opioid-induced respiratory depression.

Opioid overdose can result from excessive doses during pain therapy, or from attempted suicide or substance abuse. Any opioid may be abused for its psychoactive effects; however, morphine, meperidine, and heroin are preferred by abusers due to their potency. Although heroin is currently available as a legal analgesic in many countries, it is deemed too dangerous for therapeutic use by the FDA, and it is a major drug of abuse. Once injected or inhaled, heroin rapidly crosses the blood–brain barrier to enter the brain, where it is metabolized

TABLE 6 Opioid Antagonists

Drug	Route and Adult Dose (maximum dose where indicated)	Adverse Effects
nalmefene (Revex)	Subcutaneous/IM/IV: Use 1 mg/mL concentration Nonopioid dependent: 0.5 mg/70 kg Opioid dependent: 0.1 mg/70 kg	*Muscle and joint pains, difficulty sleeping, anxiety, headache, nervousness, withdrawal symptoms, vomiting* <u>Hepatotoxicity</u>
naloxone (Narcan)	IV: 0.4–2 mg; may be repeated every 2–3 min up to 10 mg if necessary	
naltrexone (ReVia)	PO: 25 mg followed by another 25 mg in 1 h if no withdrawal response (max: 800 mg/day)	

Note: *Italics* indicate common adverse effects. <u>Underline</u> indicates serious adverse effects.

to morphine. Thus, the effects of heroin administration are actually caused by activation of the mu and kappa receptors from its morphine metabolite. The initial effect is an intense euphoria, or rush, followed by several hours of deep relaxation.

In recent years, OxyContin has become a major drug of abuse. Because this long-acting form of oxycodone is especially beneficial to patients with chronic pain who need around-the-clock relief, it has become a first-line drug in pain management. Abusers use the drug either for its effective pain relief action or for its side effects such as relaxation or euphoria. Many of the opioid drugs are given in combination with aspirin or acetaminophen, which causes dose-limiting adverse effects. OxyContin, however, only contains oxycodone and it can be crushed by abusers and injected or snorted for an even greater "high." OxyContin is a frequent target for "doctor shoppers" who visit multiple health care providers, often reporting fictitious symptoms to obtain prescriptions. Use is increasing among all segments of the population, including teenagers. It is a potent and dangerous drug that can cause death when misused or abused.

Acute opioid intoxication is a medical emergency, with respiratory depression being the most serious medical challenge. Infusion with the opioid antagonist naloxone (Narcan) may be used to reverse respiratory depression and other acute symptoms. In cases when the patient arrives unconscious and the health care provider does not know which drug has been taken, small amounts of opioid antagonists may be given to diagnose the overdose. If an opioid antagonist fails to quickly reverse the acute symptoms, the overdose was likely due to a nonopioid substance. Doses for the opioid antagonists are listed in Table 6.

When abusing an opioid, the user usually develops tolerance to the euphoric effects of the drug and quickly escalates the dose. Following therapy with an opioid antagonist, however, the patient will become much more sensitive to the effects of opioids. If the patient returns to drug-taking behavior at the same dose used prior to opioid antagonist therapy, death may result.

Another indication for opioid antagonists is for the treatment of opioid-induced constipation or postoperative ileus. Alvimopan (Entereg) and methylnaltrexone (Relistor), both approved in 2008, act as mu receptors in the GI tract. Because they do not cross the blood–brain barrier, these drugs do not interfere with the central effects of opioids such as analgesia.

Therapeutic Effects and Uses: Naloxone was approved in 1971 to reverse the respiratory depression caused by opioid overdose. It is also used postoperatively to reverse the effects of opioids given prior to or during surgery. It has no pharmacologic actions in the absence of opioids. Off-label uses include the management of nausea, vomiting, urinary retention, or constipation induced by opioid therapy. It has also been used to reverse the acute effects of benzodiazepines and ethanol.

In administering naloxone, small doses are usually used and repeated until the patient gradually exhibits opioid withdrawal symptoms. The patient must be constantly monitored to ensure that the effects of the drug are sufficiently long to outlast the respiratory depression caused by the opioid overdose; IV doses of naloxone only last 1 hour. Maintenance of a patent airway is essential and resuscitation equipment should be immediately available. The IV route is preferred owing to its more rapid onset of action.

It is important to understand that at high doses naloxone will reverse both the toxic and therapeutic effects of opioids. Thus if the patient was using the opioid for analgesia, naloxone will reverse this effect and pain will quickly return.

Naloxone is available in fixed dose combinations with pentazocine (Talwin Nx) and buprenorphine (Suboxone), which are used to treat moderate to severe pain. The opioid agonist (pentazocine or buprenorphine) is used to provide effective analgesia. As an opioid antagonist, naloxone has no pharmacologic activity of its own, but is included to block some of the side effects of the opioid agonists and to prevent product misuse.

Mechanism of Action: Naloxone competes with opioid agonists for the mu and kappa receptors, thus antagonizing all the effects of morphine and other opioids and reversing respiratory depression and coma.

Pharmacokinetics:

Routes(s)	Subcutaneous, IM, IV
Absorption	Inactivated after absorption
Distribution	Widely distributed; crosses the placenta; may be secreted in breast milk
Primary metabolism	Hepatic
Primary excretion	Renal
Onset of action	Subcutaneous/IM: 2–5 min; IV: 1–2 min
Duration of action	IM: up to 4 h; IV: 1 h

Adverse Effects: Naloxone has no common adverse effects on its own. However, serious adverse effects that can result

---

PROTOTYPE DRUG	Naloxone (Narcan)

Classification: **Therapeutic:** Drug for opioid overdose
Pharmacologic: Opioid antagonist

from abrupt reversal of opioid depression include tachycardia, dysrhythmia, hypertension, nausea, and vomiting.

Contraindications/Precautions: Naloxone is contraindicated in patients with hypersensitivity to the drug. Opioid antagonists should be used cautiously in patients who have chronic physical dependence on opioids, because drug-induced withdrawal may be more intense than spontaneous opioid withdrawal. Naloxone should be used with caution in patients with cardiovascular disease. Naloxone may precipitate seizures in patients with seizure disorders.

Drug Interactions: When given concurrently, naloxone reverses all the effects of opioids. Use with tramadol can increase the risk for seizures.

Pregnancy: Category C.

Treatment of Overdose: Overdose with naloxone is rare.

Nursing Responsibilities:

- Assess the patient's respiratory status and administer the opioid antagonist if respirations are below 10 breaths per minute.

- Ensure that resuscitation equipment is immediately available. Be aware that the administration of this drug is an emergency situation to prevent opioid-induced respiratory arrest.

- Monitor for signs of opioid withdrawal such as cramping, vomiting, hypertension, anxiety, or return of severe pain.

- Assess the patient's pain level before drug administration and during therapy.

- Monitor vital signs and pupil size every 3 to 5 minutes. The duration of action of many opioids is longer than the duration of naloxone; repeated doses may be necessary.

- Give IV push undiluted at a rate of 0.4 mg/15 sec; or dilute and infuse via microdrip and IV pump, titrated to response.

Lifespan and Diversity Considerations:

- Use with known or suspected opioid dependency (including in neonates) produces immediate and severe withdrawal symptoms. With a mother who is an addict, administration to the infant immediately postdelivery is preferred to maternal administration during labor.

Patient and Family Education:

- Inform the patient and family why the administration of the drug is necessary.

Drugs Similar to Naloxone (Narcan)

Two additional opioid antagonists, nalmefene and naltrexone, have actions similar to those of naloxone.

Nalmefene (Revex): Approved in 1995, nalmefene is given parenterally to produce effects similar to those of naloxone but with a longer duration of action that equals that of most opioids. Like the other opioid antagonists, nalmefene will precipitate withdrawal symptoms in opioid-dependent patients within minutes after IV administration. The drug has no serious toxicity associated with it. It is a pregnancy category C drug.

Naltrexone (Depade, Embeda, ReVia, Vivitrol): Approved in 1984, naltrexone has similar effects to naloxone but is administered by the PO route. An IM form is available for patients who are unable to take the drug by the PO route. Naltrexone prevents the euphoric effects of opioids and is used primarily in drug abuse rehabilitation programs. Successful use of naltrexone in opioid rehabilitation programs is entirely dependent on patient adherence; if the patient stops taking naltrexone, the euphoric effects of opioid abuse will return. If given to opioid-dependent patients, naltrexone will precipitate withdrawal symptoms.

Naltrexone is also used to inhibit reward pathways associated with alcoholism. When it was approved for alcohol dependence in the 1990s, the trade name Trexan was changed to ReVia. A long-acting formulation of naltrexone (Vivitrol) is injected IM once monthly and is indicated for treating alcohol and opioid addiction. Naltrexone has been awarded orphan drug status by the FDA to treat symptoms of childhood autism. In 2009, a fixed dose combination of naltrexone with morphine was approved to treat moderate to severe pain. Morphine is used to provide effective analgesia, and naltrexone, which has no pharmacologic activity of its own, is included to block some of the side effects of morphine and to prevent product misuse. A black box warning states that naltrexone can cause hepatotoxicity. Patients with serious hepatic impairment should not receive naltrexone. This drug is pregnancy category C.

CONNECTION Checkpoint 29.3

Describe the symptoms of a patient undergoing acute withdrawal from opioids. How are these symptoms treated? *See Answer to Connection Checkpoint 29.3 on student resource website.*

Pharmacotherapy of Migraines

14 Migraines are a severe type of headache related to specific triggers.

Headaches are some of the most common complaints of patients. The pain and inability to concentrate causes a significant number of work-related absences and can interfere with activities of daily life. When the headaches are persistent, or manifest as migraines, drug therapy is warranted.

Why does a headache hurt? Although the skull and the brain lack pain receptors, the muscles of the scalp, face, and neck are abundantly supplied with nociceptors. These receptors can be stimulated by muscle tension, dilated blood vessels, and other headache triggers.

Of the several varieties of headaches, the most common type is the **tension headache**. This occurs when muscles of the head and neck become tight due to stress, causing a steady and lingering pain. Although quite painful, tension headaches are self-limiting and more of an annoyance than an emergency. Tension headaches can be effectively treated with OTC analgesics such as aspirin, acetaminophen, or ibuprofen. Table 7 differentiates the two common types of headaches.

TABLE 7 Differentiation of Major Headache Types

Characteristics	Vascular (Migraine) Headache	Tension Headache
Pain quality	Pulsating or throbbing	Steady pressure or tightness
Pain location	Unilateral (more often) or bilateral	Bilateral (head-band or ice tongs) pattern
Pain severity	Moderate to severe	Mild to moderate
Duration	4–72 h	Usually several hours
Precursors or triggers	Hormonal changes in women; stress or heightened emotions; bright or flickering lights; change in weather or altitude Foods: alcohol, aged cheeses, chocolate, caffeine, fermented or pickled foods, aspartame, MSG	Stress or anxiety
Associated symptoms	May be preceded by aura, nausea, vomiting, extreme sensitivity to light or sound; aggravated by physical activity	Uncommon

The most painful type of headache is the **migraine**, which is characterized by throbbing or pulsating pain, sometimes preceded by an aura. **Auras** are sensory warnings of an imminent migraine attack. Examples include flashing lights, visual blind spots, and arm or leg tingling. Nausea, vomiting, and extreme sensitivity to light and sound accompany most migraines. A positive family history is present in the majority of people who experience migraines.

Patients who get migraines appear to have blood vessels that overreact to various triggers. Triggers for migraines include foods containing nitrates or MSG, alcohol (especially red wine), perfumes, food additives, caffeine, chocolate, aspartame, and hormonal and environmental changes. Some patients can prevent or reduce the frequency of migraine attacks by avoiding known triggers.

The neurotransmitter serotonin (5-hydroxytryptamine or 5-HT) appears to be a key factor (although not the only factor) in the pathogenesis and treatment of migraines. What is the connection between serotonin levels and migraines? Although not precisely understood, the migraine "trigger" creates a spasm in the arteries at the base of the brain, reducing blood flow to the brain. During a migraine, the amount of serotonin in the brain declines and the vessels dilate; nerves surrounding the dilated vessels become inflamed. The expansion of these vessels and associated inflammation are believed to be responsible for the throbbing nature of migraine pain. As neurons in the brain generate additional serotonin, or serotonin agonist drugs are administered, the vessels dilate and pain diminishes.

PharmFACT

Migraine Statistics

- About 10% to 20% of the population experiences migraines.
- Before puberty, more boys have migraines than girls; after puberty, women are three times more likely to have migraines than men.
- Most patients who develop migraines have a first attack by age 30.
- Migraines are rare after age 50, and their presence in this age group suggests intracranial pathology. (Blanda & Wright, 2010)

15 Analgesics and triptans are the primary classes of drugs used to abort acute migraine pain.

The two primary goals of migraine pharmacotherapy are to terminate an acute migraine in progress and to prevent or reduce the frequency of the disorder. Drugs used to stop a migraine in progress are different from those used for prophylaxis. The prophylactic agents are discussed in Section 16.

Migraine pharmacotherapy is most effective if begun before the pain has reached a severe level. Drug therapy is conducted in stages based on the severity of the migraine.

- **Mild migraine (occasional headaches with no other functional impairment).** NSAIDs offer the safest and least expensive therapy; thus they are tried initially. Acetaminophen is generally not effective alone but offers additive pain relief when combined with an NSAID and caffeine. Oral serotonin (5-HT) agonists (triptans or ergot alkaloids) are initiated in persistent mild migraines that are refractory to NSAIDs.

- **Moderate migraine (moderate headaches, nausea, and some functional impairment).** Oral, intranasal, or subcutaneous serotonin (5-HT) agonists are the drugs of choice. If serotonin agonists are contraindicated or ineffective, dopamine agonists such as metoclopramide (Reglan) or prochlorperazine (Compazine) may be prescribed.

- **Severe migraine (severe headaches more than three times per month, marked nausea or vomiting, and functional impairment).** Subcutaneous, IM, or IV serotonin agonists may be indicated. A secondary choice would be a parenteral dopamine agonist, either as monotherapy or in combination with a serotonin agonist. Narcotic analgesics are effective at terminating pain from migraines that have proven to be refractory to other therapies.

The two major drug classes used to terminate migraines, the triptans and the ergot alkaloids, are both serotonin receptor agonists. About 90% of the serotonin receptors (also called serotonergic) are found in the intestine, with the remaining 10% occurring throughout the CNS and in platelets. In the CNS, serotonin is responsible for moderating diverse responses such as anger, anxiety, depression, sleep, appetite, and vomiting. At least seven receptor subtypes have been identified. Other drugs acting at serotonin receptors include certain antianxiety agents, antidepressants, antiemetics, and various hallucinogens. Doses for the triptans and ergot alkaloids are listed in Table 8.

Triptans: The first of the triptans, sumatriptan (Imitrex), was marketed in the United States in 1992. This drug was quickly followed by the introduction of the "second-generation" triptans with improved pharmacokinetic profiles: more thorough absorption, faster onset of action, and longer duration. Although all triptans have very similar actions and adverse

TABLE 8 Drugs Used to Terminate Acute Migraines

Drug	Route and Adult Dose (maximum dose where indicated)	Adverse Effects
Triptans		
almotriptan (Axert)	PO: 6.25–12.5 mg, may repeat in 2 h (max: 2 doses/24 h)	*Paresthesia, tingling, dry mouth, warming sensation, dizziness, vertigo*
eletriptan (Relpax)	PO: 20–40 mg, may repeat in 2 h (max: 80 mg/24 h)	
frovatriptan (Frova)	PO: 2.5 mg, may repeat in 2 h (max: 3 doses/24 h)	Coronary artery vasospasm, MI, cardiac arrest
naratriptan (Amerge)	PO: 1–2.5 mg, may repeat in 4 h (max: 5 mg/24 h)	
rizatriptan (Maxalt)	PO: 5–10 mg, may repeat in 2 h (max: 30 mg/24 h)	
sumatriptan (Imitrex)	PO: 25–100 mg, may repeat in 2 h (max: 200 mg/24 h)	
	Nasal: 5–20 mg, may repeat once (max: 40 mg/24 h)	
	Subcutaneous: 6 mg, may repeat in 1 h, once in 24 h	
zolmitriptan (Zomig)	PO: 2.5 mg or less, may repeat in 2 h (max: 10 mg/24 h)	
	Nasal: 5 mg, may repeat once after 2 h (max: 10 mg/24 h)	
Ergot Alkaloids		
dihydroergotamine (DHE 45, Migranal)	Nasal: 1 spray (0.5 mg) each nostril, may repeat once in 15 min (max: 3 mg/24 h, 4 mg/week)	*Weakness, nausea, vomiting, abnormal pulse, throat irritation, nasal irritation, or dysgeusia (distorted sense of taste)*
	IM/subcutaneous: 1 mg, repeat at 1 h intervals for total 3 mg (max: 6 mg/week)	
ergotamine (Ergostat; with caffeine: Cafergot; with caffeine, belladonna, pentobarbital: Cafergot P-B)	Sublingual: 2 mg, may repeat in 30 min for total 3 doses/24 h or 5 doses/week	<u>Delirium, seizures, cerebrovascular events (hemorrhage), intermittent claudication, birth defects, inhibition of lactation or cause of infant vomiting, physical dependence, withdrawal resembles migraine</u>
	PO: 2 tablets (2 mg), 1 additional tablet repeated every 30 min (max: 6 mg/attack or 10 mg/week)	
	Rectal: 2 mg, may repeat once in 1 h	

Note: Italics indicate common adverse effects. <u>Underline</u> indicates serious adverse effects.

effects, individual patients may respond more favorably, and with fewer adverse effects, to one triptan over another. The longer duration triptans are believed to be better at preventing the headache from recurring following its termination.

Triptans are selective for the 5-HT$_1$ receptor subtype, and they are thought to act by constricting certain intracranial vessels. They are effective in aborting migraines with or without auras. Although the PO forms of the triptans are most convenient, patients who experience nausea and vomiting during the migraine may require an alternate dosage form. Intranasal formulations are available and prefilled syringes of triptans may be used for patients who are able to self-administer the medication.

Triptans are not effective at preventing migraines. Other drugs, accompanied by lifestyle changes, must be used for prophylaxis (see Section 16).

Ergot alkaloids: For patients who are unresponsive to triptans, the ergot alkaloids may be used to abort migraines. They should be separated from triptan use by at least 24 hours. The first purified alkaloid, ergotamine (Ergostat), was isolated from the ergot fungus in 1920, although the actions of the ergot alkaloids had been known for thousands of years. Ergotamine is an inexpensive drug that is available in PO, sublingual, and suppository forms. Modification of the original molecule has produced a number of other pharmacologically useful drugs, such as dihydroergotamine (Migranal), which is available parenterally and as a nasal spray. Because the ergot alkaloids interact with adrenergic, dopaminergic, and serotonergic receptors, they produce multiple actions and adverse effects. The ergot alkaloids promote vasoconstriction, which terminates a migraine in progress. Adverse effects may include nausea, vomiting, weakness in the

legs, myalgia, numbness and tingling in fingers and toes, angina-like pain, and tachycardia. Toxicity may be evidenced by constriction of peripheral arteries: cold, pale, numb extremities and muscle pain. Other possible adverse effects include dizziness, drowsiness, vasoconstriction, warming sensations, tingling, lightheadedness, weakness, and neck stiffness.

Ergot alkaloids, which constrict both arteries and veins, are contraindicated in peripheral vascular disease, coronary artery disease, and severe hypertension because they decrease blood flow. Metoclopramide or prochlorperazine may be administered concurrently with ergot alkaloids to reduce or prevent nausea and vomiting. Many ergot alkaloids are pregnancy category X drugs and should not be used by women who may become pregnant. These drugs may inhibit lactation or cause vomiting in breast-fed infants. Regular daily use can cause physical dependence. Withdrawal symptoms of headache, nausea, and vomiting resemble the symptoms of migraines. Dosing and duration of use need to be restricted. Dangers of overuse and dependence should be included in patient and family teaching.

PROTOTYPE DRUG | Sumatriptan (Imitrex)

Classification: **Therapeutic:** Antimigraine agent
Pharmacologic: Serotonin (5-HT$_1$) receptor agonist

Therapeutic Effects and Uses: Available by the PO, intranasal, and subcutaneous routes, sumatriptan is used to relieve acute migraine headaches. It was the first triptan approved by the FDA in 1992. It is not effective for long-term prophylaxis of migraines; other drugs must be used for this purpose. Sumavel DosePro and Alsuma are systems that consist of a subcutaneous dose of sumatriptan with an autoinjector pen. Treximet is a fixed dose combination of sumatriptan and naproxen that was approved in 2008 for the treatment of acute migraines.

Mechanism of Action: Sumatriptan is structurally similar to serotonin. Sumatriptan activates the 5-HT_1 serotonin receptors on intracranial and extracerebral blood vessels, resulting in cranial vessel constriction and reduced transmission in trigeminal pain pathways. It has no intrinsic analgesic activity.

Pharmacokinetics:

Routes(s)	PO, intranasal, subcutaneous
Absorption	Limited bioavailability PO (14%)
Distribution	Widely distributed; crosses the placenta; secreted in breast milk; less than 21% bound to plasma protein
Primary metabolism	Hepatic
Primary excretion	60% renal; 40% feces
Onset of action	PO: 30–60 min; intranasal: 15–20 min; subcutaneous: 10–15 min
Duration of action	PO: 6–8 h; intranasal: unknown; subcutaneous: 4–6 h

Adverse Effects: Sumatriptan has infrequent adverse effects that include mild and transient dizziness or nausea, diarrhea, myalgia, and inflammation and pain at the subcutaneous injection site. Headache recurrence occurs in a large percentage of patients taking sumatriptan. Although rare, serious cardiac events have been documented with sumatriptan use. These events include coronary artery vasospasm, myocardial ischemia, dysrhythmias, and MI. These serious events are more likely to occur in patients with preexisting cardiac disease.

Contraindications/Precautions: Sumatriptan is contraindicated in patients with coronary artery disease, cerebrovascular disease, or peripheral vascular disease. This drug is not recommended for patients with uncontrolled hypertension, hypercholesterolemia, or those who have a strong family history of cardiovascular disease. Sumatriptan is contraindicated in patients with serious renal or hepatic impairment. Patients with a history of epilepsy have an increased risk for seizures when taking sumatriptan. The drug is associated with fetal deformities and demise in animal studies; it should be avoided in pregnant women. Overuse of abortive therapies for migraine headaches can lead to rebound headaches.

Drug Interactions: Sumatriptan is metabolized by monoamine oxidase and should not be used within 2 weeks of MAOIs or SSRIs. Use of sumatriptan should be avoided within 24 hours of ergot alkaloids or any other 5-HT_1 agonist due to risk of vasospastic reactions. Serotonin syndrome is possible when giving sumatriptan with other drugs that increase serotonin levels or activity, including buspirone (BuSpar), other triptans, amphetamines, sibutramine, trazodone, tricyclic antidepressants (TCAs), lithium, duloxetine, venlafaxine, or meperidine. **Herbal/Food**: St. John's wort and feverfew should be avoided during therapy with sumatriptan.

Pregnancy: Category C.

Treatment of Overdose: Few overdoses have been recorded. Treatment of overdose is supportive.

Nursing Responsibilities: Key nursing implications for patients receiving sumatriptan are included in the Nursing Practice Application for Patients Receiving Pharmacotherapy for Migraine Headaches.

Lifespan and Diversity Considerations:

- Carefully assess the older adult patient prior to and after giving the drug. Undetected cardiovascular disease may place the patient at risk for MI or other cardiovascular adverse effects.

Patient and Family Education:

- Do not use this drug if you are pregnant or plan to become pregnant, and use contraception while taking this drug. Triptans are associated with birth defects in animals.

- Do not breast-feed while using this drug without the approval of the health care provider.

- Use this drug exactly as prescribed because overuse can lead to rebound headaches.

Drugs Similar to Sumatriptan (Imitrex)

Other triptans include almotriptan, eletriptan, frovatriptan, naratriptan, rizatriptan, and zolmitriptan. All of the triptans have the same therapeutic effects and spectrum of adverse effects. All of the drugs in this class are pregnancy category C.

Almotriptan (Axert): Almotriptan was approved as an oral antimigraine drug in 2001. The drug is well absorbed and has an onset of action of 1 to 3 hours. The drug is extensively metabolized to inactive metabolites by CYP450 enzymes, and 75% is excreted via the kidneys. Drug–drug interactions with agents metabolized in the liver may occur.

Eletriptan (Relpax): Approved in 2002, eletriptan is a newer triptan with improved GI absorption and a more rapid onset of action than sumatriptan. It also has a longer duration. Less than 10% is excreted via the kidneys, making the drug safe to use in patients with renal impairment. The drug is extensively metabolized by CYP450 enzymes and thus has the potential for drug–drug interactions with agents metabolized in the liver.

Frovatriptan (Frova): Approved in 2001, frovatriptan has the same effects as sumatriptan but has a slow onset and a very long duration. The 26-hour half-life results in less headache recurrence with this drug. This drug is extensively metabolized by hepatic CYP450 enzymes, and the majority is eliminated in the feces.

Naratriptan (Amerge): Approved in 1998, this drug has a relatively slow onset of action (3 to 4 hours) but with a longer duration of action than sumatriptan. This drug is extensively metabolized to inactive metabolites by CYP450 enzymes and is excreted by the kidneys.

Rizatriptan (Maxalt): Approved in 1998, rizatriptan is absorbed more quickly than sumatriptan, with an onset of 60 to 90 minutes. It is available as PO disintegrating tablets

(Maxalt-MLT), which are allowed to dissolve on the tongue and be swallowed with saliva. Hepatic CYP450 enzymes do not significantly metabolize the drug.

Zolmitriptan (Zomig): Zolmitriptan is an oral drug that has the same effects as sumatriptan but is available in additional formulations as a nasal spray and as dissolvable tablets for sublingual (SL) use without water. This drug is metabolized to an active metabolite in the liver, which is responsible for some of its antimigraine activity. Although most adverse effects are mild and transient, zolmitriptan has the highest incidence of adverse effects in the triptan class.

16 Many drug therapies are used for migraine prophylaxis.

Prior to initiation of migraine prophylaxis, patients should attempt lifestyle changes and nonpharmacologic therapies to reduce the frequency of migraines. First and foremost, the patient needs to identify personal triggers for migraines. The nurse can help by guiding the patient through the process of assessing and identifying those personal migraine triggers. Foods are a common culprit, especially those containing nitrates or MSG. Omitting common migraine triggers from the diet is a first step in migraine prophylaxis. Other lifestyle changes that may help include adopting regular sleep patterns and meals, participating in aerobic exercise (start slowly because sudden intense activity may cause headaches), avoiding alcohol (especially red wine), and smoking cessation. Other helpful self-care measures include keeping a diary that notes when headaches start, how long they last, what provides relief, what the response is to the medication, and food intake or stress in the past 24 hours. Relaxation exercises, meditation, yoga, or progressive muscle relaxation may help. Nontraditional therapies may also be useful in preventing migraines in some patients.

Drugs for migraine prophylaxis include various classes of drugs that are discussed in other chapters of this textbook. These include beta-adrenergic blockers, calcium channel blockers, antidepressants, and antiseizure drugs. Because all of these drugs have the potential to produce adverse effects, prophylaxis is only initiated if the incidence of migraines is high and the patient is unresponsive to the drugs used to abort migraines. Example prophylactic antimigraine agents are shown in Table 9. Doses for these drugs are found in the chapters where their primary indication is presented.

TABLE 9 Drugs Used for Migraine Prophylaxis

Drug Class	Examples
Antiseizure drugs	gabapentin (Neurontin)
	topiramate (Topamax)
	valproic acid (Depakene, Depakote)
Beta-adrenergic blockers	atenolol (Tenormin)
	metoprolol (Lopressor)
	propranolol (Inderal)
	timolol (Blocadren)
Calcium channel blockers	nifedipine (Procardia)
	nimodipine (Nimotop)
	verapamil (Isoptin)
Tricyclic antidepressants	amitriptyline (Elavil)
	imipramine (Tofranil)
	protriptyline (Vivactil)
Miscellaneous	methysergide (Sansert)

Preventive treatment is recommended for headaches that occur three or more times a month. Of the various drugs, the beta-adrenergic blocker propranolol (Inderal) is one of the most commonly prescribed, although other drugs in this class have similar effectiveness. The use of beta blockers is particularly beneficial in patients with comorbid conditions such as hypertension or angina.

TCAs, especially amitriptyline (Elavil), have been used for decades to prevent migraines and are preferred for patients who may have a mood disorder or insomnia in addition to their migraines. The antimigraine action of these drugs is independent of their antidepressant action. SSRIs such as fluoxetine (Prozac) have been prescribed off-label for migraines because they exhibit fewer adverse effects than the tricyclics.

Other classes of drugs used for migraine prevention include calcium channel blockers, certain antiseizure drugs, estrogens for menstrual migraines, and miscellaneous agents such as methysergide (Sansert). An extended release form of valproic acid (Stavzor) was approved for migraine prophylaxis in 2008. OnabotulinumtoxinA (Botox), a drug often used to erase facial wrinkles, was approved to treat chronic migraines in 2010.

CONNECTIONS

Complementary and Alternative Therapies
Natural Therapies for Migraines

- Acupuncture has been found to be helpful for headache pain in clinical trials. A trained acupuncturist uses thin, disposable needles at specific points on the body to treat the pain.
- Biofeedback and relaxation training can be learned and used to stop or relieve migraine pain. Biofeedback is a relaxation technique that uses monitors to teach the patient how to respond to stress by controlling responses such as muscle tension.
- Massage and chiropractic therapy may be useful in reducing tension headaches. As stress reduction techniques, they may be useful for migraine prevention, especially by improving sleep quality.

- Riboflavin (vitamin B_2) may reduce the frequency of migraine attacks, but effects develop slowly, up to 3 months for maximum effect. Doses of 400 mg per day produce few adverse effects.
- Coenzyme Q10 may also reduce the frequency of attacks.
- Magnesium supplements may be useful in preventing migraines, especially in people who have low serum magnesium levels.

Source: Used with permission from Mayo Foundation for Medical Education & Research. All Rights Reserved.

CONNECTIONS: NURSING PRACTICE APPLICATION

Patients Receiving Pharmacotherapy for Migraine Headaches

Assessment	Potential Nursing Diagnoses
Baseline assessment prior to administration: • Understand the reason the drug has been prescribed in order to assess for therapeutic effects. • Obtain a complete health history including cardiovascular, neurologic, hepatic, or renal disease, pregnancy, or breast-feeding. Obtain a drug history including allergies, current prescription and OTC drugs, herbal preparations, caffeine, nicotine, and alcohol use. Be alert to possible drug interactions. • Obtain baseline vital signs, apical pulse, level of consciousness, and weight. • Assess level of pain. Use objective screening tools when possible (e.g., Wong-Baker FACES scale for children, numerical rating scale for adults). Assess history of pain and what has worked successfully or not for the patient in the past. • Evaluate appropriate laboratory findings (e.g., CBC, hepatic, or renal function studies). • Assess the patient's ability to receive and understand instructions. Include family and caregivers as needed.	• *Acute Pain* • *Ineffective Health Maintenance* • *Ineffective Coping* • *Deficient Knowledge* (Drug therapy)
Assessment throughout administration: • Assess for desired therapeutic effects (e.g., headache pain is decreased or absent). • Continue monitoring level of consciousness and neurologic symptoms (e.g., numbness or tingling). • Assess vital signs, especially blood pressure and pulse periodically. • Continue periodic monitoring of hepatic and renal function studies. • Assess stress and coping patterns for possible symptom correlation (e.g., existing or perceived stress, duration, coping mechanisms, or remedies). • Assess for and promptly report adverse effects: chest pain or tightness, palpitations, tachycardia, hypertension, dizziness, lightheadedness, confusion, numbness, or tingling in extremities.	

Planning: Patient Goals and Expected Outcomes

The patient will:
• Experience therapeutic effects dependent on the reason the drug is being given (e.g., absent or decreased headache pain, or prevention of acute headache pain from migraine attack).
• Be free from or experience minimal adverse effects.
• Verbalize an understanding of the drug's use, adverse effects, and required precautions.
• Demonstrate proper self-administration of the medication (e.g., dose, timing, and when to notify the provider).

Implementation

Interventions and (Rationales)	Patient-Centered Care
Ensuring therapeutic effects: • Continue assessments as above for therapeutic effects. Give the drug before the start of acute pain when possible. (Consistent use of a pain rating scale by all providers will help quantify the level of pain relief and leads to better pain control. Encourage the patient to start medication before the headache becomes severe for better control. Pain relief begins within several minutes after administration.)	• Teach the patient that pain relief, rather than merely control, is the goal of therapy. • Encourage the patient to take the drug before a headache becomes severe, and to take it consistently as ordered. • Explain the rationale behind the pain rating scale (i.e., it allows consistency among all providers). • Encourage the patient to use additional, nonmedicinal pain relief techniques (e.g., quiet, darkened, cool room).
Minimizing adverse effects: • Monitor blood pressure and pulse periodically, especially in patients at risk for undiagnosed cardiovascular disease. Cardiovascular status should be monitored frequently following the first dose given. (Triptans and ergot alkaloids cause vasoconstriction. Postmenopausal women, men over age 40, smokers, and people with other known coronary artery disease risk factors may be at greatest risk.)	• Instruct the patient to immediately report any chest pain or tightness, or throat pain that is severe or continues following drug dosage.
• Observe for changes in severity, character, or duration of headache. (Sudden severe headaches of "thunderclap" quality can signal subarachnoid hemorrhage. Headaches that differ in quality and are accompanied by such signs as fever, rash, or stiff neck may herald meningitis.)	• Instruct the patient to immediately report changes in character or duration of headache or if accompanied by additional symptoms such as fever, rash, or stiff neck.
• Continue to monitor neurologic status periodically. (Dizziness or lightheadedness may be related to headache, an adverse drug effect, or may signal cerebral ischemia.)	• Instruct the patient to immediately report increasing dizziness, lightheadedness, or blurred vision.

CONNECTIONS: NURSING PRACTICE APPLICATION *(continued)*

• Monitor dietary intake of foods that contain tyramine, caffeine, alcohol, or other food triggers. (Some foods or beverages may trigger an acute migraine. Correlating symptoms with food or beverages assists in avoiding the cause of the headache.)	• Encourage the patient to keep a food diary and correlate symptoms with specific foods or beverages. Teach the patient to avoid or limit foods containing tyramine, such as pickled foods, beer, wine, and aged cheeses, which are often known triggers for migraines.
• Encourage the patient to discuss other methods of migraine control if ergot alkaloids are required for more than short-term use. (Ergot alkaloids cause significant vasoconstriction and cause dependence. Other, safer drugs may be needed for long-term relief of migraines.)	• Instruct the patient to discuss treatment options for long-term migraine relief with the health care provider.
Patient understanding of drug therapy: • Use opportunities during administration of medications and during assessments to discuss the rationale for drug therapy, desired therapeutic outcomes, commonly observed adverse effects, parameters for when to call the health care provider, and any necessary monitoring or precautions. (Using time during nursing care helps to optimize and reinforce key teaching areas.)	• The patient should be able to state the reason for the drug, appropriate dose and scheduling, what adverse effects to observe for, and when to report them.
Patient self-administration of drug therapy: • When administering the medication, instruct the patient, family, or caregiver in the proper self-administration of drug (e.g., take the drug as prescribed when needed). (Utilizing time during nurse-administration of these drugs helps to reinforce teaching.)	• Teach the patient to take the medication before the pain becomes severe or at the first symptoms of a migraine if possible. • Teach the patient the proper administration of subcutaneous medication and have the patient or caregiver return demonstrate the technique. (Pain or redness at the injection site is common but usually disappears within an hour after the dose is taken.) • Instruct the patient that appropriate intranasal dose is one spray into one nostril unless otherwise ordered by health care provider.

Evaluation of Outcome Criteria

Evaluate effectiveness of drug therapy by confirming that patient goals and expected outcomes have been met (see "Planning").

UNDERSTANDING THE CHAPTER

Key Concepts Summary

1 Strategies for pain management have changed during the past two decades.

2 Pain is classified by its duration and its source.

3 Health care providers and patients sometimes hold myths about pain that impede optimum pain management.

4 Pain transmission processes allow multiple targets for pharmacologic intervention.

5 Nonpharmacologic interventions are utilized to reduce and augment analgesic use.

6 The overall goal of pain management is to maintain a patient pain level that allows self-care and activities of daily living.

7 Opioid analgesics exert their effects by interacting with specific receptors in the central nervous system.

8 Opioids are the drugs of choice for moderate to severe pain that cannot be controlled with other classes of analgesics.

9 Mixed agonist and antagonist opioids exhibit moderate analgesia with less risk of dependence than morphine.

10 Nonsteroidal anti-inflammatory drugs are the medications of choice for mild to moderate pain.

11 A few miscellaneous analgesics reduce pain by acting on the central nervous system.

12 Adjuvant analgesics have primary indications other than pain but can enhance analgesia.

13 The primary indication for an opioid antagonist is opioid-induced respiratory depression.

14 Migraines are a severe type of headache related to specific triggers.

15 Analgesics and triptans are the primary classes of drugs used to abort acute migraine pain.

16 Many drug therapies are used for migraine prophylaxis.

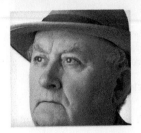

Making the PATIENT Connection

Remember the patient "Larry Smith" at the beginning of the chapter? Now read the remainder of the case study. Based on the information presented within this chapter, respond to the critical thinking questions that follow.

Larry Smith was being seen for an outpatient presurgery work-up the evening before scheduled urologic surgery. The nurse conducts a thorough history and examination related to his back pain and current pain management. His anticipated hospital stay is 2 days postsurgery.

Larry Smith is a 64-year-old male. Vital signs are blood pressure, 108/64 mmHg; pulse, 88 beats/min; respirations, 16 breaths/min. He has a well-healed midline scar on his back from lumbar vertebrae surgery, with a shorter scar over his right iliac crest. He moves a bit slowly with some limited lumbar range of motion. He

also uses a cane for ambulating any distance. He describes his pain as a constant dull ache in the lower back that increases with prolonged standing or walking. Mr. Smith also reports a feeling of "cold electricity" down both legs, with the left greater than the right, which increases with standing and walking, as well as numbness of the middle toes on his left foot. He has been using mixed opioid and nonopioid analgesics for the past 8 years and previously had used SSRI antidepressants as adjuvant for his pain. His current health care provider weaned him off Vicodin ES about a year ago. He now takes methadone 20 mg twice a day. When the pain is not relieved he uses Norco for breakthrough pain. His use of Norco is 1 to 2 per day. Constipation is an ongoing problem, requiring stool softeners and occasional laxatives.

Critical Thinking Questions

1. How should Larry's postoperative pain be managed? Is there a referral the nurse can make to facilitate effective pain management?

2. How could the nurse best communicate Larry's needs to the postoperative nursing staff?

3. What should be included in the care plan for postoperative management of analgesic adverse effects?

See Answers to Critical Thinking Questions on student resource website.

NCLEX-RN® Review

1 The nurse is monitoring the client for adverse effects associated with morphine. Which adverse effects would be the expected? Select all that apply.

1. Respiratory depression
2. Hypertension
3. Urinary retention
4. Constipation
5. Nausea

2 Several days postoperative bowel surgery, the client is eating soft food, ambulating regularly, and using hydrocodone (Vicodin) for pain. What should the nursing care plan include?

1. Monitoring vital signs for respiratory depression.
2. Inserting a urinary catheter for urinary retention.
3. Weaning pain medication to prevent addiction.
4. Increasing dietary fiber and fluids and administering a stool softener if needed.

3 A client who has migraine headaches self-administered sumatriptan (Imitrex) for the first time yesterday. Today, the client informs the nurse that after taking the medication the client began to experience chest pain. The client further states that the drug was effective in relieving the headache. The nurse should:

1. Encourage the client to continue using the drug because it was effective.
2. Advise the client to tell the health care provider about the chest pain at the next visit.
3. Caution the client to contact the health care provider to report the chest pain today and to not use the sumatriptan until talking to the health care provider.
4. Encourage the client to lie down in a quiet room and use cold packs during the next migraine.

4 A client with diabetes reports increasing pain and numbness in his legs. "It feels like pins and needles all the time, especially at night." Which drug would the nurse expect to be prescribed for this client?

1. Ibuprofen (Motrin)
2. Gabapentin (Neurontin)
3. Naloxone (Narcan)
4. Methadone

5 The emergency department nurse is caring for a client with a migraine headache. Which drug would the nurse anticipate administering to abort the client's migraine attack?

1. Morphine
2. Dihydroergotamine (Migranal)
3. Propranolol (Inderal)
4. Ibuprofen (Motrin)

6 The nurse is caring for several clients who are receiving opioids for pain relief. Which client is at the highest risk of developing hypotension, respiratory depression, and mental confusion?

1. A 23-year-old female, postoperative ruptured appendix
2. A 16-year-old male, post–motorcycle injury with lacerations
3. A 54-year-old female, post–myocardial infarction
4. An 86-year-old male, postoperative femur fracture

Additional Case Study

Rita Manson presents to the emergency department with vomiting, severe abdominal and back pain, and jaundice. Her jaundice is recent but the pain and vomiting have continued for a couple of months. Her diagnostic work-up reveals advanced pancreatic cancer with metastasis to the spine.

1. What is the drug of choice for Rita's pain management? Which route of administration would be expected initially?

2. Her prescribed pain medication is morphine sulfate 2 to 10 mg IV every 2 hours as needed for pain. Outline a nursing approach to pain management for the first 24 hours.

3. What adverse effects would the nurse expect?

4. As part of the patient's pain management, dexamethasone (Decadron) 5 mg IV is prescribed every 6 hours for 2 days. Explain the use of corticosteroids in pain management.

5. After several days, Rita expresses her concern about "becoming hooked on that narcotic." How would the nurse respond?

See Answers to Additional Case Study on student resource website.

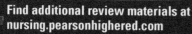

Pearson Nursing Student Resources

Find additional review materials at nursing.pearsonhighered.com

Prepare for success with additional NCLEX®-style practice questions, interactive assignments and activities, web links, animations, videos, and more!

References

Blanda, M., & Wright, J. T. (2010). *Migraine headache.* Retrieved from http://www.emedicine.com/emerg/TOPIC230.HTM

Chou, R., Fanciullo, G. J., Fine, P. G., Adler, J. A., Ballantyne, J. C., Davies, P., et al. American Pain Society-American Academy of Pain Medicine Opioids Guidelines Panel. (2009). Clinical guidelines for the use of chronic opioid therapy in chronic non-cancer pain. *The Journal of Pain, 10*(2), 113–130. doi:10.1016/j.pain.2008.10.008

Freburger, J. K., Holmes, G. M., Agans, R. P., Jackman, A. M., Darter, J. D., Wallace, A. S., et al. (2009). The rising prevalence of chronic low back pain. *Archives of Internal Medicine, 169*(3), 251–258. doi:10.1001/archinternmed.2008.543

Mayo Clinic. (n.d.). *Migraine: Alternative medicine.* Retrieved from http://www.mayoclinic.com/health/migraine-headache/DS00120/DSECTION=alternative-medicine

Voepel-Lewis, T., Zanotti, J., Danmeyer, J. A., & Merkel, S. (2010). Reliability and validity of face, legs, activity, cry, consolability behavioral tool in assessing acute pain in critically ill patients. *American Journal of Critical Care, 19*(1), 55–62. doi:10.4037/ajcc2010624

Selected Bibliography

Brennan, F., Carr, D. B., & Cousins, M. (2007). Pain management: A fundamental human right. *Anesthesia and Analgesia, 105,* 205–221. doi:10.1213/01.ane.0000268145.52345.55

Chawla, J. (2010). *Migraine headache.* Retrieved from http://emedicine.medscape.com/article/1142556-overview

Fine, P. G., & Low, C. M. (2007). *Principles of effective pain management at the end of life.* Retrieved from http://www.medscape.com/viewprogram/6079

Francis, G. J., Becker, W. J., & Pringsheim, T. M. (2010). Acute and preventative treatment of cluster headaches. *Neurology, 75*(5), 463–473. doi:10.1212/WNL.0b013e3181eb58c8

Glickman-Simon, R. (2006). *Persistent pain and palliative care.* Proceedings of the American College of Physicians 2006 Annual Session, April 6–8, 2006, Philadelphia, PA.

Gordon, D. B., Dahl, J. L., Miaskowski, C., McCarberg, B., Todd, K. H., Paice, J. A., et al. (2005). American Pain Society recommendations for improving the quality of acute and cancer pain management. *Archives of Internal Medicine, 165,* 1574–1580. doi:10.1001/archinte.165.14.1574

LeMone, P., & Burke, K. M. (2008). *Medical surgical nursing care: Critical thinking in client care* (4th ed.). Upper Saddle River, NJ: Prentice-Hall.

Merkel, S. I., Voepel-Lewis, T., Shayevitz, J. R., & Malviya, S. (1997). Practice applications of research. The FLACC: A behavioral scale for scoring postoperative pain in young children. *Pediatric Nursing, 23*(2), 293–207.

Pasternak, G. W., Inturrisi, C. E., Porreca, F., & Rowbotham, M. C. (2008). Signal transduction of pain: Implications for opioid therapy. *Medscape Education.* Retrieved from http://www.medscape.com/viewprogram/8437

Pesaturo, K. A., & Wooding, F. G. (2009). Modern management of the migraine headache. *American Journal of Lifestyle Medicine, 3*(2), 147–159. doi:10.1177/1559827608327916

Answers to NCLEX-RN® Review

1 Answer: 1, 3, 4, 5 Rationale: Common adverse effects of opioids include respiratory depression, urinary retention, constipation, and nausea. Option 2 is incorrect. Hypotension, not hypertension, is an adverse effect of opioids. Cognitive Level: Analyzing; Client Need: Physiological Integrity; Nursing Process: Evaluation

2 Answer: 4 Rationale: Opioids decrease peristalsis, and bowel surgery may produce a temporary cessation of peristalsis (paralytic ileus). Both lead to constipation. Once bowel function has returned enough for the client to start eating, constipation is still likely and needs to be prevented by increased dietary fiber and fluids, as well as taking a stool softener. Options 1, 2, and 3 are incorrect. Respiratory depression and urinary retention are not likely after several days with decreasing opioid use. Addiction is not a concern in the treatment of acute pain in this scenario. Cognitive Level: Applying; Client Need: Physiological Integrity; Nursing Process: Planning

3 Answer: 3 Rationale: Chest pain is a serious adverse effect of sumatriptan and needs to be differentiated from angina, which can also be caused by the drug. Options 1, 2, and 4 are incorrect. The client should not use the drug again until she is evaluated by her provider and she should not delay in reporting the chest pain. Reclining in a quiet room with cold packs is a nondrug treatment for migraines, but reporting the chest pain is most important at this time. Cognitive level: Applying; Client Need: Physiological Integrity; Nursing Process: Implementation

4 Answer: 2 Rationale: The client is describing neuropathic pain, which is most likely to respond to the adjuvant analgesic gabapentin, an antiseizure drug used for neuropathic pain. Options 1, 3, and 4 are incorrect. Nonopioids such as ibuprofen, or opioids such as methadone, are less effective at relieving pain that is of neurologic origin. Naloxone is an opioid antagonist and will not relieve the client's pain. Cognitive Level: Applying; Client Need: Physiological Integrity; Nursing Process: Planning

5 Answer: 2 Rationale: Ergot alkaloids such as dihydroergotamine (Migranal) are one of the two drug classes for aborting migraines. Options 1, 3, and 4 are incorrect. Morphine is an opioid agonist and is not effective in aborting migraines. Propranolol is a beta blocker and is used to prevent migraines. Ibuprofen is a nonopioid analgesic that is used to treat mild to moderate pain. Cognitive Level: Applying; Client Need: Physiological Integrity; Nursing Process: Planning

6 Answer: 4 Rationale: Older adult clients are at highest risk for hypotension, respiratory depression, and increased incidence of adverse CNS effects such as confusion. Options 1, 2, and 3 are incorrect. Most 23-year-old clients can tolerate opioids without adverse effects. Individuals who suffer from traumatic injury may receive narcotic analgesia. However, caution should be taken if the individual has also experienced any type of head injury. Opioids are often used with individuals who suffer MI. No adverse effects such as hypotension or respiratory depression are usually present if the dose is appropriate for the size of the client. Cognitive Level: Analyzing; Client Need: Physiological Integrity; Nursing Process: Evaluation

Review of the Cardiovascular System

From Chapter 31 of *Pharmacology: Connections to Nursing Practice*, Second Edition. Michael Patrick Adams, Carol Quam Urban. Copyright © 2013 by Pearson Education, Inc. All rights reserved.

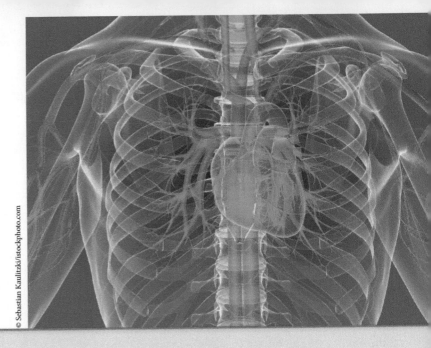

© Sebastian Kaulitzki/istockphoto.com

Review of the Cardiovascular System

Learning Outcomes

After reading this chapter, the student should be able to:

1. Describe the major structures of the cardiovascular system.
2. Identify the components of blood and their functions.
3. Construct a flowchart diagramming the primary steps of hemostasis.
4. Describe the structure of the heart and the function of the myocardium.
5. Describe the role of the coronary arteries in supplying the myocardium with oxygen.
6. Illustrate the flow of electrical impulses through the normal heart.
7. Explain the major factors affecting cardiac output.
8. Explain the effects of cardiac output, peripheral resistance, and blood volume on hemodynamics.
9. Discuss how the vasomotor center, baroreceptors, chemoreceptors, and hormones regulate blood pressure.

Chapter Outline

Structure and Function of the Cardiovascular System

Functions and Properties of Blood

Components of Blood

Hemostasis

Cardiac Structure and Function

Cardiac Muscle

Coronary Arteries

Cardiac Conduction System

Cardiac Output

Hemodynamics and Blood Pressure

Hemodynamic Factors Affecting Blood Pressure

Neural Regulation of Blood Pressure

Hormonal Influences on Blood Pressure

It is likely that the nurse will administer more cardiovascular drugs than any other class of medications. Why is this the case? First, health care providers have discovered the huge benefits of keeping blood pressure and blood lipid values within normal limits and how to prevent heart attacks and strokes. Second, the heart and vessels simply weaken over time and, as the average life span of the population increases, more pharmacotherapy will be needed to treat the cardiovascular diseases of older adults. These two goals of cardiovascular pharmacotherapeutics, prevention and treatment, are used routinely for nearly all people at some stage during their life span.

A comprehensive knowledge of cardiovascular anatomy and physiology is essential to understanding cardiovascular pharmacology. The purpose of this chapter is to offer a brief review of the components of the structure and function of the cardiovascular system that are important to pharmacotherapy. For more comprehensive treatments of these topics, the student should refer to an anatomy and physiology textbook.

Structure and Function of the Cardiovascular System

1 The cardiovascular system consists of the blood, heart, and blood vessels.

The three major components of the cardiovascular system are the blood, heart, and blood vessels, as shown in Figure 1. These three components work as an integrated whole to transport various substances throughout the body, providing the necessary life substances essential to all cells. Disruption of this flow for even brief periods can have serious, if not mortal, consequences. The functions of the cardiovascular system are diverse and include the following:

- Transport of nutrients and wastes
- Pumping of blood
- Regulation of blood pressure
- Regulation of acid–base balance
- Regulation of fluid balance
- Regulation of body temperature
- Protection against invasion by microbes

It must be clearly understood that the cardiovascular system can only function with the cooperation of other body systems. For example, consider the role of the autonomic nervous system in controlling heart rate and blood vessel diameter. The kidneys are intimately involved in assisting the cardiovascular system with fluid and acid–base balance. The respiratory system must bring oxygen to the blood and remove carbon dioxide from it. The student should view the cardiovascular system as an important part of the body's ability to maintain overall homeostasis.

Functions and Properties of Blood

2 Blood consists of formed elements and plasma.

Blood is a fluid tissue that consists of solid, formed elements suspended in plasma. The solid, formed elements of the blood are the erythrocytes, leukocytes, and platelets. When combined, the formed elements comprise about 45% of the composition of blood.

The most numerous blood cells are erythrocytes, which comprise 99.9% of the formed elements. Carrying the iron-containing protein hemoglobin, the erythrocytes are responsible for transporting oxygen to the tissues and carbon dioxide from the tissues to the lungs. Without a nucleus, a single erythrocyte can carry as many as one billion molecules of oxygen. Erythrocyte homeostasis is controlled by **erythropoietin**, a hormone secreted by the kidney in response to low oxygen levels in the blood. Once secreted, erythropoietin stimulates the body's production of erythrocytes. Insufficient numbers of erythrocytes or structural defects such as sickle shapes lead to anemia, which is a common indication for pharmacotherapy.

Although small in number, leukocytes serve an essential role in the body's defense against infection. Unlike erythrocytes, which are all identical, there are several types of leukocytes, each serving a different function. For example, neutrophils are the most common leukocyte and they respond to bacterial infections through phagocytosis of the microbes. The second most common leukocyte, the lymphocyte, is the key cell in the immune response that responds by secreting antibodies (B lymphocytes) or secreting cytokines (T lymphocytes) that rid the body of the microbe. Homeostasis of leukocytes is controlled by different **colony-stimulating factors (CSF)**. Once secreted, CSFs activate existing white blood cells to fight an infection and increase the production of leukocytes. Too few leukocytes, called leukopenia, will make

Key Terms

action potentials

afterload

antidiuretic hormone (ADH)

atrial natriuretic peptide (ANP)

atrial reflex

automaticity

baroreceptors

cardiac output (CO)

chemoreceptors

coagulation

colony-stimulating factors (CSF)

contractility

ectopic foci

erythropoietin

extrinsic pathway

fibrin

fibrinogen

hemopoiesis

hemostasis

inotropic agents

intrinsic pathway

myocardium

peripheral resistance

preload

prothrombin

reflex tachycardia

renin-angiotensin-aldosterone system (RAAS)

sinus rhythm

stroke volume

thrombin

thrombopoietin

vasomotor center

venous return

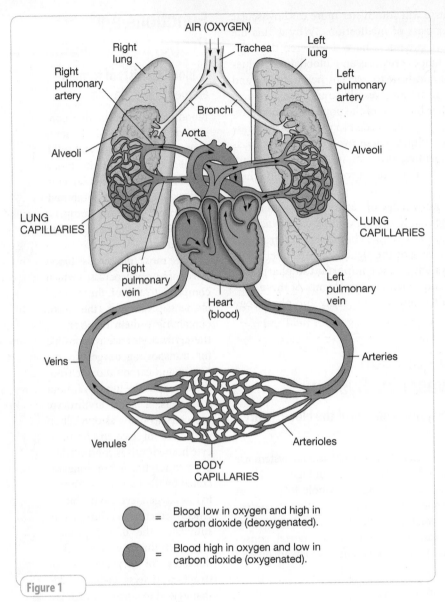

AIR (OXYGEN)

Right lung

Trachea

Left lung

Right pulmonary artery

Left pulmonary artery

Bronchi

Aorta

Alveoli

Alveoli

LUNG CAPILLARIES

LUNG CAPILLARIES

Right pulmonary vein

Left pulmonary vein

Heart (blood)

Veins

Arteries

Venules

Arterioles

BODY CAPILLARIES

= Blood low in oxygen and high in carbon dioxide (deoxygenated).

= Blood high in oxygen and low in carbon dioxide (oxygenated).

Figure 1

The cardiovascular system.

the patient susceptible to infection. Too many leukocytes, called leukocytosis, is a sign of infection, inflammation, or perhaps leukemia. Lymphocyte activation, CSFs, and enhancing body defenses are important topics in pharmacology.

The final formed elements of the blood are thrombocytes or platelets, which are actually fragments of larger cells called megakaryocytes. Platelets stick to the walls of damaged blood vessels to begin the process of blood coagulation, which prevents excessive bleeding from sites of injury. Abnormally low numbers of platelets, or thrombocytopenia, can result in serious delays in blood clotting. Platelet homeostasis is controlled by the hormone **thrombopoietin**, which promotes the formation of additional platelets.

The production and maturation of blood cells, called **hemopoiesis**, or hematopoiesis, occurs in red bone marrow. It is here that primitive stem cells of the blood, which have the capacity to develop into any blood cell type, become committed to becoming an erythrocyte, leukocyte, or platelet. This process occurs continuously throughout the life span and is subject to various homeostatic controls as well as chemical and physical agents. For example, ionizing radiation and a large number of drugs have the potential to adversely affect bone marrow and cause myelosuppression. Myelosuppression is a very serious adverse effect that reduces the number of erythrocytes, leukocytes, and thrombocytes, leaving patients susceptible to anemia, infection, and bleeding. Many agents used to treat cancer and those given to reduce the possibility of transplant rejection can produce profound myelosuppression as a dose-limiting adverse effect.

Plasma is the fluid portion of blood that consists of water and various proteins, electrolytes, lipoproteins, carbohydrates, and other regulatory substances. The primary proteins in plasma are albumins (54%), globulins (38%), and fibrinogen (7%). Albumin is the primary regulator of blood osmotic pressure (also called oncotic pressure), which determines the movement of fluids among the vascular, interstitial, and cellular compartments or spaces. Globulins, also known as immunoglobulins or antibodies, are important in protecting the body from foreign agents such as bacteria or viruses. Fibrinogen is a critical protein in the coagulation of blood. The liver synthesizes over 90% of the plasma proteins; therefore, patients with serious hepatic impairment will have deficiencies in coagulation and in maintaining body defenses.

Normal fluid balance in the body is achieved by maintaining the proper amount of plasma in the blood. Too little water in plasma results in dehydration, whereas too much causes edema and hypertension. Various organs help to maintain normal fluid balance, including the kidneys, gastrointestinal (GI) tract, and skin. The pharmacotherapy of fluid and electrolyte imbalances is an important topic in pharmacology.

CONNECTION Checkpoint 31.1

What role does plasma protein play in the distribution of drugs? *See Answer to Connection Checkpoint 31.1 on student resource website.*

PharmFACT

To maintain homeostasis, the body must make 3 million erythrocytes every second. Red blood cells are so numerous that they comprise approximately one third of all cells in the body (Martini, Nath, & Bartholomew, 2012).

3 Hemostasis is a complex process involving multiple steps and a large number of enzymes and factors.

The process of **hemostasis** is complex, involving 13 different clotting factors that contribute to the stoppage of blood flow. Hemostasis occurs in a series of sequential steps, sometimes referred to as a cascade. Hemostasis is an essential mechanism that the body uses to prevent excessive bleeding following injury. Medications can be used to modify several of these steps, either to speed up or delay the clotting process.

When a blood vessel is injured, the clotting process is initiated. The vessel spasms, causing constriction, which slows blood flow to the injured area. Platelets have an affinity for the damaged vessel: They become sticky and adhere to each other and to the injured area. The clumping of platelets, or aggregation, is facilitated by adenosine diphosphate (ADP), the enzyme thrombin, and thromboxane A_2. Platelet receptor sites and von Willebrand's factor make adhesion possible. The aggregated platelets disintegrate to initiate a platelet binding cascade. Blood flow is further slowed, thus allowing the process of **coagulation**, which is the formation of an insoluble clot, to occur. The basic steps of hemostasis are shown in Figure 2.

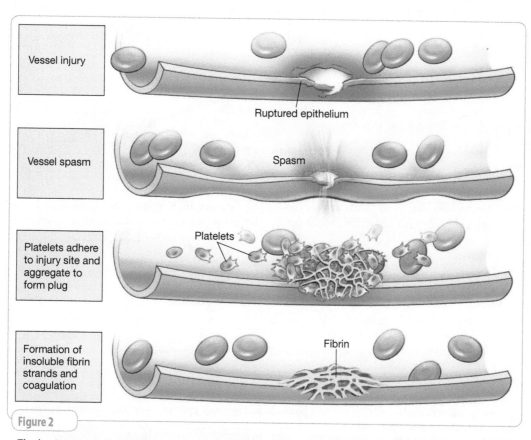

Vessel injury

Ruptured epithelium

Vessel spasm

Spasm

Platelets adhere to injury site and aggregate to form plug

Platelets

Formation of insoluble fibrin strands and coagulation

Fibrin

Figure 2

The basic steps in hemostasis.

When collagen is exposed at the site of injury, the damaged cells initiate the coagulation cascade. Coagulation itself occurs when fibrin threads create a meshwork that fortifies the blood constituents so that clots can develop. During the cascade, various plasma proteins that are circulating in an inactive state are converted to their active forms. Two separate pathways, along with numerous biochemical processes, lead to coagulation. The **intrinsic pathway** is activated in response to injury and takes several minutes to complete. The **extrinsic pathway** is activated when blood leaks out of a vessel and enters tissue spaces. The extrinsic pathway is less complex and is completed within seconds. The two pathways share some common steps and the outcome is the same—the formation of the fibrin clot. The steps in each pathway are shown in Figure 3.

Near the end of the common pathway, a chemical called prothrombin activator (called Active X in Figure 3) is formed.

The prothrombin activator converts the clotting factor **prothrombin** to an enzyme called **thrombin**. Thrombin then converts **fibrinogen**, a plasma protein, to long strands of **fibrin**. The fibrin strands provide a framework to anchor the clot. Thus two of the factors essential to clotting, thrombin and fibrin, are only formed after injury to the vessels. The fibrin strands form an insoluble web over the injured area to stop blood loss. Normal blood clotting occurs in about 6 minutes.

It is important to note that several clotting factors, including thromboplastin and fibrinogen, are proteins made by the liver that are constantly circulating through the blood in an inactive form. Vitamin K, which is made by bacteria residing in the large intestine, is required for the liver to make four of the clotting factors. Because of the crucial importance of the liver in creating these clotting factors, patients with serious hepatic disorders often have abnormal coagulation.

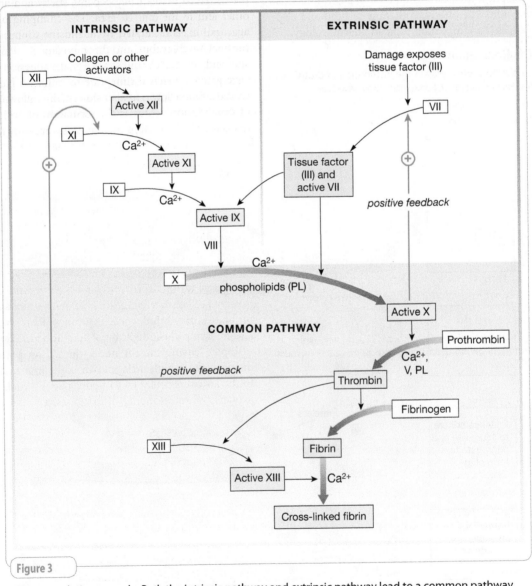

Figure 3

The coagulation cascade. Both the intrinsic pathway and extrinsic pathway lead to a common pathway and eventually a dense fibrin clot.

Source: From SILVERTHORN, DEE UNGLAUB, HUMAN PHYSIOLOGY: AN INTEGRATED APPROACH, 5th Ed., © 2010. Reprinted and electronically reproduced by permission of Pearson Education, Inc., Upper Saddle River, New Jersey.

Cardiac Structure and Function

4 The heart is responsible for pumping blood throughout the circulatory system.

The heart is the hardest working organ in the body, pumping blood from before birth to the last minute of life. With the massive, continuous workload, it is not surprising that this organ weakens over time and that heart disease is the leading cause of death in the United States. The heart is a frequent target for pharmacotherapy.

The heart may be thought of as a thick, specialized muscle. The muscular layer, called the **myocardium**, is the thickest of the heart layers and is responsible for the physical pumping action of the heart. The thickness of the myocardium varies throughout the different regions of the heart in proportion to its function. Because the ventricles perform the most work, the myocardium is thickest there. Cardiac muscle is a highly specialized tissue that is unlike either skeletal muscle or smooth muscle. Extensive branching networks of cellular structures connect cardiac muscle cells to each other, allowing the entire myocardium to contract as a coordinated whole.

Should cardiac cells, or myocytes die, the body is unable to replace them with new cardiac muscle cells. If a large area becomes deprived of oxygen and undergoes necrosis, the cells are replaced by fibrotic scar tissue and cardiac function may be impaired. The different regions of the heart may not contract in a coordinated manner because conduction of the electrical potential may skip over spots on the myocardium where no conduction occurs. This can result in heart failure or dysrhythmias, which are frequent indications for pharmacotherapy.

The heart has four chambers that receive blood prior to being pumped, as illustrated in Figure 4b. These chambers differ in size, depending on their function. The left ventricle is the largest, because it must hold enough blood to pump to all body tissues. During heart failure, the size of the left ventricle and the thickness of the myocardial layer in this chamber can increase in size in patients, which is a condition known as left ventricular hypertrophy.

PharmFACT

The heart pumps about 8,000 liters of blood every day, which is enough to fill forty, 55-gallon drums or 8,800 quart-size containers (Martini et al., 2012).

5 The coronary arteries bring essential nutrients to the myocardium.

Working continuously around the clock, the heart requires a bountiful supply of oxygen and other nutrients. These are provided by the right and left coronary arteries and their branches, as shown in Figure 4a. The coronary arteries must have the ability to rapidly adapt to the heart's needs for oxygen. For example, during exercise the heart rate and strength of contraction markedly increase, and the coronary arteries must be able to quickly dilate to provide oxygen to meet this increased workload placed on the myocardium.

As critical vessels, the coronary arteries serve a major role in maintaining body health. Should these arteries be unable to deliver essential nutrients, the myocardium will be affected either immediately, such as during intense exercise, or slowly, over a period of many years. The coronary arteries are subject to atherosclerosis, a buildup of fatty plaque, which narrows the lumen and restricts the amount of blood supply reaching the myocardium. If allowed to progress, the narrowing results in chest pain on exertion, a condition known as angina pectoris.

The coronary arteries are important targets for pharmacotherapy. Reducing lipid levels in the blood can decrease the risk of atherosclerosis of the coronary arteries (and other arteries). Drugs can be used to reduce angina pain and decrease the risk of mortality following a heart attack. There are also drugs that reduce the cardiac workload in patients with heart failure so that the heart does not require as much oxygen from the coronary arteries.

6 The cardiac conduction system keeps the heart beating in a synchronized manner.

For the heart to function properly, the atria must contract simultaneously, sending their blood into the ventricles. Following atrial contraction, the right and left ventricles then must contract simultaneously. Lack of synchronization of the atria and ventricles or of the right and left sides of the heart may have profound consequences. Proper timing of chamber contractions is made possible by the cardiac conduction system, a branching network of specialized cardiac muscle cells that sends a synchronized, electrical signal across the myocardium. These electrical impulses, or **action potentials**, carry the signal for the cardiac muscle cells to contract and must be coordinated precisely for the chambers to beat in a synchronized manner. The cardiac conduction system is illustrated in Figure 5.

Control of the cardiac conduction system begins in a small area of tissue in the wall of the right atrium known as the sinoatrial (SA) node or cardiac pacemaker. The SA node has the property of **automaticity**, which is the ability to spontaneously generate an action potential. The SA node generates a new action potential approximately 75 times per minute under resting conditions. This is referred to as the normal **sinus rhythm**. The SA node is greatly influenced by the activity of the sympathetic and parasympathetic divisions of the autonomic nervous system.

Upon leaving the SA node, the action potential travels quickly across both atria and through internodal pathways to the atrioventricular (AV) node. The AV node also has the property of automaticity, although less so than the SA node. Should the SA node malfunction, the AV node has the ability to spontaneously generate action potentials and continue the heart's contraction at a rate of 40 to 60 beats per minute. Compared to other areas in the heart, impulse conduction through the AV node is slow. This allows the atria sufficient time to completely contract and empty their blood before the ventricles receive their signal to contract. If the ventricles should contract prematurely, the AV valves will close and the atria will be prevented from completely emptying their contents.

As the action potential leaves the AV node, it travels rapidly to the AV bundle or bundle of His. The pathway between the AV node and the bundle of His is the only electrical connection between the atria and the ventricles. The impulse is

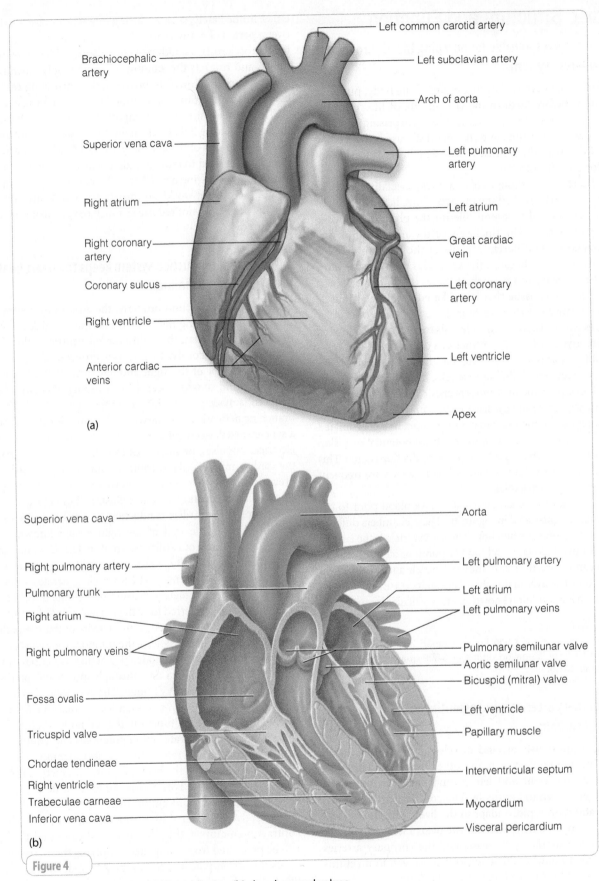

Left common carotid artery

Brachiocephalic artery

Left subclavian artery

Arch of aorta

Superior vena cava

Left pulmonary artery

Right atrium

Left atrium

Right coronary artery

Great cardiac vein

Coronary sulcus

Left coronary artery

Right ventricle

Anterior cardiac veins

Left ventricle

Apex

(a)

Superior vena cava

Aorta

Right pulmonary artery

Left pulmonary artery

Pulmonary trunk

Left atrium

Right atrium

Left pulmonary veins

Right pulmonary veins

Pulmonary semilunar valve

Aortic semilunar valve

Bicuspid (mitral) valve

Fossa ovalis

Left ventricle

Tricuspid valve

Papillary muscle

Chordae tendineae

Right ventricle

Interventricular septum

Trabeculae carneae

Myocardium

Inferior vena cava

Visceral pericardium

(b)

Figure 4

The heart: (a) coronary arteries and veins; (b) chambers and valves.

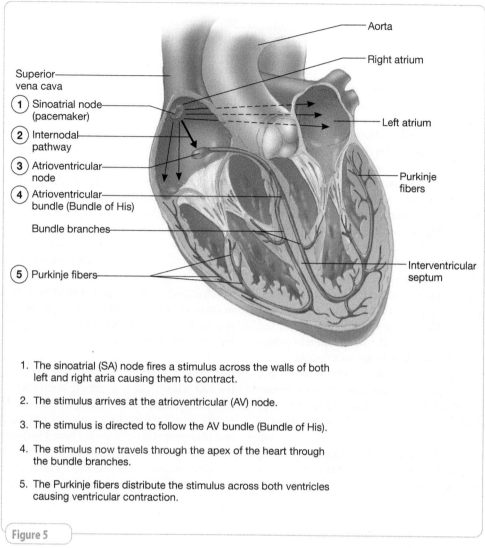

Superior vena cava

1. Sinoatrial node (pacemaker)
2. Internodal pathway
3. Atrioventricular node
4. Atrioventricular bundle (Bundle of His)

Bundle branches

5. Purkinje fibers

Aorta

Right atrium

Left atrium

Purkinje fibers

Interventricular septum

1. The sinoatrial (SA) node fires a stimulus across the walls of both left and right atria causing them to contract.

2. The stimulus arrives at the atrioventricular (AV) node.

3. The stimulus is directed to follow the AV bundle (Bundle of His).

4. The stimulus now travels through the apex of the heart through the bundle branches.

5. The Purkinje fibers distribute the stimulus across both ventricles causing ventricular contraction.

Figure 5

The cardiac conduction system.

conducted down the right and left bundle branches to the Purkinje fibers, which rapidly carry the action potential to all regions of the ventricles almost simultaneously. Should the SA and AV nodes become nonfunctional, cells in the AV bundle and Purkinje fibers can continue to generate myocardial contractions at a rate of about 30 beats per minute.

Although action potentials normally begin at the SA node and spread across the myocardium in a coordinated manner, other regions of the heart may also initiate beats. These areas, known as **ectopic foci** or *ectopic pacemakers*, may send impulses across the myocardium that competes with those from the normal conduction pathway. The timing and synchronization of atrial and ventricular contractions may be affected. Although healthy hearts occasionally experience an extra beat without incident, ectopic foci in diseased hearts have the potential to cause dysrhythmias, or disorders of cardiac rhythm. The events associated with the cardiac conduction system are recorded on an electrocardiogram (ECG).

It is important to understand that the underlying purpose of the cardiac conduction system is to keep the heart beating in a regular, synchronized manner so that cardiac output can be maintained. Dysrhythmias that profoundly affect cardiac output have the potential to produce serious, if not mortal, consequences. These types of dysrhythmias require pharmacologic intervention.

7 Cardiac output is determined by stroke volume and heart rate.

To understand how medications act on the heart and to predict the consequences of pharmacotherapy, it is essential to have a comprehensive knowledge of normal cardiac physiology. This includes a thorough understanding of factors that determine the amount of blood pumped by the heart and the forces acting on the chambers.

The amount of blood pumped by each ventricle per minute is the **cardiac output (CO)**. The average CO is 5 L/minute. CO may be calculated by multiplying stroke volume by the heart rate.

CO = stroke volume (mL/beat) × heart rate (beats/minute)

Stroke volume: **Stroke volume** is the amount of blood pumped by a ventricle in a single contraction. What types of factors might cause a ventricle to eject more blood during a contraction? To understand these factors, a simple comparison to a rubber band is useful. If you stretch a small rubber band 2 inches, it will snap back with a certain force. Stretching the band 4 inches will cause it to snap back with greater force. The force of the snap will continue to increase up to a certain limit, after which the rubber band has been stretched as far as possible and has reached maximum force (or it breaks!).

Cardiac muscle fibers are analogous to rubber bands. If you fill the chambers with more blood, the fibers will have more stretch and will "snap back" with greater force. This is known as Starling's law of the heart: The strength (force) of contraction, or **contractility**, is proportional to the muscle fiber length (stretch). The contractility determines the amount of blood ejected per beat, or the stroke volume. The degree to which the ventricles are filled with blood and the myocardial fibers are stretched just prior to contraction is called **preload**. Up to a physiological limit, drugs that increase preload and contractility will increase the CO. In addition to preload, the force of contraction can be increased by activation of beta$_1$-adrenergic receptors in the autonomic nervous system.

What causes the chambers to fill up with more blood, become stretched (more preload), and contract with greater force? Although several factors affect preload, the most important is **venous return**: the volume of blood returning to the heart from the veins. Giving a drug that constricts veins will increase venous return to the heart, as will simply increasing the total amount of blood in the vascular system (increased blood volume). Drugs or other mechanisms that constrict veins or increase blood volume will therefore increase stroke volume and CO. Conversely, drugs that dilate veins or reduce blood volume will lower CO.

Factors that increase cardiac contractility are called positive **inotropic agents**. Examples of positive inotropic agents include epinephrine, norepinephrine, thyroid hormone, and dopamine. Factors that decrease cardiac contractility are called negative inotropic agents. Examples include quinidine and beta-adrenergic antagonists such as propranolol.

A second primary factor affecting stroke volume is afterload. In order for the left ventricle to pump blood out of the heart, it must overcome a substantial "back pressure" in the aorta. **Afterload** is the systolic pressure in the aorta that must be overcome for blood to be ejected from the left ventricle. As afterload increases, the heart pumps less blood, and stroke volume (and thus CO) decreases. The most common cause of increased afterload is an increase in systemic blood pressure, or hypertension (HTN). HTN creates an increased workload on the heart, which explains why patients with chronic HTN are more likely to experience heart failure. Antihypertensive drugs create less afterload, increase stroke volume, and result in less workload for the heart. Preload and afterload are illustrated in Figure 6.

Heart rate: Heart rate is the second primary factor determining CO. Heart rate is generally controlled by the autonomic nervous system, which makes the minute-by-minute adjustments demanded by the circulatory system. Both sympathetic and parasympathetic fibers are found in the SA node, and heart rate is determined by which fibers are firing at a greater rate at any given moment. Circulating hormones such as epinephrine and thyroid hormone also affect heart rate. In theory, drugs

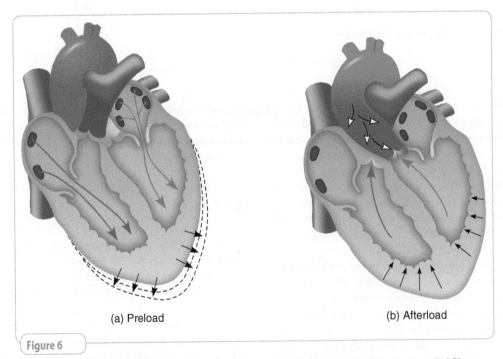

(a) Preload

(b) Afterload

Figure 6

(a) Preload is the degree to which the ventricles are filled with blood and the myocardial fibers are stretched just prior to contraction. (b) Afterload is the systolic pressure in the aorta that must be overcome for blood to be ejected from the left ventricle.

that increase heart rate will increase CO, although compensatory mechanisms may prevent this effect (see Section 8). In addition, a very rapid heart rate may not give the chambers sufficient time to completely fill, thus reducing CO.

CONNECTION Checkpoint 31.2

Predict what effect the following would have on heart rate: sympathomimetics, parasympathomimetics, adrenergic agonists, and anticholinergics. *See Answer to Connection Checkpoint 31.2 on student resource website.*

Hemodynamics and Blood Pressure

8 The primary factors responsible for blood pressure are cardiac output, peripheral resistance, and blood volume.

The homeostatic regulation of blood pressure is a key topic in pharmacology because HTN is so prevalent in the population. Regulation of blood pressure is complex with many diverse factors, both local and systemic, interacting to maintain adequate blood flow to the tissues. The three primary factors that regulate arterial blood pressure—CO, peripheral resistance, and blood volume are shown in Figure 7. The following simple formula should be memorized (as well as understood) because it will help the student predict the actions and adverse effects of many classes of cardiovascular medications:

$$\text{Blood pressure} = \text{CO} \times \text{peripheral resistance}$$

CO is determined by heart rate and stroke volume as discussed in Section 7. From the preceding equation, it is easy to see that as CO increases, blood pressure also increases. This is important to pharmacology because medications that change the CO, stroke volume, or heart rate have the potential to influence a patient's blood pressure.

As blood flows at high speeds through the vascular system, it exerts force against the walls of the vessels. Although the endothelial lining of the blood vessel is extremely smooth, friction reduces the velocity of blood flow. Further friction is encountered as the stream of fast-moving blood narrows to enter smaller vessels, divides into two channels (arteries), or encounters fatty deposits on the vessel walls (plaque). Blood flow may become turbulent, which is a chaotic, tumbling motion that greatly increases friction. The friction that blood encounters in the arteries is called **peripheral resistance**. Arteries have smooth muscle in their walls, which can control the total peripheral resistance. For example, if arteries constrict, their inside diameter or lumen will become smaller and create more resistance and higher blood pressure. A large number of medications affect vascular smooth muscle. Some of these agents cause vessels to constrict, thus raising blood pressure, whereas others relax smooth muscle, thereby opening the lumen and lowering blood pressure.

An additional factor responsible for blood pressure is the total amount of blood in the vascular system, or blood volume. Although the average person maintains a relatively constant blood volume of approximately 5 L, this can change due to many regulatory factors, certain disease states, and pharmacotherapy. More fluid in the vascular system increases venous pressure and venous return to the heart, thus increasing CO and arterial blood pressure. Drugs are frequently used to adjust blood volume. For example, infusion of intravenous (IV) fluids quickly increases blood volume and raises blood pressure. This is used to advantage when treating hypotension due to shock. On the other hand, diuretics cause fluid loss through urination, thus decreasing blood volume and lowering blood pressure.

PharmFACT

It is estimated that all the blood vessels in an adult stretch through about 60,000 miles of internal body landscape (Marieb & Hoehn, 2010).

9 Neural regulation of blood pressure includes baroreceptor and chemoreceptor reflexes.

It is critical for the body to maintain a normal range of blood pressure, and for it to be able to safely and rapidly change pressure as it proceeds through daily activities such as sleep and

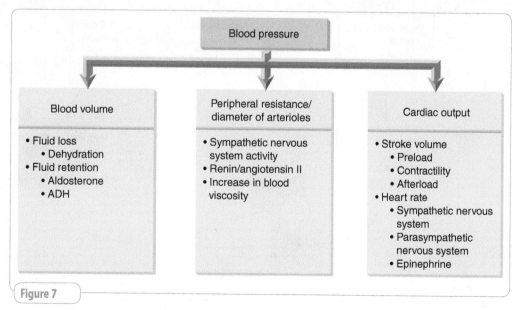

Figure 7

The primary factors affecting blood pressure.

exercise. Hypotension can cause dizziness and lack of adequate urine formation, whereas extreme HTN can cause vessels to rupture and result in ischemia of critical organs. Figure 8 illustrates how the body maintains homeostasis during periods of blood pressure change.

The central and autonomic nervous systems are intimately involved in regulating blood pressure. On a minute-to-minute basis, blood pressure is regulated by a cluster of neurons in the medulla oblongata called the **vasomotor center**. Sensory receptors in the aorta and the internal carotid artery provide the vasomotor center with vital information on conditions in the vascular system. **Baroreceptors** have the ability to sense pressure within large vessels, whereas **chemoreceptors** recognize levels of oxygen, carbon dioxide, and the acidity or pH in the blood. The vasomotor center reacts to information from baroreceptors and chemoreceptors by raising or lowering blood pressure accordingly. Nerves travel from the vasomotor center to the arteries, where the smooth muscle is directed to either constrict (raise blood pressure) or relax (lower blood pressure). Sympathetic outflow from the vasomotor center stimulates alpha$_1$-adrenergic receptors on arterioles, causing vasoconstriction. Alpha$_2$-adrenergic agonists can also decrease blood pressure by their central effects on the vasomotor center.

The baroreceptor reflex is an important mechanism used by the body for making rapid adjustments to blood pressure. If pressure in the vascular system increases, the baroreceptors in the aortic arch and carotid sinus trigger reflexes that constrict the arterioles and veins and accelerate the heart rate. Together, these actions return blood pressure to normal levels within seconds.

Drugs that raise or lower blood pressure can trigger the baroreceptor reflex. For example, antihypertensives administered by the IV route cause an immediate reduction in blood pressure that is recognized by the baroreceptors. The baroreceptors respond by attempting to return blood pressure back to the original levels. The resulting accelerated heart rate, or **reflex tachycardia**, may cause the patient to experience palpitations. The baroreceptors are not able to offer a continuous or sustained reduction in blood pressure. Continued administration of an antihypertensive drug will "overcome" the reflex.

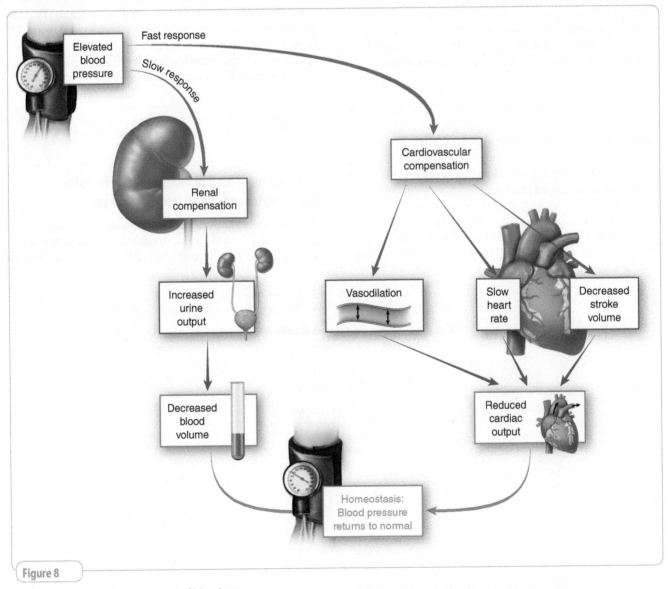

Figure 8

Cardiovascular and renal control of blood pressure.

In addition, with aging or certain disease states such as diabetes, the baroreceptor response may be diminished.

Another example of the baroreceptor reflex occurs when baroreceptors in the right atrium are triggered. These receptors recognize excess stretching of the right atrium, such as might occur when large amounts of IV fluids are administered. The **atrial reflex** causes the heart rate and CO to increase until the backlog of venous blood (or IV fluid) is distributed throughout the body.

The chemoreceptor reflex can also significantly affect blood pressure. Sensors in the carotid sinus and near the aortic arch recognize levels of oxygen and carbon dioxide and the acidity (pH) in the blood. Triggering these chemoreceptors activates the sympathetic nervous system and causes heart rate and CO to increase. The purpose of this reflex is to circulate blood faster so that the respiratory system can remove excess carbon dioxide (which returns pH to normal levels) and add more oxygen to the blood.

CONNECTION Checkpoint 31.3

Many autonomic drugs dilate or constrict blood vessels. Which class of autonomic drugs is most commonly prescribed for HTN? *See Answer to Connection Checkpoint 31.3 on student resource website.*

10 Hormones may have profound effects on blood pressure.

Several hormones affect blood pressure, and certain classes of medications are given to either enhance or block the actions of these hormones. For example, injection of the catecholamines

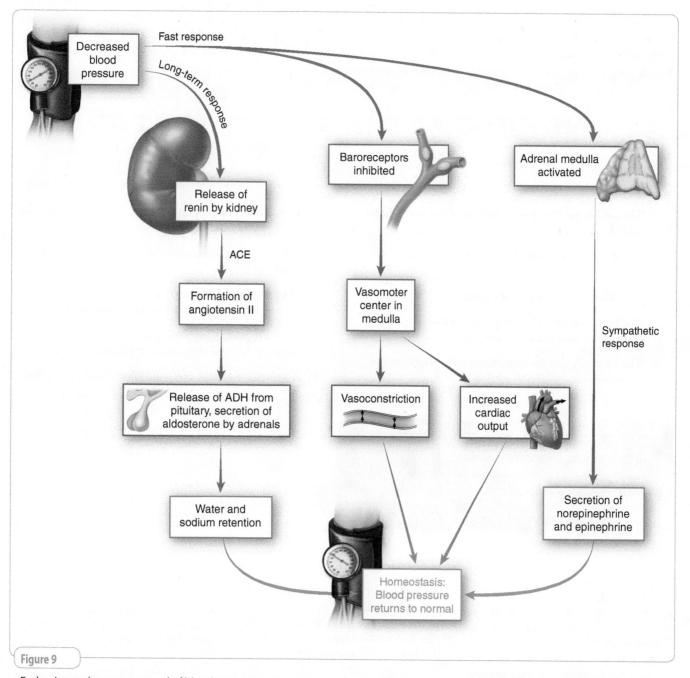

Figure 9

Endocrine and nervous control of blood pressure.

epinephrine or norepinephrine will immediately raise blood pressure, which is essential for patients experiencing shock.

Antidiuretic hormone (ADH) is a hormone released by the posterior pituitary gland when blood pressure falls or when the osmotic pressure of the blood increases. ADH, also known as vasopressin, is a potent peripheral vasoconstrictor that quickly increases blood pressure. The hormone also acts on the kidneys to conserve water and increase blood volume, thereby causing blood pressure to increase.

The **renin-angiotensin-aldosterone system (RAAS)** is particularly important in the drug therapy of HTN. As blood pressure falls, the enzyme renin is released by the kidneys. Through a two-step pathway, angiotensin II is formed, which subsequently increases CO and constricts arterioles to return blood pressure to original levels. Angiotensin II also promotes the release of aldosterone from the adrenal gland, which causes sodium and water retention. Drugs that block the RAAS are key drugs in the treatment of HTN and heart failure.

Atrial natriuretic peptide (ANP) is a hormone that is secreted by specialized cells in the right atrium when large increases in blood volume produce excessive stretch on the atrial wall. ANP has multiple effects, all of which attempt to return blood pressure to original levels. Sodium ion transport in the kidney is affected, resulting in enhanced sodium and water excretion. The release of ADH and aldosterone is suppressed by ANP. In addition, ANP reduces sympathetic outflow from the central nervous system, resulting in dilation of peripheral arteries. A summary of the various nervous and hormone factors influencing blood pressure is shown in Figure 9.

UNDERSTANDING THE CHAPTER

Key Concepts Summary

1 The cardiovascular system consists of the blood, heart, and blood vessels.

2 Blood consists of formed elements and plasma.

3 Hemostasis is a complex process involving multiple steps and a large number of enzymes and factors.

4 The heart is responsible for pumping blood throughout the circulatory system.

5 The coronary arteries bring essential nutrients to the myocardium.

6 The cardiac conduction system keeps the heart beating in a synchronized manner.

7 Cardiac output is determined by stroke volume and heart rate.

8 The primary factors responsible for blood pressure are cardiac output, peripheral resistance, and blood volume.

9 Neural regulation of blood pressure includes baroreceptor and chemoreceptor reflexes.

10 Hormones may have profound effects on blood pressure.

Pearson Nursing Student Resources

Find additional review materials at nursing.pearsonhighered.com

Prepare for success with additional NCLEX®-style practice questions, interactive assignments and activities, web links, animations, videos, and more!

References

Marieb, E. N., & Hoehn, K. (2010). *Human anatomy and physiology* (8th ed.). San Francisco, CA: Benjamin Cummings.

Martini, F. H., Nath, J. L., & Bartholomew, E. F. (2012). *Fundamentals of human anatomy and physiology* (9th ed.). San Francisco, CA: Benjamin Cummings.

Silverthorn, D. U. (2010). *Human physiology: An integrated approach* (5th ed.). San Francisco, CA: Benjamin Cummings.

Selected Bibliography

Krogh, D. (2011). *Biology: A guide to the natural world* (5th ed.). San Francisco, CA: Benjamin Cummings.

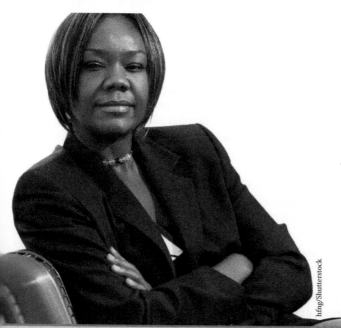

"My mother had it and my grandmother had it too. Now, I'm told that I have it. My doctor says my cholesterol level is too high."

Patient "Belinda Cummings"

hfng/Shutterstock

Pharmacotherapy of Hyperlipidemia

Chapter Outline

Types of Lipids and Lipoproteins

Measurement and Control of Serum Lipids

Drugs for Dyslipidemias

HMG-CoA Reductase Inhibitors

PROTOTYPE **Atorvastatin (Lipitor)**

Bile Acid Sequestrants

PROTOTYPE **Cholestyramine (Questran)**

Niacin

Fibric Acid Agents

PROTOTYPE **Gemfibrozil (Lopid)**

Cholesterol Absorption Inhibitors

Learning Outcomes

After reading this chapter, the student should be able to:

1. Summarize the link between high blood cholesterol, low-density lipoprotein levels, and atherosclerosis.

2. Compare and contrast the different types of lipids.

3. Illustrate how lipids are transported through the blood.

4. Compare and contrast the clinical importance of the different types of lipoproteins.

5. Give examples of how cholesterol and low-density lipoprotein levels can be controlled with nonpharmacologic means.

6. For each of the classes shown in the chapter outline, identify the prototype and representative drugs and explain the mechanism(s) of drug action, primary indications, contraindications, significant drug interactions, pregnancy category, and important adverse effects.

7. Categorize antihyperlipidemic drugs based on their classification and mechanism of action.

8. Explain the nurse's role in the safe administration of drugs for lipid disorders.

9. Apply the nursing process to care for patients receiving pharmacotherapy for lipid disorders.

From Chapter 32 of *Pharmacology: Connections to Nursing Practice*, Second Edition. Michael Patrick Adams, Carol Quam Urban. Copyright © 2013 by Pearson Education, Inc. All rights reserved.

Key Terms

apoprotein

atherosclerosis

dyslipidemia

high-density lipoprotein
(HDL)

HMG-CoA
reductase

hypercholesterolemia

hyperlipidemia

hypertriglyceridemia

lecithins

lipoproteins

low-density lipoprotein
(LDL)

phospholipids

reverse cholesterol
transport

rhabdomyolysis

steroids

sterol nucleus

triglycerides

very low-density
lipoprotein
(VLDL)

Research during the 1970s and 1980s brought about a nutritional revolution as new knowledge about lipids and their relationships to obesity and cardiovascular disease allowed people to make more intelligent lifestyle choices. Since then advances in the diagnosis of lipid disorders have helped to identify those people at greatest risk for cardiovascular disease and those most likely to benefit from pharmacologic intervention. As a result of this knowledge and from advancements in pharmacology, the incidence of death due to most cardiovascular diseases has been declining, although cardiovascular disease remains the leading cause of death in the United States.

Types of Lipids and Lipoproteins

1 Lipids are classified as triglycerides, phospholipids, or sterols.

There are three types of lipids that are important to human physiology, as illustrated in Figure 1. The most common types are **triglycerides** or neutral fats, which form a large family of different lipids, all having three fatty acids attached to a chemical backbone of glycerol. Triglycerides are the major storage form of fat in the body and the only type of lipid that serves as an important energy source. They account for 90% of the total lipids in the body.

A second class, the **phospholipids**, is formed when a phosphorous group replaces one of the fatty acids in a triglyceride. This class of lipids is essential to building plasma membranes. The best known phospholipids are **lecithins**, which are found in high concentration in egg yolks and soybeans. Once promoted as a natural treatment for high cholesterol levels, controlled studies have not shown lecithin to be of benefit for this disorder. Likewise, lecithin has been proposed as a remedy for nervous system diseases such as Alzheimer's disease and bipolar disorder, but there is no definitive evidence to support these claims.

The third class of lipids, the **steroids**, is a diverse group of substances having a common **sterol nucleus** or ring structure. Cholesterol is the most widely known of the steroids, and its role in promoting **atherosclerosis** has been clearly demonstrated. Atherosclerosis is the presence of plaque—a fatty, fibrous material within the walls of the coronary arteries. Unlike the triglycerides that provide fuel for the body, cholesterol is a vital component of plasma membranes and serves as a building block for essential biochemicals, including vitamin D,

bile acids, cortisol, estrogen, and testosterone. Although clearly essential for life, the body needs only minute amounts of cholesterol because the liver is able to synthesize adequate amounts from other chemicals. It is not necessary, nor desirable, to provide excess cholesterol in the diet. The dietary sources of cholesterol are obtained solely from animal products; humans do not absorb the sterols produced by plants. The American Heart Association recommends less than 300 mg of dietary cholesterol per day.

2 Lipoproteins are important predictors of cardiovascular disease.

Because lipid molecules are not soluble in plasma, they must be specially packaged for transport through the blood. To accomplish this, the body forms complexes called **lipoproteins**, which consist of various amounts of cholesterol, triglycerides, and phospholipids bound to carrier proteins. The protein component is called an **apoprotein** (*apo-* means "separated from" or "derived from"). The four apoproteins important to lipid transport are known as A-I, A-II, A-IV, and B-100.

Lipoproteins are classified according to their composition, size, and weight or density, which come primarily from the amount of apoprotein present in the complex. Each type varies in lipid and apoprotein makeup and serves a different function in transporting lipids from the sites of synthesis and absorption to the sites of utilization. For example, **high-density lipoprotein (HDL)** contains the most apoprotein, up to 50% by weight. The highest amount of cholesterol is carried by **low-density lipoprotein (LDL)**. Figure 2 illustrates the three basic lipoproteins and their compositions.

To understand the pharmacotherapy of lipid disorders, it is important to know the functions of the major lipoproteins and their roles in transporting cholesterol. LDL transports cholesterol from the liver to the tissues and organs, where it is used to build plasma membranes or to synthesize other steroids. Once in the tissues it can also be stored for later use. Storage of cholesterol in the lining of blood vessels, however, is not desirable because it contributes to plaque buildup. LDL is often called "bad" cholesterol because this lipoprotein contributes significantly to plaque deposits and coronary artery disease (CAD). Sixty to seventy percent of the cholesterol circulating in the blood is found in LDL.

Very low-density lipoprotein (VLDL) is the primary carrier of triglycerides in the blood. VLDLs account for virtually all triglycerides being transported from the liver to storage in adipose tissue. Through a series of steps, VLDL is reduced in size to become LDL. Lowering LDL levels in the blood has been shown to decrease the incidence of CAD.

HDL is manufactured in the liver and small intestine and assists in the transport of excess cholesterol away from the body tissues and back to the liver for metabolism in a process known as **reverse cholesterol transport**. The cholesterol component of the HDL is then broken down to unite with bile, which is subsequently excreted in the feces. Excretion via bile is the only route the body uses to remove cholesterol. Because HDL transports cholesterol for destruction and removes it from the body, it is considered "good" cholesterol. Patients

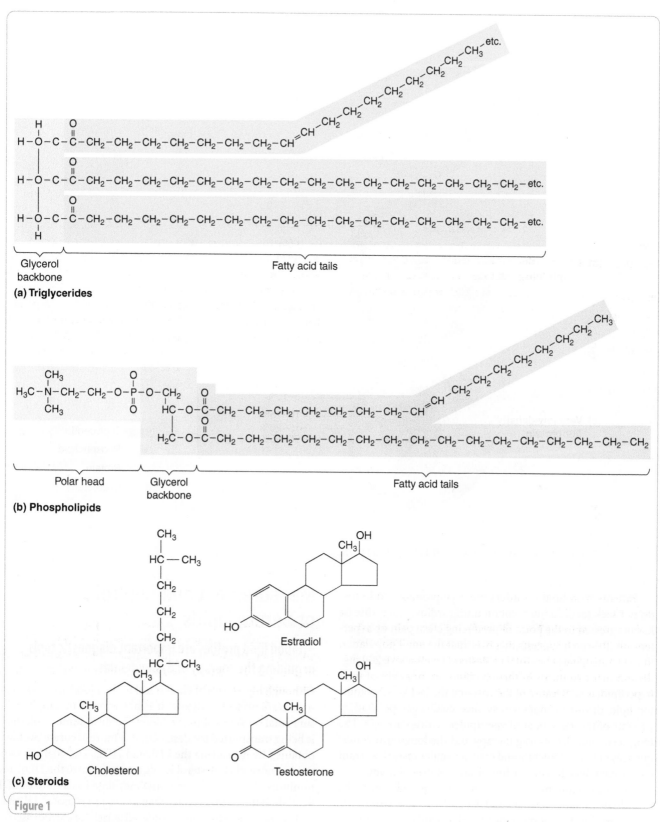

(a) Triglycerides

Glycerol backbone

Fatty acid tails

(b) Phospholipids

Polar head

Glycerol backbone

Fatty acid tails

(c) Steroids

Estradiol

Cholesterol

Testosterone

Figure 1

Chemical structure of lipids.

with insufficient amounts of HDL are at risk for atherosclerosis, even if their total cholesterol levels are normal.

Several terms are used to describe lipid disorders. **Hyperlipidemia** is the general term meaning high levels of lipids in the blood. The term hyperlipidemia, however, does not specify which lipid is elevated. Elevated blood cholesterol, or **hypercholesterolemia**, is the type of hyperlipidemia that is most familiar to the general public. **Dyslipidemia** is the term that refers to abnormal (excess or deficient) levels of lipoproteins. Some patients exhibit an increase in triglyceride levels known as **hypertriglyceridemia**.

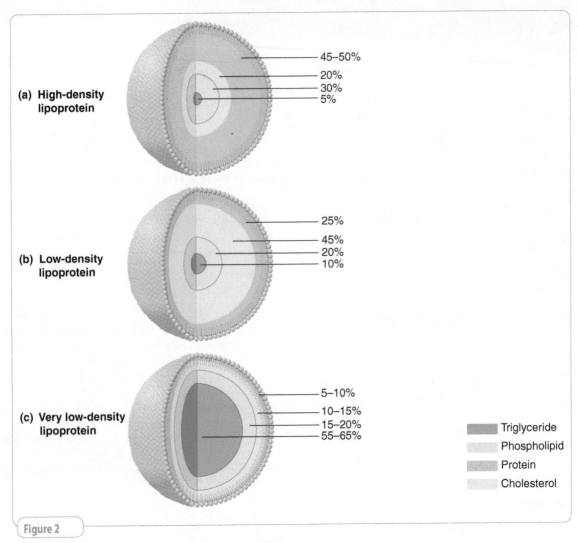

(a) **High-density lipoprotein**

45–50%
20%
30%
5%

(b) **Low-density lipoprotein**

25%
45%
20%
10%

(c) **Very low-density lipoprotein**

5–10%
10–15%
15–20%
55–65%

- Triglyceride
- Phospholipid
- Protein
- Cholesterol

Figure 2

Composition of lipoproteins: (a) HDL; (b) LDL; (c) VLDL.

Patients with lipid disorders are asymptomatic and often do not seek medical intervention until cardiovascular disease has progressed to the point of producing chest pain or hypertension. Research suggests that over half the adult population in the United States has total cholesterol levels above 200 mg/dL and that two thirds of these patients are unaware of their hyperlipidemia. Because of the cost and the lack of symptoms for lipid disorders, nurses may face challenges persuading patients of the value of antihyperlipidemic drug therapy. The long-term benefits of drug therapy and the long-term consequences of hyperlipidemia and cardiovascular disease warrant consistent education on the importance of drug therapy.

Hyperlipidemia may be inherited or acquired. Certainly, diets high in saturated fats and lack of exercise contribute greatly to the development of hyperlipidemia and resulting cardiovascular diseases. However, genetics determines one's ability to metabolize lipids and contributes to high lipid levels in substantial numbers of patients. Some genetic dyslipidemias can be so severe as to cause CAD and death due to myocardial infarction (MI) in early childhood (Citkowitz, 2011). For most patients, dyslipidemias are the result of a combination of genetic and environmental (lifestyle) factors.

Measurement and Control of Serum Lipids

3 Blood lipid profiles are important diagnostic tools in guiding the therapy of dyslipidemias.

Although high levels of cholesterol in the blood are associated with cardiovascular disease, it is not enough to simply measure total cholesterol in the blood. Because some cholesterol is being transported for destruction, a more accurate profile is obtained by measuring the LDL and HDL. The goal in maintaining normal cholesterol levels is to maximize the HDL and minimize the LDL. This is sometimes stated as a ratio of LDL to HDL. If the ratio is greater than 5 (five times more LDL than HDL), the male patient is considered at risk for cardiovascular disease. The normal ratio in women is slightly lower at 4.5.

Scientists have further divided LDL into subclasses of lipoproteins. For example, one variety found in LDL, called *lipoprotein (a)*, has been strongly associated with plaque formation and heart disease. It is likely that further research will find other varieties with the expectation that drugs will be designed to be more selective toward the "bad" lipoproteins. Table 1

Treating the Diverse Patient   Cultural Dietary Habits

When different cultural groups prepare food in the way they have been taught by older family members, it can be difficult to change dietary cholesterol intake. For example, traditional Latin American cooking may include the use of lard for preparation of frijoles and biscochitos and for frying tortillas. Foods prepared in traditional ways in the southern and south central United States often include large amounts of lard, butter, or oil. Examples include fried okra, fried catfish, and chicken-fried steak. To encourage patients to maintain healthy eating habits while enjoying their cultural cuisine, it is important to offer alternative ideas for preparing traditional foods rather than restricting such foods altogether. For example, healthy oils low in saturated fat may be substituted for saturated fats in cooking. Many new ethnic cookbooks are now available with recipes offering low-fat alternatives to traditional cooking

methods. They provide tasty alternatives that help reduce overall fat intake. In addition, the Food and Nutrition Information Center of the U.S. Department of Agriculture offers multiple ethnic food pyramids. Oldways, an international nonprofit group, perhaps best known for its development of the Mediterranean food pyramid, offers dietary guidance and Latino, Asian, Mediterranean, and Vegetarian Food Pyramids.

The nurse should assist patients to evaluate their current dietary intake, especially when cultural diets are followed, to be sure that adequate amounts of fat-soluble vitamins and proteins are taken, along with lowered fat intake. Because the fibric acid agents may affect antidiabetic medications, the nurse can also help the patient with diabetes and family members to select culturally desirable foods that will aid in the stabilization of blood glucose as well.

TABLE 1   Standard Laboratory Lipid Profiles

Type of Lipid	Laboratory Value (mg/dL)	Standard
Serum cholesterol	Less than 200	Desirable
	200–240	Moderate risk
	Greater than 240	High risk
Low-density lipoproteins (LDLs)	Less than 100	Optimal
	100–129	Near or above optimal
	130–159	Moderate risk
	160–189	High risk
	Greater than 190	Very high risk
High-density lipoproteins (HDLs)	Less than 35	High risk
	35–45	Moderate risk
	46–59	Low risk
	Greater than 60	Desirable
Serum triglycerides	Less than 149	Desirable
	150–199	Borderline high risk
	200–499	High risk
	Greater than 500	Very high risk

gives the desirable, borderline, and high laboratory values for each of the major lipids and lipoproteins. These values change periodically as additional research becomes available on the association between heart disease and lipid levels.

Establishing treatment guidelines for dyslipidemia has been difficult because the condition itself has no symptoms and the progression to cardiovascular disease may take decades. Based on many years of research, the National Cholesterol Education Program (NCEP), a panel of experts of the National Heart, Lung, and Blood Institute, has published recommended treatment guidelines for dyslipidemia. The guidelines are based on accumulated evidence that reducing borderline high cholesterol levels can result in fewer heart at-

tacks and decreased mortality. It is estimated that for every 1% reduction in LDL, there is a 1% reduction in the possibility of an acute coronary event such as an MI. For example, lowering LDL levels by 25%, which is possible through lifestyle changes and medications, can reduce the risk of heart attack by 25%. Changes in HDL are claimed to be even more protective; each 1% increase in HDL may decrease the risk of MI by as much as 2%.

Based on this research, optimal levels of LDL cholesterol have been lowered from 130 mg/dL to 100 mg/dL. HDL cholesterol is now at least 60 mg/dL compared to 35 mg/dL a decade before. In addition, the NCEP guidelines recommend that high cholesterol levels be treated more aggressively in patients with diabetes because it is the most common systemic disease associated with dyslipidemia. These guidelines will likely lead to more widespread use of antihyperlipidemics, which are already the most widely prescribed drug class in the United States.

Blood lipid profiles are used to classify the different patterns of hyperlipidemias observed in clinical practice. These patterns are shown in Table 2. The specific type of dyslipidemia exhibited by patients is considered when planning therapy. For example, Type I requires dietary restrictions and does not respond well to pharmacotherapy. Whereas the remaining types respond to the statins, the hypertriglyceridemias may respond better to therapy with fibric acid agents (fibrates).

4 Lipid levels can often be controlled through therapeutic lifestyle changes.

Therapeutic lifestyle changes (TLCs) should always be included in any treatment plan for reducing blood lipid levels. Many patients with borderline high-risk laboratory values can control their dyslipidemia entirely through nonpharmacologic means. It is important to note that all the TLCs for reducing blood lipid levels also apply to cardiovascular disease in general. Because many patients who take lipid-lowering drugs have underlying cardiovascular disease, these lifestyle changes are particularly important.

TABLE 2 Types of Dyslipidemias

Name	Laboratory Findings	Features
Type I Exogenous hyperlipidemia	Triglycerides increased three times Chylomicrons increased Cholesterol normal	Rare condition, usually occurring in childhood
Type IIa Familial hypercholesterolemia	LDL and cholesterol increased Triglycerides and VLDL normal	Common condition, may occur at any age
Type IIb Combined familial hyperlipidemia Carbohydrate-induced hypertriglyceridemia	LDL, VLDL, cholesterol, and triglycerides increased	May occur at any age but more commonly in adults
Type III Dysbetalipoproteinemia	Chylomicrons, VLDL, cholesterol, and triglycerides increased	Uncommon condition, occurs in middle-aged adults
Type IV Endogenous hyperlipidemia Carbohydrate-induced hypertriglyceridemia	VLDL and triglycerides increased Cholesterol normal or elevated Glucose intolerance Hyperuricemia	Most common dyslipidemia, occurs in middle-aged adults; associated with obesity, excessive alcohol intake, tobacco use, and other lifestyle factors
Type V Mixed hyperlipidemia Carbohydrate and fat-induced hypertriglyceridemia	LDL, VLDL, cholesterol, and chylomicrons increased Triglycerides increased three times Glucose intolerance Hyperuricemia	Uncommon type, may begin in childhood and manifest in adults

Patients should be taught that all drugs used for hyperlipidemia have adverse effects and that maintaining normal lipid values without pharmacotherapy should be a therapeutic goal. Pharmacotherapy should only be initiated after attempts to lower lipid levels with TLCs fail. Following are the most important lipid-reduction lifestyle interventions:

- Monitor blood lipid levels regularly, as recommended by the health care provider.
- Maintain weight at an optimal level.
- Implement a medically supervised exercise plan.
- Reduce dietary saturated fats and cholesterol.
- Increase soluble fiber in the diet, as found in oat bran, apples, beans, grapefruit, and broccoli.
- Eliminate tobacco use.

The single most important lifestyle factor contributing to dyslipidemia is a high amount of saturated fat in the diet. Nutritionists recommend that the intake of dietary fat be limited to less than 30% of the total caloric intake. Cholesterol intake should be reduced as much as possible and not exceed 200 mg/day. It is interesting to note that restriction of dietary cholesterol alone will not result in a significant reduction in blood cholesterol levels. In fact, cutting back on cholesterol consumption may actually increase the amount of circulating cholesterol. How is this possible? The liver reacts to a low cholesterol diet by making more cholesterol and by inhibiting its excretion whenever saturated fats are present. Saturated fats are the building blocks that the liver uses for making cholesterol. Patients must therefore reduce saturated fat in their diet to less than 7% of total calories, in addition to reducing cholesterol consumption, in order to control the amount made by the liver and to ultimately lower blood cholesterol levels.

The NCEP recommends a dietary intake of plant sterols as a means to reduce blood cholesterol levels. Plant sterols, also called phytosterols or stanols, are lipids used by plants to construct their cell membranes. The structure of plant sterols is very similar to that of cholesterol. When ingested, the plant sterols compete with cholesterol for absorption in the digestive tract. When the body absorbs the plant sterols, cholesterol is excreted from the body, less cholesterol is delivered to the liver, and serum LDL (the "bad" cholesterol) levels fall. Rich, natural sources of plant sterols include wheat, corn, rye, oats, and rice, as well as nuts and olive oil. In recent years, plant sterols have been added to commercial products such as margarines, salad dressings, certain cereals, and some fruit juices.

To be of benefit in reducing high serum cholesterol, nutritionists recommend a daily intake of plant sterols of 2 to 3 grams. Cholesterol levels can be reduced by 10% to 15% after just a couple of months of sufficient plant sterol intake.

Drugs for Dyslipidemias

5 The statins are the most effective drugs for reducing blood lipid levels.

In the late 1970s substances were isolated from various species of fungi that were found to inhibit cholesterol production in human cells in the laboratory. This class of drugs, known as the statins, has revolutionized the treatment of lipid disorders. Statins can produce a dramatic 20% to 40% reduction in LDL cholesterol levels. In addition to dropping the LDL cholesterol level in the blood, statins can lower triglyceride and VLDL levels and raise the level of "good" HDL cholesterol. These

Lifespan Considerations   Pediatric Dyslipidemias and Lipid-Lowering Drugs

Many people consider dyslipidemia to be a condition that occurs with advancing age. Dyslipidemias are also a concern for some pediatric patients, and multiple research studies have demonstrated that the early stages of atherosclerosis begin in childhood. With the increasing childhood obesity epidemic, there is concern that dyslipidemias, cardiovascular disease, and metabolic syndrome will occur at younger and younger ages. In 2007, the American Heart Association (AHA) published guidelines that recommend the use of the statin drugs for select children at risk for hyperlipidemia (McCrindle et al., 2007). Risk factors include overweight or obese children, family history of dyslipidemias or premature cardiovascular disease, hypertension, smoking or passive smoke exposure, and known lipid disorders (e.g., low HDL or high LDL level).

The AHA also recommended that statins ideally should be prescribed after age 10, or after menarche in girls. Subsequent research studies have demonstrated the safety of statins in the pediatric population but no long-term studies have been done, and the drugs are recommended for short-term use. It was also noted that for girls past the age of first menarche, teaching about pregnancy prevention and the risks of taking statins while breast-feeding should be included in patient education.

effects have been shown to reduce the incidence of serious cardiovascular-related events by 25% to 30%.

Cholesterol is manufactured in the liver by a series of more than 25 metabolic steps, beginning with acetyl CoA, a two-carbon unit that is produced from the breakdown of fatty acids (Figure 3). Of the many enzymes involved in this complex pathway, **HMG-CoA reductase** (3-hydroxy-3-methylglutaryl coenzyme A reductase) serves as the primary regulatory enzyme for cholesterol biosynthesis. Under normal conditions, this enzyme is controlled through negative feedback. High levels of LDL cholesterol in the blood will shut down production of HMG-CoA reductase, thus turning off the cholesterol synthesis pathway. Pharmacotherapy Illustrated 1 shows some of the steps in the biosynthesis of cholesterol and the importance of HMG-CoA reductase.

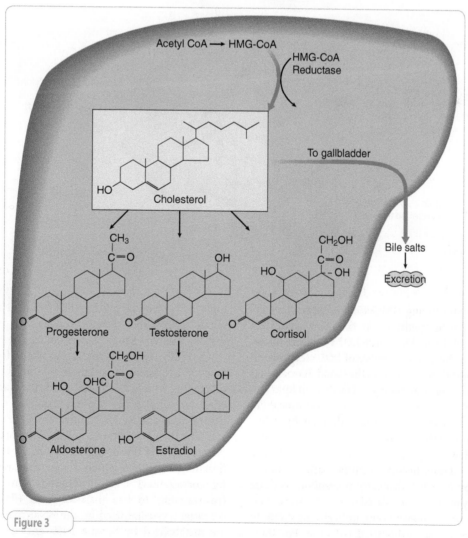

Figure 3

Cholesterol biosynthesis and excretion.

PHARMACOTHERAPY ILLUSTRATED

1

Mechanisms of Action of Lipid-Lowering Drugs

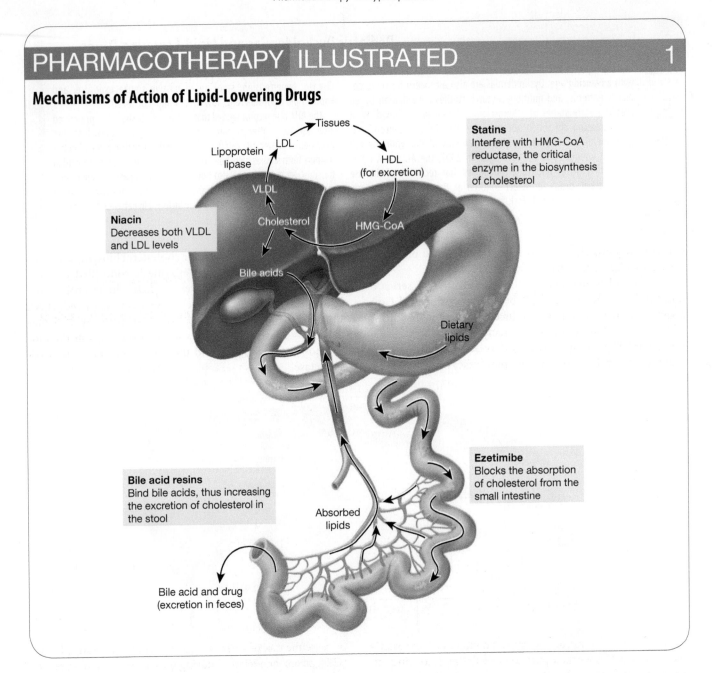

Statins
Interfere with HMG-CoA reductase, the critical enzyme in the biosynthesis of cholesterol

Niacin
Decreases both VLDL and LDL levels

Bile acid resins
Bind bile acids, thus increasing the excretion of cholesterol in the stool

Ezetimibe
Blocks the absorption of cholesterol from the small intestine

Tissues

LDL

Lipoprotein lipase

HDL (for excretion)

VLDL

Cholesterol

HMG-CoA

Bile acids

Dietary lipids

Absorbed lipids

Bile acid and drug (excretion in feces)

The statins act by inhibiting HMG-CoA reductase, resulting in less cholesterol biosynthesis. As the liver makes less cholesterol, it responds by making more LDL receptors on the surface of liver cells. The greater number of LDL receptors on liver cells removes additional LDL from the blood. Blood levels of both LDL and cholesterol are reduced. The drop in lipid levels is not permanent, however, so patients must continue these drugs for the remainder of their lives or until their hyperlipidemia can be controlled through dietary or lifestyle changes.

Statins clearly slow the progression of CAD and reduce mortality in patients with a history of cardiovascular disease. This type of therapy is called *secondary* prevention, because the patient is already at risk for increased mortality. The data is less clear regarding *primary* prevention: administering statins to patients with no history of cardiovascular disease. For these patients the risk of adverse drug effects and cost of the medication

must be carefully weighed against potential benefits. Some, but not all, studies show benefits for primary prevention and this will likely remain a topic of continuing research.

Currently, seven statins are available for treating various types of dyslipidemias, and these are listed in Table 3. Although differences among the statins exist, their actions and adverse effects are similar. Lovastatin, pravastatin, and simvastatin are natural agents derived from fungi and have a different chemical structure than the synthetic statins. There are also differences in potency among the drugs. For example, the maximum daily dose for pitavastatin is only 4 mg, whereas the dose is 80 mg for atorvastatin. The half-lives of the statins vary from 20 hours (rosuvastatin) to less than an hour (fluvastatin). Whereas pravastatin is eliminated by the renal route, the other statins are metabolized by hepatic P450 enzymes. In patients with renal disease, dosage adjustment is required for lovastatin,

TABLE 3 Drugs for Dyslipidemias

Drug	Route and Adult Dose (maximum dose where indicated)	Adverse Effects
HMG-CoA Reductase Inhibitors		
atorvastatin (Lipitor)	PO: 10–20 mg once daily (max: 80 mg/day)	*Headache, dyspepsia, abdominal cramping, myalgia, back pain, rash, pruritus*
fluvastatin (Lescol)	PO: 20 mg daily (max: 80 mg/day)	
lovastatin (Mevacor)	PO: 10–20 mg once daily (max: 80 mg/day immediate release; 60 mg/day extended release)	Rhabdomyolysis, severe myositis, elevated hepatic enzymes
pitavastatin (Livalo)	PO: 1–4 mg daily (max: 4 mg/day)	
pravastatin (Pravachol)	PO: 10–40 mg daily (max: 80 mg/day)	
rosuvastatin (Crestor)	PO: 5–40 mg daily (max: 80 mg/day)	
simvastatin (Zocor)	PO: 5–40 mg daily (max: 80 mg/day)	
Bile Acid Sequestrants		
cholestyramine (Questran)	PO; 4-8 g bid-qid (max; 32 g/day)	*Constipation, nausea, vomiting, abdominal pain, bloating, dyspepsia*
colesevelam (WelChol)	PO: 1.9 g bid (max: 4.4 g/day)	
colestipol (Colestid)	PO: 5–20 g/day in divided doses (30 g/day granules or 16 g/day tablets)	Gastrointestinal (GI) tract obstruction, vitamin deficiencies due to poor absorption
Fibric Acid Agents		
clofibrate (Atromid-S)	PO: 2 g/day in two to four divided doses	*Abdominal pain, rash, myalgia, fatigue, flulike symptoms, dyspepsia, nausea, vomiting, asthenia*
fenofibrate (TriCor)	PO: 54 mg/day (max: 160 mg/day)	
fenofibric acid (Trilipix)	PO: 45–135 mg once daily	Cholelithiasis, pancreatitis
gemfibrozil (Lopid)	PO: 600 mg bid (max: 1,500 mg/day)	
Other Agents		
ezetimibe and simvastatin (Vytorin)	PO: 10 mg/10 mg or 10 mg/20 mg every evening (max: 10 mg/80 mg)	*Arthralgia, fatigue, abdominal pain, diarrhea*
		Anaphylaxis, rhabdomyolysis
ezetimibe (Zetia)	PO: 10 mg daily (max: 10 mg/day)	*Nasopharyngitis, myalgia, upper respiratory tract infection, arthralgia, diarrhea*
		Anaphylaxis, rhabdomyolysis
niacin (Niaspan)	Hyperlipidemia: PO: 1.5–3 g daily in divided doses (max: 6 g/day)	*Flushing, nausea, pruritus, headache, bloating, diarrhea*
	Niacin deficiency: PO: 10–20 mg daily	Dysrhythmias

Note: Italics indicate common adverse effects. Underline indicates serious adverse effects.

pravastatin, simvastatin, and rosuvastatin but not for fluvastatin or atorvastatin. Despite these pharmacokinetic differences, in clinical practice the choice of statin is often guided by the experience of the prescriber and the response of each individual patient.

All the statins are given orally (PO) and are tolerated well by most patients. Adverse effects are rarely severe enough to cause discontinuation of therapy. Minor adverse effects include headache, abdominal cramping, diarrhea, muscle or joint pain, and heartburn.

Severe myopathy and rhabdomyolysis are rare, although they are serious adverse effects of the statins. **Rhabdomyolysis** is a breakdown of muscle fibers usually due to muscle trauma or ischemia. The mechanism by which statins cause this disorder is unknown. During rhabdomyolysis, the contents of muscle cells spill into the systemic circulation, causing potentially fatal acute renal failure. Macrolide antibiotics such as erythromycin, azole antifungals, fibric acid agents, and certain immunosuppressants should be avoided during statin therapy, because these interfere with statin metabolism and increase the risk of severe myopathy. Levels of creatine kinase (CK), an enzyme released during muscle injury, should be obtained if myopathy is suspected. If CK levels become elevated during therapy, the drug should be immediately discontinued. Statins may be discontinued if muscle weakness persists even without CK elevation. Nurses should urge all patients who develop unexplained muscle or joint pain during statin therapy to immediately report this to the prescriber.

Statins are pregnancy category X drugs because teratogenic effects have been reported in laboratory animals exposed to these agents. Statins should not be used in patients who may become pregnant, are pregnant, or who are breast-feeding.

Because cholesterol biosynthesis in the liver is higher at night, statins with short half-lives such as lovastatin should be administered in the evening. The other statins have longer half-lives and are effective regardless of the time of day they are taken.

Much research is ongoing to determine the other therapeutic effects of the drugs in the statin class. For example, statins block the vasoconstrictive effect of the A-beta protein, a significant chemical associated with Alzheimer's disease. Cholesterol and A-beta protein had very similar effects on blood vessels, both causing vasoconstriction. Preliminary research suggests that the statins may protect against dementia by inhibiting this protein, thus slowing dementia caused by blood vessel constriction. Research also suggests that the statins may have the ability to lower the incidence of colorectal cancer. The mechanism of this effect is unknown. Several attempts have been made to move low doses of certain statins to over-the-counter (OTC) status; however, the U.S Food and Drug Administration (FDA) has not approved these applications.

PROTOTYPE DRUG | Atorvastatin (Lipitor)

Classification: **Therapeutic:** Antihyperlipidemic
Pharmacologic: HMG-CoA reductase inhibitor, statin

Therapeutic Effects and Uses: Approved in 1996, atorvastatin was initially approved to treat hypercholesterolemia. Following several years of use, it became evident that the drug also prevents cardiovascular events in high-risk patients. After 2 to 4 weeks of therapy, atorvastatin lowers LDL and VLDL cholesterol as well as triglycerides. It appears to lower LDL cholesterol levels greater than most other statins—as much as 60%. Atorvastatin may also be prescribed for the treatment of familial hypercholesterolemia. All patients receiving this drug should be placed on a cholesterol-lowering diet, because this will enhance the drug's therapeutic effects. The primary goal in atorvastatin therapy is to reduce the risk of MI and stroke.

To decrease gastrointestinal (GI) discomfort, atorvastatin may be administered with food. It produces the same degree of LDL cholesterol reduction regardless of the time of day it is taken. Because atorvastatin is not excreted by the kidneys, no adjustment in dosage is necessary in patients with renal impairment. Extensive metabolism to active metabolites gives atorvastatin a long duration of action.

Mechanism of Action: Atorvastatin acts by inhibiting HMG-CoA reductase, the primary regulatory enzyme in cholesterol biosynthesis. As the liver makes less cholesterol, it responds by making more LDL receptors, removing LDL cholesterol from the blood. Blood levels of both LDL and cholesterol are reduced.

Pharmacokinetics:

Route(s)	PO
Absorption	Rapidly absorbed but only 30% reaches the circulation; food reduces absorption
Distribution	Widely distributed; crosses the placenta and is secreted in breast milk; 98% bound to plasma proteins
Primary metabolism	Hepatic; extensively metabolized to active metabolites
Primary excretion	Biliary
Onset of action	2 weeks for lipid-lowering effect; peak plasma level: 1–2 h
Duration of action	Half-life: 14 h (20–30 h for active metabolites)

Adverse Effects: Most patients tolerate atorvastatin well and only 2% or fewer discontinue the drug due to adverse effects. Common adverse effects include headache, intestinal cramping, diarrhea, and constipation. The most serious adverse effect is rhabdomyolysis. Therapy is generally discontinued in patients reporting unexplained muscle pain, weakness, fever, or fatigue due to the potential for rhabdomyolysis.

Contraindications/Precautions: Patients with hepatic impairment should be monitored carefully, because the liver extensively metabolizes atorvastatin and the drug has been associated with a small risk of liver failure. Liver enzyme tests may become elevated during therapy, although this does not necessarily indicate liver damage. Because atorvastatin is pregnancy category X, pregnancy testing should be conducted prior to treatment in women of childbearing years, and these patients should be advised to take precautions to prevent pregnancy during therapy. Atorvastatin is contraindicated during lactation because the drug is secreted in breast milk.

Drug Interactions: Because atorvastatin is a substrate for hepatic CYP3A4, it has the potential to interact with many other drugs. For example, it may increase digoxin levels by 20% as well as increase levels of norethindrone and ethinyl estradiol (oral contraceptives). Erythromycin may increase atorvastatin levels by as much as 40%. Risk of rhabdomyolysis increases with concurrent administration of atorvastatin with macrolide antibiotics, cyclosporine, and azole antifungals. The risk of myopathy increases when atorvastatin is administered concurrently with fibric acid agents or niacin. Atorvastatin may increase serum transaminase and CK levels. **Herbal/Food:** Grapefruit juice inhibits the metabolism of statins, allowing them to reach high serum levels. Because HMG-CoA reductase inhibitors decrease the synthesis of Coenzyme Q10 (CoQ10), patients may benefit from CoQ10 supplements.

Pregnancy: Category X.

Treatment of Overdose: No specific therapy is available; patients are treated symptomatically.

Nursing Responsibilities: Key nursing implications for patients receiving atorvastatin are included in the Nursing Practice Application for Patients Receiving Pharmacotherapy for Hyperlipidemia.

Lifespan and Diversity Considerations:
- Monitor hepatic function laboratory values more frequently with the older adult, because normal physiological changes related to aging may affect the drug's metabolism and/or excretion.
- Because atorvastatin is metabolized through the P450 system pathways, monitor ethnically diverse populations more frequently to ensure optimal therapeutic effects and minimize adverse effects.

Patient and Family Education:
- Take this medication in the evening with food or before going to bed because cholesterol biosynthesis in the liver is higher at night.
- Immediately report the following symptoms to the health care provider: unexplained muscle pain, weakness, or

tenderness, especially with fever; yellowing of the skin or eyes; stomach pain with nausea, loss of appetite, or vomiting; or skin rash or hives.

- Avoid grapefruit and grapefruit juice because these may lead to an interaction with potentially dangerous effects.

- Consult with the health care provider when using statins with erythromycin, cyclosporine, antifungals, niacin, cholestyramine, or birth control pills.

- Immediately notify the health care provider of any known or suspected pregnancy, because statins can cause birth defects. Discontinue use if confirmed pregnant.

- Do not breast-feed while taking statins, unless approved by the health care provider.

Drugs Similar to Atorvastatin (Lipitor)

Other statins include fluvastatin, lovastatin, pitavastatin, pravastatin, rosuvastatin, and simvastatin.

Fluvastatin (Lescol): Approved in 1993, fluvastatin is a synthetic statin that has the shortest half-life of all the drugs in this class. Because the kidneys excrete less than 5% of a PO dose, dosage adjustment for patients with renal impairment is not necessary. Fewer drug interactions are expected with fluvastatin because it is not metabolized through the hepatic P450 system. It is approved for hypercholesterolemia and several other types of dyslipidemia. In 2003, the indications were expanded to include prevention of major cardiac events such as cardiac death and nonfatal MI. An extended release formulation, called Lescol-XL, is available. The drug may be administered without regard to meals. Fluvastatin is well tolerated and its adverse effects are similar to those of atorvastatin. It is contraindicated in patients with severe hepatic impairment and in patients who are pregnant. Fluvastatin is a pregnancy category X drug.

Lovastatin (Mevacor): Approved in 1987, lovastatin, a natural substance derived from fungi, was the first HMG-CoA reductase inhibitor marketed. Lovastatin is a prodrug with no intrinsic activity of its own, but the liver converts it to several active metabolites. This drug may achieve a 20% to 40% reduction in LDL cholesterol. Lovastatin is more effective if administered in the evening and should be taken on an empty stomach to maximize absorption. Although only 10% of this drug is excreted by the kidneys, dosage adjustment for patients with renal impairment is recommended. Lovastatin was originally approved for hypercholesterolemia; however, its indications have been expanded to include slowing the progression of coronary atherosclerosis and prevention of MI and stroke. An extended release form is available (Altoprev), as is a fixed-dose combination product with lovastatin and niacin (Advicor). Adverse effects are the same as those of other drugs in this class. It is contraindicated in patients with severe hepatic impairment and in patients who are pregnant. Lovastatin is a pregnancy category X drug.

Pitavastatin (Livalo): Approved in 2009, pitavastatin is one of the newest drugs in the statin class. It is indicated for patients with primary hyperlipidemia and mixed dyslipidemia as an adjunctive therapy to diet to reduce elevated total cholesterol, LDL, apolipoprotein B, and triglycerides, and to increase HDL. It may be administered with or without food and without regard to the time of day. It has similar effectiveness and adverse effects as other statins. Because it is only minimally metabolized by CYP enzymes, it may exhibit fewer drug–drug interactions than some of the other statins. However, like other drugs in this class, hepatic enzymes should be evaluated regularly and there is a small risk of myopathy. This drug is pregnancy category X and patients should be advised not to breast-feed during pitavastatin therapy.

Pravastatin (Pravachol): Like lovastatin, pravastatin is a natural substance derived from fungi. Twenty percent of the drug is excreted by the kidneys, and dosage adjustment for patients with renal impairment is recommended. Like fluvastatin, it is not metabolized through the hepatic P450 system; thus fewer drug interactions are expected. The drug may be taken without regard to meals and is slightly more effective if administered in the evening. Approved in 1991, pravastatin is approved for primary hypercholesterolemia, slowing the progression of coronary atherosclerosis and the prevention of MI and stroke. Unlabeled uses include other types of dyslipidemias. Pravigard PAC is a copackage that contains separate aspirin and pravastatin tablets in various dosage strengths. Adverse effects are the same as those of other drugs in this class. It is contraindicated in patients with hepatic impairment and in those who are pregnant. Pravastatin is a pregnancy category X drug.

Rosuvastatin (Crestor): Approved in 2003, rosuvastatin is a second-generation statin that contains a sulfur group. This drug is the most potent, has the longest half-life in its class (20 hours), and is capable of lowering LDL cholesterol by as much as 65%. Rosuvastatin is not a prodrug and it undergoes minimal hepatic metabolism. This drug may be administered with or without food and without regard to time of day. It is approved for hypercholesterolemia, hypertriglyceridemia, and for slowing the progression of coronary atherosclerosis. Adverse effects are the same as those of other drugs in this class. Rosuvastatin is a pregnancy category X drug.

Simvastatin (Zocor): Approved in 1991, simvastatin is a natural substance derived from fungi. Like lovastatin, simvastatin is an inactive prodrug that is changed to active metabolites by the liver. The drug can lower LDL cholesterol levels by as much as 47%. Although the kidneys excrete only 13% of the drug, dosage adjustment for patients with significant renal impairment is recommended. The drug may be taken with or without food but should be administered in the evening for maximum effectiveness. It is approved for hypercholesterolemia, for hypertriglyceridemia, slowing the progression of coronary atherosclerosis, and prevention of MI and stroke. Adverse effects are the same as those of other drugs in this class. Simvastatin is contraindicated in patients with hepatic impairment and in those who are pregnant. This is a pregnancy category X drug.

CONNECTION Checkpoint 32.1

Several of the statins are prodrugs. What type of dosage adjustment should be made if these statin prodrugs are prescribed for a patient with hepatic cirrhosis? If a dosage adjustment is not made, what types of adverse effects might you observe? *See Answer to Connection Checkpoint 32.1 on student resource website.*

About 10% of adolescents ages 12 through 19 are estimated to have total blood cholesterol levels of 200 mg/dL or above. Female adolescents have significantly higher "bad" cholesterol levels than do boys of the same age (American Heart Association, n.d.).

6 Bile acid sequestrants are often combined with statins to reduce LDL cholesterol levels.

Bile acids contain a high concentration of cholesterol and are secreted by the liver to emulsify fats in the small intestine. After performing their digestive function, bile acids are reabsorbed in the ileum and sent back to the liver to again become part of bile. This mechanism is known as enterohepatic circulation. In effect, the cholesterol in bile acids is recycled, with only small amounts leaving the body in the feces.

Prior to the discovery of the statins, the primary means of lowering blood cholesterol was through the use of bile acid sequestrants or resins. The bile acid sequestrants bind to bile acids, forming a large complex that cannot be reabsorbed from the small intestine. The enterohepatic circulation of cholesterol is interrupted and the bound bile acids and cholesterol are eliminated in the feces. The liver responds to the loss of cholesterol by making more LDL receptors, which removes LDL cholesterol from the blood in a mechanism similar to that of the statins.

The bile acid resins are capable of producing a 20% drop in LDL cholesterol, which is generally less response than can be obtained from the statins. They are no longer considered first-line drugs for dyslipidemia, although they are sometimes combined with statins for patients who are unable to achieve sufficient response from the statins alone.

The bile acid sequestrants tend to cause more frequent adverse effects than statins. Because they are not absorbed into the systemic circulation, adverse effects are limited to the GI tract, causing symptoms such as abdominal pain, bloating, diarrhea, steatorrhea, and constipation. In addition to binding bile acids, these agents can bind drugs such as digoxin and warfarin and increase the potential for drug–drug interactions.

Bile acid sequestrants also interfere with the absorption of vitamins and minerals, and nutritional deficiencies may occur with extended use. Other medications and vitamins should be taken at least 1 hour before or 4 hours after taking a bile acid sequestrant to avoid drug interactions.

Bile acid sequestrants may cause a transient increase in triglyceride levels. This effect is particularly prominent and often sustained in patients with preexisting hypertriglyceridemia. Because of this, the bile acid sequestrants are generally not prescribed for patients with elevated triglycerides.

PROTOTYPE DRUG	Cholestyramine (Questran)

Classification: **Therapeutic:** Antihyperlipidemic
Pharmacologic: Bile acid sequestrant

Therapeutic Effects and Uses: Approved in 1966, cholestyramine is indicated for the reduction of elevated serum cholesterol in patients with primary hypercholesterolemia (elevated LDL) who do not respond adequately to dietary modifications alone. Cholestyramine monotherapy slows the progression and increases the rate of regression of coronary atherosclerosis. A secondary indication is to relieve pruritus associated with partial biliary obstruction. It is available as a powder that is mixed with fluid before being taken once or twice daily. The drug should be mixed with 60 to 180 mL of water, noncarbonated beverages, highly liquid soups, or pulpy fruits (applesauce, crushed pineapple) to prevent esophageal irritation. The patient should swallow the medication immediately after stirring. If taken with too small a fluid volume or if not completely swallowed, the drug can swell in the throat or esophagus to cause an obstruction.

It may take 30 days or longer for cholestyramine to produce its maximum effect. To avoid interference with absorption, cholestyramine should not be taken at the same time as vitamins or other medications. An off-label indication for cholestyramine is diarrhea caused by *Clostridium difficile*, although antibiotics are the drugs of first choice.

Complementary and Alternative Therapies   Coenzyme Q10

Description: Coenzyme Q10 (CoQ10) is a lipid-soluble vitamin-like substance found in most animal cells. It is an essential component in the cell's mitochondria for producing adenosine triphosphate (ATP) energy. Because the heart requires high levels of ATP, a sufficient level of CoQ10 is especially important to that organ.

History and Claims: The applications of CoQ10 to treating disease are relatively recent, with the agent being claimed to be an antioxidant and having benefited patients with heart failure in the mid-1960s. Subsequent reports have claimed that CoQ10 may be beneficial in angina pectoris, dysrhythmias, periodontal disease, immune disorders, neurologic disease, obesity, diabetes mellitus, and cancers.

Standardization: The dose of CoQ10 varies widely. Typical doses range from 100 to 200 mg/day.

Evidence: As with most dietary supplements, controlled research studies with CoQ10 are often lacking and give conflicting results. Supplementation with CoQ10 may be important to patients taking the HMG-CoA reductase inhibitors (statins) because these drugs significantly lower blood levels of CoQ10 (Suzuki et al., 2008). Coenzyme Q10 and cholesterol share the same metabolic pathways. Inhibition of the enzyme HMG-CoA reductase concurrently decreases CoQ10 levels. Many of the adverse effects of statins, including muscle weakness and rhabdomyolysis, are due to the decrease in CoQ10 levels; supplementation with CoQ10 may improve myopathy symptoms.

Foods richest in this substance are pork, sardines, beef heart, salmon, broccoli, spinach, and nuts. Elderly people appear to have an increased need for CoQ10. Although CoQ10 can be synthesized by the body, many amino acids and other substances are required for this synthesis; thus patients with nutritional deficiencies may need supplementation.

Mechanism of Action: Cholestyramine binds to bile acids, forming an insoluble complex containing cholesterol that is excreted in the feces. Cholestyramine lowers LDL cholesterol levels by increasing LDL receptors on hepatocytes.

Pharmacokinetics:

Route(s)	PO
Absorption	Not absorbed
Distribution	Not distributed; acts locally in the alimentary canal
Primary metabolism	Not metabolized
Primary excretion	Feces
Onset of action	1–2 days
Duration of action	2–4 weeks

Adverse Effects: Cholestyramine is not absorbed or metabolized once it enters the intestine; thus it does not produce systemic adverse effects. Common GI-related adverse effects include constipation, bloating, belching, and nausea. Serious adverse effects include obstruction of the GI tract, hyperchloremic acidosis, and malabsorption syndrome. Chronic use may cause increased bleeding due to hypoprothrombinemia associated with vitamin K deficiency.

Contraindications/Precautions: Cholestyramine should be used cautiously in patients with GI disorders such as peptic ulcer disease, hemorrhoids, inflammatory bowel diseases, or chronic constipation, because bile acid sequestrants may worsen or aggravate these conditions. This drug should not be used in patients with complete biliary obstruction. Bile acid resins should be used with caution in patients with hypertriglyceridemia because they may increase serum triglyceride concentrations. They are absolutely contraindicated if serum triglycerides rise above 400 mg/dL. Although cholestyramine use is safe during pregnancy because it is not absorbed, precautions must be taken to ensure that this drug is not interfering with vitamin absorption, especially folic acid.

Drug Interactions: Cholestyramine can bind to other drugs and interfere with their absorption, causing reduced effects. This interaction has been reported for digoxin, penicillins, iron supplements, thyroid hormone, and thiazide diuretics, although it has the potential to occur with any drug administered PO. Cholestyramine may indirectly increase the effects of warfarin by binding to vitamin K, decreasing its absorption and lowering the levels of vitamin K in the body. The absorption of raloxifene can be reduced as much as 60% if coadministered with cholestyramine. To reduce the possibility of absorption interference, cholestyramine should be administered 1 hour before or 4 hours after other PO medications.
Herbal/Food: Cholestyramine may block the absorption of iron and fat-soluble vitamins in food.

Pregnancy: Category B.

Treatment of Overdose: No specific therapy is available; patients are treated symptomatically.

Nursing Responsibilities: Key nursing implications for patients receiving cholestyramine are included in the Nursing Practice Application for Patients Receiving Pharmacotherapy for Hyperlipidemia.

Lifespan and Diversity Considerations:
- Because of normal changes in bowel tone related to aging, monitor bowel sounds in the older adult and monitor for the development of constipation. A stool softener or laxative agent may be required.
- Monitor the older adult for signs of increased bruising. Long-term use of the drug interferes with vitamin K synthesis, increasing the chance of bleeding.

Patient and Family Education:
- Completely dissolve cholestyramine powder or granules thoroughly because they are irritating to mucous membranes and may cause esophageal impaction if administered dry. Drink an additional cup of liquid after taking the dose to help prevent constipation.
- Take other medications 1 hour before or 4 hours after administration of bile sequestrants.
- Increase intake of fluids and maintain a high-fiber diet to prevent constipation. Report constipation to the health care provider. GI symptoms usually subside after the first month of therapy.

Drugs Similar to Cholestyramine (Questran)

Other bile acid sequestrants include colesevelam and colestipol.

Colesevelam (WelChol): Approved in 2000, colesevelam is a bile acid-binding agent that is claimed to have more bile acid-binding capacity than the older resins. The drug has the capacity to reduce LDL cholesterol by as much as 20%. It may be administered as monotherapy or concurrently with statins to achieve greater efficacy. At least 2 weeks of therapy may be necessary before maximum therapeutic response is achieved. In 2008, colesevelam was approved as an adjunct to diet, exercise, and antidiabetic drugs to improve glycemic control in patients with type 2 diabetes. It is not approved for patients with type 1 diabetes. The most common adverse reactions with colesevelam are constipation, dyspepsia, and nausea. Colesevelam can interfere with the absorption of other medications and should be administered 4 hours after other PO drugs. Like cholestyramine, colesevelam can increase serum triglyceride levels and is contraindicated in patients with triglyceride levels greater than 500 mg/dL. The large tablets can cause dysphagia or esophageal obstruction; thus this drug should be used with caution in patients with swallowing disorders. An oral suspension, dissolved in 4 to 8 ounces of water, is available for patients who have difficulty swallowing the tablets. This drug is pregnancy category B.

Colestipol (Colestid): Approved in 1977, colestipol acts by the same mechanism as cholestyramine, has the same effectiveness in lowering LDL cholesterol, and exhibits the same adverse effects. Other drugs should be administered at least 1 hour before or 4 to 6 hours after a dose of colestipol to prevent interference with absorption. Maximum therapeutic effects may take as long as a month to appear. Because the drug can increase serum triglycerides, it should not be administered to patients with hypertriglyceridemia. Colestipol is rarely used as monotherapy. In addition to its use in treating elevated HDL cholesterol, colestipol may be used off-label to treat digoxin overdose, diarrhea, and pruritus associated with biliary obstruction. This drug is pregnancy category B.

PharmFACT

Familial hypercholesterolemia affects 1 in 500 people and is a genetic disease that predisposes people to premature CAD (Citkowitz, 2011).

7 Niacin can reduce triglycerides and LDL cholesterol levels, but adverse effects limit its usefulness.

Niacin, also called nicotinic acid, is a B-complex vitamin (B_3). Its ability to lower lipid levels, however, is unrelated to its role as a vitamin because much higher doses are needed to produce its antihyperlipidemic effects. For lowering cholesterol, the usual dose is 2 to 3 g per day. When taken as a vitamin, the dose is only 25 mg per day.

The primary action of niacin (Niaspan) is to decrease the production of VLDL, which lowers serum triglyceride levels. Because LDL is synthesized from VLDL, the patient also experiences a reduction in LDL cholesterol levels. Niacin also has the desirable effect of increasing HDL levels, although this effect does not appear to be significant in reducing mortality from cardiovascular disease. As with other lipid-lowering drugs, maximum therapeutic effects may take a month or longer to achieve.

Although effective at reducing LDL cholesterol by 20%, niacin produces more adverse effects than the statins. Intense flushing and hot flashes occur in almost every patient. Taking one aspirin tablet 30 minutes prior to niacin administration can reduce uncomfortable flushing in many patients. In addition, a variety of uncomfortable GI effects such as nausea, excess gas, and diarrhea are commonly reported. Paresthesias, such as tingling in the extremities, may also occur.

More serious adverse effects such as hepatotoxicity and gout are possible but uncommon. Patients with elevated liver enzymes or a history of liver disease should use an alternate drug to lower lipids. In patients predisposed to gout, niacin may increase uric acid levels and precipitate acute gout.

Niacin is not usually prescribed for patients with diabetes mellitus because the drug can raise fasting glucose levels. When beginning therapy, patients with diabetes should monitor their blood glucose levels more frequently until the effect of niacin is determined.

Because of the high incidence of adverse effects, niacin is most often used in lower doses in combination with a statin or bile acid sequestrant; the beneficial effects of these drugs are additive. Combining niacin with lovastatin can reduce LDL cholesterol by as much as 45%. The two drugs are combined in a fixed-dose formulation marketed as Advicor. In 2008 the FDA approved Simcor, a combination of niacin and simvastatin to lower LDL levels.

Because supplemental niacin is available without a prescription, patients should be instructed not to attempt self-medication with this drug. One form of niacin that is available OTC as a vitamin supplement, called nicotinamide, has no lipid-lowering effects. If niacin is to be used to lower cholesterol, it should be done under medical supervision.

8 Fibric acid agents lower triglyceride levels but have little effect on LDL cholesterol.

The first fibric acid agent, clofibrate (Atromid-S), was widely prescribed until a 1978 study determined that it did not reduce mortality from cardiovascular disease. In fact, clofibrate was found to increase overall mortality, compared to a control group. Although this drug is no longer marketed in the United States, three other fibric acid agents, fenofibrate (TriCor), fenofibric acid (Trilipix), and gemfibrozil (Lopid), are sometimes used for patients with high triglyceride levels. They are preferred drugs for treating severe hypertriglyceridemia (Types IV and V hyperlipidemia), although they have little effect on LDL cholesterol. Combining a fibric acid agent with a statin results in greater decreases in triglyceride levels than either drug used alone. The mechanism of action of the fibric acid agents is largely unknown. Doses for the fibric acid agents are listed in Table 3.

The most common adverse effects of the fibrates are abdominal pain, nausea, and vomiting. Taking these medications with meals usually diminishes GI distress. Clofibrate has a tendency to concentrate bile and cause gallbladder disease. This increase in gallbladder disease has not been seen with other fibric acid agents, but drugs in this class are generally not used in patients with preexisting gallbladder or biliary disease.

PROTOTYPE DRUG   Gemfibrozil (Lopid)

Classification: **Therapeutic:** Antihyperlipidemic
Pharmacologic: Fibric acid agent (fibrate)

Therapeutic Effects and Uses: Approved in 1981, gemfibrozil lowers serum triglycerides and LDL cholesterol. It is most effective in patients who present with hypertriglyceridemia and VLDL. Effects of gemfibrozil include up to a 50% reduction in VLDL with an increase in HDL. It is less effective than the statins at lowering LDL; thus it is not used as monotherapy. It is considered a second-line therapy that is used when statins are ineffective or not well tolerated.

Mechanism of Action: The exact mechanism of action of gemfibrozil is unknown. The drug inhibits the breakdown of stored fat, or lipolysis, in adipose tissue. By inhibiting the uptake of free fatty acids by the liver, hepatic production of triglycerides is decreased. The drug may also increase the excretion of cholesterol in the feces.

Pharmacokinetics:

Route(s)	PO
Absorption	Well absorbed
Distribution	Unknown; distribution across the placenta or secretion in breast milk is unknown; 99% bound to plasma protein
Primary metabolism	Hepatic; undergoes enterohepatic recirculation
Primary excretion	Primarily renal, 6% in feces
Onset of action	1–2 h
Duration of action	Half-life: 1.5 h

Adverse Effects: The most common adverse effects of gemfibrozil are GI related, such as abdominal cramping, diarrhea, nausea, and dyspepsia. Nervous system effects include headache, dizziness, peripheral neuropathy, and diminished libido. Serious adverse effects include cholelithiasis, anemia, and eosinophilia.

Contraindications/Precautions: Gemfibrozil may worsen or cause biliary disease; thus it is contraindicated in patients with preexisting gallbladder disease or serious liver impairment. Because it is excreted by the kidneys, the drug should be used cautiously in patients with renal impairment.

Drug Interactions: Although antihyperlipidemic agents from different drug classes are sometimes combined to produce an enhanced effect, the use of gemfibrozil with statins increases the risk of myositis and rhabdomyolysis. CK levels should be regularly monitored during combined therapy and the combination immediately discontinued if myopathy is suspected. In most cases the risk of rhabdomyolysis, which may be fatal, outweighs the potential benefits of combined statin and gemfibrozil therapy.

Concurrent use of gemfibrozil with PO anticoagulants may increase the risk of bleeding because the fibrate displaces warfarin from its plasma protein binding sites. If a patient is taking warfarin, dosages should be lowered. More frequent monitoring of prothrombin time (PT) and international normalized ratio (INR) is necessary until stabilization occurs.

Gemfibrozil may enhance the hypoglycemic effects of antidiabetic agents. Serum glucose levels must be carefully monitored because the dosage of the antidiabetic drug may require adjustment. **Herbal/Food:** No significant interactions.

Pregnancy: Category C.

Treatment of Overdose: No specific therapy is available; patients are treated symptomatically.

Nursing Responsibilities: Key nursing implications for patients receiving gemfibrozil are included in the Nursing Practice Application for Patients Receiving Pharmacotherapy for Hyperlipidemia.

Lifespan and Diversity Considerations:

- Monitor the older adult for development of dizziness. Assist with ambulation as needed to prevent falls.

- Monitor for the development of gallbladder disease, particularly in Hispanic or Native American patients. Research has demonstrated a higher risk of gallbladder disease in these ethnic groups.

Patient and Family Education:

- Inform the health care provider if you have other medical problems such as gallbladder disease, gallstones, kidney disease, or liver disease.

- Do not breast-feed while taking this drug without approval of the health care provider.

Drugs Similar to Gemfibrozil (Lopid)

Drugs similar to gemfibrozil include fenofibrate and fenofibric acid.

Fenofibrate (Antara, TriCor, others) and fenofibric acid (Trilipix): Fenofibrate is indicated as supplemental therapy to diet to reduce elevated LDL, total cholesterol, triglycerides, and apo B and to increase HDL in patients with primary hypercholesterolemia, hypertriglyceridemia and mixed dyslipidemia. Approved in 1993, fenofibrate may reduce serum triglycerides by as much as 30%. One advantage of the fenofibrate formulations over gemfibrozil is that they may be taken once daily rather than twice a day. Several fenofibrate formulations, which vary in strength, bioavailability, and whether the drug should be administered with a meal, are available. These forms are not interchangeable. The most recent formulation, Trilipix, was approved in 2008 for concurrent therapy with statins. The most frequent adverse effects are GI related, such as nausea, vomiting, dyspepsia, constipation, flatulence, and abdominal pain. Liver tests should be performed periodically to monitor for elevated serum transaminases. Myopathy and rhabdomyolysis have been reported and the risks for these adverse effects are increased when fibrates are coadministered with a statin. Rash and photosensitivity are other adverse effects. This drug is pregnancy category C.

CONNECTION Checkpoint 32.2

What changes in physiology occur with aging that may require decreased starting dosages for antihyperlipidemic agents? *See Answer to Connection Checkpoint 32.2 on student resource website.*

Cholesterol Absorption Inhibitors

9 Cholesterol absorption inhibitors are the newest class of drugs for hyperlipidemia.

In the early 2000s, a class of drugs was discovered that inhibits the absorption of cholesterol. Ezetimibe (Zetia) is the only drug in this class.

Cholesterol is absorbed from the intestinal lumen by cells in the jejunum of the small intestine. Ezetimibe blocks this absorption by as much as 50%, causing less cholesterol to enter the blood. Unlike the statins, the drug does not inhibit cholesterol synthesis in the liver or increase the excretion of bile acid.

When given as monotherapy, ezetimibe produces a modest reduction in LDL of about 20%. Adding a statin to the therapeutic regimen reduces LDL by an additional 15% to 20%. The drug produces a slight drop in serum triglycerides. Ezetimibe is available as a single tablet with a once-daily dosing regimen. Vytorin is a fixed-dose combination tablet containing ezetimibe and simvastatin.

Serious adverse effects from ezetimibe are uncommon. Nasopharyngitis, myalgia, upper respiratory tract infection, arthralgia, and diarrhea are the most common adverse effects, although these rarely require discontinuation of therapy. Because it is extensively metabolized in the liver, patients with significant hepatic impairment should receive other antihyperlipidemic agents. Ezetimibe is pregnancy category C.

Because bile acid sequestrants inhibit the absorption of ezetimibe, these drugs should not be taken together. In addition, ezetimibe and statins should not be given concurrently to patients with serious hepatic impairment or with elevated serum transaminase levels.

CONNECTIONS: NURSING PRACTICE APPLICATION

Patients Receiving Pharmacotherapy for Hyperlipidemia

Assessment	Potential Nursing Diagnoses
Baseline assessment prior to administration: • Understand the reason the drug has been prescribed in order to assess for therapeutic effects. • Obtain a complete health history including cardiovascular, musculoskeletal (preexisting conditions that might result in muscle or joint pain), GI (peptic ulcer disease, hemorrhoids, inflammatory bowel disease, chronic constipation, gallbladder disease, dysphagia or esophageal strictures), and the possibility of pregnancy. Obtain a drug history including allergies, current prescription and OTC drugs, herbal preparations, and alcohol use. Be alert to possible drug interactions. • Evaluate appropriate laboratory findings, especially liver function studies, lipid profiles, and CK. • Assess the patient's ability to receive and understand instructions. Include the family or caregiver as needed.	• *Imbalanced Nutrition: More than Body Requirements* • *Ineffective Health Maintenance* (Individual or Family) • *Chronic Pain*, related to drug-induced myopathy • *Deficient Knowledge* (Drug Therapy)
Assessment throughout administration: • Assess for desired therapeutic effects (e.g., lowered total cholesterol and LDL levels, increased HDL levels). • Continue periodic monitoring of lipid profiles, liver function studies, CK, and uric acid levels. • Assess for adverse effects: musculoskeletal discomfort, nausea, vomiting, abdominal cramping, or diarrhea. Immediately report any severe musculoskeletal pain, unexplained muscle tenderness accompanied by fever, inability to perform activities of daily living (ADLs) due to musculoskeletal weakness or pain, unexplained numbness or tingling of extremities, yellowing of the sclera or skin, severe constipation, straining with passing of stools, or tarry stools.	

Planning: Patient Goals and Expected Outcomes

The patient will:
- Experience therapeutic effects (e.g., lowered total cholesterol and LDL, increased HDL, normal liver enzymes).
- Be free from or experience minimal adverse effects.
- Verbalize an understanding of the drug's use, adverse effects, and required precautions.
- Demonstrate proper self-administration of the medication (e.g., dose, timing, and when to notify the provider).

Implementation

Interventions and (Rationales)	Patient-Centered Care

Ensuring therapeutic effects:
• Follow appropriate administration guidelines. (Many of the lipid-lowering drugs have specific administration requirements. For best results, they should be taken at night when cholesterol biosynthesis is at its highest.)
	• Teach the patient to take the drug following appropriate guidelines as follows:
	  • **Statins:** Take with the evening meal; avoid grapefruit and grapefruit juice, which could inhibit the drug's metabolism, leading to toxic levels.
	  • **Bile acid resins:** Take before meals with plenty of fluids, mixing powders or granules thoroughly with liquid. Take other medications 1 h before or 4 h after the bile acid resin is taken.
	  • **Niacin:** Take with cold water to decrease the sensation of flushing associated with the drug. Take one adult-strength (325-mg) aspirin 30 min before the niacin dose.
	  • **Fibric acid agents:** Take with a meal.

• Encourage appropriate lifestyle changes: lowered fat intake, increased exercise, limited alcohol intake, and smoking cessation. Provide for dietitian consultation as needed. (Healthy lifestyle changes will support and minimize the need for drug therapy.)	• Encourage the patient and family to adopt a healthy lifestyle of low-fat food choices, increased exercise, decreased alcohol consumption, and smoking cessation. • Encourage increased intake of foods rich in omega-3 and coenzyme Q10: fish such as salmon and sardines, nuts, extra-virgin olive and canola oils, beef, chicken, and pork. Supplementation may be needed; instruct the patient to seek the advice of a health care provider before taking supplements.
Minimizing adverse effects: • Continue to monitor periodic liver function tests and CK levels. (Abnormal liver function tests or increased CK levels may indicate drug-induced adverse hepatic effects or myopathy and should be reported.)	• Instruct the patient on the need to return periodically for laboratory work.

CONNECTIONS: NURSING PRACTICE APPLICATION *(continued)*

- Continue to assess for drug-related symptoms which may indicate adverse effects are occurring. (Lipid-lowering drugs often adversely affect the liver but may also cause drug-specific adverse effects.)
- Assess for the possibility of increased adverse effects when a combination of lipid-lowering agents is used. (Lipid-lowering agents may be combined for better effects, but this increases the risk of adverse effects.)

- Teach the patient the importance of reporting signs or symptoms related to adverse drug effects as follows:
  - **Statins:** Report unusual or unexplained muscle tenderness, increasing muscle pain, numbness or tingling of extremities, or effects that hinder normal ADLs.
  - **Bile acid resins:** Report severe nausea, heartburn, constipation, or straining with passing stools. Any tarry stools or yellowing of the sclera or skin should also be reported.
  - **Niacin:** Report flank, joint, or stomach pain, or yellowing of the sclera or skin.
  - **Fibric acid agents:** Report unusual bleeding or bruising, right upper quadrant pain, muscle cramping, or changes in the color of the stool. Diabetics on PO medications may need a change in their dosage and should monitor their glucose more frequently in early therapy.
- Instruct patients taking a combination of lipid-lowering drugs to be alert to symptoms related to adverse effects of *both* drugs, as above.

- If long-term therapy is used, ensure adequate intake of fat-soluble vitamins (A, D, E, K) and folic acid in the diet or consider supplementation. (Lipid-lowering drugs may cause depletion or diminished absorption of these nutrients.)

- Instruct the patient, family, or caregiver about foods high in folic acid and fat-soluble vitamins, and about the need to consult with the health care provider about the need for vitamin and folic acid supplementation while on long-term therapy.

Patient understanding of drug therapy:
- Use opportunities during administration of medications and during assessments to discuss the rationale for drug therapy, desired therapeutic outcomes, commonly observed adverse effects, parameters for when to call the health care provider, and any necessary monitoring or precautions. (Using time during nursing care helps to optimize and reinforce key teaching areas.)

- The patient, family, or caregiver should be able to state the reason for the drug, appropriate dose and scheduling, what adverse effects to observe for and when to report them, and the anticipated length of medication therapy.

Patient self-administration of drug therapy:
- When administering the medication, instruct the patient, family, or caregiver in proper self-administration of the drug, e.g., during the evening meal. (Utilizing time during nurse-administration of these drugs helps to reinforce teaching.)

- The patient, family, or caregiver is able to discuss appropriate dosing and administration needs.

Evaluation of Outcome Criteria

Evaluate the effectiveness of drug therapy by confirming that patient goals and expected outcomes have been met (see "Planning").

UNDERSTANDING THE CHAPTER

Key Concepts Summary

1 Lipids are classified as triglycerides, phospholipids, or sterols.

2 Lipoproteins are important predictors of cardiovascular disease.

3 Blood lipid profiles are important diagnostic tools in guiding the therapy of dyslipidemias.

4 Lipid levels can often be controlled through therapeutic lifestyle changes.

5 The statins are the most effective drugs for reducing blood lipid levels.

6 Bile acid sequestrants are often combined with statins to reduce LDL cholesterol levels.

7 Niacin can reduce triglycerides and LDL cholesterol levels, but adverse effects limit its usefulness.

8 Fibric acid agents lower triglyceride levels but have little effect on LDL cholesterol.

9 Cholesterol absorption inhibitors are the newest class of drugs for hyperlipidemia.

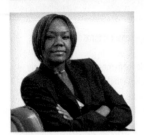

Making the PATIENT *Connection*

Remember the patient "Belinda Cummings" at the beginning of the chapter? Now read the remainder of the case study. Based on the information presented within this chapter, respond to the critical thinking questions that follow.

Belinda Cummings is a 39-year-old black female who feels fine. However, she recently had her cholesterol level checked at her church's health fair where she was told that it exceeded the normal value. As directed, she made an appointment and saw her health care provider for a checkup.

During the office visit, the nurse collects Belinda's social and health history. Belinda's vital signs are within normal limits, except her blood pressure is elevated (142/90 mmHg). She is also slightly overweight and has been on a low-carbohydrate diet for 1 week. Her favorite foods are potato chips and all dairy products, especially cheese. She admits to smoking less than a pack of cigarettes per day and occasionally drinks a glass of wine with dinner. Belinda is divorced and has one teenage son.

A series of laboratory and diagnostic tests is completed during the visit. Belinda's physical exam is normal, and there are no ECG abnormalities. The blood tests are unremarkable with the exception of the lipid profile.

	Patient Value	Normal Range
Total Cholesterol	240 mg/dL	Less than 200
Triglycerides	199 mg/dL	Less than 150
HDL Cholesterol	30 mg/dL	Greater than 60
LDL Cholesterol	184	Less than 100
Cholesterol-to-HDL Ratio	6.6	Less than 4.5

The patient is placed on a standard cholesterol-lowering diet and prescribed atorvastatin (Lipitor) 10 mg daily. Belinda is instructed to return to the office in 1 month for a follow-up visit.

Critical Thinking Questions

1. How would you respond to Belinda when she asks you, "Is high cholesterol due to heredity or from what I eat?"

2. What health teaching should you provide the patient about ways to reduce high blood lipid levels?

3. Create a list of potential adverse effects that this patient should be taught to watch for related to the medication.

See Answers to Critical Thinking Questions on student resource website.

NCLEX-RN® Review

1. The client taking atorvastatin (Lipitor) reports weakness and fatigue, pain in the shoulders, and aching joints. The nurse initially assesses the client for which condition?
   1. Rhabdomyolysis
   2. Renal failure
   3. Rheumatoid arthritis
   4. Hepatic insufficiency

2. A client is receiving cholestyramine (Questran) for elevated low-density lipoprotein levels. Which adverse effect should the nurse include in the care plan to monitor the client?
   1. Orange-colored urine
   2. Abdominal pain
   3. Sore throat and fever
   4. Decreased capillary refill

3. The provider orders colestipol (Colestid) in combination with atorvastatin (Lipitor) for a client with elevated low-density lipoprotein levels. The nurse collaborates with the prescriber about which data related to the client?
   1. Past history of peptic ulcer disease
   2. Recent myocardial infarction
   3. Laboratory value for serum sodium of 136 mEq/L
   4. Allergies to foods high in tyramine

4. Which assessment findings discovered by the nurse would be an expected adverse effect associated with niacin therapy? Select all that apply.
   1. Fever and chills
   2. Intense flushing and hot flashes
   3. Tingling of the fingers and toes
   4. Dry mucous membranes
   5. Hypoglycemia

5. The community health nurse visits a client who has been prescribed lovastatin (Mevacor). Which statement, if made by the client, indicates that further teaching is necessary concerning this drug therapy?
   1. "I should try to maintain my body weight at an optimal level."
   2. "Most clients with lipid disorders don't have any symptoms."
   3. "The best time for me to take this medication is before I go to bed."
   4. "I will take my drug with beverages that contain grapefruit juice."

6. The nurse is caring for a client receiving gemfibrozil (Lopid) for hyperlipidemia. The nurse would validate the order with the prescriber if the client reported a history of which of the following? Select all that apply.
   1. Gallbladder disease
   2. Angina
   3. Hypertension
   4. Diabetes
   5. Renal disease

Additional Case Study

David Hamilton has been taking cholestyramine (Questran) for elevated blood lipid levels for 2 years. He presents today in your clinic for a routine follow-up visit that will include a lipid profile test. He states that he has been somewhat consistent with his cholesterol-lowering diet and attempting to get "a little more" exercise. You are the nurse caring for David.

1. Outline key concepts related to health promotion activities that you would want to be sure David understands.

2. What adverse effects related to Questran should David watch for?

3. If David's triglyceride levels increase or remain consistently high, what drug group(s) might be prescribed?

See Answers to Additional Case Study on student resource website.

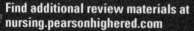

Pearson Nursing Student Resources

Find additional review materials at **nursing.pearsonhighered.com**

Prepare for success with additional NCLEX®-style practice questions, interactive assignments and activities, web links, animations, videos, and more!

References

American Heart Association. (n.d.). *Youth and cardiovascular diseases—Statistics.* Retrieved from http://www.americanheart.org/downloadable/heart/1059110431975FS11YTH3REV7-03.pdf

Citkowitz, E. (2011). Familial hypercholesterolemia. *Medscape Reference.* Retrieved from http://emedicine.medscape.com/article/121298-overview

McCrindle, B. W., Urbina, E. M., Dennison, B.A., Jacobson, M.S., Steinberger, J., Rocchini, A. P.,... Daniels, S. R. (2007). Drug therapy of high-risk lipid abnormalities in children and adolescents. *Circulation, 115,* 1948–1967. doi:10.1161/circulationaha.107.181946

Suzuki, T., Nozawa, T., Sobajima, M., Igarashi, N., Matsuki, A., Fujii, N., & Inoue, H. (2008). Atorvastatin-induced changes in plasma coenzyme Q10 and brain natriuretic peptide in patients with coronary artery disease. *International Heart Journal, 49*(4), 423–433.

Selected Bibliography

Bersot, T. P. (2011). Drug therapy for hypercholesterolemia and dyslipidemia. In L. L. Brunton, B. A. Chabner, & B. C. Knollman (Eds.), *The pharmacological basis of therapeutics* (12th ed., pp. 877–908). New York, NY: McGraw-Hill.

Citkowitz, E. (2009). Hypercholesterolemia, familial. *Medscape Reference.* Retrieved from http://emedicine.medscape.com/article/121298-overview

Eiland, L. S., & Luttrell, P. K. (2010). Use of statins for dyslipidemia in the pediatric population. *Journal of Pediatric Pharmacology and Therapeutics, 15*(3), 160–172.

Florentin, M., Liberopoulos, E. N., Mikhailidis, D.P., & Elisaf, M.S. (2008). Fibrate-associated adverse effects beyond muscle and liver toxicity. *Current Pharmaceutical Design, 14*(6), 574–587. doi:10.2174/138161208783885362

Marcoff, L., & Thompson, P. (2007). The role of coenzyme Q10 in statin-associated myopathy: A systematic review. *Journal of the American College of Cardiology, 49*(23), 2231–2237. doi:10.1016/j.jacc.2007.02.049

Menown, I. B. A., Murtagh, G., Maher, V., Cooney, M. T., Graham, I. M., & Tomkin, G. (2009). Dyslipidemia therapy update: The importance of full lipid profile assessment. *Advances in Therapy, 17*(7), 711–718. doi:10.1007/s12325-009-0052-3

Oldways. (n.d.). Traditional diets and Oldways' four pyramids. Retrieved from http://www.oldwayspt.org/eating-well/introduction-traditional-diet-pyramids

Ray, K. K., Seshasai, S. R. K., Jukema, W., & Sattar, N. (2010). Statins and all-cause mortality in high-risk primary prevention: A meta-analysis of 11 randomized controlled trials involving 65,229 participants. *Archives of Internal Medicine, 170*(12):1024–1031. doi:10.1001/archinternmed.2010.182

Spratt, K.A. (2010). Treating dyslipidemia: Reevaluating the data using evidence-based medicine. *Journal of the American Osteopathic Association, 110*(4), 6–11.

Steinberger, J., & Kelly, A. S. (2008). Challenges of existing pediatric dyslipidemia guidelines: Call for reappraisal. *Circulation, 117,* 9–10. doi:10.1161/circulationaha.107.743104

Taylor, F., Ward, K., Moore, T. H. M., Burke, M., Davey-Smith, G., Casas J-P., & Ebrahim, S. (2011). Statins for the primary prevention of cardiovascular disease. *Cochrane Database of Systematic Reviews, 1,* CD004816. doi:10.1002/14651858.CD004816.pub4

U.S. Department of Agriculture, Food and Nutrition Information Center. (2010). Retrieved from http://fnic.nal.usda.gov/nal_display/index.php?info_center=4&tax_level=3&tax_subject=256&topic_id=1348&level3_id=5732

Answers to NCLEX-RN® Review

1 Answer: 1   Rationale: Rhabdomyolysis is a serious adverse effect of the statins. Early signs include unexplained fatigue or muscle weakness, pain in joints or muscles, and an increase in CK level. Options 2, 3, and 4 are incorrect. The weakness, fatigue, and pain that the client is experiencing are not symptoms of renal failure or hepatic insufficiency. In rheumatoid arthritis, pain is often present, but tends to be greatest in the mornings and associated with red, hot, swollen joints. Cognitive Level: Analyzing; Client Need: Physiological Integrity; Nursing Process: Evaluation

2 Answer: 2   Rationale: One of the most serious adverse effects of cholestyramine is obstruction of the GI tract. Options 1, 3, and 4 are incorrect. Cholestyramine does not cause orange urine, sore throat and fever, or affect capillary refill. Cognitive Level: Applying; Client Need: Physiological Integrity; Nursing Process: Planning

3 Answer: 1   Rationale: Although there are few contraindications to using bile acid sequestrants such as colestipol, they should be used cautiously in clients with GI disorders such as peptic ulcer disease. Options 2, 3, and 4 are incorrect. MI is not a contraindication for the use of bile acid sequestrants. Bile acid sequestrant agents do not affect serum sodium levels, and clients allergic to foods high in tyramine may be prescribed bile acid sequestrants. Cognitive Level: Applying; Client Need: Physiological Integrity; Nursing Process: Implementation

4 Answer: 2, 3   Rationale: Intense flushing and hot flashes occur in almost every client who is taking niacin. Tingling of the extremities may also occur. Options 1, 4, and 5 are incorrect. Neither fever and chills nor dry mucous membranes are associated adverse effects of niacin therapy. Niacin may cause an *increase* in fasting blood glucose, especially in people with diabetes. Cognitive Level: Analyzing; Client Need: Physiological Integrity; Nursing Process: Evaluation

5 Answer: 4   Rationale: Grapefruit juice inhibits the metabolism of statins such as lovastatin, allowing them to reach high serum levels. Options 1, 2, and 3 are incorrect. Most clients with lipid disorders are asymptomatic. A client should be instructed that maintenance of optimal body weight will help reduce unhealthy lipid levels. Because cholesterol biosynthesis in the liver is higher at night, statins are usually best taken in the evening. Cognitive Level: Applying; Client Need: Health Promotion and Maintenance; Nursing Process: Evaluation

6 Answer: 1, 4, 5   Rationale: Fibric acid agents (fibrates) such as gemfibrozil may cause or worsen gallbladder disease and may enhance the hypoglycemic effects of antidiabetes drugs. Because it is excreted through the kidneys, it may be used cautiously in clients with renal impairment, but the order should be validated with the provider before giving if the client has a history of renal impairment. Options 2 and 3 are incorrect. Angina and hypertension may indicate the existence of atherosclerosis and arteriosclerosis, both of which are indications for a lipid-lowering drug. Cognitive Level: Applying; Client Need: Physiological Integrity; Nursing Process: Implementation

Drugs Affecting the Renin-Angiotensin-Aldosterone System

From Chapter 34 of *Pharmacology: Connections to Nursing Practice*, Second Edition. Michael Patrick Adams, Carol Quam Urban. Copyright © 2013 by Pearson Education, Inc. All rights reserved.

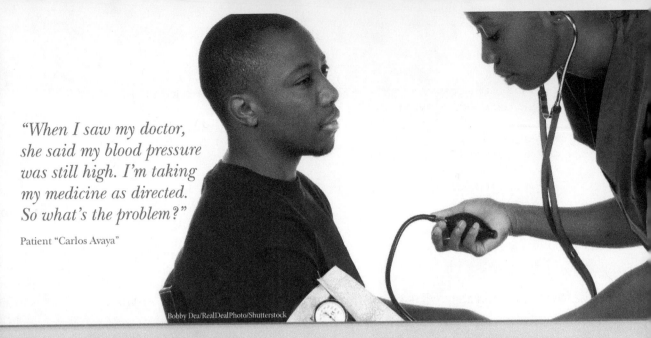

"When I saw my doctor, she said my blood pressure was still high. I'm taking my medicine as directed. So what's the problem?"

Patient "Carlos Avaya"

Bobby Dea/RealDealPhoto/Shutterstock

Drugs Affecting the Renin-Angiotensin-Aldosterone System

Learning Outcomes

After reading this chapter, the student should be able to:

1. Illustrate the steps in the renin-angiotensin-aldosterone pathway.

2. Identify the primary physiological factors that control renin secretion.

3. Explain the two primary functions of angiotensin-converting enzyme.

4. Describe multiple mechanisms by which angiotensin II raises blood pressure.

5. Explain how the actions of aldosterone can lead to high blood pressure.

6. Identify the specific steps in the renin-angiotensin-aldosterone system that can be blocked by medications.

7. For each of the classes shown in the chapter outline, identify the prototype and representative drugs and explain the mechanism(s) of drug action, primary indications, contraindications, significant drug interactions, pregnancy category, and important adverse effects.

8. Apply the nursing process to care for patients receiving drugs that affect the renin-angiotensin-aldosterone system.

Chapter Outline

Components of the Renin-Angiotensin-Aldosterone System

Physiological Effects of the Renin-Angiotensin-Aldosterone System

Drugs Affecting the Renin-Angiotensin-Aldosterone System

Angiotensin-Converting Enzyme (ACE) Inhibitors

PROTOTYPE **Lisinopril (Prinivil, Zestril)**

Angiotensin II Receptor Blockers (ARBs)

PROTOTYPE **Losartan (Cozaar)**

Aldosterone Antagonists

The renin-angiotensin-aldosterone system (RAAS) is a key homeostatic mechanism controlling blood pressure and fluid balance. The RAAS is presented early in the study of cardiovascular pharmacology because the drugs affecting this pathway are frequently used to treat hypertension (HTN) and heart failure (HF). This chapter examines components of the RAAS and describes how drugs affecting this system are used for therapeutic benefit.

Components of the Renin-Angiotensin-Aldosterone System

1 The formation of angiotensin II requires two enzymatic steps.

In the mid-1900s, scientists discovered a peptide circulating in the blood that caused profound vasoconstriction. Named angiotensin (*angio* = blood vessel; *tensin* = pressure), high levels of this substance were found in people with HTN. Thus began the search for components of what is now called the renin-angiotensin-aldosterone system.

We now know that there are several forms of angiotensin. **Angiotensin II** is the vasopressor substance originally isolated by scientists in the 1900s. The formation of angiotensin II requires two key enzymatic steps, and an understanding of these steps is critical to learning the pharmacology of drugs affecting the RAAS. The RAAS is illustrated in Figure 1.

Step 1—Formation of angiotensin I: **Angiotensinogen** is a protein synthesized by the liver that is continuously circulating in the bloodstream. In the blood, angiotensinogen is split by the enzyme renin to form **angiotensin I.** Neither angiotensinogen nor angiotensin I has any significant biologic activity; they simply serve as precursors to angiotensin II.

Step 2—Formation of angiotensin II: Angiotensin I travels through the circulation until it encounters angiotensin-converting enzyme (ACE), which cleaves two amino acids to form angiotensin II. ACE is located on the membrane surface of the blood vessel endothelium. Because the lung possesses such an extensive number of capillaries, it is the primary organ responsible for converting angiotensin I to angiotensin II. Angiotensin II is one of the most potent natural vasoconstrictors known; it is approximately 40 times more potent at raising blood pressure than norepinephrine.

2 Renin secretion is controlled by the juxtaglomerular cells of the kidney and the sympathetic nervous system.

Because renin is responsible for the first step in the RAAS pathway, it is a major factor in determining the amount of angiotensin II produced in the body. Therefore, factors affecting the secretion of renin are important to understanding the pharmacotherapy associated with this system.

Renin is an enzyme that is synthesized, stored, and secreted by specialized cells in the kidney known as **juxtaglomerular (JG) cells.** Found in the afferent arteriole that supplies blood to the glomerulus, JG cells are specialized smooth muscle cells that act as pressure sensors. As blood pressure falls, there is less pressure on the JG cells, which respond by releasing renin to the circulation. The increase in renin ultimately leads to larger amounts of circulating angiotensin II, which returns blood pressure to normal. The release of renin is caused by factors that lower blood pressure, such as a loss of blood volume due to dehydration or hemorrhage. Through negative feedback, increased blood pressure is sensed by the JG cells, which then turn off renin secretion.

Key Terms

angioedema

angiotensin I

angiotensin II

angiotensinogen

bradykinin

cardiac remodeling

juxtaglomerular (JG) cells

macula densa

renin

renin-angiotensin-aldosterone system (RAAS)

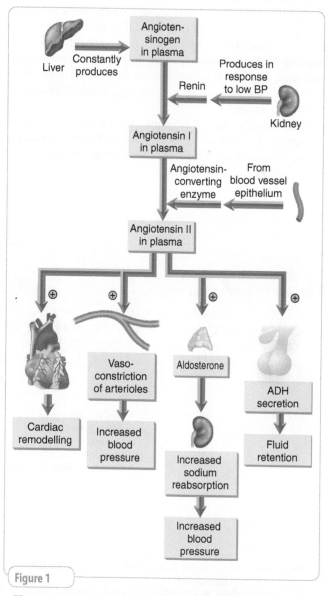

Figure 1

The renin-angiotensin-aldosterone pathway.

169

To the Community — Angiotensin-Converting Enzyme Inhibitors and Hyperkalemia

CONNECTIONS

The development of hyperkalemia is uncommon in patients taking ACE inhibitors, occurring in less than 30% of patients. While it is more common in patients with diabetes and renal disease, other patients taking ACE inhibitors may also be at risk. Potassium supplements or potassium-sparing diuretics should be stopped when a patient is started on ACE inhibitors, but other drugs and substances may also cause hyperkalemia. Salt substitutes often contain potassium chloride instead of sodium chloride and the additional potassium may cause hyperkalemia if the patient mistakenly thinks that because it's a salt substitute, it can be used liberally as a healthy replacement to table salt.

Other drugs that have been known to increase the risk of hyperkalemia when given concurrently with ACE inhibitors include NSAIDs, beta blockers, heparin, ketoconazole, trimethoprim, pentamidine, and immunosuppressants such as cyclosporine and tacrolimus. In addition to diabetes or renal disease, severe HF, volume depletion, or advanced age also place the patient at risk. Prior to starting ACE inhibitors, a thorough personal and drug history should be taken to screen for any condition or medication that may lead to hyperkalemia development. Frequent testing for potassium levels may be required if the patient is on required concurrent medications that raise the risk. The patient should be educated to avoid salt substitutes that contain potassium chloride.

Several other important factors control the release of renin. Adjacent to the JG cells in the distal convoluted tubule of the nephron is a specialized cluster of cells called the macula densa. The macula densa is in a perfect location to sense the flow rate and the concentration of sodium ions (osmolality) in the filtrate. As blood pressure falls, blood flow through the kidney diminishes and the flow rate of renal tubular filtrate slows. The **macula densa** recognizes the slow flow rate (and less sodium) and sends a chemical message to the JG cells to release more renin. The renin release forms more angiotensin II and blood pressure rises.

Anatomically, the JG cells and the macula densa are in proximity, as shown in Figure 2. The JG cells and the macula densa are sometimes considered a single anatomic unit called the juxtaglomerular apparatus.

CONNECTION Checkpoint 34.1

Substances that lower blood pressure may trigger reflex tachycardia. Explain the mechanism involved in this reflex. *See Answer to Connection Checkpoint 34.1 on student resource website.*

A third mechanism for controlling the release of renin is more direct: activation of the sympathetic nervous system. JG cells contain beta$_1$-adrenergic receptors, which are activated by the classic fight-or-flight response of the sympathetic nervous system. The release of renin helps to raise blood pressure when dealing with a stressful or harmful situation.

To summarize, factors that promote the release of renin by JG cells will raise blood pressure. The three primary factors causing an increase are decreased pressure in blood flowing through the kidney, decreased tubular flow rate (or fewer

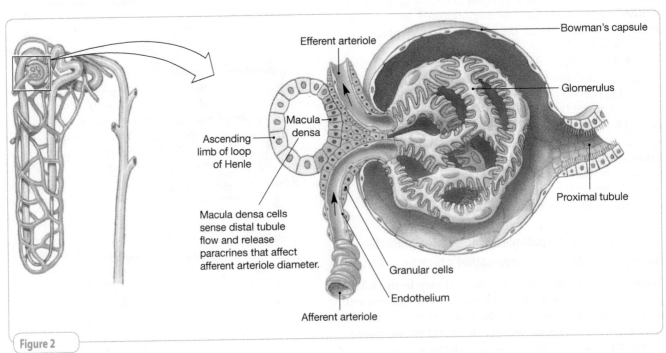

Figure 2

The macula densa and the juxtaglomerular (JG) cells. Osmoreceptors in the macula densa sense low sodium levels, which signals the JG cells to release renin.

Source: From SILVERTHORN, DEE UNGLAUB, HUMAN PHYSIOLOGY: AN INTEGRATED APPROACH, 5th Ed., © 2010. Reprinted and Electronically reproduced by permission of Pearson Education, Inc., Upper Saddle River, New Jersey.

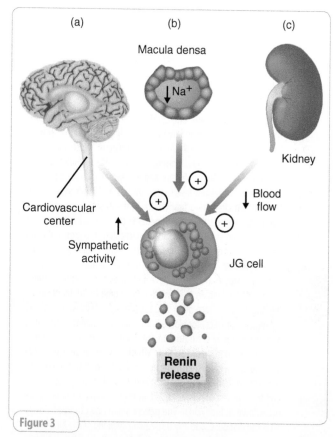

(a)   (b)   (c)

Macula densa

↓Na⁺

Kidney

Cardiovascular
center

↑
Sympathetic
activity

↓ Blood
flow

+

+

+

JG cell

Renin
release

Figure 3

Overview of factors affecting renin release: (a) activation of the sympathetic nervous system; (b) low osmolarity in the macula densa; (c) low blood flow through the kidney.

sodium ions) sensed by the macula densa, and activation of the sympathetic nervous system. Conversely, the factors that decrease renin secretion lower blood pressure. These factors are illustrated in Figure 3.

Increasing renin secretion will not always cause an increase in blood pressure. Remember that RAAS is a two-step pathway, and both steps are essential to produce a physiological response. Section 3 examines this second step.

CONNECTION Checkpoint 34.2

Other than JG cells, in what organ are beta₁-adrenergic receptors predominantly located? What is the response of that organ when these receptors are activated? *See Answer to Connection Checkpoint 34.2 on student resource website.*

3 Angiotensin-converting enzyme is responsible for the formation of angiotensin II.

Once angiotensin I is formed, its conversion to angiotensin II by ACE is almost instantaneous. This is because ACE lies on the membranes of blood vessels and has immediate access to angiotensin I as soon as it is formed. A single pass of the blood through lung capillaries converts most of the circulating angiotensin I to angiotensin II.

In addition to its role in the formation of angiotensin II, ACE has a second function important to homeostasis and pharmacotherapy. ACE is one of several enzymes that break

down **bradykinin**, a natural mediator of inflammation and pain. Bradykinin has many of the same effects as histamine, including increasing arteriolar vasodilation and vascular permeability, and is likely responsible for some of the adverse effects of the ACE inhibitor medications. When referring to its actions on bradykinin, ACE is sometimes called kininase II; *kininase* is the general term for an enzyme that breaks down kinins. ACE and kininase II refer to the identical enzyme.

Pharmacologically, ACE is an important enzyme in the RAAS because it serves as a target molecule for drugs in the ACE inhibitor class of medications. Inhibition of ACE will prevent the formation of angiotensin II, thus interrupting the RAAS pathway. These medications also inhibit kininase II, thus preventing the breakdown of bradykinin. Accumulation of bradykinin in certain tissues can cause several adverse effects of ACE inhibitors, such as angioedema and cough.

Physiological Effects of the Renin-Angiotensin-Aldosterone System

4 Angiotensin II has multiple effects on the cardiovascular system that raise blood pressure and affect cardiac function.

The final product of the two-step renin-angiotensin pathway is angiotensin II. Angiotensin II has several important physiological effects important to homeostasis and to pharmacotherapy.

Direct vasoconstriction: Angiotensin II acts directly on vascular smooth muscle to cause vasoconstriction and increased systemic blood pressure. This effect is rapid; formation of angiotensin II results in a nearly instantaneous increase in blood pressure. This vasopressor action of angiotensin II is much greater on arterioles compared to veins; arterioles serving the kidneys are especially sensitive to this vasopressor action.

Increased sympathetic nervous system activity: Angiotensin II activates the sympathetic nervous system by causing the release of norepinephrine from sympathetic nerve terminals. The adrenal medulla is also affected by angiotensin II, which responds by releasing additional epinephrine to the circulation. Furthermore, through largely unknown mechanisms, angiotensin II increases sympathetic outflow from the brain. All three of these actions increase peripheral resistance and raise blood pressure.

Alteration of cardiovascular structure: Angiotensin II causes hypertrophy of myocardial cells (myocytes) and promotes collagen deposits in the cardiac matrix, essentially forming scar-like tissue in the heart. These changes are known as **cardiac remodeling**. The hypertrophy, fibrosis, and remodeling of cardiac structure have been correlated with increased morbidity and mortality associated with heart disease. In blood vessels, angiotensin II causes the release of multiple chemical mediators of atherosclerosis, accelerating the deposition of fatty plaque on the walls of the vessels. Increased plaque deposits lead to an increased risk for myocardial infarction (MI) and stroke.

CONNECTION Checkpoint 34.3

What effect would you expect angiotensin II formation to have on cardiac output and afterload? *See Answer to Connection Checkpoint 34.3 on student resource website.*

Release of aldosterone and effects on the renal tubule: Angiotensin II has two primary effects on the kidney that promote an increase in blood pressure. First, angiotensin II has a direct effect on the nephron that increases Na^+ and Cl^- reabsorption in the proximal tubule. Second, angiotensin II indirectly affects sodium reabsorption by stimulating the adrenal cortex to synthesize and secrete additional amounts of the hormone aldosterone. Aldosterone acts on the distal and collecting tubules of the nephron to increase Na^+ reabsorption and K^+ and H^+ excretion. The enhanced sodium reabsorption from both direct and indirect actions of angiotensin II causes the body to retain water, thus increasing blood volume and raising blood pressure. Aldosterone is a key component of the RAAS.

Unlike its immediate and direct effects on sympathetic nerves, the actions of angiotensin II on the kidney develop more slowly. This slow vasopressor response is believed to be responsible for producing a sustained elevation of blood pressure and a gradual decline of renal function.

Students often think of angiotensin II as a "bad actor" because it can create HTN and cause the damaging effects of cardiac remodeling. Remember, however, that the cardiovascular and renal effects of angiotensin II serve an essential homeostatic function. Should blood pressure fall, the increased synthesis and production of angiotensin II help return blood pressure to normal levels to maintain blood flow to vital organs. When the body is subjected to chronically elevated levels of angiotensin II, however, the once vital reflex pathway becomes a detriment to the body.

5 The renin-angiotensin-aldosterone pathway offers multiple points for drug intervention.

Having learned details of the different components in the short pathway leading from angiotensinogen to angiotensin II, the student should recognize several potential mechanisms by which drugs could intervene:

- **ACE inhibitors.** These are the first and, thus far, the largest and most important class of agents modifying the RAAS. ACE inhibitors block the conversion of angiotensin I to angiotensin II.

- **Angiotensin receptor blockers.** After angiotensin II is formed, it must interact with its receptors on target cells to cause its biologic actions. There are two receptor subtypes, known as AT_1 and AT_2 receptors. Blocking AT_1 receptors prevents angiotensin from raising blood pressure and from causing cardiac remodeling. Angiotensin receptor blockers are medications that intervene at this step in the RAAS by blocking the AT_1 receptor. The role of the AT_2 receptor in physiology is largely unknown but is an area of active research.

- **Aldosterone antagonists.** Much of the blood pressure increase resulting from the formation of angiotensin II is caused by its stimulation of aldosterone secretion. Two drugs are available that block receptors for aldosterone

To the Community

Angiotensin-Converting Enzyme Inhibitors and Angioedema

Angioedema is the development of edema of the mouth, lips, tongue, pharynx, larynx, and epiglottis that may be fatal if respiratory distress occurs secondary to the swelling of the upper airway. Less commonly, intestinal edema may also occur, causing a sudden onset of abdominal pain, vomiting, and diarrhea. Angioedema is associated with ACE inhibitors and appears to be related to the increase in bradykinin levels when ACE is no longer available to break down circulating bradykinin. While angioedema occurs in approximately less than 1% of patients taking ACE inhibitors, it is more common in African Americans, particularly those of Caribbean descent, and in older adults. In 50% of patients, angioedema occurs after the first dose of an ACE inhibitor, although it may occur anytime during therapy. Patients who have had a previous episode of angioedema after taking an ACE inhibitor are at greater risk for developing angioedema from other ACE inhibitors. It may also be caused by angiotensin-receptor blockers, although less commonly. Itching and urticaria may occur prior to the development of angioedema, but are not good predictors as to whether or not angioedema will develop. Immediate treatment may include administration of epinephrine, antihistamines (both H_1 and H_2 blockers), corticosteroids, and fresh frozen plasma. The ACE in fresh plasma accelerates the breakdown of bradykinin. The patient should be observed closely after the first dose, and any subsequent swelling of the facial, oral, or pharynx areas should be immediately reported to the provider.

in the kidney, thus preventing the aldosterone-induced increase in blood pressure.

- **Renin inhibitors.** In 2007, the FDA approved the first renin inhibitor. Aliskiren (Tekturna) is approved to treat HTN as monotherapy or in combination with other antihypertensives. It is likely that other renin inhibitors will be submitted for FDA approval in the future.

Drugs Affecting the Renin-Angiotensin-Aldosterone System

6 ACE inhibitors are key drugs in the pharmacotherapy of hypertension and heart failure.

First detected in the venom of pit vipers in the 1960s, inhibitors of ACE have been approved for HTN since the 1980s. Since then drugs in this class have become first-line agents in the treatment of HTN and HF. Doses for the ACE inhibitors are listed in Table 1.

ACE inhibitors block the conversion of angiotensin I to angiotensin II. The decline in angiotensin II levels causes blood pressure to decrease because there is less sympathetic activation and, thus, lower peripheral resistance. In addition, the decreased aldosterone secretion reduces blood volume, which also contributes to blood pressure reduction.

Research studies have clearly demonstrated that ACE inhibitors can slow the progression of HF and reduce mortality from

TABLE 1 ACE Inhibitors

Drug	Route and Adult Dose (maximum dose where indicated)	Adverse Effects
benazepril (Lotensin)	PO: 10–40 mg in one to two divided doses (max: 40 mg/day)	*Headache, dry cough, dizziness, orthostatic hypotension, rash*
captopril (Capoten)	PO: 6.25–25 mg tid (max: 450 mg/day)	
enalapril (Vasotec)	PO: 5–40 mg in one to two divided doses (max: 40 mg/day)	Angioedema, acute renal failure, first-dose phenomenon, fetal toxicity
fosinopril (Monopril)	PO: 5–40 mg once daily (max: 40 mg/day)	
lisinopril (Prinivil, Zestril)	PO: 10 mg daily (max: 80 mg/day)	
moexipril (Univasc)	PO: 7.5–30 mg once daily (max: 30 mg/day)	
perindopril (Aceon)	PO: 4 mg once daily (max: 16 mg/day for HTN; 4 mg/day for HF)	
quinapril (Accupril)	PO: 10–20 mg once daily (max: 80 mg/day)	
ramipril (Altace)	PO: 2.5–20 mg daily (max: 20 mg/day)	
trandolapril (Mavik)	PO: 1–4 mg once daily (max: 8 mg/day)	

Note: *Italics* indicate common adverse effects. <u>Underline</u> indicates serious adverse effects.

this disease. This is likely due to both the reduction in systemic blood pressure and a reversal of the angiotensin II-induced structural changes in the heart. Because of their relative safety, they have replaced digoxin (Lanoxin) as the first-line drugs for the treatment of chronic HF. Indeed, unless specifically contraindicated, all patients with HF usually receive an ACE inhibitor.

Research has also indicated a clear benefit for administering ACE inhibitors to patients who have experienced a recent MI. If therapy is begun immediately after the infarction and continued for several weeks, these drugs lower the mortality associated with an acute MI. The mechanism by which these drugs improve the outcome following an acute MI involves reduced peripheral vascular resistance, improved perfusion, and a direct action on the myocardium that reduces the cardiac workload.

ACE inhibitors may also be prescribed as prophylaxis therapy in patients at high risk for an adverse cardiovascular event. ACE inhibitors can reduce the incidence of a stroke or MI in these high-risk patients. They may also prevent or delay the progression of renal disease and retinopathy in patients with diabetes.

At least 11 ACE inhibitors have been approved and all have very similar indications and adverse effect profiles. All drugs in this class are approved to treat HTN, although only a few are approved for HF and acute MI, and for prophylaxis of cardiovascular disease. With the exception of enalaprilat, ACE inhibitors are administered orally (PO), and nearly all offer the convenience of once-daily dosing. Many of the ACE inhibitors are prodrugs, which are converted to active metabolites by enzymes in the liver. Most ACE inhibitors are excreted by the kidneys; thus dose reductions may be required in patients with significant renal impairment.

The low incidence of serious adverse effects is a major contributing factor to the widespread use of the ACE inhibitors. Orthostatic hypotension following the first few doses of the drug can be severe in patients who are on low-sodium diets or who have HF. Drug therapy is sometimes begun with very low doses and increased gradually to avoid orthostatic hypotension. Hyperkalemia may occur during ACE inhibitor therapy; however, this is predominantly a major concern only for patients with diabetes, those with renal impairment, and

those who are taking potassium supplements or potassium-sparing diuretics. Persistent, dry cough is an annoying adverse effect that occurs in 5% to 20% of patients taking ACE inhibitors. This adverse effect is likely due to a buildup of bradykinin in the lung. Drugs in this class have minimal or no effect on serum glucose or uric acid levels.

Though rare, the most serious adverse effect of ACE inhibitors is the development of **angioedema**, a rapid swelling of the throat, face, larynx, and tongue that can lead to airway obstruction and death. When it does occur, angioedema most often develops within a few hours after the first dose, although it may occur after several days of ACE inhibitor therapy. Accumulation of bradykinin is thought to be responsible. Treatment of angioedema is to discontinue the drug immediately and maintain the airway until the effects of the drug wear off.

PharmFACT

ACE inhibitors are especially useful in patients with diabetes. Although these drugs do not directly lower blood glucose, they do increase the body's sensitivity to insulin by increasing insulin release and improving glucose uptake in peripheral tissues. Because of this action, ACE inhibitors are sometimes used off-label to prevent new-onset type 2 diabetes (Solski & Longyhore, 2008).

PROTOTYPE DRUG Lisinopril (Prinivil, Zestril)

Classification: **Therapeutic:** Antihypertensive
Pharmacologic: ACE inhibitor

Therapeutic Effects and Uses: Approved for the treatment of HF, HTN, and acute MI, lisinopril is one of the most frequently prescribed medications. Approved in 1987, it may be used as monotherapy or it may be combined with other agents: Fixed-dose combinations of lisinopril and hydrochlorothiazide (a diuretic) are marketed for HTN as Prinzide and Zestoretic. Unlike many drugs in this class, lisinopril is active itself; it is not a prodrug. Treatment of migraines is an off-label indication for lisinopril.

Although captopril was the first drug that was marketed in this class, lisinopril is more widely prescribed because it has

173

a longer duration of action that allows for once-daily dosing. Like other ACE inhibitors, 2 to 3 weeks of therapy may be required to achieve maximum therapeutic outcomes.

Mechanism of Action: Lisinopril binds to and inhibits the action of ACE, thus preventing the conversion of angiotensin I to angiotensin II. The decrease in serum angiotensin II reduces aldosterone secretion, which results in less sodium and water retention. In patients with HTN, blood pressure is reduced with minimal effect on heart rate, stroke volume, or cardiac output.

Pharmacokinetics:

Route(s)	PO
Absorption	25–30% absorbed from the gastrointestinal (GI) tract
Distribution	Small amount crosses the blood–brain barrier; crosses the placenta; limited amounts are secreted in breast milk; not bound to plasma protein
Primary metabolism	Not metabolized
Primary excretion	Renal
Onset of action	1 h; peak effect: 6–8 h
Duration of action	24 h; half-life: 12 h

Adverse Effects: Lisinopril is well tolerated and adverse effects are uncommon and transient. The most common adverse effects are cough, headache, dizziness, orthostatic hypotension, and rash. Hyperkalemia occurs in about 2% to 4% of patients taking ACE inhibitors, although this usually resolves during therapy. Patients with HF or renal impairment or who are taking potassium supplements or potassium-sparing diuretics are at highest risk for hyperkalemia. Rare, though serious adverse effects include angioedema, agranulocytosis, and hepatotoxicity. **Black Box Warning**: Fetal injury and death may occur when ACE inhibitors are taken during pregnancy. When pregnancy is detected, they should be discontinued as soon as possible.

Contraindications/Precautions: Lisinopril should be used with extreme caution in patients with hyperkalemia because they may experience serious and even fatal dysrhythmias. Patients with a history of angioedema should not receive lisinopril. Caution should be used in treating patients with serious renal impairment: Dosage should be reduced. Lisinopril is contraindicated during pregnancy.

Drug Interactions: Indomethacin and other nonsteroidal anti-inflammatory drugs (NSAIDs) interact with lisinopril to decrease antihypertensive activity. The combination of lisinopril and NSAIDs may also worsen preexisting renal disease. Because of synergistic hypotensive action, concurrent therapy with diuretics and other antihypertensives such as ACE inhibitors should be carefully monitored. When taken with potassium supplements or potassium-sparing diuretics, hyperkalemia may result. Lisinopril may increase lithium levels and toxicity. **Herbal/Food**: Hawthorn should not be taken concurrently with lisinopril due to the possibility of additive hypotensive action.

Pregnancy: Categories C (first trimester) and D (second and third trimesters).

Treatment of Overdose: Overdose will cause hypotension, which may be treated with normal saline or a vasopressor. The drug may also be removed by hemodialysis.

Nursing Responsibilities: Key nursing implications for patients receiving lisinopril are included in the Nursing Practice Application for Patients Receiving Angiotensin-Converting Enzyme Inhibitor and Angiotensin Receptor Blocker Therapy.

Lifespan and Diversity Considerations:

- Monitor for the development of angioedema in older adults, African American patients, and patients who have previously experienced angioedema with an ACE inhibitor, because these patients are at higher risk.
- Monitor potassium levels frequently in the older adult who is at greater risk for the development of hyperkalemia while on these drugs.

Patient and Family Education:

- Monitor blood pressure regularly as directed by the health care provider. Maintain a written log of blood pressure readings, and present it at follow-up visits.
- Immediately report any swelling of the face, mouth, lips, or tongue, hoarseness, or sudden trouble with breathing.
- Avoid salt substitutes that contain potassium chloride.
- Immediately inform the health care provider of any known or suspected pregnancy because these drugs can cause birth defects.
- Do not breast-feed while taking this drug without approval of the health care provider.

Drugs Similar to Lisinopril (Prinivil, Zestril)

In addition to lisinopril, there are nine other ACE inhibitors on the market. All have very similar actions and adverse effects.

Benazepril (Lotensin): Approved in 1991, benazepril is approved only for HTN, although an off-label indication is HF. It is a prodrug that is metabolized by hepatic enzymes to its active form, benazeprilat. It has a long duration of action that allows for once-daily dosing and is excreted by the kidneys. Orthostatic hypotension is the most common adverse effect, especially after the first dose. Other adverse effects, contraindications, and indications are the same as lisinopril. Lotensin HCT is a fixed-dose combination of benazepril and hydrochlorothiazide. Lotrel is a combination of benazepril with amlodipine. This drug is pregnancy category C (first trimester) and D (second and third trimesters).

Captopril (Capoten): Captopril, the first ACE inhibitor marketed in 1981, is approved for HTN, HF, left ventricular dysfunction after an acute MI, and diabetic nephropathy. It has a short half-life, which requires multiple daily doses for some patients. The drug should be taken on an empty stomach, because food reduces its bioavailability. Neutropenia and agranulocytosis have occurred during captopril use. Other adverse effects, contraindications, and indications are the same as those of lisinopril. Capozide is a fixed-dose combination of captopril and hydrochlorothiazide. This is a pregnancy category D drug.

Enalapril (Vasotec): Approved in 1985, enalapril is indicated for HTN, HF, and asymptomatic left ventricular dysfunction in post-MI patients. Like most drugs in this class, it has an extended half-life and is excreted by the kidneys. It has a shorter half-life than some other ACE inhibitors and may require twice-daily dosing. Enalapril is a prodrug, being converted by hepatic enzymes to enalaprilat, which is its active form. The most frequent adverse effect is hypotension, which can be especially troublesome in patients with HF. Adverse effects, contraindications, and indications are the same as lisinopril. Enalaprilat (Vasotec IV) is available as a drug for severe HTN and is the only ACE inhibitor administered parenterally. Vaseretic is a fixed-dose combination of enalapril and hydrochlorothiazide. Both enalapril and enalaprilat are pregnancy category D drugs.

Fosinopril (Monopril): Approved in 1991, fosinopril is approved for HTN and HF. It is a prodrug that is metabolized by hepatic enzymes to its active form, fosinoprilat. An extended half-life allows for once-daily dosing, and it may be taken without regard to meals. It is excreted by both the liver and kidneys, and does not require a dosage adjustment in patients with renal impairment. The most common adverse effects of fosinopril are orthostatic hypotension, dizziness, and headache. Monopril HCT is a fixed-dose combination of Monopril and hydrochlorothiazide. This drug is pregnancy category C (first trimester) and D (second and third trimesters).

Moexipril (Univasc): Approved in 1995, moexipril is indicated only for HTN. It is a prodrug that is metabolized to its active form, moexiprilat, by hepatic enzymes. An extended half-life allows for once-daily dosing. This drug should be taken on an empty stomach, because food reduces its bioavailability by 40% to 50%. It is excreted by the kidneys, and dosage should be reduced in patients with renal impairment. Dizziness is one of the most common adverse effects. Adverse effects, contraindications, and indications are the same as lisinopril. Uniretic is a fixed-dose combination of moexipril and hydrochlorothiazide. Moexipril is a pregnancy category D drug.

Perindopril (Aceon): Approved in 1993, perindopril is approved for HTN and the prophylaxis of cardiovascular events such as MI in patients with coronary artery disease. HF is an off-label use. It is a prodrug that is metabolized by hepatic enzymes to its active form, perindoprilat. It is excreted by the kidneys, and its long half-life allows for once- or twice-daily dosing. Food may reduce the bioavailability of the drug by as much as 35%. Cough and dizziness are the most frequent adverse effects of perindopril. Other adverse effects, contraindications, and indications are the same as those of lisinopril. This is a pregnancy category D drug.

Quinapril (Accupril): Approved in 1991, quinapril is indicated for HTN and as adjunctive therapy for HF in combination with diuretics or digoxin. It is a prodrug that is metabolized by hepatic enzymes to its active form, quinaprilat, and may be dosed either once or twice daily. Because the kidney contributes to about 96% of the excretion of the drug, doses should be reduced in patients with renal impairment. Adverse effects are generally mild and transient, and include dizziness, cough,

and diarrhea. Other adverse effects, contraindications, and indications are the same as those of lisinopril. Accuretic is a fixed-dose combination of quinapril and hydrochlorothiazide. This is a pregnancy category D drug.

Ramipril (Altace): Approved in 1991, ramipril is indicated for HTN, HF following an MI, and to reduce mortality and stroke in high-risk patients with left ventricular dysfunction after an acute MI. It is a prodrug that is metabolized by hepatic enzymes to its active form, ramiprilat. Excretion is predominantly renal, and dosage should be reduced in patients with serious renal impairment. It may be administered without regard to meals. The most common adverse effects are orthostatic hypotension, dizziness, and headache. Other adverse effects, contraindications, and indications are the same as those of lisinopril. This is a pregnancy category D drug.

Trandolapril (Mavik): Approved in 1996, trandolapril is indicated for HTN and HF following an MI, and to reduce the mortality in high-risk patients with left ventricular dysfunction after an acute MI. It is a prodrug that is metabolized by hepatic enzymes to trandolaprilat, its active form. It has an extended half-life that permits once-daily dosing, and may be administered without regard to meals. Unlike other ACE inhibitors, a large amount of trandolapril (66%) is excreted in the feces. Dosages should be lowered in patients with hepatic or renal impairment. The most common adverse effects are cough, dizziness, and fatigue. Other adverse effects, contraindications, and indications are the same as those of lisinopril. Tarka is a fixed-dose combination of trandolapril and the calcium channel blocker verapamil SR, which is prescribed for HTN. This is a pregnancy category D drug.

CONNECTION Checkpoint 34.4

Knowing that ACE inhibitors decrease sympathetic activation, what type of interaction (additive or antagonistic) would you expect from the autonomic drugs epinephrine and propranolol? *See Answer to Connection Checkpoint 34.4 on student resource website.*

7 Angiotensin II receptor blockers act by inhibiting the AT₁ receptor and are used for hypertension and heart failure.

While pharmacologists were examining the mechanism of action of the ACE inhibitors in the 1980s and developing new drugs in this class, research continued on the other enzymes and components of the RAAS. The receptors for angiotensin II in smooth muscle, known as AT_1 and AT_2, were discovered, and a new class of drugs, the angiotensin II receptor blockers (ARBs), was developed. The ARBs are selective for AT_1-type receptors. Unlike the ACE inhibitors, ARBs do not prevent the formation of angiotensin II, but they do effectively prevent it from activating their target receptors. Doses for the ARBS are listed in Table 2.

The ARBs cause vasodilation, with a resultant reduction in peripheral resistance and fall in blood pressure, by blocking angiotensin II receptors in arteriolar smooth muscle. The blockade of AT_1 receptors in the adrenal gland prevents secretion of aldosterone and promotes increased Na^+ and excretion of water by the kidneys. Blockade of AT_1 receptors in the heart prevents the

CONNECTIONS: NURSING PRACTICE APPLICATION

Patients Receiving Angiotensin-Converting Enzyme Inhibitor and Angiotensin Receptor Blocker Therapy

Assessment	Potential Nursing Diagnoses
Baseline assessment prior to administration: • Understand the reason the drug has been prescribed in order to assess for therapeutic effects. • Obtain a complete health history including cardiovascular (MI, HF), diabetes, renal disease, and the possibility of pregnancy. Obtain a drug history including allergies, current prescription and over-the-counter (OTC) drugs, herbal preparations, and alcohol use. Be alert to possible drug interactions. • Evaluate appropriate laboratory findings, electrolytes, especially potassium level, liver function studies, and lipid profiles. • Obtain baseline weight, vital signs (especially blood pressure and pulse), breath sounds, and cardiac monitoring (e.g., ECG, cardiac output) if appropriate. Assess for location, character, and amount of edema, if present. • Assess the patient's ability to receive and understand instructions. Include the family and caregivers as needed. **Assessment throughout administration:** • Assess for desired therapeutic effects (e.g., lowered blood pressure within established limits). • Continue periodic monitoring of electrolytes, especially potassium. • Assess for adverse effects: headache, cough, orthostatic hypotension, fatigue or weakness, lightheadedness or dizziness, symptoms of hyperkalemia, sexual dysfunction, or impotence. Angioedema should be immediately reported to the health care provider.	• *Decreased Cardiac Output* • *Activity Intolerance* • *Sexual Dysfunction* • *Deficient Knowledge* (Drug Therapy) • *Risk for Decreased Cardiac Tissue Perfusion*, related to adverse drug effects • *Risk for Falls*, related to adverse drug effects • *Risk for Injury*, related to adverse drug effects • *Risk for Imbalanced Nutrition: More than Body Requirements* (Potassium), related to potassium intake resulting in adverse drug effects

Planning: Patient Goals and Expected Outcomes

The patient will:

• Experience therapeutic effects dependent on the reason the drug is being given (e.g., decreased blood pressure to established parameters).
• Be free from or experience minimal adverse effects.
• Verbalize an understanding of the drug's use, adverse effects, and required precautions.
• Demonstrate proper self-administration of the medication (e.g., dose, timing, and when to notify the provider).

Implementation

Interventions and (Rationales)	Patient-Centered Care
Ensuring therapeutic effects: • Continue frequent assessments as above for therapeutic effects. (Blood pressure and pulse should be within normal limits or within parameters set by the health care provider.)	• Teach the patient, family, or caregiver how to monitor pulse and blood pressure. Ensure proper use and functioning of any home equipment obtained.
• Encourage appropriate lifestyle changes: lowered fat intake, increased exercise, limited alcohol intake, and smoking cessation. Provide for dietitian consultation as needed. (Healthy lifestyle changes will support and minimize the need for drug therapy.)	• Encourage the patient to adopt a healthy lifestyle of low-fat food choices, increased exercise, decreased alcohol consumption, and smoking cessation.
Minimizing adverse effects: • Continue to monitor vital signs. Take the blood pressure lying, sitting, and standing to detect orthostatic hypotension. Be particularly cautious with the first few doses of the drug and with older adults who are at increased risk for hypotension. (ACE inhibitors and ARBs cause vasodilation, resulting in lowered blood pressure. A first-dose effect may occur with a significant drop in blood pressure with the first few doses. Orthostatic hypotension may increase the risk of falls and injury.)	• Instruct the patient to take the first dose of the new prescription in the evening before bed and to be cautious during the next few doses until drug effects are known. • Teach the patient to rise from lying or sitting to standing slowly to avoid dizziness or falls. • Instruct the patient to stop taking the medication if the blood pressure is 90/60 mmHg or below, or per parameters set by the health care provider, and promptly notify the provider.
• Continue to monitor periodic electrolyte levels, especially potassium, hepatic and renal function laboratory values, and ECG as appropriate. (Hyperkalemia may occur and may increase the risk of dysrhythmias.)	• Instruct the patient on the need to return periodically for laboratory work. • Advise the patient to carry a wallet identification card or wear medical identification jewelry indicating ACE inhibitor/ARB therapy.
• Ensure patient safety, especially in the older adult. Observe for lightheadedness or dizziness. Monitor ambulation until the effects of the drug are known. (Dizziness from orthostatic hypotension may occur.)	• Instruct the patient to call for assistance prior to getting out of bed or attempting to walk alone, and to avoid driving or other activities requiring mental alertness or physical coordination until the effects of the drug are known.

CONNECTIONS: NURSING PRACTICE APPLICATION *(continued)*

• Monitor for persistent dry cough or increasing cough severity. (ACE inhibitors increase bradykinin levels, which results in a dry cough. A change in the severity of the cough may indicate another disease process or may result in the need to consider other medications.)	• Teach the patient to anticipate a dry cough that may persist and to use nonmedicinal measures to treat (e.g., OTC cough lozenges or hard candy or increased fluid intake). • Instruct the patient that if the cough becomes troublesome when in a supine position, sleep with the head elevated on additional pillows. • Advise the patient to consult with the health care provider about the use of antihistamines to treat a persistent cough unrelieved by nonmedicinal measures. • Instruct the patient to promptly report any change in the severity or frequency of a cough. Any cough accompanied by shortness of breath, fever, or chest pain should be reported immediately because it may indicate more severe pathologic conditions.
• Monitor for hyperkalemia. (Reduced aldosterone levels may cause hyperkalemia, especially in patients with diabetes or impaired kidney function.)	• Instruct the patient on the signs of hyperkalemia (nausea, irregular heartbeat, profound fatigue or muscle weakness, and slow or faint pulse), and to report them immediately. • Teach the patient to avoid salt substitutes containing potassium chloride, consuming snacks advertised as "electrolyte-fortified," specialized sports drinks that contain high levels of potassium, or excessive intake of foods high in potassium different from their normal diet.
Patient understanding of drug therapy: • Use opportunities during the administration of medications and during assessments to discuss the rationale for the drug therapy, desired therapeutic outcomes, commonly observed adverse effects, parameters for when to call the health care provider, and any necessary monitoring or precautions. (Using time during nursing care helps to optimize and reinforce key teaching areas.)	• The patient, family, or caregiver should be able to state the reason for the drug, appropriate dose and scheduling, what adverse effects to observe for and when to report them, and the anticipated length of medication therapy.
Patient self-administration of drug therapy: • When administering the medication, instruct the patient, family, or caregiver in proper self-administration of the drug, e.g., take the first dose of the new prescription at bedtime. (Utilizing time during nurse-administration of these drugs helps to reinforce teaching.)	• The patient, family, or caregiver is able to discuss appropriate dosing and administration needs.

Evaluation of Outcome Criteria

Evaluate the effectiveness of drug therapy by confirming that patient goals and expected outcomes have been met (see "Planning").

TABLE 2 Angiotensin II Receptor Blockers, Aldosterone Antagonists, and Renin Inhibitors

Drug	Route and Adult Dose (maximum dose where indicated)	Adverse Effects
Angiotensin II Receptor Blockers		
azilsartan (Edarbi)	PO: 40–80 mg once daily	*Headache, dizziness, orthostatic hypotension, rash, diarrhea* Angioedema, acute renal failure, first-dose phenomenon, fetal toxicity and neonatal mortality
candesartan (Atacand)	PO: Start at 16 mg/day for HTN and 4 mg/day for HF (max: 32 mg/day)	
eprosartan (Teveten)	PO: 600 mg/day or 400 mg PO qid–bid (max: 800 mg/day)	
irbesartan (Avapro)	PO: 150–300 mg/day (max: 300 mg/day)	
losartan (Cozaar)	PO: 25–50 mg in one to two divided doses (max: 100 mg/day)	
olmesartan medoxomil (Benicar)	PO: 20–40 mg/day	
telmisartan (Micardis)	PO: 40 mg/day (max: 80 mg/day	
valsartan (Diovan)	PO: 80 mg/day (max: 320 mg/day)	
Aldosterone Antagonists		
eplerenone (Inspra)	PO: Start with 25–50 mg/day (max: 100 mg/day for HTN; 50 mg/day for HF)	*Minor hyperkalemia, headache, fatigue, gynecomastia (spironolactone)* Dysrhythmias (from hyperkalemia), dehydration, hyponatremia, agranulocytosis and other blood dyscrasias
spironolactone (Aldactone)	PO: 50–100 mg/day in single or divided doses (max: 400 mg/day)	
Renin Inhibitor		
aliskiren (Tekturna)	PO: 150 mg/day (max: 300 mg/day)	*Diarrhea, hypotension, cough* Angioedema

Note: Italics indicate common adverse effects. <u>Underline</u> indicates serious adverse effects.

destructive effects of angiotensin-induced cardiac remodeling. Although they act by a different mechanism, ARBs essentially produce the same pharmacologic actions as the ACE inhibitors.

The indications for ARBs are the same as those for the ACE inhibitors. All are approved to treat HTN, and they are often combined with drugs from other classes. Valsartan (Diovan) and candesartan (Atacand) were subsequently approved to treat HF. Some are approved to treat MI and are used for the prophylaxis of stroke. All are administered orally and have prolonged half-lives that permit once-daily dosing. A few are prodrugs, and most are extensively bound to plasma proteins.

Are the ARBs identical to the ACE inhibitors? Not exactly. Unlike the ACE inhibitors, they do not cause cough, and angioedema is less common. This is because ARBs do not promote the accumulation of bradykinin, as do the ACE inhibitors. ARBs can, however, cause dizziness, hypotension, and hyperkalemia, especially in patients with renal impairment or who are concurrently taking potassium supplements or potassium-sparing diuretics.

If ARBs have the same pharmacologic actions and an improved safety profile, why have they not replaced the ACE inhibitors? The answer is because the ACE inhibitors are generally less expensive, and health care providers have much more clinical experience prescribing them. Because the ARBs are newer, a significant body of research has not yet accumulated that demonstrates clear benefits over the ACE inhibitors. Because of these factors, the ARBs are usually reserved for patients unable to tolerate the adverse effects of ACE inhibitors.

PROTOTYPE DRUG	Losartan (Cozaar)

Classification: Therapeutic: Antihypertensive
Pharmacologic: Angiotensin II receptor blocker

Therapeutic Effects and Uses: Approved for the treatment of HTN, stroke prophylaxis in patients with left ventricular hypertrophy, and the prevention of type 2 diabetic nephropathy, losartan was the first ARB marketed in 1995. An off-label use is for HF. Although losartan undergoes extensive first-pass metabolism and has a short half-life, it is metabolized to an active intermediate that exerts more prolonged action, allowing for once-daily dosing. Its actions include vasodilation and reduced blood volume, due to the drug blocking the release of aldosterone by angiotensin II. Hyzaar is a fixed-dose combination of losartan and hydrochlorothiazide.

Mechanism of Action: Losartan selectively blocks angiotensin AT_1 receptors, resulting in a decline in blood pressure. The blockade of angiotensin II receptors prevents cardiac remodeling and deterioration of renal function in patients with diabetes.

Pharmacokinetics:

Route(s)	PO
Absorption	Well absorbed from the GI tract
Distribution	Does not appear to cross the blood–brain barrier or the placenta, or to be secreted in breast milk; approximately 99% bound to protein
Primary metabolism	Hepatic: extensive first-pass metabolism; converted to active metabolite
Primary excretion	35% renal, 60% in feces
Onset of action	Peak effect: 6 h
Duration of action	Half-life: 1.5–2 h (losartan), 6–9 h (active metabolite)

Adverse Effects: The incidence of adverse effects of losartan is very low. The most common adverse effects are headache, dizziness, nasal congestion, fatigue, and insomnia. Serious adverse effects include angioedema and acute renal failure. **Black Box Warning:** Fetal injury and death may occur when ARBs are taken during pregnancy. When pregnancy is detected, they should be discontinued as soon as possible.

Contraindications/Precautions: Losartan is contraindicated in patients with prior hypersensitivity to the drug. Because ARBs exhibit the same teratogenic effects as ACE inhibitors, they should not be used during pregnancy and lactation. Caution should be used in treating patients with serious renal or hepatic impairment and dosage may need to be reduced. Patients with a history of angioedema should be monitored carefully. Patients with hypovolemia are at high risk of symptomatic hypotension during therapy. Hypovolemia should be corrected prior to administration of losartan.

Drug Interactions: The drug interactions of losartan and other ARBs are similar to those of the ACE inhibitors. Indomethacin and other NSAIDs may decrease the antihypertensive activity of losartan. When taken concurrently with potassium supplements or potassium-sparing diuretics, care must be taken to avoid hyperkalemia. Concurrent use of losartan with diuretics and other antihypertensives may cause additive hypotensive effects. Use with alcohol may also add to the hypotensive effects of losartan. Losartan may increase lithium levels and toxicity. **Herbal/Food:** Hawthorn should not be taken concurrently with losartan due to the possibility of additive hypotensive action.

Pregnancy: Categories C (first trimester) and D (second and third trimesters).

Treatment of Overdose: Overdose will cause hypotension, which may be treated with an infusion of normal saline or a vasopressor. The drug is not removed by hemodialysis.

Nursing Responsibilities: Key nursing implications for patients receiving losartan are included in the Nursing Practice Application for Patients Receiving Angiotensin-Converting Enzyme Inhibitor and Angiotensin Receptor Blocker Therapy.

Lifespan and Diversity Considerations:

- Use special caution when administering losartan to the older patient who is at greater risk for hypotension, dizziness, and falls. Provide assistance with ambulation as needed.

- Monitor for the development of angioedema in older adults, African American patients, and patients who have previously experienced angioedema with an ACE inhibitor, because these patients are at higher risk.

Patient and Family Education:

- Monitor blood pressure regularly as directed by the health care provider. Maintain a written log of blood pressure readings and present it at follow-up visits.
- Immediately report any swelling of the face, mouth, lips, or tongue, hoarseness, or sudden trouble with breathing.
- Avoid salt substitutes that contain potassium chloride.
- Immediately inform the health care provider of any known or suspected pregnancy, because these drugs can cause birth defects.
- Do not breast-feed while taking this drug without approval of the health care provider.

Drugs Similar to Losartan (Cozaar)

In addition to losartan, seven other ARBs available. They all have similar indications, actions and adverse effects.

Azilsartan medoxomil (Edarbi): The newest of the ARBS, azilsartan was approved in 2011 for the treatment of HTN, either as monotherapy or in combination with other antihypertensives. Azilsartan medoxomil is a prodrug that is converted to its active form (azilsartan) when it is absorbed across the GI tract. It appears to lower blood pressure faster than other drugs in its class. The drug is well tolerated, with diarrhea being the most frequent adverse effect. Caution should be used in treating volume or salt-depleted patients because transient hypotension may occur. This drug is pregnancy category C (first trimester) and D (second and third trimesters).

Candesartan (Atacand): Approved in 1998, candesartan is indicated for HTN and HF in patients with left ventricular dysfunction. It is a prodrug that is metabolized to its active form during its absorption from the GI tract. Optimal therapeutic effects may take up to 4 weeks. The drug is 99% protein bound and is primarily excreted in the bile (66%). Adverse effects are generally mild and include headache and dizziness. Other adverse effects, contraindications, and indications are the same as those of losartan. Atacand HCT is a fixed-dose combination of candesartan and hydrochlorothiazide. This drug is pregnancy category D.

Eprosartan (Teveten): Approved in 1997, eprosartan is indicated only for HTN. It is mostly unmetabolized and primarily excreted in the feces (90%). Optimum blood pressure reduction may require 2 to 3 weeks of therapy. The most common adverse effects are headache, dizziness, arthralgia, and fatigue. Other adverse effects, contraindications, and indications are the same as those of losartan. Teveten HCT is a fixed-dose combination of eprosartan and hydrochlorothiazide. This drug is pregnancy category D.

Irbesartan (Avapro): Approved in 1997, irbesartan is indicated for HTN and type 2 diabetic nephropathy. The drug is 90% protein bound and is primarily excreted in the feces (80%). Adverse effects are generally mild and include diarrhea, dyspepsia, arthralgia, and fatigue. Other adverse effects, contraindications, and indications are the same as those of losartan. Avalide is a fixed-dose combination of irbesartan and hydrochlorothiazide. This drug is pregnancy category D.

Olmesartan medoxomil (Benicar): Approved in 2002, olmesartan is indicated only for HTN. It is a prodrug that is metabolized to its active form during its absorption from the GI tract. Olmesartan is 99% protein bound and excreted equally in urine and the feces. The drug is administered once daily and optimal blood pressure reduction may require 2 weeks of therapy. The drug exhibits few adverse effects, with dizziness being the most common complaint. Other adverse effects, contraindications, and indications are the same as those of losartan. There are three fixed-dose combinations of olmesartan: Benicar HCT (with hydrochlorothiazide), Azor (with amlodipine), and Tribenzor (with amlodipine and hydrochlorothiazide). This drug is pregnancy category D.

Telmisartan (Micardis): Approved in 1998, telmisartan is indicated only for HTN. An off-label use is for the treatment of renal dysfunction in patients with diabetic nephropathy.

CONNECTIONS

Complementary and Alternative Therapies   Hawthorn

Description: Hawthorn (*Crataegus*) is a thorny shrub or small tree that is widespread in North America, Europe, and Asia. Leaves, flowers, and berries of the plant are dried or extracted in liquid form.

History and Claims: Hawthorn, sometimes called May bush, was used in ancient Greece. In traditional Chinese medicine, hawthorn is used as a digestive aid. European and American interest in the herb began in the late 1800s. It has been widely used in European countries to treat HTN and HF. The berries may be consumed raw or made into jellies, juices, and alcoholic beverages. Some cultures believe that the shrub is magical, and it is used in religious rites to ward off evil spirits.

Standardization: Active ingredients in hawthorn include flavonoids and procyanidins. A typical dose is 4.5 to 6 g of dried leaves or flowers or 160 to 900 mg of extract per day.

Evidence: Hawthorn has been well studied (National Center for Complementary and Alternative Medicine, 2010). Positive inotropic action, improved exercise tolerance, and vasodilation have been documented. Some studies also report its ability to lower blood lipids. Hawthorn has been used to lower blood pressure but is slow in onset, taking 4 weeks or longer before a small effect is experienced. Hawthorn may work by inhibition of ACE or reduction of cardiac workload. Hawthorn has few adverse effects at normal doses. This product should be used with caution in patients taking cardiac glycosides and other prescription medications for cardiovascular disease. Because hypotension may occur, frequent blood pressure measurements should be taken when using this therapy.

It is mostly unmetabolized, 99% protein bound, and excreted primarily in the feces. Initial doses should be reduced in patients with hepatic impairment. The drug is well tolerated and serious adverse effects are uncommon. Adverse effects, contraindications, and indications are the same as those of losartan. Fixed-dose combinations include Micardis HCT (with hydrochlorothiazide) and Twynsta (with amlodipine). This drug is pregnancy category D.

Valsartan (Diovan): Approved in 1996, valsartan is indicated for HTN, HF, and MI when the patient is unable to tolerate an ACE inhibitor. It undergoes hepatic metabolism, is 95% protein bound, and is eliminated in the feces. Because food can reduce drug absorption by as much as 40%, the drug should be given on an empty stomach. Headache and dizziness are the two most common adverse effects. Other adverse effects, contraindications, and indications are the same as those of losartan. Fixed-dose combinations include Diovan HCT (with hydrochlorothiazide), Exforge (with amlodipine), and Valturna (with aliskiren). This drug is pregnancy category D.

8 Aldosterone antagonists block the biologic effects of aldosterone in the renal tubule.

As described in Section 3, angiotensin II causes the release of aldosterone, which subsequently contributes to increased blood pressure due to sodium and water retention. Receptors for aldosterone are located in the distal tubule and collecting ducts of the nephron. Two drugs are available that block these receptors in the kidney, thus inhibiting the physiological actions of aldosterone. Both spironolactone (Aldactone) and eplerenone (Inspra) are used to treat edema and HTN. Doses for these drugs are listed in Table 2.

Spironolactone is an aldosterone antagonist that has been used for its diuretic action for many decades. By binding to aldosterone receptors, spironolactone produces a mild diuresis by promoting Na^+ and Cl^- excretion. Because it has little or no effect on the excretion of potassium, spironolactone is also classified as a potassium-sparing diuretic and is featured as a prototype diuretic. Spironolactone produces only a mild diuresis; it is often combined with drugs from other diuretic classes when used for HTN. It is also useful in treating primary aldosteronism, a rare condition in which the body produces an overabundance of aldosterone, usually due to a tumor of the adrenal gland. Spironolactone has been shown to reduce morbidity, mortality, and dysrhythmias associated with HF.

The primary concern with spironolactone is potassium retention, which can result in serious hyperkalemia. Some patients experience GI-related adverse effects such as nausea, vomiting, and diarrhea. Because spironolactone has a similar chemical structure to steroid hormones, it sometimes causes endocrine adverse effects in males, such as gynecomastia and erectile dysfunction. Females may experience menstrual irregularities, and breast tenderness.

Eplerenone (Inspra) is a newer aldosterone antagonist that has a very different chemical structure than spironolactone. It is more selective for aldosterone receptors and has a very low incidence of endocrine-related adverse effects. Like spironolactone, hyperkalemia is a potentially serious adverse effect. Headache and dizziness are common adverse effects. Eplerenone is approved to treat HTN and HF and to reduce morbidity and mortality associated with post-MI in patients with left ventricular dysfunction.

UNDERSTANDING THE CHAPTER

Key Concepts Summary

1 The formation of angiotensin II requires two enzymatic steps.

2 Renin secretion is controlled by the juxtaglomerular cells of the kidney and the sympathetic nervous system.

3 Angiotensin-converting enzyme is responsible for the formation of angiotensin II.

4 Angiotensin II has multiple effects on the cardiovascular system that raise blood pressure and affect cardiac function.

5 The renin-angiotensin-aldosterone pathway offers multiple points for drug intervention.

6 ACE inhibitors are key drugs in the pharmacotherapy of hypertension and heart failure.

7 Angiotensin II receptor blockers act by inhibiting the AT_1 receptor and are used for hypertension and heart failure.

8 Aldosterone antagonists block the biologic effects of aldosterone in the renal tubule.

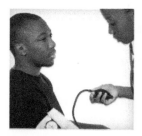

Making the PATIENT Connection

Remember the patient "Carlos Avaya" at the beginning of the chapter? Now read the remainder of the case study. Based on the information presented within this chapter, respond to the critical thinking questions that follow.

Carlos Avaya is a 26-year-old single man who was diagnosed with primary HTN 4 months ago. Carlos has been taking losartan (Cozaar) 50 mg daily PO and has been faithful in taking the medication as prescribed. When Carlos was told that his blood pressure was still elevated during this clinic visit, he was obviously distressed and concerned.

The health care team begins to investigate external factors that may be causing his blood pressure to remain elevated. Carlos has never smoked or used alcohol. He does not like to exercise but participates in a weekly game of soccer at the nearby community center. He denies being overly stressed with work or home life. Furthermore, he claims that he rarely salts his food.

The nurse asks Carlos to describe a typical day. During the description the nurse notices a concerning pattern. Because Carlos lives alone, he frequently cooks for himself. He admits that he enjoys salty foods such as pretzels and popcorn. He denies having consumed either prior to the visit to the clinic. However, to Carlos, cooking a meal involves preparing canned processed foods and frozen dinners. He never reads food labels. Without recording a complete dietary history, the nurse is able to determine that Carlos's intake of sodium-rich foods is quite extensive.

Critical Thinking Questions

1. In your own words, how would you describe how losartan (Cozaar) works to reduce blood pressure?

2. Considering the adverse effects of losartan (Cozaar), when would you instruct Carlos to notify the prescriber?

3. In addition to teaching Carlos about his losartan (Cozaar), what additional health teaching should he receive?

See Answers to Critical Thinking Questions on student resource website.

NCLEX-RN® Review

1. The community health nurse teaches a client at home. Lisinopril (Prinivil) has been prescribed for the client. Which statement, if made by the client, indicates that further teaching is necessary?

   1. "I should notify my health care provider of symptoms of hypotension such as dizziness or fainting."
   2. "I should avoid the use of salt substitute containing potassium."
   3. "If a dose is missed, I will take it as soon as possible but not too close to the next dose."
   4. "Too much calcium in my diet will elevate my blood pressure."

2. The client states, "I always keep my lisinopril (Prinivil) on my kitchen window sill. It helps me to remember to take it." The nurse's response would be based on which pharmacologic concept about heat and moisture?

   1. They cause the medicine to break down.
   2. They enhance the strength of the drug.
   3. They crystallize the medication.
   4. They convert the medicine to toxic metabolites.

3. A client is hospitalized for uncontrolled hypertension and is receiving enalapril (Vasotec). The nurse should notify the health care provider if the client exhibits:

   1. Dry mucous membranes.
   2. A decline in systolic blood pressure.
   3. Nonproductive cough.
   4. A reduction of diastolic blood pressure.

4. The nurse is caring for a client with chronic hypertension. The client is receiving losartan (Cozaar) daily. Which client manifestations would the nurse conclude is an adverse effect of this medication?

   1. Irritability and tremors
   2. Headache and dizziness
   3. Sleepiness and slurred speech
   4. Pruritus and rash

5. Irbesartan (Avapro) is prescribed for each of the following clients. A nurse should question the order for which client? A client who has:

   1. Severe dehydration from diuretic therapy.
   2. Long-term diabetes mellitus.
   3. A systolic blood pressure of 162.
   4. A 5-year history of heart failure.

6. The nurse determines that the client does not understand an important principle in self-administration of benazepril (Lotensin) when the client makes which statement?

   1. "I will learn to monitor my own blood pressure and write down all my daily measurements."
   2. "While taking this medication, I should avoid over-the-counter medications for colds, sinus, or appetite control."
   3. "This drug will not impair thinking and reaction time. I don't need to wait to start driving my car."
   4. "Drinking alcohol while on this medication can lower my blood pressure and lead to dizziness and faintness."

Additional Case Study

Ella Daniels, a middle-aged African American woman, takes spironolactone (Aldactone) for HTN. As the nurse responsible for providing her with health information, you plan to talk with her about this drug.

1. How does the mechanism of action of spironolactone differ from that of lisinopril (Prinivil, Zestril)?

2. What are the main precautions specific to Aldactone that should be included in the teaching plan?

See Answers to Additional Case Study on student resource website.

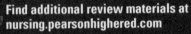

Pearson Nursing Student Resources

Find additional review materials at nursing.pearsonhighered.com

Prepare for success with additional NCLEX®-style practice questions, interactive assignments and activities, web links, animations, videos, and more!

References

National Center for Complementary and Alternative Medicine. (2010). *Herbs at a glance: Hawthorn.* Retrieved from http://nccam.nih.gov/health/hawthorn

Silverthorn, D. U. (2010). *Human physiology: An integrated approach* (5th ed.). San Francisco, CA: Pearson/Benjamin Cummings.

Solski, L. V., & Longyhore, D. S. (2008). Prevention of type 2 diabetes with angiotensin converting enzyme inhibitors. *American Journal of Health-System Pharmacists, 65*(10), 935–940. doi:10.2146/ajhp070388

Selected Bibliography

Benjamin, R., Szwejkowski, B. R., Rekhraj, S., Hj Elder, D., & Struthers, A. D. (2011). Update on heart failure. *British Journal of Diabetes and Vascular Disease 11*(1), 25–30. doi:10.1177/1474651410397246

Brugts, J. J., Danser, A. H. J., de Maat, M. P. M., den Uil, C. A., Boersma, E., Ferrari, R., & Simoons, M. L. (2008). Pharmacogenetics of ACE inhibition in stable coronary artery disease: Steps towards tailored drug therapy. *Current Opinion in Cardiology, 23*(4), 296–301. doi:10.1097/HCO.0b013e3283007ba6

Cohen, D. L., & Townsend, R. R. (2008). Can an angiotensin receptor blocker be used in a patient in whom angioedema developed with an angiotensin-converting enzyme inhibitor? *The Journal of Clinical Hypertension, 10*(12), 949–950. doi:10.1111/j.1751-7176.2008.00042.x

Fitzgerald, M. A. (2011). Hypertension treatment update: Focus on direct renin inhibition. *Journal of the American Academy of Nurse Practitioners, 23*(5), 239–248. doi:10.1111/j.1745-7599.2010.00589.x

Holdiness, A., Monahan, K., Minor, D., & de Shazo, R. D. (2011). Renin angiotensin aldosterone system blockade: Little to no rationale for ACE inhibitor and ARB combinations. *American Journal of Medicine, 124*(1), 15–19. doi:10.1016/j.amjmed.2010.07.021

Linus, S. L. (2008). Are two better than one? Angiotensin-converting enzyme inhibitors plus angiotensin receptor blockers for reducing blood pressure and proteinuria in kidney disease. *Clinical Journal of the American Society of Nephrology, 3*(Suppl. 1), S17–S23. doi:10.2215/CJN.03270807

Miller, N. H. (2010). Cardiovascular risk reduction with renin-angiotensin aldosterone system blockade. *Nursing Research and Practice, vol. 2010,* Article ID 101749, 7 pages. doi:10.1155/2010/101749

Parfrey, P. S. (2008). Inhibitors of the renin angiotensin system: Proven benefits, unproven safety. *Annals of Internal Medicine, 148*(1), 76–77.

U.S. Department of Health and Human Services. (2010). *Dietary guidelines for Americans.* Retrieved from http://www.health.gov/DietaryGuidelines

Answers to NCLEX-RN® Review

1 Answer: 4 Rationale: Lisinopril does not affect serum calcium levels, causing an elevated blood pressure. Options 1, 2, and 3 are incorrect. Common adverse effects for lisinopril are cough, headache, dizziness, and orthostatic hypotension. These symptoms should be reported to the prescriber. Salt substitutes usually contain potassium chloride and should be avoided to reduce the risk of hyperkalemia. Clients on this medication should be instructed to stay on regular doses of blood pressure medication. If a dose is missed, take it as soon as possible but not too close to the next dose. Never take a double dose. Cognitive Level: Analyzing; Client Need: Health Promotion and Maintenance; Nursing Process: Evaluation

2 Answer: 1 Rationale: Lisinopril should be stored in a dry place at room temperature, because heat and moisture may cause drug breakdown. Options 2, 3, and 4 are incorrect. Heat and moisture do not enhance the strength of the drug, crystallize the medication, or convert the medication to toxic metabolites. Cognitive Level: Analyzing; Client Need: Health Promotion and Maintenance; Nursing Process: Evaluation

3 Answer: 3 Rationale: ACE inhibitors such as enalapril also prevent the breakdown of bradykinin. Accumulation of bradykinin in certain tissues such as the lungs can cause adverse effects as manifested by a nonproductive cough, and may require an antihistamine for treatment. Options 1, 2, and 4 are incorrect. Dry mucous membranes are not adverse effects related to ACE inhibitors. The expected outcome associated with ACE inhibitors is a decline in blood pressure, and the nurse should expect both systolic and diastolic pressures to be reduced. Cognitive Level: Applying; Client Need: Physiological Integrity; Nursing Process: Implementation

4 Answer: 2 Rationale: The most common adverse effects of losartan are headache, dizziness, nasal congestion, and insomnia. Options 1, 3, and 4 are incorrect. Irritability, tremors, sleepiness, slurred speech, pruritus, or rash are not common adverse effects associated with losartan. Cognitive Level: Analyzing; Client Need: Physiological Integrity; Nursing Process: Evaluation

5 Answer: 1 Rationale: Clients with severe dehydration may experience hypovolemia and are at high risk of life-threatening hypotension. Options 2, 3, and 4 are incorrect. Irbesartan may be prescribed for the prevention of diabetic nephropathy, HTN, and as an off-label use for heart failure. Cognitive Level: Applying; Client Need: Physiological Integrity; Nursing Process: Implementation

6 Answer: 3 Rationale: Clients receiving benazepril should avoid driving or engaging in other potentially hazardous activities until the effects of the drug are known. Benazepril may cause adverse effects that impair thinking and reaction time. Options 1, 2, and 4 are incorrect. The client or family should be taught methods of home blood pressure measurement and maintenance of a blood pressure log while taking benazepril. OTC medications for colds, sinus, fever, asthma, or appetite control should be avoided because they may increase blood pressure. The consumption of alcohol while taking benazepril can lower blood pressure, which will lead to dizziness and fainting. Cognitive Level: Analyzing; Client Need: Health Promotion and Maintenance; Nursing Process: Evaluation

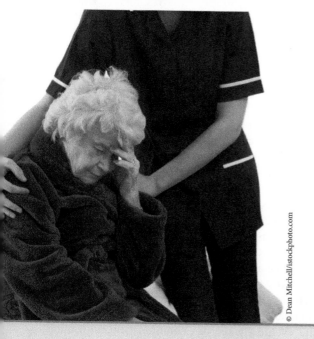

"I feel terrible. I have no energy and I feel as weak as a kitten. Lately, I don't even feel like getting out of bed in the mornings. I try to take my medications just as I was told to do."

Patient "Katherine Crosland"

© Dean Mitchell/istockphoto.com

Diuretic Therapy and the Pharmacotherapy of Renal Failure

Chapter Outline

Review of Renal Physiology

Pharmacotherapy in Patients with Renal Failure

Diuretic Therapy

Loop (High-Ceiling) Diuretics

PROTOTYPE **Furosemide (Lasix)**

Thiazide and Thiazide-Like Diuretics

PROTOTYPE **Hydrochlorothiazide (Microzide)**

Potassium-Sparing Diuretics

PROTOTYPE **Spironolactone (Aldactone)**

Osmotic Diuretics

PROTOTYPE **Mannitol (Osmitrol)**

Carbonic Anhydrase Inhibitors

PROTOTYPE **Acetazolamide (Diamox)**

Learning Outcomes

After reading this chapter, the student should be able to:

1. Explain the role of the urinary system in maintaining fluid, electrolyte, and acid–base homeostasis.

2. Explain the physiological processes that change the composition of filtrate as it travels through the nephrons.

3. Describe the adjustments in pharmacotherapy that must be considered in patients with renal failure.

4. Identify indications for diuretics.

5. Compare and contrast the loop, thiazide, potassium-sparing, osmotic, and carbonic anhydrase inhibitor diuretics.

6. Describe the nurse's role in the pharmacologic management of renal failure and in diuretic therapy.

7. For each of the classes shown in the chapter outline, identify the prototype and representative drugs and explain the mechanism(s) of drug action, primary indications, contraindications, significant drug interactions, pregnancy category, and important adverse effects.

8. Apply the nursing process to care for patients who are receiving diuretics or other drugs for renal failure.

From Chapter 35 of *Pharmacology: Connections to Nursing Practice*, Second Edition. Michael Patrick Adams, Carol Quam Urban. Copyright © 2013 by Pearson Education, Inc. All rights reserved.

Key Terms

carbonic anhydrase

diuretic

filtrate

glomerular filtration
rate (GFR)

glomerulus

natriuresis

nephrons

osmotic pressure

reabsorption

renal failure

secretion

symporter

The kidneys serve an amazing role in maintaining proper homeostasis. By filtering a volume equivalent to all of the body's extracellular fluid every 100 minutes, the kidneys are able to make immediate adjustments to fluid volume, electrolyte composition, and acid–base balance. Failure of the kidneys to adjust to changing internal conditions of the body may result in dire consequences, and pharmacotherapy is often used to correct these imbalances. This chapter examines diuretics, agents that increase urine output, and other drugs used to treat patients with renal dysfunction.

PharmFACT

More than 16,000 kidney transplants are performed annually. Approximately 10,500 of these patients receive organs from deceased donors, and 6,000 receive organs from living donors. Over 80,500 people are on the waiting list for kidney transplants (Axelrod et al., 2010).

Review of Renal Physiology

1 The kidneys are major organs of excretion and body homeostasis.

When most people think of the kidneys, they think of excretion. Although this is certainly true, the kidneys have many other essential homeostatic functions. The kidneys are the primary organs for regulating fluid balance, electrolyte composition, and the pH of body fluids. They also secrete the enzyme renin, which helps to regulate blood pressure, and erythropoietin, a hormone that stimulates red blood cell production. In addition, the kidneys are responsible for the production of calcitriol, the active form of vitamin D, which helps maintain bone homeostasis. It is not surprising that our overall health is strongly dependent on the proper functioning of the kidneys.

The urinary system consists of two kidneys, two ureters, one urinary bladder, and a urethra. Blood enters the kidneys through the large renal arteries, bringing 25% of the total cardiac output to the kidneys each minute. After a series of branches, blood enters the **nephrons**, the functional units of the kidney. Once in the nephron, the artery forms the **glomerulus**, a specialized capillary containing pores. Each kidney contains over 1 million nephrons.

As blood travels at high pressure through the glomerulus, the fluid portion of the blood is filtered through the glomerular pores and collected by Bowman's capsule, the first portion of the collecting system of the nephron. Together, the glomerulus and Bowman's capsule are called the renal corpuscle. During filtration, not all substances in the blood reach Bowman's capsule. Plasma proteins and the formed elements of the blood—the erythrocytes, leukocytes, and platelets—are too large to pass through the pores of the glomerulus and thus continue circulating through the bloodstream. Water and other small molecules in plasma, however, readily pass through the glomerular pores and enter the next section of the nephron.

The fluid filtered into Bowman's capsule is called **filtrate**. Essentially, the initial composition of filtrate may be thought of as plasma minus proteins. After leaving Bowman's capsule, the filtrate enters the proximal tubule, travels through the loop of Henle and, subsequently, the distal tubule. The proximal and distal tubules are twisted and highly convoluted, which greatly increases the length of the nephron, allowing for enhanced processing of substances in the filtrate. The filtrate eventually reaches common collecting ducts, which empty into increasingly larger collecting structures inside the kidney. Fluid leaving the collecting ducts and entering subsequent portions of the kidney is called urine. Approximately 1 mL of urine is produced each minute. Parts of the nephron and their functions are illustrated in Figure 1.

Many drugs are small enough to pass through the glomerulus and enter the filtrate. If the drug is bound to plasma proteins, however, it will be too large and will continue circulating in the blood. Plasma proteins such as albumin are also too large to pass through the filter and will not be present in the filtrate or in the urine of healthy patients. The appearance of excess plasma proteins in urine (proteinuria or albuminuria) is a sign of kidney pathology. For example, during glomerulonephritis the glomeruli become inflamed and the size of the pores increases, allowing larger substances such as proteins to enter the filtrate.

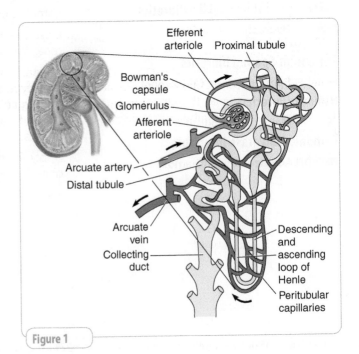

Figure 1

The nephron.

2 The composition of filtrate changes dramatically as a result of the processes of reabsorption and secretion.

The filtrate's composition changes dramatically as it makes its long journey through the nephron. Some substances in the filtrate cross the tubule walls to reenter the blood; this process is known as tubular **reabsorption**. Water is the most important molecule reabsorbed in the tubule. For every 180 L of water entering the filtrate each day, approximately 178.5 L are reabsorbed, leaving only 1.5 L to be excreted in the urine. Over 65% of the filtered sodium is reabsorbed in the proximal tubule, and 25% in the loop of Henle. Glucose, amino acids, and essential ions such as chloride, calcium, and bicarbonate are also reabsorbed.

Hormones can markedly affect the degree of reabsorption in the renal tubule. This is important to pharmacology because many drugs either enhance or block the effects of hormones on tubular processes. Aldosterone, for example, exerts a major effect on the tubule by stimulating sodium reabsorption in the distal portions of the nephron. Under the influence of aldosterone, potassium excretion is increased because this ion is "exchanged" for sodium ions, which are reabsorbed. Antidiuretic hormone (ADH) also affects kidney function, increasing water reabsorption by making the collecting ducts become more permeable to water. The formation of urine is indeed a dynamic process that undergoes continuous modification as the filtrate travels down the tubule.

Certain ions and molecules too large to pass through Bowman's capsule may still enter the urine by crossing from the blood to the filtrate using a process known as tubular **secretion**. The tubule contains molecular pumps for organic acids and bases. Acidic drugs secreted in the proximal tubule include penicillin G, ampicillin, sulfisoxazole, nonsteroidal anti-inflammatory drugs (NSAIDs), and furosemide. Basic drugs include procainamide, epinephrine, dopamine, neostigmine, and trimethoprim. Potassium, phosphate, hydrogen, and ammonium ions also enter the filtrate through active secretion. The amounts of selected substances reabsorbed, secreted, and excreted are shown in Table 1.

Reabsorption and secretion are critical to the pharmacokinetics of drugs. Some drugs are reabsorbed, whereas others are secreted into the filtrate. For example, approximately 90% of a dose of penicillin G enters the urine through secretion. When the kidney is diseased, reabsorption and secretion mechanisms are impaired and serum drug levels may be dramatically affected. Figure 2 illustrates the possible fates of drugs entering the glomerulus.

TABLE 1 Substances Filtered, Reabsorbed, and Excreted by the Kidneys

Substance	Filtered	Reabsorbed	Excreted
Water	180 L	178–179 L	1–2 L
Glucose	162 g	162 g	0 g
Proteins	2 g	1.9 g	0.1 g
Ions			
Sodium	579 g	575 g	4 g
Potassium	29.6 g	29.6 g	2 g
Bicarbonate	275 g	274.97 g	0.03 g
Metabolic Waste Products			
Creatine	1.6 g	0 g	1.6 g
Urea	54 g	24 g	30 g
Uric acid	8.5 g	7.7 g	0.8 g

Pharmacotherapy in Patients with Renal Failure

3 Renal failure may significantly impact the success of pharmacotherapy.

Renal failure is a condition characterized by a decrease in the kidneys' ability to maintain electrolyte and fluid balance and excrete waste products. Renal failure may be intrinsic to the kidney itself or result from disorders of other body systems. The primary treatment goals for a patient with renal failure are to maintain blood flow through the kidneys and adequate urine output so that metabolic wastes can be removed from the body.

PharmFACT

More than 526,000 Americans are treated for kidney failure each year, and about 87,000 die annually from causes related to the disease. Type 2 diabetes and hypertension account for about 85% of all new cases each year (National Kidney Foundation, n.d.).

The most basic diagnostic test of kidney function is a urinalysis, which examines urine for the presence of blood cells, proteins, pH, specific gravity, ketones, glucose, and microorganisms. The urinalysis can detect proteinuria and albuminuria, which are the primary measures of structural kidney damage. Although easy to perform, the urinalysis is nonspecific: Many diverse diseases and conditions can cause abnormal urinalysis values. Serum creatinine is an additional measure for detecting kidney disease. To provide a more definitive diagnosis, diagnostic imaging such as computed tomography, sonography, or magnetic resonance imaging may be necessary. Renal biopsy may be performed to obtain a more specific diagnosis.

The best marker for estimating kidney function is the **glomerular filtration rate (GFR)**, which is the volume of water filtered through the Bowman's capsules per minute. The GFR can be used to predict the onset and progression of kidney failure and it indicates the ability of the kidneys to excrete drugs from the body. A progressive decline in GFR

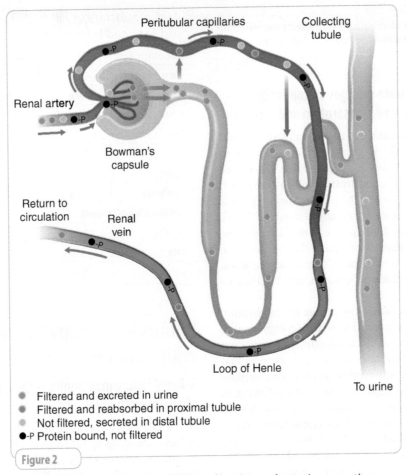

Peritubular capillaries

Collecting tubule

Renal artery

Bowman's capsule

Return to circulation

Renal vein

Loop of Henle

To urine

- Filtered and excreted in urine
- Filtered and reabsorbed in proximal tubule
- Not filtered, secreted in distal tubule
- -P Protein bound, not filtered

Figure 2

Fates of drugs entering the glomerulus: filtration, reabsorption, secretion, and excretion.

indicates a reduction in the number of functioning nephrons. As nephrons "die," however, the remaining healthy ones have the ability to compensate by increasing their filtration capacity. Because of this, patients with significant kidney damage may be asymptomatic until 50% or more of the nephrons have become nonfunctional and the GFR has fallen to less than half its normal value.

Renal failure may be classified as acute or chronic, depending on its onset. Acute renal failure requires immediate treatment because retention of nitrogenous waste products in the body such as urea and creatinine can result in death if left untreated. The most common cause of acute renal failure is renal hypoperfusion, the lack of sufficient blood flow through the kidneys. Hypoperfusion can lead to permanent destruction of kidney cells and nephrons. To correct this type of renal failure, the cause of the hypoperfusion must be quickly identified and corrected. Potential causes include heart failure (HF), dysrhythmias, hemorrhage, toxins, and dehydration. Pharmacotherapy with nephrotoxic drugs can also lead to either acute or chronic renal failure. It is good practice for the nurse to remember common nephrotoxic drugs, which are listed in Table 2, so that kidney function may be continuously monitored during therapy with these agents.

Chronic renal failure occurs over a period of months or years. Over half of the patients with chronic renal failure

TABLE 2 Nephrotoxic Drugs	
Drug or Class	Indication/Classification
aminoglycosides	Antibiotics
amphotericin B (Amphotec, AmBisome)	Systemic antifungal
angiotensin-converting enzyme (ACE) inhibitors	Hypertension, HF
cisplatin (Platinol), carboplatin (Paraplatin)	Antineoplastic
cyclosporine (Neoral, Sandimmune), tacrolimus (Prograf)	Immunosuppressant
foscarnet (Foscavir)	Antiviral
nonsteroidal anti-inflammatory drugs (NSAIDs)	Inflammation and pain
pentamidine (NebuPent, Pentam)	Anti-infective (*Pneumocystis*)
radiographic intravenous (IV) contrast agents	Diagnosis of kidney and vascular disorders

have long-standing hypertension (HTN) or diabetes mellitus. Due to the long, gradual development of chronic renal failure and its nonspecific symptoms, the condition may go undetected for many years. By the time the disease is diagnosed, the renal impairment may be irreversible. In end-stage

TABLE 3 Pharmacologic Management of Renal Failure

Complication	Pathogenesis	Selected Therapies
Anemia	Kidneys are unable to synthesize sufficient erythropoietin for red blood cell production.	epoetin alfa (Procrit, Epogen)
Hyperkalemia	Kidneys are unable to adequately excrete potassium.	Dietary restriction of potassium; polystyrene sulfate (Kayexalate) with sorbitol
Hyperphosphatemia	Kidneys are unable to adequately excrete phosphate.	Dietary restriction of phosphate; phosphate binders such as calcium carbonate (Os-Cal 500, others), calcium acetate (Calphron, PhosLo), lanthanum carbonate (Fosrenol), or sevelamer (Renagel)
Hypervolemia	Kidneys are unable to excrete sufficient sodium and water, leading to water retention.	Dietary restriction of sodium; loop diuretics in acute conditions, thiazide diuretics in mild conditions
Hypocalcemia	Hyperphosphatemia leads to loss of calcium.	Usually corrected by reversing the hyperphosphatemia, but additional calcium supplements may be necessary
Metabolic acidosis	Kidneys are unable to adequately excrete metabolic acids.	Sodium bicarbonate or sodium citrate

renal disease (ESRD), dialysis and kidney transplantation become treatment alternatives.

Pharmacotherapy of renal failure attempts to cure the cause of the dysfunction. Diuretics are given to increase urine output, and cardiovascular drugs are administered to treat underlying HTN or HF. Dietary management is often necessary to prevent worsening of renal impairment. Depending on the stage of the disease, dietary management may include restriction of protein and reduction of dietary sodium, potassium, phosphorous, and magnesium intake. For patients with diabetes, control of blood glucose through intensive insulin therapy may reduce the risk of renal damage. See Table 3 for a summary of selected pharmacologic agents used to prevent and treat the complications of renal failure.

The nurse serves a key role in assessing and providing interventions for patients with renal failure. Once a diagnosis has been established, all nephrotoxic medications should be either discontinued or used with extreme caution. Because the kidneys excrete most drugs or their metabolites, many medications will require a significant dosage reduction in patients with moderate to severe renal failure. The importance of this cannot be overemphasized: Administering the "average" dose to a patient in severe renal failure can have mortal consequences.

Diuretic Therapy

4 Diuretics are used to treat hypertension, heart failure, accumulation of edema fluid, and renal failure.

By simple definition, a **diuretic** is a drug that increases the rate of urine flow. When used therapeutically for HTN, HF, renal failure, or removal of edema fluid, however, diuretics do much more than increase urine flow. These drugs change the rate of excretion of specific electrolytes, most importantly sodium and chloride. The goal of most diuretic therapy is to reduce extracellular fluid volume, so that abnormal fluid retention by the body may be reversed. Excretion of excess fluid in the body is particularly desirable in the following conditions:

- HTN
- Heart failure
- Renal failure
- Liver failure or cirrhosis
- Pulmonary edema

The most common mechanism by which diuretics act is by blocking sodium ion (Na^+) reabsorption in the nephron, thus

CONNECTIONS

Lifespan Considerations   Diuretic Therapy

Children

Diuretics in children are often used in the treatment of fluid overload such as occurs with HF or renal failure. The degree of kidney maturation and function depend on the age of the child and will affect the pharmacodynamics of the diuretic chosen. Pharmacokinetic factors also play a role. For examples, premature and term infants have differences in gastric pH, gastric emptying, and peristalsis, which can affect absorption. Total body water and plasma protein binding differences may affect the distribution of the drug. Safety of therapy in children has not been empirically established for all diuretics, and parents or caregivers are encouraged to discuss the potential risks and benefits with the health care provider before their child begins taking these drugs.

Geriatric Patients

Diuretics are one of the most common classes of drugs prescribed for older adults. Older adults have a higher frequency and intensity of adverse effects such as lightheadedness, dizziness, and fainting (syncope) as a result of the dehydration, hypovolemia (decrease in circulating blood volume), and deficiencies of calcium, potassium, sodium, and magnesium caused by the diuretic. In active older adults, diuretics may cause urge incontinence that may interfere with the ability or desire to participate in social activities in which restroom facilities are not nearby. If not taken early in the day, diuretics may affect sleep patterns due to frequent urination at night. The use of diuretics in older adults requires comprehensive patient, family, or caregiver education and ongoing assessment to ensure patient safety and optimal therapeutic effects.

sending more Na$^+$ to the urine (**natriuresis**). The human body is particularly sensitive to sodium imbalances and dietary intake must be balanced with excretion mechanisms. For example, a 1% increase in sodium reabsorption (retention) could potentially cause a 1.8-L net gain of water each day, which is equivalent to 4 lb of body weight. On the other hand, even small decreases in sodium reabsorption can cause net losses of sodium from the body, resulting in volume depletion and circulatory collapse. These examples illustrate the need for patients to monitor their weight daily when taking diuretics.

Natriuresis results in two other important effects. Chloride ions (Cl$^-$) follow sodium, potentially causing a net loss of chloride from the body and possible hypochloremia. In addition, because water molecules travel passively with sodium ions, blocking the reabsorption of Na$^+$ increases the total volume of urination, or diuresis. The amount of diuresis produced by a diuretic is directly related to the amount of sodium reabsorption that is blocked: Those that block the most sodium are the most effective at increasing urine output. Diuretics also affect the renal excretion of ions such as magnesium, potassium, phosphate, calcium, and bicarbonate. It is important to remember that imbalances may occur in virtually any electrolyte during diuretic therapy.

Diuretics are classified into five major groups, based on differences in their chemical nature and mechanism of action. The sites in the nephron at which the various diuretics act are shown in Pharmacotherapy Illustrated 1.

- **Loop or high-ceiling.** These drugs prevent the reabsorption of Na$^+$ in the loop of Henle; thus, they are called loop diuretics. Because there is an abundance of Na$^+$ in the filtrate within the loop of Henle, drugs in this class are capable of producing large increases in urine output.

- **Thiazides.** The largest diuretic class, the thiazides act by blocking Na$^+$ in the distal tubule. Because most Na$^+$ has already been reabsorbed from the filtrate by the time it reaches this part of the nephron, the thiazides produce less diuresis than loop diuretics.

- **Potassium-sparing.** The third major class is named potassium-sparing diuretics, because they have minimal effect on potassium ion (K$^+$) excretion. These agents produce a mild diuresis.

- **Osmotic.** These agents are relatively inert drugs that change the osmolality of filtrate, causing water to remain in the

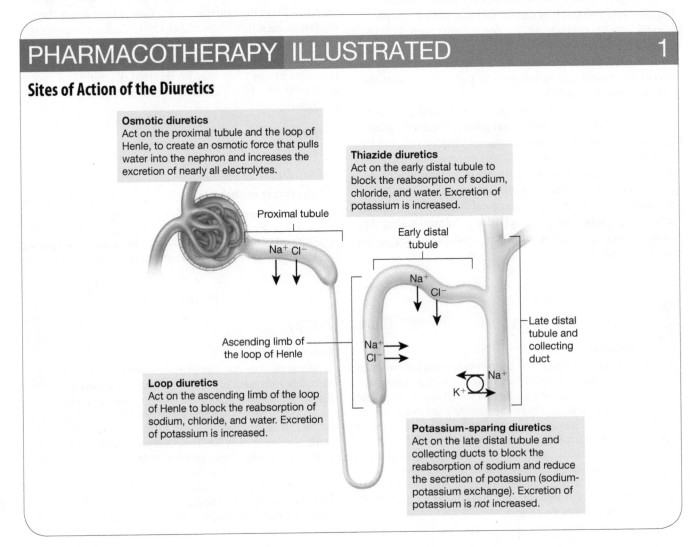

PHARMACOTHERAPY ILLUSTRATED   1

Sites of Action of the Diuretics

Osmotic diuretics
Act on the proximal tubule and the loop of Henle, to create an osmotic force that pulls water into the nephron and increases the excretion of nearly all electrolytes.

Thiazide diuretics
Act on the early distal tubule to block the reabsorption of sodium, chloride, and water. Excretion of potassium is increased.

Proximal tubule

Na$^+$ Cl$^-$

Early distal tubule

Na$^+$

Cl$^-$

Ascending limb of the loop of Henle

Na$^+$
Cl$^-$

Late distal tubule and collecting duct

Na$^+$

K$^+$

Loop diuretics
Act on the ascending limb of the loop of Henle to block the reabsorption of sodium, chloride, and water. Excretion of potassium is increased.

Potassium-sparing diuretics
Act on the late distal tubule and collecting ducts to block the reabsorption of sodium and reduce the secretion of potassium (sodium-potassium exchange). Excretion of potassium is *not* increased.

nephron for excretion. These drugs are very effective but are rarely prescribed because they can produce potentially serious adverse effects.

- **Carbonic anhydrase inhibitors.** These agents block the enzyme in the nephron responsible for bicarbonate reabsorption. They produce a weak diuresis and are rarely used.

It is common practice to combine two or more drugs in the pharmacotherapy of HTN and fluid retention disorders. Diuretics are often a component of fixed-dose combinations with drugs from other classes. The primary rationales for combination therapy are that the incidence of adverse effects is decreased and the pharmacologic effects (such as diuresis or blood pressure reduction) may be enhanced. For patient convenience, some of these drugs are available in single-tablet formulations. Examples of single-tablet diuretic combinations include the following:

- **Aldactazide.** Hydrochlorothiazide and spironolactone
- **Apresazide.** Hydrochlorothiazide and hydralazine
- **Dyazide.** Hydrochlorothiazide and triamterene
- **Moduretic.** Hydrochlorothiazide and amiloride.

Loop (High-Ceiling) Diuretics

5 The most effective diuretics are the loop diuretics that block sodium reabsorption in the loop of Henle.

The most effective diuretics, the loop or high-ceiling diuretics, act by blocking the reabsorption of sodium and chloride in the loop of Henle. This occurs when the drug inhibits the molecule responsible for transporting sodium and chloride from the filtrate to the blood, known as the Na^+-K^+-$2Cl^-$ symporter. A **symporter** is a membrane protein that transports two molecules at the same time. When the loop diuretics block this symporter, sodium and chloride are prevented from being reabsorbed, and diuresis is increased. All loop diuretics have an additional action that is responsible for a major adverse effect of drugs in this class: increasing potassium

excretion. An illustration showing the effects caused when this symporter is inhibited is shown in Figure 3.

All loop diuretics are available for either oral (PO) or parenteral administration and are extensively bound by plasma proteins. They have relatively short half-lives, and extended release preparations are not available. When given intravenously (IV), loop diuretics have the ability to cause large amounts of fluid to be excreted by the kidney in a very short time. Loop diuretics are used to reduce the edema associated with HF, hepatic cirrhosis, or chronic renal failure. Furosemide and torsemide are also approved for HTN, although their short half-lives make them less suitable for this indication than thiazide diuretics. Occasionally, loop diuretics are given to speed the renal excretion of a drug that has been overdosed or a toxin that has been accidentally ingested. Doses of the loop diuretics are listed in Table 4.

The rapid excretion of large amounts of fluid has the potential to produce serious adverse effects, including dehydration and electrolyte imbalances. Signs of dehydration include thirst, dry mouth, weight loss, and headache. Dizziness and fainting can result from the fall in blood pressure caused by the rapid fluid loss. Potassium depletion can be serious and result in dysrhythmias. Potassium supplements are often prescribed concurrently with these diuretics to prevent hypokalemia. Potassium loss is of particular concern to those concurrently taking digoxin (Lanoxin), because hypokalemia predisposes these patients to dysrhythmias. Significant loss of sodium, magnesium, and calcium is also possible, especially with large doses. Continuous use of loop diuretics in postmenopausal women may affect bone metabolism due to excessive calcium loss. Loop diuretics can cause gout in some patients due to hyperuricemia—the accumulation of uric acid in the blood.

Although rare, loop diuretics may cause ototoxicity, which may manifest as tinnitus, vertigo, or deafness. Use of other ototoxic drugs such as the aminoglycoside antibiotics should be avoided during loop diuretic therapy due to the potential for additive hearing impairment. Because of the potential for serious adverse effects, the loop diuretics are normally prescribed for patients with moderate to severe fluid retention such as

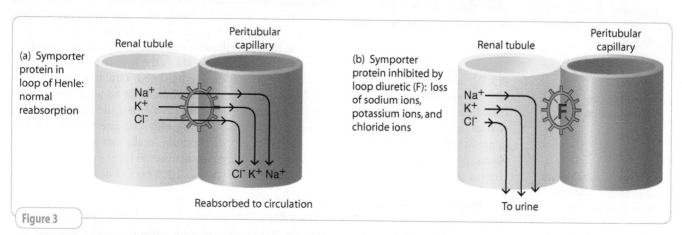

Figure 3

Symporter protein in the loop of Henle: (a) normal reabsorption of inhibition of the Na^+, K^+, and Cl^-; (b) inhibition of symporter by furosemide causes excretion of Na^+, K^+, Cl^-.

TABLE 4 Loop Diuretics

Drug	Route and Adult Dose (maximum dose where indicated)	Adverse Effects
bumetanide (Bumex)	PO: 0.5–2 mg/day, may repeat at 4- to 5-h intervals if needed (max: 10 mg/day) IV/IM: 0.5–1 mg over 1–2 min, repeated every 2–3 h prn (max: 10 mg/day)	*Minor hypokalemia, orthostatic hypotension, tinnitus, nausea, diarrhea, dizziness, fatigue*
ethacrynic acid (Edecrin)	PO: 50–100 mg one to two times/day; may increase by 25–50 mg prn (max: 400 mg/day) IV: 0.5–1 mg/kg or 50 mg (max: 100 mg/dose)	<u>Serious hypokalemia, blood dyscrasias, dehydration, ototoxicity, electrolyte imbalances, circulatory collapse</u>
furosemide (Lasix)	PO: 20–80 mg in one or more divided doses (max: 600 mg/day) IV/IM: 20–40 mg in one or more divided doses (max: 600 mg/day)	
torsemide (Demadex)	PO/IV: 10–20 mg/day (max: 200 mg/day)	

Note: Italics indicate common adverse effects. <u>Underline</u> indicates serious adverse effects.

acute pulmonary edema, or when thiazide diuretics have failed to achieve therapeutic goals.

Furosemide (Lasix)

Classification: **Therapeutic:** Antihypertensive
Pharmacologic: Loop- or high-ceiling-type diuretic

Therapeutic Effects and Uses: An established diuretic approved in 1966, furosemide is frequently used in the treatment of acute edema associated with liver cirrhosis, renal impairment, or HF because it has the ability to remove large amounts of edema fluid from the patient in a short time. When given IV, diuresis begins within 5 minutes, providing patients quick relief from their distressing symptoms. Unlike the thiazide diuretics, furosemide is able to increase urine output even when blood flow to the kidneys is diminished, which makes it of particular value in patients with low cardiac output or renal failure. It is also approved for HTN, although it is not generally a drug of choice for this indication because of its short half-life and potential for serious adverse effects.

Mechanism of Action: Furosemide prevents the reabsorption of sodium and chloride by blocking the Na^+-K^+-$2Cl^-$ symporter in the loop of Henle. Because this is the region of the nephron that normally filters the bulk of sodium, furosemide can exert a profound diuresis. The extensive diuresis results in the increased urinary excretion of sodium, chloride, potassium, and hydrogen ions.

Pharmacokinetics:

Route(s)	PO, IV, intramuscular (IM)
Absorption	60% absorbed PO
Distribution	Distributes to most tissues; crosses the placenta; secreted in breast milk; 95% bound to plasma protein
Primary metabolism	Hepatic (small amounts)
Primary excretion	Renal
Onset of action	PO: 30–60 min; IV: 5 min; IM: 10–30 min
Duration of action	PO: 6–8 h; IV: 2 h; IM: 4–8 h

Adverse Effects: The greatest concerns during furosemide therapy are excessive fluid loss and electrolyte imbalances. Hypovolemia may cause orthostatic hypotension and syncope. Imbalances may occur in any or all electrolytes, causing symptoms such as tachycardia, dysrhythmias, nausea, and vomiting. Ototoxicity is rare but may result in permanent hearing deficit. Hyperuricemia caused by the drug may cause exacerbations of gout. In patients with hypokalemia and hypochloremia, furosemide may induce metabolic alkalosis.

Contraindications/Precautions: Contraindications include hypersensitivity to furosemide or sulfonamide antibiotics, anuria, hepatic coma, or severe fluid or electrolyte depletion. Because furosemide is extremely potent, fluid loss must be carefully monitored to avoid possible dehydration and hypotension. Any preexisting hypovolemia or hypotension should be corrected before furosemide therapy is initiated. Loop diuretics can impair glucose tolerance: Serum glucose levels should be assessed in patients with diabetes mellitus.

Drug Interactions: Hypokalemia from the use of furosemide may cause dysrhythmias in patients taking digoxin; therefore, combination therapy with furosemide and digoxin should be avoided or carefully monitored. Concurrent use with corticosteroids, amphotericin B, or other potassium-depleting drugs can result in hypokalemia. When given with lithium, elimination of lithium is decreased, causing a higher risk of toxicity. Furosemide may diminish the hypoglycemic effects of sulfonylureas and insulin. Concurrent use with NSAIDs can result in a diminished diuretic effect. Additive hypotension will occur if furosemide is given concurrently with antihypertensives, including thiazide diuretics. Use of ethanol should be restricted because it may add to the hypotensive and diuretic actions of furosemide. **Herbal/Food:** Oral aloe can decrease the levels of potassium and should not be used concurrently with loop diuretics. Use with hawthorn could result in additive hypotensive effects. Ginseng may decrease the effectiveness of loop diuretics. High sodium intake can reduce the effectiveness of diuretics; patients should be placed on a sodium-restricted intake of 1,500 to 2,300 mg per day.

Treatment of Overdose: Overdose with furosemide can cause serious hypotension, fluid loss, and electrolyte imbalances. Treatment is supportive, with replacement of fluids and electrolytes and the possible administration of a vasopressor.

Pregnancy: Category C.

Nursing Responsibilities: Key nursing implications for patients receiving furosemide are included in the Nursing Practice Application for Patients Receiving Diuretic Therapy.

Lifespan and Diversity Considerations:

- Use extreme caution when administering the drug to the older adult who is at greater risk for hypotension, dizziness, and falls. Provide assistance with ambulation as needed.

- Monitor potassium levels frequently in the older adult who is at greater risk for the development of hypokalemia while on diuretics.

- Because of pharmacokinetic differences, exercise additional caution when administering furosemide to infants and very young children. Additional monitoring, such as audiology, may be ordered.

Patient and Family Education:

- Monitor blood pressure regularly. Maintain a written log of blood pressure readings and present it at follow-up visits.

- Eat potassium-rich foods daily (e.g., bananas, oranges, peaches, or dried dates) to reduce or prevent potassium depletion.

- Avoid prolonged exposure to direct sun because furosemide may cause the skin to be more sensitive to sunlight.

- Immediately report any changes in hearing or balance.

- If diabetic, monitor blood glucose levels frequently at the beginning of therapy and during dosage adjustments.

- Do not breast-feed while taking this drug without approval of the health care provider.

Drugs Similar to Furosemide (Lasix)

Furosemide is the most commonly prescribed drug in this class. Other loop diuretics include bumetanide, ethacrynic acid, and torsemide.

Bumetanide (Bumex): Approved in 1983, bumetanide is indicated for ascites and the treatment of peripheral edema, usually associated with HF or renal failure. This drug is available by the PO, IV, and IM routes and is 40 times more potent than furosemide but has a shorter duration of action. It may be used in acute clinical situations when furosemide has proven ineffective in patients with severe renal impairment. Like furosemide, bumetanide can cause electrolyte imbalances, hypotension, and dehydration. Unlike furosemide and torsemide, bumetanide is not approved for HTN, although it may be used off-label for that indication. This drug is pregnancy category C.

Ethacrynic acid (Edecrin): Approved in 1967, ethacrynic acid is indicated for the treatment of edema, usually associated with heart, liver, or renal failure. Given by either the oral or IV route, ethacrynic acid is the only loop diuretic that does not contain a sulfur group in its structure; thus it can safely be used in patients allergic to sulfonamides. Of the loop diuretics, ethacrynic acid causes the most severe hearing loss, which may be irreversible. The patient must be carefully monitored to prevent excessive electrolyte and fluid losses. Although ethacrynic acid is not approved for HTN, it may be prescribed off-label for this indication. This drug is pregnancy category B.

Torsemide (Demadex): Approved in 1993, torsemide is indicated for the treatment of HTN and edema, usually associated with heart, liver, or renal failure. Given by either the oral or IV route, torsemide is twice as potent as furosemide and has a longer half-life, which offers the advantage of once-a-day dosing. The incidence of ototoxicity with torsemide is very low, and the risk of hypokalemia is less than that of other drugs in this class. At higher doses, however, torsemide carries the same potential risks as furosemide and other loop diuretics, including electrolyte imbalances and hypovolemia. Torsemide is contraindicated in patients with sensitivity to sulfonylureas. This drug is pregnancy category B.

Thiazide and Thiazide-Like Diuretics

6 The thiazides are the most commonly prescribed class of diuretics.

The thiazides comprise the largest and most commonly prescribed class of diuretics. Like the loop diuretics, the thiazides block a symport protein in the renal tubule wall that is responsible for reabsorbing sodium and chloride ions from the filtrate. However, the thiazides block a different symport protein, and in a different location than the loop diuretics. The thiazides act on the Na^+Cl^- symporter in the distal tubule to block Na^+ reabsorption and increase K^+ and water excretion. The thiazides are less effective than the loop diuretics because over 90% of the Na^+ has already been reabsorbed by the time the filtrate reaches the distal tubule. There are simply fewer Na^+ to block; thus the maximum diuresis produced by thiazides is less than the loop diuretics.

The primary indication for thiazide diuretics is the treatment of mild to moderate HTN. Mild HTN can often be controlled with only a thiazide diuretic, whereas moderate to severe HTN requires two or more antihypertensive agents. Thiazides are also indicated for edema due to mild to moderate heart, liver, and renal failure. They are not effective in patients with severe organ impairment because their ability to produce a diuresis diminishes as blood flow through the kidneys is reduced. Doses of the thiazide diuretics are listed in Table 5.

Thiazides are available only by the PO route with the exception of chlorothiazide (Diuril, Diurigen), which is also available parenterally. All the thiazide diuretics have equivalent effectiveness and safety profiles. They differ, however, in their potency and duration of action. For example, metolazone (Zaroxolyn) is 10 times more potent than hydrochlorothiazide (Microzide). At therapeutic doses all thiazides produce the same level of diuresis.

Three drugs in Table 5, chlorthalidone (Hygroton), indapamide (Lozol), and metolazone (Zaroxolyn), are not true thiazides because they do not contain the two-ring structure that chemically defines a thiazide. However, these drugs block the same symport protein and have the same pharmacologic effects as thiazides. They are sometimes called "thiazide-like" and are always considered along with the true thiazides because of their similar mechanism of action, indications, and adverse effects.

TABLE 5 Thiazide and Thiazide-Like Diuretics

Drug	Route and Adult Dose (maximum dose where indicated)	Adverse Effects
Short Acting		
chlorothiazide (Diuril)	PO: 250 mg–1 g/day once or twice daily in divided doses IV: 250 mg–1 g/day in one to two divided doses (max: 2 g/day)	*Minor hypokalemia, fatigue* Serious hypokalemia, electrolyte depletion, dehydration, hypotension, hyponatremia, hyperglycemia, coma, blood dyscrasias
hydrochlorothiazide (Microzide)	PO: 25–100 mg/day as single or divided dose (max: 50 mg/day for HTN; 100 mg/day for edema)	
Intermediate Acting		
bendroflumethiazide and nadolol (Corzide)	PO: 1 tablet/day (40–80 mg nadolol and 5 mg bendroflumethiazide)	
metolazone (Zaroxolyn)	PO: 2.5–10 mg once daily (max: 5 mg/day for HTN; 20 mg/day for edema)	
Long Acting		
chlorthalidone (Hygroton)	PO: 50–100 mg/day (max: 50 mg/day for HTN; 200 mg/day for edema)	
indapamide (Lozol)	PO: 1.25–2.5 mg once daily (max: 5 mg/day)	
methyclothiazide (Enduron)	PO: 2.5–5 mg once daily (max: 5 mg/day for HTN; 10 mg/day for edema)	

Note: Italics indicate common adverse effects. Underline indicates serious adverse effects.

The adverse effects of thiazides are similar to those of the loop diuretics, though their frequency is less and they do not cause ototoxicity. Dehydration and excessive loss of sodium, potassium, or chloride ions may occur with overtreatment: Hypokalemia and hypochloremia can cause metabolic alkalosis. Concurrent therapy with digoxin requires careful monitoring to avoid dysrhythmias caused by excessive potassium loss. Potassium supplements are sometimes prescribed during thiazide therapy to prevent hypokalemia. Patients with diabetes should be aware that thiazide diuretics sometimes raise blood glucose levels. Like the loop diuretics, thiazides can increase serum levels of uric acid, although this is only clinically significant in patients with a history of gout.

PROTOTYPE DRUG | Hydrochlorothiazide (Microzide)

Classification: **Therapeutic:** Antihypertensive
Pharmacologic: Thiazide-type diuretic

Therapeutic Effects and Uses: Approved in 1959, hydrochlorothiazide (sometimes abbreviated HCTZ) is the most widely prescribed diuretic for HTN. Like many diuretics, it produces few adverse effects and is effective at producing a 10- to 20-mmHg reduction in blood pressure. Patients with severe HTN or a compelling condition such as HF, postmyocardial infarction (post-MI), high risk for coronary artery disease, diabetes, chronic kidney disease, or recurrent stroke prevention may require the addition of a second drug from a different class to control the disease.

Hydrochlorothiazide is approved to treat ascites, edema, HF, HTN, and nephrotic syndrome. Off-label indications include premenstrual syndrome (PMS), diabetes insipidus, hypercalciuria, and nephrolithiasis. Hydrochlorothiazide is the most common agent found in fixed-dose combination drugs for HTN.

Mechanism of Action: Hydrochlorothiazide acts on the distal tubule to decrease the reabsorption of Na^+. This results in less water reabsorption, increased diuresis, and removal of edema fluid. Blood volume decreases and blood pressure falls. Increasing the amount of sodium in the distal tubule also increases potassium excretion via a sodium–potassium exchange mechanism.

Pharmacokinetics:

Route(s)	PO
Absorption	Variable; incompletely absorbed
Distribution	Distributed to most tissues; crosses the placenta and is secreted in breast milk
Primary metabolism	Not metabolized
Primary excretion	Renal
Onset of action	2 h; peak effect: 4 h
Duration of action	6–12 h; half-life: 45–120 min

Adverse Effects: Hydrochlorothiazide is generally well tolerated and exhibits few serious adverse effects. Hypotension may cause dizziness or headache. Electrolyte imbalances such as hypochloremia, hypomagnesemia, hypokalemia, and hyponatremia may occur. Dysrhythmias due to hypokalemia may be serious if not prevented by maintaining normal serum potassium levels, usually by the administration of potassium supplements during therapy. Hydrochlorothiazide may precipitate gout attacks due to its tendency to cause hyperuricemia. Blood dyscrasias such as leukopenia, agranulocytosis, and aplastic anemia are rare, though serious, adverse effects.

Contraindications/Precautions: Contraindications include anuria and prior hypersensitivity to thiazide diuretics or sulfonamide antibiotics. Because hydrochlorothiazide can cause glycosuria and hyperglycemia, serum glucose levels must be carefully monitored in patients with diabetes. Preexisting hypovolemia or hypotension should be corrected before thiazide therapy is initiated because diuretics can worsen these conditions. Hydrochlorothiazide should not be used in jaundiced neonates because it can cause hyperbilirubinemia.

Drug Interactions: When given concurrently with other antihypertensives, additive effects on blood pressure usually occur. Thiazides may reduce the effectiveness of anticoagulants, sulfonylureas, and antidiabetic drugs, including insulin. Cholestyramine and colestipol bind to and decrease the absorption of HCTZ, thus reducing its effectiveness. Hydrochlorothiazide increases the risk of renal toxicity from NSAIDs. Corticosteroids and amphotericin B increase potassium loss when given with HCTZ. Hypokalemia caused by HCTZ may increase digoxin toxicity and the possibility of dysrhythmias. Hydrochlorothiazide decreases the excretion of lithium and can lead to lithium toxicity. Because thiazides decrease the renal excretion of calcium, concurrent administration with calcium supplements may lead to hypercalcemia. **Herbal/Food:** Ginkgo biloba may produce a paradoxical increase in blood pressure. Oral aloe can decrease levels of potassium and should not be used concurrently with thiazide diuretics. Use with hawthorn could result in additive hypotensive effects. High sodium intake can reduce the effectiveness of diuretics; patients should be placed on a sodium-restricted diet of 1,500 to 2,300 mg per day.

Treatment of Overdose: Overdose is manifested as electrolyte depletion, which is treated with infusions of fluids containing electrolytes. Infusion of fluids also prevents dehydration and hypotension.

Pregnancy: Category B.

Nursing Responsibilities: Key nursing implications for patients receiving hydrochlorothiazide are included in the Nursing Practice Application for Patients Receiving Diuretic Therapy.

Lifespan and Diversity Considerations:

- Use caution when administering the drug to the older adult who is at greater risk for hypotension, dizziness, and falls. Provide assistance with ambulation as needed.

- Monitor potassium levels frequently in the older adult who is at greater risk for the development of hypokalemia while on diuretics.

- Because of pharmacokinetic differences, exercise additional caution when administering hydrochlorothiazide to infants and very young children.

Patient and Family Education:

- Monitor blood pressure regularly as directed by the health care provider. Maintain a written log of blood pressure readings and present it at follow-up visits.

- If diabetic, monitor blood glucose levels frequently at the beginning of therapy and during dosage adjustments.

- Eat potassium-rich foods daily (e.g., bananas, oranges, peaches, or dried dates) to reduce or prevent potassium depletion.

- Avoid direct contact with sunlight because photosensitivity may occur 10 to 14 days after initial sun exposure.

- Do not breast-feed while taking this drug without the approval of the health care provider.

Drugs Similar to Hydrochlorothiazide (Microzide)

Many thiazide and thiazide-like diuretics are available. They may be grouped into subclasses based on their relative duration of action.

Short-acting thiazides: This group includes chlorothiazide (Diuril) and hydrochlorothiazide (Microzide). These drugs have a rapid onset of 1 to 2 hours with a duration of action of 6 to 12 hours. Chlorothiazide is available by the IV route for patients who are unable to take PO thiazides.

Intermediate-acting thiazides: This group includes metolazone (Zaroxolyn) and Corzide, a fixed-dose combination of bendroflumethiazide (a thiazide) with nadolol (a beta-adrenergic blocker). These drugs have an onset time of about 2 hours with a duration of action of 12 to 24 hours.

Long-acting thiazides: This group includes chlorthalidone (Hygroton), indapamide (Lozol), and methyclothiazide (Enduron). These agents have a 2-hour onset with a duration of action ranging from 24 to 72 hours.

CONNECTION Checkpoint 35.3

The use of lithium is often contraindicated when a patient is taking diuretics. Identify the indications for lithium and explain how the use of a diuretic can lead to lithium toxicity. *See Answer to Connection Checkpoint 35.3 on student resource website.*

Potassium-Sparing Diuretics

7 Potassium-sparing diuretics have low effectiveness but can help prevent hypokalemia.

As discussed in Sections 5 and 6, hypokalemia is a potentially serious adverse effect of the loop and thiazide diuretics. The therapeutic advantage of the potassium-sparing diuretics is that increased diuresis can be obtained without affecting blood potassium levels. The potassium-sparing diuretics are listed in Table 6. There are two distinct subclasses of potassium-sparing diuretics: sodium ion channel inhibitors and aldosterone antagonists.

Sodium ion channel inhibitors: In the distal tubule, Na^+ is reabsorbed from the filtrate through sodium ion channels. As the sodium ion in the filtrate travels across the renal tubule cell and returns to the bloodstream, potassium ion moves in the opposite direction. In other words, as sodium ion is reabsorbed, potassium ion is secreted.

Triamterene (Dyrenium) and amiloride (Midamor) block the Na^+ channel, causing sodium to stay in the filtrate. Because water always follows sodium ions, additional water remains in the filtrate and ultimately leaves in the urine. When the sodium ion channel is blocked, another important action occurs: Potassium ion is not secreted to the filtrate. The body, therefore, does not lose potassium, as is the case with the thiazide and loop diuretics. Because most of the sodium ion has already been removed before the filtrate reaches the distal tubule, these potassium-sparing diuretics produce only a mild diuresis. Drugs in this class are rarely prescribed alone, but they may be used in combination with thiazide or loop diuretics to

	TABLE 6 Potassium-Sparing Diuretics	
Drug	**Route and Adult Dose** (maximum dose where indicated)	**Adverse Effects**
Sodium Channel Inhibitors		
amiloride (Midamor)	PO: 5–10 mg/day (max: 20 mg/day)	*Minor hyperkalemia, headache, fatigue, gynecomastia (spironolactone)*
triamterene (Dyrenium)	PO: 50–100 mg bid (max: 300 mg/day)	
Aldosterone Antagonists		<u>Dysrhythmias (from hyperkalemia), dehydration, hyponatremia, agranulocytosis, and other blood dyscrasias</u>
eplerenone (Inspra)	PO: 25–50 mg once daily (max: 100 mg/day for HTN; 50 mg/day for HF)	
spironolactone (Aldactone)	PO: 25–100 mg one to two times/day (max: 400 mg/day)	

Note: Italics indicate common adverse effects; <u>Underline</u> indicates serious adverse effects.

minimize loss of potassium ions in the pharmacotherapy of HTN or edema.

Aldosterone antagonists: Aldosterone is the primary mineralocorticoid hormone secreted by the adrenal gland. The physiological targets, or membrane receptors (MRs), for aldosterone are located in the distal tubule and collecting ducts of the nephron. Once bound to its receptors, the MR–aldosterone complex causes the renal tubule cells to synthesize more Na^+ channels, thereby allowing for more reabsorption of Na^+ from the filtrate. Simply stated, aldosterone increases sodium reabsorption.

Spironolactone (Aldactone) and eplerenone (Inspra) prevent the formation of the MR–aldosterone complex and are called aldosterone antagonists. By blocking the actions of aldosterone, these drugs enhance the excretion of sodium and the retention of potassium. Like the sodium ion channel inhibitors, spironolactone and eplerenone produce only a weak diuresis, and they are normally combined with drugs from other classes when treating HTN or edema. Spironolactone, has also been found to significantly reduce mortality in patients with HF and, because of this important beneficial effect, its use has increased. The aldosterone antagonists are also used to treat hyperaldosteronism, a rare disorder in which a tumor of the adrenal gland secretes large amounts of aldosterone.

Using potassium supplements or adding potassium-rich foods to the diet when taking these medications may lead to life-threatening hyperkalemia. Signs and symptoms of hyperkalemia include muscle weakness, ventricular tachycardia, or fibrillation. Other minor adverse effects of the drugs include headache, dizziness, nausea, and vomiting. Spironolactone binds to progesterone and androgen receptors, resulting in a small incidence of adverse effects such as gynecomastia, menstrual abnormalities, and impotence. Gynecomastia, abnormal enlargement of the breasts in males, appears to be related to dosage level and duration of therapy; it may persist after the drug is discontinued. The incidence of adverse reproductive system effects is lower with eplerenone.

PROTOTYPE DRUG	Spironolactone (Aldactone)

Classification: **Therapeutic:** Antihypertensive
Pharmacologic: Potassium-sparing diuretic/ aldosterone antagonist

Therapeutic Effects and Uses: Approved in 1960, spironolactone is the most frequently prescribed potassium-sparing diuretic.

The most common indication for spironolactone is mild HTN. Because it does not cause potassium depletion, the drug is particularly useful in patients who are at high risk for hypokalemia. However, spironolactone does such an efficient job of retaining potassium that hyperkalemia may develop, especially if the patient is taking potassium supplements or is concurrently receiving angiotensin-converting enzyme (ACE) inhibitors. When serum potassium levels are monitored carefully and maintained within normal values, serious adverse effects from spironolactone are uncommon.

Spironolactone is approved for the management of edema and sodium retention associated with HF, nephrotic syndrome, and liver disease. It is particularly useful in treating edema or ascites in patients with hepatic cirrhosis, because it counteracts the large amount of aldosterone secreted by these patients. Spironolactone may also be used for the short-term, preoperative treatment of primary hyperaldosteronism. An off-label indication is to improve survival and reduce hospitalizations in patients with severe HF. Other off-label indications include treatment of minor edema associated with PMS, polycystic ovary, and hirsutism in females. It is available in tablet form and as a fixed-dose combination with hydrochlorothiazide (Microzide).

Mechanism of Action: Spironolactone acts by inhibiting the actions of aldosterone in the distal tubule and collecting ducts of the nephron. When the actions of aldosterone are blocked by spironolactone, sodium, chloride, and water excretion are increased and the body retains potassium.

Pharmacokinetics:

Route(s)	PO
Absorption	Rapid absorption; 73% absorbed
Distribution	Distributed to most tissues; crosses the placenta; secreted in breast milk; more than 90% bound to plasma protein
Primary metabolism	Hepatic and renal; converted to active metabolites
Primary excretion	Renal (40–57%) and biliary (35–40%)
Onset of action	2–3 days; may take 2 weeks for maximum effect
Duration of action	2–3 days; half-life: 1.3–2.4 h for parent compound, and 18–23 h for active metabolites

Adverse Effects: Hyperkalemia induced by spironolactone can cause life-threatening cardiac dysrhythmias. Signs and symptoms associated with spironolactone-induced hyperkalemia include muscle weakness, paresthesia, fatigue, bradycardia, flaccid paralysis of the extremities, and shock. In men, spironolactone can cause gynecomastia, impotence, and diminished libido. Women may experience menstrual irregularities, hirsutism, and breast tenderness. Fertility may decrease during therapy. Agranulocytosis and other blood dyscrasias are rare adverse effects. **Black Box Warning:** Spironolactone produces tumors in laboratory animals; unnecessary use of the drug should be avoided.

Contraindications/Precautions: Contraindications include anuria, severe renal impairment, pregnancy, and hyperkalemia. Older patients and those with renal insufficiency or diabetes mellitus are at greatest risk for hyperkalemia. At high doses, spironolactone produces teratogenic effects in laboratory animals; thus it should not be used during pregnancy. A major metabolite of spironolactone is secreted in breast milk; thus this drug should not be given to lactating patients.

Drug Interactions: When combined with ammonium chloride, acidosis may occur. Aspirin and other salicylates may decrease the diuretic effect of the medication. Concurrent use with digoxin may decrease the effects of digoxin. When taken with potassium supplements, ACE inhibitors, angiotensin-receptor blockers (ARBs), or the potassium salts of other drugs (such as penicillin G potassium), severe hyperkalemia and possible dysrhythmias may result. Concurrent use with other antihypertensives will result in an additive hypotensive effect. **Herbal/Food:** Licorice extract contains a substance with aldosterone-like actions and should be avoided. Use with hawthorn may result in hypotension.

Treatment of Overdose: Acute overdoses produce drowsiness, mental confusion, rash, nausea, vomiting, dizziness, or diarrhea. The most serious symptoms of spironolactone overdose are related to hyperkalemia. If severe, therapies are administered to counteract the hyperkalemia. These include IV calcium chloride, IV sodium bicarbonate, or the administration of glucose with rapid-acting insulin. Cationic exchange resins such as sodium polystyrene sulfonate (Kayexalate) may be administered.

Pregnancy: Category D.

Nursing Responsibilities: Key nursing implications for patients receiving spironolactone are included in the Nursing Practice Application for Patients Receiving Diuretic Therapy.

Lifespan and Diversity Considerations:
- Use caution when administering the drug to the older adult who is at greater risk for hypotension, dizziness, and falls. Provide assistance with ambulation as needed.
- Monitor potassium levels frequently in the older adult who is at greater risk for the development of hyperkalemia while on potassium-sparing diuretics.
- Because of pharmacokinetic differences, exercise additional caution when administering spironolactone

to infants and very young children. Educate parents or caregivers about the possibility of gynecomastia and that it is usually reversible after the drug is stopped.

Patient and Family Education:
- Monitor blood pressure regularly. Maintain a written log of blood pressure readings and present it at follow-up visits.
- Immediately report nausea, fatigue, muscle weakness, tingling, slow heartbeat, or weak pulse which are potential symptoms of hyperkalemia.
- Breast enlargement or tenderness may occur with the drug and is usually reversible once the drug is stopped.
- Avoid excessive intake of high-potassium foods or salt substitutes that contain potassium chloride. Never take over-the-counter (OTC) potassium supplements without approval of the health care provider.
- Do not breast-feed while taking this drug without approval of the health care provider.

Drugs Similar to Spironolactone (Aldactone)

The three other potassium-sparing diuretics include amiloride, eplerenone, and triamterene.

Amiloride (Midamor): Approved in 1981, amiloride is an oral Na^+ channel inhibitor with weak diuretic activity whose major indication is HTN. It is also used to treat peripheral edema due to HF and to reverse hypokalemia. When combined with a thiazide diuretic, additive hypotensive action is achieved, and potassium balance is maintained. It should not be used as monotherapy or in combination with other potassium-sparing diuretics because hyperkalemia may develop. Contraindications and adverse effects are similar to those of spironolactone, including the risk of severe hyperkalemia in patients receiving other potassium-containing drugs. Moduretic is a fixed-dose combination of amiloride and hydrochlorothiazide. Amiloride is pregnancy category B.

Eplerenone (Inspra): Approved in 2002, eplerenone is an aldosterone antagonist administered by the oral route that was initially approved for HTN. Later, post-MI management of HF was added as an indication. Research has not shown eplerenone to be more effective than spironolactone, but it is more expensive. Two to four weeks of therapy are required to achieve maximum therapeutic effects. Eplerenone is more selective for the aldosterone receptor than spironolactone, and it has the advantage of producing a lower incidence of endocrine-related adverse effects such as gynecomastia, impotence, or menstrual irregularities. Like other drugs in this class, however, the development of hyperkalemia is a potentially serious adverse effect. Eplerenone is sometimes referred to as a selective aldosterone receptor antagonist. This drug is pregnancy category B.

Triamterene (Dyrenium): Approved in 1964, triamterene is an oral drug that acts by the same mechanism as amiloride and has the same indications and adverse effects. It is a relatively weak diuretic and is sometimes used to manage hypokalemia

TABLE 7 Miscellaneous Diuretics

Drug	Route and Adult Dose (maximum dose where indicated)	Adverse Effects
Carbonic Anhydrase Inhibitors		
acetazolamide (Diamox)	PO: 250–375 mg/day (max: 1,500 mg/day)	*Electrolyte imbalances, fatigue, nausea, vomiting, dizziness*
	IM/IV: 250–375 mg/day	Dehydration, blood dyscrasias, pancytopenia, flaccid paralysis, hemolytic anemia, aplastic anemia
methazolamide (Neptazane)	PO: 50–100 mg bid–tid (max: 300 mg/day)	
Osmotic Type		
glycerin	PO: 1–1.8 g/kg, 1–2 h before ocular surgery	*Electrolyte imbalances, fatigue, nausea, vomiting, dizziness*
mannitol (Osmitrol)	IV: 100 g infused over 2–6 h	Hyponatremia, edema, convulsions, tachycardia
urea (Ureaphil)	IV: 1–1.5 g/kg over 1–2.5 h	

Note: Italics indicate common adverse effects. Underline indicates serious adverse effects.

in patients who are unable to tolerate potassium supplements. Triamterene is rarely used as monotherapy and should not be used concurrently with other potassium-sparing diuretics due to the potential for hyperkalemia. Dyazide is a fixed-dose combination of triamterene and hydrochlorothiazide. This drug is pregnancy category C.

CONNECTION Checkpoint 35.4

Explain why patients who are taking an ACE inhibitor should probably not receive an aldosterone antagonist. *See Answer to Connection Checkpoint 35.4 on student resource website.*

Osmotic Diuretics

8 Osmotic diuretics cause diuresis by increasing the osmolality of the filtrate.

The osmotic diuretics, shown in Table 7, are a small class of drugs that are reserved for very specific indications. Unlike the thiazides and loop diuretics that block transport proteins, osmotic diuretics are mostly inert and act by raising the osmolality, which is a measure of the amount of dissolved particles, or solutes in a solution. This in turn increases the **osmotic pressure**, which creates a force that moves substances between compartments. Osmotic diuretics cause water to shift compartments by creating a difference in osmotic pressure across a membrane or between two body compartments.

When given IV, osmotic diuretics are filtered at the glomerulus and readily enter the renal filtrate. Once in the tubule, they remain unchanged. As normal sodium and water reabsorption progresses in the proximal tubule, the diuretic remains behind, and its concentration in the tubule begins to increase. The osmolality of the filtrate increases due to the presence of the osmotic diuretic in the tubule. This osmotic force draws water into the filtrate, resulting in increased diuresis.

A second action of osmotic diuretics is their ability to raise the osmolality of the plasma. This creates an osmotic force that moves water from the intracellular and extravascular spaces to the plasma. The increased volume of water in the plasma is filtered by the kidney, resulting in enhanced diuresis. This action is used to advantage in the treatment of two conditions where fluid has accumulated in extravascular spaces. For example, following a traumatic head injury, fluid accumulates in the brain, causing dangerously high intracranial pressure. Osmotic diuretics create an osmotic force that promotes the fluid to leave the brain and enter the blood, thus reducing cerebral edema. A second example is high intraocular pressure caused by excess fluid accumulation in the eye (glaucoma). Osmotic diuretics can cause the fluid to leave the eye and enter the blood, thus relieving the high intraocular pressure.

Osmotic diuretics are rarely the drugs of first choice due to their potential toxicity. Mannitol and urea are given by the IV route under controlled conditions where the patient can be closely monitored. Although as diuretics they are useful in increasing urine output, they are contraindicated in patients with severe renal impairment. The rapid movement of water from the extravascular spaces to the blood can result in severe dehydration in the tissues, and cause a serious fluid overload in patients with severe HF. Electrolyte imbalances, especially hyponatremia, may occur with these agents.

PROTOTYPE DRUG Mannitol (Osmitrol)

Classification: Therapeutic: Drug for renal failure
Pharmacologic: Osmotic diuretic

Therapeutic Effects and Uses: Approved in 1944, mannitol is a parenteral diuretic primarily used to increase urine output in patients experiencing oliguria from acute renal failure. In addition, by its ability to increase the osmolality of plasma, this drug is able to "pull" fluid out of extravascular spaces; thus it is used to reduce intracranial pressure following head trauma and to lower intraocular pressure in patients with acute glaucoma. Reduction in the amount and pressure of cerebrospinal fluid can occur as quickly as 15 minutes after initiating the infusion; intraocular pressure reduction may take up to an hour. Mannitol may be administered concurrently with nephrotoxic drugs such as cisplatin (an antineoplastic drug) to speed them through the kidney and reduce damage to the walls of the renal tubules.

Mannitol has nondrug uses as a sweetener and food stabilizer. When taken orally, it is absorbed so slowly that it has no effect on insulin levels, making it an alternative sweetener in foods for patients with diabetes. The drug has a laxative effect when taken in large quantities.

Mechanism of Action: Administered by the IV route, mannitol is filtered by the glomerulus of the kidney but is incapable of being reabsorbed from the renal tubule. This creates an osmotic gradient, resulting in decreased water and Na^+ reabsorption and increased diuresis.

Pharmacokinetics:

Route(s)	IV
Absorption	Does not cross biologic membranes
Distribution	Remains in extracellular space; does not cross the blood–brain barrier
Primary metabolism	Hepatic (small amounts)
Primary excretion	Renal
Onset of action	1–3 h
Duration of action	4–6 h; half-life: 100 min

Adverse Effects: Electrolyte imbalances, either deficiencies or excesses, can occur during mannitol therapy. For example, as mannitol draws fluid from the intravascular spaces, hyperkalemia or hypernatremia may occur. However, mannitol also increases the excretion of sodium and potassium ions, which can result in hypokalemia or hyponatremia. The same holds true for fluid balance. As mannitol draws fluid into the extracellular spaces, peripheral edema, HF, or pulmonary edema may occur. As diuresis progresses, the patient may become hypovolemic and dehydrated. Other adverse effects include fatigue, nausea, vomiting, dizziness, convulsions, and tachycardia.

Contraindications/Precautions: Contraindications include anuria, severe HF, organic central nervous system (CNS) disease or intracranial bleeding, severe dehydration, and shock. A test dose may be given to patients with oliguria to determine renal function. Function is considered satisfactory if urine flow is at least 30 to 50 mL/h over 2 to 3 hours following an IV test dose of 0.2 g/kg. If this response is not achieved, the kidneys are too impaired to administer a full dose of mannitol.

There is evidence that high doses of mannitol may open the blood–brain barrier by temporarily shrinking the endothelial cells that line the barrier. Should this happen, mannitol will enter the brain (bringing water with it) and increase intracranial pressure. Extreme precautions must be taken when treating patients with high intracranial pressure. Experimentally, mannitol is used to intentionally open the blood–brain barrier to deliver higher doses of various drugs, such as antineoplastic agents, directly to the brain.

Drug Interactions: Because of its intense diuretic effect, mannitol can increase the excretion of many drugs. This results in a decreased effect for drugs such as lithium, imipramine, salicylates, barbiturates, and potassium supplements. **Herbal/Food:** Unknown.

Pregnancy: Category C.

Treatment of Overdose: Overdose will result in a shift of fluid to the vascular compartment, resulting in HF and pulmonary edema. Intense diuresis may cause significant electrolyte imbalances, especially hyponatremia. There is no specific antidote and treatment is supportive to the presenting symptoms.

Nursing Responsibilities: Key nursing implications for patients receiving mannitol are included in the Nursing Practice Application for Patients Receiving Diuretic Therapy.

Lifespan and Diversity Considerations:
- Use caution when administering the drug to the older adult who is at greater risk for hypotension, dizziness, and falls. Provide assistance with ambulation as needed.
- Monitor electrolyte levels frequently in the older adult who is at greater risk for developing imbalances due to renal changes associated with aging.
- Use extreme caution when administering mannitol to infants and very young children. Carefully monitor for signs of HF or increased intracranial pressure, especially in preterm infants.

Patient and Family Education:
- Family or caregivers should immediately report any evidence of confusion to the health care provider.
- Do not breast-feed while taking this drug without approval of the health care provider.

Drugs Similar to Mannitol (Osmitrol)

Other osmotic diuretics include glycerin and urea. Drugs in this class are infrequently used.

Glycerin: Also known as glycerol, glycerin is an osmotic diuretic given for a large number of indications. When given by the oral route, glycerin creates an osmotic gradient like mannitol that can reduce intraocular and intracranial pressure. As a laxative suppository, glycerin draws water into the colon, creating more bulk and promoting defecation. It is used in a variety of OTC products as an emollient or lubricant, including toothpaste, shaving cream, hair products, soaps, and skin care products. Like mannitol, it tastes sweet and is used as a food additive to sweeten and keep products moist. Contraindications for oral use include hypovolemia, HF, or intestinal obstruction. This drug is pregnancy category C.

Urea (Ureaphil): Urea is a small molecule that is a natural waste product of nitrogen metabolism in the body. Approved in 1966 as a drug, it is given IV to create an osmotic gradient that reduces cerebral edema and intraocular pressure. Contraindications and adverse effects are similar to those of mannitol. It is also available topically to rehydrate the skin or to remove excess keratin. Urea has a large number of industrial uses, including its use in fertilizer, hair products, deicing agents, and bath oils, and even as a flavor enhancer in cigarettes. This drug is pregnancy category C.

Carbonic Anhydrase Inhibitors

9 Carbonic anhydrase inhibitors are weak diuretics that have specific indications.

Carbonic anhydrase is an essential enzyme that helps regulate acid–base balance in the body. Carbonic anhydrase converts CO_2 to carbonic acid (H_2CO_3), which immediately dissociates to bicarbonate ion (HCO_3^-). Note that these reactions are reversible.

$$CO_2 + H_2O \longleftrightarrow H_2CO_3 \longleftrightarrow HCO_3^- + H^+$$

Carbonic acid is present in multiple tissues. In red blood cells, it converts CO_2 (an acidic, poorly soluble gas) to bicarbonate, which can be transported to the lungs, reconverted to CO_2, and exhaled. In the mucosa of the stomach, carbonic anhydrase is responsible for forming gastric acid (H^+). For this chapter, the most important action of carbonic anhydrase occurs in the renal tubule cells.

In the kidney tubules, carbonic anhydrase is necessary for the formation and reabsorption of bicarbonate ion, which is essential for maintaining proper acid–base balance. Sodium ions are reabsorbed with bicarbonate ion in the proximal tubule using a symporter protein.

Several drugs that inhibit carbonic anhydrase are available. Blocking carbonic anhydrase prevents bicarbonate formation and reabsorption in the renal tubule. Without bicarbonate ion, sodium reabsorption does not occur, more water remains in the filtrate, and diuresis is promoted. The reduction in plasma bicarbonate eventually causes metabolic acidosis, which tends to reverse the diuretic action of this drug.

Although once used as diuretics, the carbonic anhydrase inhibitors are now rarely prescribed for that purpose because they produce only a weak, short-lived diuresis and can contribute to metabolic acidosis. Carbonic anhydrase inhibitors that are given by the oral route include acetazolamide (Diamox) and methazolamide (Neptazane). Methazolamide is only approved for reducing intraocular pressure in patients with open-angle glaucoma. Acetazolamide (Diamox), also used to decrease intraocular fluid pressure, has several other indications. Two drugs in this class, dorzolamide (Trusopt) and brinzolamide (Azopt), are administered topically to the eye for open-angle glaucoma.

PROTOTYPE DRUG | Acetazolamide (Diamox)

Classification: **Therapeutic:** Drug for edema, antiglaucoma agent
Pharmacologic: Carbonic anhydrase inhibitor

Therapeutic Effects and Uses: Given by either the oral or parenteral route, acetazolamide produces a mild diuresis and is occasionally used to reduce edema fluid in patients with HF. An older drug approved in 1953, it has largely been replaced by thiazide diuretics.

Acetazolamide also has applications as an anticonvulsant for treating absence seizures and in treating motion sickness. It has been used to acclimatize people to high altitudes to prevent or treat acute mountain sickness. It accomplishes this by increasing the renal excretion of bicarbonate, which accumulates in the body because of the hyperventilation that occurs at high altitude. Acetazolamide is effective in treating open-angle glaucoma and for preoperative treatment of acute closed-angle glaucoma, although it is not a drug of first choice for these disorders.

Mechanism of Action: Acetazolamide produces its diuretic effect by inhibiting carbonic anhydrase activity in the proximal renal tubule, causing increased excretion of sodium and bicarbonate. In the eye, the inhibition of carbonic anhydrase reduces the rate of aqueous humor formation and consequently lowers intraocular pressure.

Pharmacokinetics:

Route(s)	PO, IV
Absorption	75% absorbed when given with food
Distribution	Distributed to most tissues; crosses the placenta, and is secreted in breast milk
Primary metabolism	Not metabolized
Primary excretion	Renal
Onset of action	PO: 90 min; IV: 2 min
Duration of action	PO: 8–12 h; PO extended release: 18–24 h; IV: 15 min; half-life: 2.4–5.8 h

Adverse Effects: Acetazolamide can cause various electrolyte imbalances, including hyperchloremia and hypokalemia. Gastrointestinal adverse effects include nausea, vomiting, diarrhea, and anorexia. CNS effects may occur, such as dizziness, fatigue, and numbness in the extremities, lips, or facial muscles. Metabolic acidosis may result from excess bicarbonate loss.

Contraindications/Precautions: Acetazolamide is contraindicated in patients who have hypersensitivity to sulfonamides and similar drugs such as thiazide diuretics. Other contraindications include severe renal or hepatic impairment and adrenocortical insufficiency. Patients with preexisting electrolyte imbalances such as hyponatremia, hypokalemia, or hypochloremic acidosis should be treated with caution because acetazolamide may worsen these conditions.

Drug Interactions: The potential for hypokalemia is greatest early in the course of acetazolamide therapy and is accelerated by amphotericin B and corticosteroids. Because acetazolamide alkalinizes the urine, the renal excretion of many drugs may be decreased, including tricyclic antidepressants, procainamide, amphetamines, ephedrine, and quinidine. Renal excretion of lithium and phenobarbital may be increased. High-dose aspirin therapy can compete with tubular secretory mechanisms with acetazolamide, causing the CA inhibitor to accumulate to toxic levels. **Herbal/Food:** Unknown.

Pregnancy: Category C.

Treatment of Overdose: Overdose with acetazolamide results in metabolic acidosis, which may be treated by administering sodium bicarbonate. Electrolyte depletion and dehydration are treated with infusions of fluids containing electrolytes.

Nursing Responsibilities: Key nursing implications for patients receiving acetazolamide are included in the Nursing Practice Application for Patients Receiving Diuretic Therapy.

Lifespan and Diversity Considerations:
- Use caution when administering the drug to the older adult who is at greater risk for hypotension, dizziness, and falls. Provide assistance with ambulation as needed.

Patient and Family Education:
- Maintain adequate fluid intake (1.5–2.5 L/24 h; 1 liter is approximately equal to 1 quart) to reduce the risk of kidney stones.

- Immediately report numbness, tingling, burning, drowsiness, visual problems, sore throat or mouth, unusual bleeding, fever, and skin or urinary problems to the health care provider.

- Do not breast-feed while taking this drug without approval of the health care provider.

Drugs Similar to Acetazolamide (Diamox)

The other oral carbonic anhydrase inhibitor is methazolamide (Neptazane), which is used as a systemic antiglaucoma agent rather than a diuretic.

Complementary and Alternative Therapies — Dandelion

Description: The common dandelion, *Taraxacum officinale*, is found worldwide and is considered a weed by homeowners and gardeners; however, this plant has both culinary and medicinal uses.

History and Claims: Medicinal applications of dandelion have been recorded as early as the 10th century by Arab health care providers, and the plant was introduced by the Celts when Roman legions invaded Britain. Native Americans used the plant to treat heartburn and kidney disease. Leaves of the plant are rich in vitamin A, potassium, minerals, and fiber and have been eaten raw in salads or cooked like spinach as a major nutritional source. The dandelion root has been dried and used to treat a large variety of conditions, including constipation, liver ailments, bronchitis, gout, and arthritis, although there is insufficient evidence to suggest it is effective for these conditions (National Center for Complementary and Alternative Medicine, 2010). The plant is also sold as a diuretic to ease premenstrual fluid retention.

Standardization: Dandelion is available in tea, liquid, or tablet form. Standardization is generally based on the amount of dandelion in grams (2–12 g/day).

Evidence: Research evidence to support most uses of dandelion is lacking, and data regarding the use of dandelion as a diuretic are conflicting. When taken in moderation, dandelion is safe and is a significant source of vitamins and minerals. High doses of dandelion should be discouraged due to potential interactions with prescription medications.

CONNECTIONS: NURSING PRACTICE APPLICATION

Patients Receiving Diuretic Therapy

Assessment	Potential Nursing Diagnoses
Baseline assessment prior to administration: • Understand the reason the drug has been prescribed in order to assess for therapeutic effects. • Obtain a complete health history including cardiovascular disease, diabetes, pregnancy, or breast-feeding. Obtain a drug history including allergies, current prescription and OTC drugs, herbal preparations, use of digoxin, lithium, or antihypertensive drugs, and alcohol use. Be alert to possible drug interactions. • Evaluate appropriate laboratory findings such as electrolytes, glucose, CBC, hepatic or renal function studies, uric acid levels, and lipid profiles. • Obtain baseline weight, vital signs (especially blood pressure and pulse), breath sounds, and cardiac monitoring (e.g., ECG, cardiac output) if appropriate. Assess for location, character, and amount of edema, if present. Assess baseline hearing and balance. • Assess the patient's ability to receive and understand instructions. Include the family and caregivers as needed.	• *Deficient Fluid Volume* • *Fatigue* • *Decreased Cardiac Output* • *Deficient Knowledge* (Drug Therapy) • *Risk for Falls*, related to hypotension and dizziness associated with adverse drug effects • *Risk for Injury*, related to hypotension and dizziness associated with adverse drug effects • *Risk for Urge Incontinence*
Assessment throughout administration: • Assess for desired therapeutic effects (e.g., adequate urine output or lowered blood pressure if given for HTN). • Continue periodic monitoring of electrolytes, glucose, CBC, lipid profiles, liver function studies, creatinine, and uric acid levels. • Assess for and promptly report adverse effects: hypotension, palpitations, dizziness or lightheadedness, musculoskeletal weakness or cramping, nausea, vomiting, abdominal cramping, diarrhea, or headache. Immediately report tinnitus or hearing loss, loss of balance or incoordination, severe hypotension accompanied by reflex tachycardia, dysrhythmias, decreased urine output, or weight gain or loss over 1 kg (2.2 lb) in a 24-h period.	

(continued)

CONNECTIONS: NURSING PRACTICE APPLICATION *(continued)*

Planning: Patient Goals and Expected Outcomes

The patient will:

* Experience therapeutic effects dependent on the reason the drug is being given (e.g., decreased blood pressure).
* Be free from or experience minimal adverse effects.
* Verbalize an understanding of the drug's use, adverse effects and required precautions.
* Demonstrate proper self-administration of the medication (e.g., dose, timing, and when to notify the provider).

Implementation

Interventions and (Rationales)	Patient-Centered Care
Ensuring therapeutic effects: • Continue frequent assessments as above for therapeutic effects: urine output is increased, blood pressure and pulse are within normal limits or within the parameters set by the health care provider. (Diuresis may be moderate to extreme depending on the type of diuretic given. Blood pressure should be within normal limits without the presence of reflex tachycardia.) • Daily weights should remain at or close to baseline weight. (An increase in weight over 1 kg (2.2 lb) per day may indicate excessive fluid gain. A decrease of over 1 kg (2.2 lb) per day may indicate excessive diuresis and dehydration.)	• Teach the patient, family, or caregiver how to monitor the pulse and blood pressure. Ensure proper use and functioning of any home equipment obtained. • Have the patient weigh self daily and record weight along with blood pressure and pulse measurements.
Minimizing adverse effects: • Continue to monitor vital signs. Take blood pressure lying, sitting, and standing to detect orthostatic hypotension. Be particularly cautious with the older adult who is at increased risk for hypotension. (Diuretics reduce circulating blood volume, resulting in lowered blood pressure. Orthostatic hypotension may increase the risk of falls and injury.)	• Teach the patient to rise from lying or sitting to standing slowly to avoid dizziness or falls. • Instruct the patient to stop taking the medication if blood pressure is 90/60 mmHg or below, or is below the parameters set by the health care provider, and promptly notify the provider.
• Continue to monitor electrolytes, glucose, CBC, lipid profiles, liver function studies, creatinine, and uric acid levels. (Most diuretics cause loss of Na^+ and K^+ and may increase lipid, glucose, and uric acid levels.)	• Instruct the patient on the need to return periodically for laboratory work and to inform laboratory personnel of diuretic therapy when providing blood or urine samples. • Advise the patient to carry a wallet identification card or wear medical identification jewelry indicating diuretic therapy.
• Continue to monitor hearing and balance, reporting persistent tinnitus or vertigo promptly. (Ototoxicity of cranial nerve VIII may occur, especially with loop diuretics.)	• Have the patient report persistent tinnitus or balance or coordination problems immediately.
• Ensure patient safety, especially in the older adult. Observe for lightheadedness or dizziness. Monitor ambulation until effects of drug are known. (Dizziness from orthostatic hypotension may occur.)	• Instruct the patient to call for assistance prior to getting out of bed or attempting to walk alone, and to avoid driving or other activities requiring mental alertness or physical coordination until the effects of the drug are known.
• Weigh the patient daily and report weight gain or loss of 1 kg (2.2 lb) or more in a 24-h period. Measure intake and output in the hospitalized patient. (Daily weight is an accurate measure of fluid status and takes into account intake, output, and insensible losses. Diuresis is indicated by output significantly greater than intake.)	• Have the patient weigh self daily, ideally at the same time of day, and record weight along with blood pressure and pulse measurements. Have the patient report weight loss or gain of more than 1 kg (2.2 lb) in a 24-h period. • Advise the patient to continue to consume enough liquids to remain adequately, but not overly hydrated. Drinking when thirsty, avoiding alcoholic beverages, and ensuring adequate but not excessive salt intake will assist in maintaining normal fluid balance. • Teach the patient that excessive heat conditions contribute to excessive sweating and fluid and electrolyte loss. Extra caution is warranted in these conditions.
• Monitor nutritional status and encourage appropriate intake to prevent electrolyte imbalances. (Electrolyte imbalances may occur dependent on the type of diuretic used. Most diuretics cause Na^+ and K^+ loss. Potassium-sparing diuretics may result in Na^+ loss but K^+ increase.)	• Instruct patients taking potassium-wasting diuretics (e.g., thiazide, thiazide-like, and loop diuretics) to consume foods high in potassium: fresh fruits such as strawberries and bananas, dried fruits such as apricots and prunes, vegetables and legumes such as tomatoes, beets, and dried beans, juices such as orange, grapefruit, or prune, and fresh meats. • Instruct patients taking potassium-sparing diuretics to avoid foods high in potassium such as above, not to use salt substitutes (which often contain potassium salts), and to consult with a health care provider before taking vitamin and mineral supplements or specialized sports beverages. (Typical OTC sports beverages, e.g., Gatorade and Powerade, may have lesser amounts of potassium but have high carbohydrate amounts that may lead to increased diuresis, diarrhea, and the potential for dehydration from the hyperosmolarity.)

CONNECTIONS: NURSING PRACTICE APPLICATION (continued)

• Observe for signs of hypokalemia or hyperkalemia. Use with caution in patients taking corticosteroids, ACE inhibitors, ARBs, digoxin, or lithium. Report symptoms to the health care provider promptly. (Thiazide, thiazide-like, and loop diuretics can cause hypokalemia; potassium-sparing diuretics may cause hyperkalemia. Symptoms of *hypokalemia* include muscle weakness or cramping, and palpitations. Symptoms of *hyperkalemia* include irritability or anxiety, fatigue, palpitations, nausea, and abdominal cramping. Concurrent use with corticosteroids may increase the risk of hypokalemia. Concurrent use with ACE inhibitors or ARBs may increase the risk of hyperkalemia. Concurrent use with digoxin increases the risk of potentially fatal dysrhythmias and with lithium may cause toxic levels of the drug.)	• Instruct the patient to report signs and symptoms of hypokalemia or hyperkalemia immediately to the health care provider. • Teach the patient to follow recommended dietary intake of high- or low-potassium foods as appropriate to the type of diuretic taken to avoid hypokalemia or hyperkalemia.
• Observe for signs of hyperglycemia. Use with caution in patients with diabetes. (Thiazide, thiazide-like, and loop diuretics may cause hyperglycemia, especially in diabetics.)	• Instruct the patient to report signs and symptoms of diabetes mellitus (e.g., polydipsia, polyphagia) or elevated blood glucose to the health care provider. Patients with diabetes may need to monitor their blood glucose levels more frequently until the effects of the diuretic are known.
• Observe for symptoms of gout. (Diuretics may cause hyperuricemia, which may result in gout-like symptoms including warmth, pain, tenderness, swelling, and redness around the joints, especially great toes, hand joints, elbows, and around ears, tophi (nodules), arthritis-like symptoms, and limited movement in affected joints.)	• Instruct the patient to report signs and symptoms of gout promptly to the health care provider. • Teach gout-prone patients to increase fluid intake, avoid shellfish, organ meats (e.g., liver, kidneys), alcohol, and high-fructose beverages.
• Observe for sunburning if prolonged sun exposure has occurred. (Many diuretics cause photosensitivity and an increased risk of sunburning.)	• Instruct patients to wear sunscreen and protective clothing if prolonged sun exposure is anticipated.
• Observe for signs of infection. (Some diuretics may decrease white blood cell counts and the body's ability to fight infection. Agranulocytosis is a possible adverse effect of diuretic therapy.)	• Instruct the patient to report any flulike symptoms: shortness of breath, fever, sore throat, malaise, joint pain, or profound fatigue.
Patient understanding of drug therapy: • Use opportunities during administration of medications and during assessments to discuss the rationale for the drug therapy, desired therapeutic outcomes, commonly observed adverse effects, parameters for when to call the health care provider, and any necessary monitoring or precautions. (Using time during nursing care helps to optimize and reinforce key teaching areas.)	• The patient, family, or caregiver should be able to state the reason for the drug, appropriate dose and scheduling, what adverse effects to observe for and when to report them, and the anticipated length of medication therapy.
Patient self-administration of drug therapy: • When administering the medication, instruct the patient, family, or caregiver in proper self-administration of the drug, e.g., early in the day to prevent disruption of sleep from nocturia. (Utilizing time during nurse-administration of these drugs helps to reinforce teaching.)	• The patient, family, or caregiver is able to discuss appropriate dosing and administration needs.

Evaluation of Outcome Criteria

Evaluate the effectiveness of drug therapy by confirming that patient goals and expected outcomes have been met (see "Planning").

UNDERSTANDING THE CHAPTER

Key Concepts Summary

1 The kidneys are major organs of excretion and body homeostasis.

2 The composition of filtrate changes dramatically as a result of the processes of reabsorption and secretion.

3 Renal failure may significantly impact the success of pharmacotherapy.

4 Diuretics are used to treat hypertension, heart failure, accumulation of edema fluid, and renal failure.

5 The most effective diuretics are the loop diuretics that block sodium reabsorption in the loop of Henle.

6 The thiazides are the most commonly prescribed class of diuretics.

7 Potassium-sparing diuretics have low effectiveness but can help prevent hypokalemia.

8 Osmotic diuretics cause diuresis by increasing the osmolality of the filtrate.

9 Carbonic anhydrase inhibitors are weak diuretics that have specific indications.

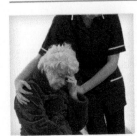

Making the PATIENT Connection

Remember the patient "Katherine Crosland" at the beginning of the chapter? Now read the remainder of the case study. Based on the information presented within this chapter, respond to the critical thinking questions that follow.

Katherine Crosland, a 79-year-old widow, has lived alone for the past 5 years. Although her son and daughters all reside in distant locations, they check on her at least weekly by telephoning. Katherine is fairly independent; however, she does not drive, and is dependent on a neighbor to get her groceries and medications.

Three years ago, Katherine was hospitalized for an MI, which resulted in heart failure. She is adherent with her medications, which include digoxin (Lanoxin) 0.125 mg daily, furosemide (Lasix) 20 mg/day, and potassium supplements (K-Dur) 20 mEq daily.

Recently Katherine's neighbor went on an extended, out-of-town trip. Katherine was certain that she had enough of her medicine to last through that time. However, before the neighbor returned, Katherine discovered she had miscalculated her potassium supplement and only had enough for 10 days. Katherine figured that because the potassium was only a "supplement," she would be able to wait until her neighbor returned to get the medication refilled.

Today, she presents to the clinic with generalized weakness and fatigue. She has lost 3.6 kg (8 lb) since her last clinic visit 6 weeks ago. Her blood pressure is 104/62 mmHg, her heart rate is 98 beats/min, and she has a slightly irregular, respiratory rate of 20 breaths/min, and body temperature is 36.2°C (97.2°F). The blood specimen collected for diagnostic studies showed several outstanding findings such as a serum sodium level of 150 mEq/L and potassium level of 3.2 mEq/L. Katherine is diagnosed with dehydration and hypokalemia induced by diuretic therapy.

Critical Thinking Questions

1. Discuss fluid and electrolyte imbalances related to the following diuretic therapies:
   a. Loop diuretics
   b. Thiazide diuretics
   c. Potassium-sparing diuretics
   d. Osmotic diuretics

2. What relationship exists between this patient's diuretic therapy, digoxin therapy, and hypokalemia?

3. What patient education should the nurse provide about diuretic therapy?

See Answers to Critical Thinking Questions on student resource website.

NCLEX-RN® Review

1. The nurse is teaching a group of clients with cardiac conditions who are taking diuretic therapy. The nurse explains that individuals prescribed furosemide (Lasix) should:
   1. Avoid consuming large amounts of cabbage, cauliflower, and kale.
   2. Rise slowly from sitting or lying positions.
   3. Count their pulse for 1 full minute before taking the medication.
   4. Restrict fluid intake to no more than 1,000 mL in a 24-hour period.

2. The client who is receiving bumetanide (Bumex) is instructed to watch for symptoms associated with electrolyte imbalances. Which condition would the client most likely experience?
   1. Hyponatremia
   2. Hypokalemia
   3. Hyperkalemia
   4. Hypocalcemia

3. While preparing a client for discharge, which of the following statements should the nurse include in the instructions regarding the client's new prescription of hydrochlorothiazide (Microzide)?
   1. "There are no limitations on the amount of salt and fluid intake."
   2. "Ingest vitamin K-rich foods daily, such as green, leafy vegetables and broccoli."
   3. "Report muscle cramps or weakness to the health care provider."
   4. "Antihypertensive drugs taken concurrently may produce sleepiness."

4. Clients prescribed spironolactone (Aldactone) are often at risk for electrolyte imbalance. The nurse assesses for this adverse effect because this drug may cause the body to:
   1. Retain potassium.
   2. Release magnesium.
   3. Excrete potassium.
   4. Bind calcium.

5 Which nursing measures should be a nursing priority for a client when beginning mannitol (Osmitrol)?

1. Keep the urinal or bedpan available for clients with limited mobility.
2. Assess for hypokalemia and encourage foods high in potassium.
3. Monitor intake and output ratio, and weigh the client daily.
4. Monitor blood pressure and assess for level of consciousness.

6 The nurse is monitoring a client receiving acetazolamide (Diamox). Which acid–base imbalance is a potential risk for this client?

1. Metabolic acidosis
2. Metabolic alkalosis
3. Respiratory acidosis
4. Respiratory alkalosis

Additional Case Study

During a recent visit to the clinic, Miles Davenport learned that his antihypertensive medication was not maintaining his blood pressure at the desired level. The nurse practitioner prescribed spironolactone (Aldactone) 50 mg twice daily in addition to his regular antihypertensive medications.

1. Discuss the mechanism of action for spironolactone.
2. Prepare a list of foods that should be eaten sparingly while taking spironolactone.
3. List the symptoms of hyperkalemia that Miles needs to know to manage his disease and medications.

See Answers to Additional Case Study on student resource website.

Pearson Nursing Student Resources

Find additional review materials at
nursing.pearsonhighered.com

Prepare for success with additional NCLEX®-style practice questions, interactive assignments and activities, web links, animations, videos, and more!

References

Axelrod, D. A., McCullough, K. P., Brewer, E. D., Becker, B. N., Segev, D. L., & Rao, P. S. (2010). Kidney and pancreas transplantation in the United States, 1999–2008: The changing face of living donation. *American Journal of Transplantation, 10*(4 part 2), 987–1002. doi:10.1111/j.1600-6143.2010.03022.x

National Center for Complementary and Alternative Medicine. (2010). *Herbs at a glance: Dandelion.* Retrieved from http://nccam.nih.gov/health/dandelion

National Kidney Foundation. (n.d.). *Key facts about chronic kidney disease (CKD).* Retrieved from http://www.kidney.org/news/newsroom/fs_new/keyFactsCKD.cfm

Selected Bibliography

Brandimarte, F., Mureddu, G. F., Boccanelli, A., Cacciatore, G., Brandimarte, C., Fedele, F., & Gheorghiade, M. (2010). Diuretic therapy in heart failure: Current controversies and new approaches for fluid removal. *Journal of Cardiovascular Medicine, 11*(8), 563–570. doi:10.2459/JCM.0b013e3283376bfa

Charlesworth, J. A., Gracey, D. M., & Pussell, B. A. (2008). Adult nephrotic syndrome: Non-specific strategies for treatment. *Nephrology, 13*(1), 45–50. doi:10.1111/j.1440-1797.2007.00890.x

Martin, R. K. (2010). Acute kidney injury: Advances in definition, pathophysiology, and diagnosis. *AACN Advanced Critical Care, 21*(4), 350–356. doi:10.1097/NCI.0b013e3181f9574b

Moser, M., & Feig, P. U. (2009). Fifty years of thiazide diuretic therapy for hypertension. *Archives of Internal Medicine, 169*(20), 1851–1856. doi:10.1001/archinternmed.2009.342

Reilly, R. F., & Jackson, E. K. (2011). Diuretics. In L. L. Brunton, B. A. Chabner, & B. C. Knollman (Eds.), *The pharmacological basis of therapeutics* (12th ed., pp. 671–720). New York, NY: McGraw-Hill.

St. Peter, W. (2010). Improving medication safety in chronic kidney disease patients on dialysis through medication reconciliation. *Advances in Chronic Kidney Disease, 17*(5), 413–419. doi:10.1053/j.ackd.2010.06.001

Schiffrin, E. L., Lipman, M. L., & Mann, J. F. E. (2007). Chronic kidney disease: Effects on the cardiovascular system. *Circulation, 116*(1), 85–97. doi:10.1161/CIRCULATIONAHA.106.678342

Schütz, K., Carle, R., & Schieber, A. (2006). Taraxacum—A review on its phytochemical and pharmacological profile. *Journal of Ethnopharmacology, 107*(3), 313–323.

van der Vorst, M. M. J., Kist, J. E., van der Heijiden, A. J., & Burggraaf, J. (2006). Diuretics in pediatrics. *Paediatric Drugs, 8*(4), 245–264.

Answers to NCLEX-RN® Review

1 Answer: 2   Rationale: As a diuretic, furosemide may dramatically reduce the client's circulating blood volume, thus producing episodes of orthostatic hypotension. Clients may minimize this effect by rising slowly from sitting or lying positions. Options 1, 3, and 4 are incorrect. Cabbage, cauliflower, and kale are high in vitamin K, but furosemide does not restrict the consumption of these foods. Monitoring pulse rate during administration of furosemide is advised to monitor for reflex tachycardia secondary to hypotension, but it is not required that it be taken before the dose or for one full min. Due to the potential for significant diuresis, fluids should not be restricted unless ordered by the health care provider. Cognitive Level: Applying; Client Need: Physiological Integrity; Nursing Process: Implementation

2 Answer: 2   Rationale: Loop diuretics such as bumetanide cause a significant loss of potassium. Hypokalemia is often the most predominant electrolyte imbalance. Options 1, 3, and 4 are incorrect. Hyponatremia is unlikely with the administration of bumetanide because it promotes sodium loss. Hyperkalemia is inconsistent with the administration of bumetanide due to the increase in potassium excretion. If elevated potassium levels are present in these clients, other etiologies should be investigated. Bumetanide does not cause hypocalcemia but may cause hypercalciuria with an increased risk of calcium-based kidney stones. Cognitive Level: Analyzing; Client Need: Physiological Integrity; Nursing Process: Evaluation

3 Answer: 3   Rationale: Muscle cramps and weakness may indicate hypokalemia and should be reported to the health care provider. Options 1, 2, and 4 are incorrect. Many clients taking diuretic therapy are instructed to monitor the intake of both sodium and water to maintain adequate but not excessive amounts. Clients should ingest foods high in potassium, not vitamin K. Thiazide diuretics and antihypertensive drugs are not known to cause sleepiness when taken together. Cognitive Level: Applying; Client Need: Physiological Integrity; Nursing Process: Implementation

4 Answer: 1   Rationale: Spironolactone is a potassium-sparing diuretic and may cause hyperkalemia. Options 2, 3, and 4 are incorrect. This drug does not have a direct effect on magnesium and does not cause hypokalemia. It does not have calcium-binding effects. Cognitive Level: Applying; Client Need: Physiological Integrity; Nursing Process: Assessment

5 Answer: 4   Rationale: In the early stages of the administration of mannitol, fluid is drawn into extracellular spaces and vascular compartments. Pulmonary and peripheral edema may occur, and increased intracranial pressure may also occur along with an early change in level of consciousness. Options 1, 2, and 3 are incorrect. Keeping a urinal or bedpan nearby, monitoring electrolytes, including potassium, and recording I&O and daily weight are important nursing interventions but are not the main nursing priority in the early administration of mannitol. Cognitive Level: Applying; Client Need: Physiological Integrity; Nursing Process: Implementation

6 Answer: 1   Rationale: Clients receiving acetazolamide are at risk for metabolic acidosis due to excess bicarbonate loss. Options 2, 3, and 4 are incorrect. Metabolic alkalosis is characterized by a deficit of bicarbonate, and is not an adverse effect of acetazolamide (Diamox). Acetazolamide does not cause respiratory acidosis. Respiratory alkalosis is also not an expected adverse effect of acetazolamide. Cognitive Level: Analyzing; Client Need: Physiological Integrity; Nursing Process: Evaluation

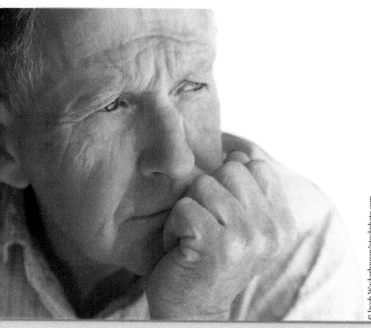

"I am doing everything my doctor has advised me to do to control my hypertension. My doctor has prescribed several different types of drugs over the last few months. My blood pressure is still elevated. What else can I do?"

Patient "Elmer Foley"

© Jacob Wackerhausen/istockphoto.com

Pharmacotherapy of Hypertension

Chapter Outline

Learning Outcomes

After reading this chapter, the student should be able to:

1. Explain how hypertension is classified.

2. Summarize the long-term consequences of untreated hypertension.

3. Compare and contrast the roles of nonpharmacologic and pharmacologic methods in the management of hypertension.

4. Describe general principles guiding the pharmacotherapy of hypertension.

5. Identify drug classes used in the primary and alternate management of hypertension.

6. Describe the pharmacologic management of hypertensive emergencies.

7. For each of the classes shown in the chapter outline, identify the prototype and representative drugs and explain the mechanism(s) of drug action, primary indications, contraindications, significant drug interactions, pregnancy category, and important adverse effects.

8. Apply the nursing process to care for patients receiving antihypertensive drugs.

From Chapter 37 of *Pharmacology: Connections to Nursing Practice*, Second Edition. Michael Patrick Adams, Carol Quam Urban. Copyright © 2013 by Pearson Education, Inc. All rights reserved.

Diseases affecting the heart and blood vessels are the most frequent causes of death in the United States. Hypertension (HTN) or high blood pressure is the most common of the cardiovascular diseases. According to the American Heart Association, chronic HTN affects one in every three Americans and contributes to over 326,000 deaths in the United States each year (Centers for Disease Control and Prevention, 2011). Although mild HTN can be controlled with lifestyle modifications, moderate to severe HTN requires pharmacotherapy.

Because nurses encounter so many patients with this disease, it is critical for the nurse to understand the underlying principles of antihypertensive therapy. By improving public awareness of HTN and teaching the importance of early intervention, the nurse can contribute significantly to reducing cardiovascular mortality.

PharmFACT

Among people with HTN, about 25% are unaware of their condition. African American men have the highest rate of HTN (over 50%), and this population has a death rate from hypertension that is three times higher than that of white males (American Heart Association, 2011).

Definition and Classification of Hypertension

1 Hypertension is classified by stages, based on the degree of elevation of systolic and diastolic blood pressure.

Hypertension (HTN) is defined as the consistent elevation of systemic arterial blood pressure. The diagnosis of chronic HTN is made after repeated blood pressure measurements. A patient with a sustained systolic blood pressure of greater than 140 mmHg or diastolic pressure of greater than 90 to 99 mmHg after multiple assessments are conducted over several clinic visits is said to have HTN.

When most people use the word *hypertension*, they are referring to systemic HTN, that which is measured routinely by a conventional blood pressure cuff on the upper arm over the brachial artery. Systemic HTN is a general measurement of arterial blood pressure in the body. Localized HTN may also occur. For example, patients with cirrhosis of the liver often develop portal HTN, which occurs in the portal vein and its branches serving the liver. Pulmonary HTN occurs in the pulmonary artery and its branches and is most often observed in patients with left-sided heart failure. These localized types of HTN respond to many of the same antihypertensive drugs used for systemic HTN.

To develop guidelines for treatment, many attempts have been made to further define HTN. In 2003, the National High Blood Pressure Education Program Coordinating Committee of the National Heart, Lung, and Blood Institute at the National Institutes of Health determined the need for new guidelines that addressed the relationship between blood pressure and the risk of cardiovascular disease. This committee issued *The Seventh Report of the Joint National Committee on Prevention, Detection, Evaluation, and Treatment of High Blood Pressure* (JNC-7), which has become the standard for treating HTN. The recommendations from the JNC-7 report are summarized in Table 1.

In addition to classifying HTN into three categories (prehypertension, stage 1, and stage 2), the JNC-7 report issued remarkable data regarding the disease:

- The risk of cardiovascular disease beginning at 115/75 mmHg doubles with each additional increment of 20/10 mmHg.

- Individuals with a systolic blood pressure of 120 to 139 mmHg or a diastolic blood pressure of 80 to 89 mmHg should be considered as prehypertensive. These patients should be strongly encouraged by the nurse to adopt health-promoting lifestyle modifications to prevent cardiovascular disease.

- Patients with prehypertension are at increased risk for progression to HTN; those in the 130 to 139/80 to 89 mmHg blood pressure range are at twice the risk to develop HTN as those with lower values.

TABLE 1 Recommendations for Treating Hypertension

CLASSIFICATION OF HYPERTENSION		INITIAL ANTIHYPERTENSIVE THERAPY	
Blood Pressure Classification	Systolic/Diastolic Blood Pressure (mmHg)	Without Compelling Indication*	With Compelling Indication*
Normal	119/79 or less	No antihypertensive indicated	No antihypertensive indicated
Prehypertension	120–139/80–89		
Stage 1 hypertension	140–159/90–99	Thiazide diuretic (for most patients)	Other antihypertensives, as needed
Stage 2 hypertension	160 or higher/100 or higher	Two-drug combination antihypertensive (for most patients)	

*Compelling indications include heart failure, post–myocardial infarction, high risk for coronary artery disease, diabetes, chronic kidney disease, and recurrent stroke prevention.
Source: From *JNC-7 Express: The Seventh Report of the Joint National Committee on Prevention, Detection Evaluation and Treatment of High Blood Pressure,* U.S. Department of Health and Human Services, National Institutes of Health, National Heart, Lung, and Blood Institute, National High Blood Pressure Education Program Coordinating Committee, 2003, Bethesda, MD: Author. Retrieved from http://www.nhlbi.nih.gov/guidelines/hypertension/express.pdf

Average blood pressure changes throughout the life span, gradually and continuously rising from childhood through adulthood. Normal blood pressure at one age may be considered abnormal in someone older or younger. HTN affects approximately 30% of those over 50 years old, 64% of men over age 65, and 75% of women over age 75.

Etiology and Pathogenesis of Hypertension

2 Failure to properly manage hypertension can lead to stroke, heart failure, or myocardial infarction.

Hypertension is a complex disease that is caused by a combination of genetic and environmental factors. Approximately 30% to 40% of HTN is thought to be due to genetic factors. Scientists have discovered specific genes that appear to predispose a patient to HTN. These genes control critical activities such as renal sodium and water transport and the renin-angiotensin-aldosterone system. As discussed in Section 3, environmental factors related to diet and exercise also play an important role in the development of HTN.

For the large majority of hypertensive patients, no specific cause can be identified. HTN having no identifiable cause is called idiopathic, essential, or **primary hypertension**, and accounts for 90% of all cases. Although patients with primary HTN may not be cured, the disease can be managed such that the risk of serious, long-term consequences can be reduced.

In some cases, a specific cause of the HTN can be identified. This type, called **secondary hypertension**, accounts for 10% of all patients with HTN. Certain diseases, such as Cushing's syndrome, hyperthyroidism, chronic renal impairment, pheochromocytoma, and arteriosclerosis are associated with elevated blood pressure. Certain drugs are also associated with HTN, including corticosteroids, oral contraceptives, estrogen, erythropoietin, and sibutramine. The therapeutic goal for secondary HTN is to treat or remove the underlying condition that is causing the blood pressure elevation. In many cases, correcting the comorbid condition will cure the associated HTN.

Research has clearly demonstrated that failure to control HTN can result in serious consequences. Prolonged or improperly controlled HTN damages blood vessels, particularly small arteries and arterioles. As it progresses, the walls of the arteries gradually thicken, in an attempt to protect the vessels against injury from the increased pressure. The injured vessel walls become inflamed, increasing the permeability of the vessels and causing additional thickening of their walls. Eventually, the lumen of the artery permanently narrows, reducing blood flow to vital tissues. HTN accelerates atherosclerosis, and will worsen conditions such as coronary artery disease (CAD).

Hypertension may exist for years, indeed decades, before becoming symptomatic. As the disease progresses, however, the risk of target-organ damage increases. Because sustained HTN may affect any artery in the body, damage may be widespread and symptoms vary greatly according to which vessels are affected.

The heart is a primary organ damaged by chronic HTN. Hypertension increases afterload, forcing the heart to work harder to pump blood to the tissues. The heart is subjected to chronic pressure overload, resulting in left ventricular hypertrophy. If untreated, this excessive workload eventually causes the heart to fail and the lungs to fill with fluid, a condition known as congestive heart failure (CHF).

Further damaging the heart is the effect of HTN on the coronary vessels. Hypertension accelerates the deposition of atherosclerotic plaque, creating or worsening CAD. This places the patient at greater risk of dysrhythmias, angina pectoris, and myocardial infarction (MI). Heart failure and MI are the most common causes of death in hypertensive patients.

The brain is also a major target organ for hypertensive damage. Occlusion of the small vessels supplying blood and oxygen to the brain can cause transient ischemic attacks and stroke. These neurologic events are common in hypertensive patients and are a major cause of disability.

Because a large percentage of blood pumped per minute circulates through the kidneys, chronic HTN creates major stress on these organs. As the small arteries supplying the kidney become injured, inflamed, and atherosclerotic, the patient's renal function gradually declines. Poorly managed HTN is an important contributor to kidney failure and end-stage kidney disease.

Hypertension is a major cause of visual impairment, which can occur when vessels in the eye become atherosclerotic. Although patients may remain asymptomatic for many years, small hemorrhages that affect vision may occur. Symptoms of retinal damage range from subtle vision changes to blindness. Retinopathy is particularly serious in patients who present with diabetes as a comorbid condition with HTN.

The importance of treating this disorder in the prehypertensive stage cannot be overstated. The long-term damage to target organs caused by HTN may be irreversible if the disease is allowed to progress unchecked. This is especially critical in people with diabetes and those with chronic kidney disease, as these patients are particularly susceptible to the long-term consequences of HTN.

Nonpharmacologic Management of Hypertension

3 Therapeutic lifestyle changes can reduce blood pressure and lessen the need for antihypertensive medications.

When a patient is first diagnosed with HTN, a comprehensive medical history is necessary to determine if the disease can be controlled by nonpharmacologic means. Therapeutic lifestyle changes should be recommended for all patients with prehypertension or HTN. Of greatest importance is maintaining optimum weight, since obesity is closely associated with dyslipidemia (abnormal serum lipid levels) and HTN. A 5- to 9-kg (11- to 20-lb) weight loss often produces a measurable decrease in blood pressure, even in patients who are obese. Combining a medically supervised weight loss program with proper nutrition can delay the progression from prehypertension to HTN.

CONNECTIONS

Complementary and Alternative Therapies   Grape Seed Extract

Description: Grape seed extract is obtained from the seeds of the types of grapes that are usually used in the process of winemaking.

History and Claims: Grapes and grape seeds have been used for medicinal purposes for thousands of years. The primary use of the extract has been to treat cardiovascular conditions such as HTN, high blood cholesterol, atherosclerosis, and to generally improve circulation. Some claim that it improves wound healing, prevents cancer, and lowers the risk for the long-term consequences of diabetes. The drug is being examined for its effects on Alzheimer's disease.

Standardization: The grape seeds are crushed and placed into tablet, capsule, or liquid forms. Typical doses are 50 to 300 mg/day. Standardization is based on percentage of polyphenols. The seeds also contain a high concentration of essential fatty acids and vitamin E.

Evidence: Thousands of studies have been conducted on the polyphenols contained in this supplement. Grape seed extract has antioxidant properties (University of Maryland Medical Center, 2010). In general, antioxidants improve wound healing and repair cellular injury. Preliminary evidence suggests it may have some benefit in repairing blood vessel damage that could lead to atherosclerosis and HTN (National Center for Complementary and Alternative Medicine, 2010). Controlled, long-term studies on the effects of grape seed extracts on HTN have not been conducted. It has few adverse effects. Caution should be used if taking anticoagulant drugs, because increased bleeding may result. Overall, the benefits of grape seed extract are no different than those of a diet balanced with natural antioxidants (and an occasional glass of red wine).

In some cases, implementing positive lifestyle changes may eliminate the need for pharmacotherapy altogether. Even if medication is required to manage the HTN, positive lifestyle changes may allow dosages to be minimized, thus lowering the potential for drug adverse effects. The nurse plays a vital role in educating patients about controlling their HTN. Because all blood pressure medications have potential adverse effects, it is important for patients to attempt to control their disease though nonpharmacologic means, to the greatest extent possible. Nonpharmacologic methods for controlling HTN include the following:

- Limit intake of alcohol.
- Restrict sodium consumption.
- Reduce intake of saturated fat and cholesterol, and increase consumption of fruits and vegetables.
- Increase aerobic physical activity.
- Discontinue use of all tobacco products.
- Explore measures for dealing with excessive stress.
- Maintain optimum weight

Pharmacologic Management of Hypertension

4 The choice of antihypertensive medication is determined by the degree of hypertension and the presence of other medical conditions.

The goal of antihypertensive therapy is to reduce the morbidity and mortality associated with chronic HTN. Research has confirmed that keeping blood pressure within normal limits reduces the risk of hypertension-related target-organ damage.

The pharmacologic management of HTN is individualized to the patient's risk factors, comorbid medical conditions, and degree of blood pressure elevation. Patient responses to antihypertensive medications vary widely because of the many complex genetic and environmental factors affecting blood pressure.

Nine different drug classes are used to treat HTN. Each class has specific benefits and characteristic adverse effects.

The mechanisms of action of antihypertensive agents are summarized in Figure 1. Although many effective drugs are available, and the data supporting the benefits of therapy are strong, HTN remains a challenging disorder to treat successfully. Choice of therapy is often based on the clinician's experience. Although antihypertensive treatment varies, there are several principles that guide pharmacotherapy.

Initial Drug of Choice

The JNC-7 report recommends thiazide diuretics as initial drugs for the management of mild to moderate HTN. Clinical research has clearly demonstrated that thiazide diuretics reduce HTN-related morbidity and mortality. Patients with a compelling condition, however, may benefit from a second drug, either in combination with the thiazide or in place of the thiazide. The JNC-7 report lists the following as compelling conditions: heart failure, post–MI, high risk for CAD, diabetes, chronic kidney disease, and recurrent stroke prevention.

In most cases, low doses of the initial drug are prescribed and the patient is reevaluated after an appropriate time period. As therapy continues, dosage is adjusted to maintain optimum blood pressure. The following drug classes are considered primary antihypertensive agents:

- Diuretics
- Angiotensin-converting enzyme (ACE) inhibitors
- Angiotensin II receptor blockers (ARBs)
- Calcium channel blockers (CCBs)
- Beta-adrenergic antagonists

Adding Drugs to the Antihypertensive Regimen

If the patient does not respond to the initial medication, a drug from a different antihypertensive class may be added to the regimen. Prescribing two antihypertensives concurrently results in additive or synergistic blood pressure reduction, and is common practice when managing resistant HTN. This is often necessary when the patient has a compelling condition,

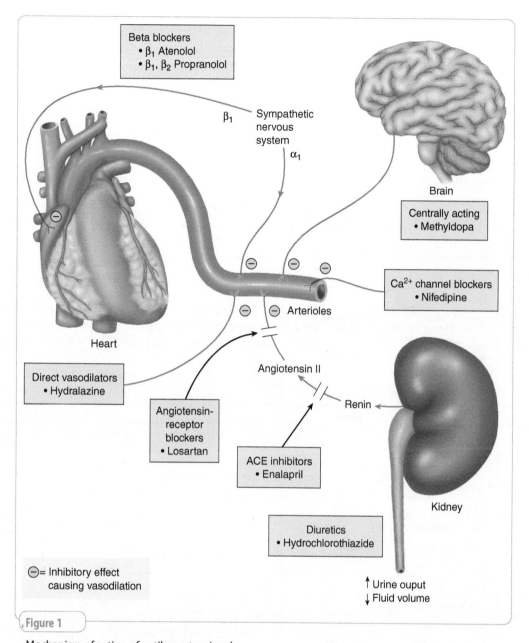

Figure 1

Mechanism of action of antihypertensive drugs.

or when sustained blood pressure is particularly high. The advantage of using two drugs is that lower doses of each may be used, resulting in fewer adverse effects and better patient adherence. Drug manufacturers sometimes combine two drugs into a single pill or capsule for dosing convenience and to improve patient adherence. The majority of these combinations include a thiazide diuretic, usually hydrochlorothiazide (HCTZ). Selected combination antihypertensives are shown in Table 2.

Certain antihypertensive classes cause a higher incidence of adverse effects and are generally prescribed when primary agents do not produce a satisfactory response. In some cases, research studies have not demonstrated a firm link between drug use and lowered morbidity or mortality. The alternative antihypertensive drug classes include the following:

- Alpha$_1$-adrenergic antagonists
- Alpha$_2$-adrenergic agonists
- Direct-acting vasodilators
- Peripheral adrenergic antagonists

Enhancing Patient Adherence

Because chronic HTN may produce no identifiable symptoms for as long as 10 to 20 years, many people are not aware of their condition. Convincing patients to change established lifestyle habits, spend money on medication, and take drugs on a regular basis when they are feeling healthy is a difficult task for the nurse. Patients with limited income or who do not have health insurance are at high risk for not purchasing the drugs after receiving a prescription. The prescriber should consider generic forms of these drugs to reduce costs and increase adherence.

Further reducing adherence to the regimen is the occurrence of adverse drug effects. Some of the antihypertensive drugs cause embarrassing adverse effects such as impotence,

TABLE 2 Selected Combination Medications for Hypertension

Trade Name	Thiazide Diuretic	Adrenergic Agent	Potassium-Sparing Diuretic	ACE Inhibitor or Angiotensin II Blocker	Other
Accuretic	hydrochlorothiazide			quinapril	
Aldactazide	hydrochlorothiazide		spironolactone		
Apresazide	hydrochlorothiazide				hydralazine
Avalide	hydrochlorothiazide			irbesartan	
Azor				olmesartan	amlodipine
Benicar HCT	hydrochlorothiazide			olmesartan	
Capozide	hydrochlorothiazide			captopril	
Corzide	bendroflumethiazide	nadolol			
Diovan HCT	hydrochlorothiazide			valsartan	
Dyazide	hydrochlorothiazide		triamterene		
Exforge				valsartan	amlodipine
Hyzaar	hydrochlorothiazide			losartan	
Inderide	hydrochlorothiazide	propranolol			
Lexxel				enalapril	felodipine
Lopressor HCT	hydrochlorothiazide	metoprolol			
Lotensin HCT	hydrochlorothiazide			benazepril	
Lotrel				benazepril	amlodipine
Minizide	polythiazide	prazosin			
Tarka				trandolapril	verapamil
Tekalmo					amlodipine & aliskiren
Tekturna HCT	hydrochlorothiazide				aliskiren
Tenoretic	chlorthalidone	atenolol			
Teveten HCT	hydrochlorothiazide			eprosartan	
Timolide	hydrochlorothiazide	timolol			
Tribenzor	hydrochlorothiazide			olmesartan	amlodipine
Uniretic	hydrochlorothiazide			moexipril	
Vaseretic	hydrochlorothiazide			enalapril	
Zestoretic	hydrochlorothiazide			lisinopril	
Ziac	hydrochlorothiazide	bisoprolol			

which may go unreported. Others cause fatigue and generally make patients feel sicker than they were before therapy was initiated. The nurse should teach the patient the importance of treating the disease to avoid serious long-term consequences. Furthermore, the nurse should teach patients to report adverse effects so that dosage can be adjusted, or the drug changed, so the treatment may continue without interruption. Simple adjustments to the dosage or changing the selected drug can often eliminate the adverse effects causing nonadherence.

Antihypertensives in African Americans

The incidence of HTN is significantly higher in African Americans than in other ethnic groups. As expected from this high incidence, African Americans experience greater target-organ damage than other populations. In an effort to reduce the high morbidity and mortality risks, aggressive antihypertensive therapy may be necessary to overcome resistant HTN in African Americans.

Some studies have suggested that certain antihypertensive drug classes are less effective in African Americans. For example monotherapy with ACE inhibitors, angiotensin II receptor blockers, or beta-adrenergic antagonists does not reduce blood pressure as much in African Americans compared to other ethnic groups. Thiazide diuretics and calcium channel blockers seem to provide the greatest blood pressure reduction in this population. Some health care providers recommend initiating therapy with two drugs to ensure an adequate response.

Although African Americans present a special challenge in controlling HTN, the fundamental principles and guidelines for effective clinical practice apply to all ethnic groups: early treatment, therapeutic lifestyle changes, and keeping blood pressure within established limits.

Treating the Diverse Patient   Personalized Medicine in the Era of BiDil

BiDil, a fixed-dose combination of hydralazine and isosorbide dinitrate, became available in 2005 and was marketed to African Americans after research demonstrated it was particularly effective in treating HTN in that population. Since that time, many articles have been written, research conducted, and questions raised about the efficacy, ethics, and legality of marketing a medication strictly to one population, especially based on race or ethnicity (Seguin, Hardy, Singer, & Daar, 2008).

The incidence of HTN is higher in African Americans than other populations and not all antihypertensive drugs work as well in all populations. Prior to the release of BiDil, some health care providers recommended initiating therapy with two drugs to ensure adequate response. The combination of a thiazide diuretic and calcium channel blocker seemed to provide adequate control of HTN in African Americans. Was a "new

and improved" fixed-combination medication needed? Postmarketing research seems to suggest that BiDil is an effective drug for controlling HTN in its target population. With concerns about the bioequivalence of the drugs when given separately, BiDil seems to provide clear benefit (Tam, Sabolinski, Worcel, Packer, & Cohn, 2007). The questions raised by the approval of a "race-based drug" have advanced the era of pharmacogenomics. Recognizing that race or outward appearance is not a sensitive indicator of genotype and ancestry has also highlighted the need to recruit more diverse patients into clinical drug trials. It has also raised important questions about how genotypes can be identified and how they affect pharmacodynamics. BiDil has proven its clinical effectiveness and it has also launched an era toward more personalized medicine.

Drug Classes for Hypertension

5 Diuretics are often drugs of first choice for treating mild to moderate hypertension.

Diuretics were the first class of medications used to treat HTN in the 1950s. Despite the many advances in drug therapy, diuretics are still considered first-line drugs for this disease because they are very effective at controlling mild to moderate HTN with few serious adverse effects. Although sometimes used as monotherapy, they are frequently prescribed with other antihypertensive medications to enhance their effectiveness. The following section is a brief summary of their application to the treatment of HTN.

Although dozens of diuretics are available for the treatment of HTN, all produce a similar result: the reduction of blood volume through the urinary excretion of water and electrolytes. Reducing blood volume places less pressure on the arterial walls, thereby decreasing peripheral resistance and lowering systemic blood pressure. The mechanism by which diuretics increase the excretion of water and electrolytes, specifically where and how the kidney is affected, differs among the various classes of diuretics.

Whenever a medication changes urine flow or composition, dehydration and electrolyte depletion are possible. Dehydration may manifest as increased thirst or poor skin turgor. Excessive sodium loss (hyponatremia) is a concern for all diuretics. Potassium loss (hypokalemia) is of particular concern for loop and thiazide diuretics. The potassium-sparing diuretics such as triamterene (Dyrenium) have fewer tendencies to cause hypokalemia. Drug classes for HTN are shown in Table 3.

Thiazide and thiazide-like diuretics: Thiazide and thiazide-like diuretics have been the mainstay for the pharmacotherapy of HTN for decades. The thiazide diuretics are inexpensive, and most are available in generic formulations. They are safe drugs, with excessive urinary potassium loss being the primary adverse effect. Because hypokalemia can induce serious dysrhythmias in susceptible patients, careful laboratory monitoring of serum potassium is necessary. Patients should increase their amount of dietary potassium, and potassium supplements may be prescribed. These diuretics may also cause hyperglycemia; therefore, blood glucose levels should

be monitored in patients with diabetes. Because thiazides may increase blood lipids, these agents should be used cautiously in patients with existing hyperlipidemia. Hydrochlorothiazide (Microzide) is sometimes abbreviated as HCTZ.

Potassium-sparing diuretics: Although potassium-sparing diuretics such as spironolactone (Aldactone) and triamterene (Dyrenium) produce only a modest diuresis, their primary advantage is they do not cause potassium depletion. They are especially beneficial when the patient is at risk of developing hypokalemia due to a medical condition or the use of thiazide or loop diuretics. The primary concern when using potassium-sparing diuretics is the possibility of retaining too much potassium, which can cause serious dysrhythmias. Patients with diabetes and those with renal impairment are particularly susceptible to hyperkalemia. Patients should be instructed to avoid excess potassium in their diet, including salt substitutes containing KCl, and not to use potassium supplements during therapy. Concurrent use with an ACE inhibitor or angiotensin II receptor blocker significantly increases the potential for development of hyperkalemia.

Loop (high-ceiling) diuretics: The loop diuretics such as furosemide (Lasix) and bumetanide (Bumex) cause greater diuresis, and have the potential to produce a higher reduction in blood pressure than the thiazides or potassium-sparing diuretics. Although this makes them very effective at reducing blood pressure, they are not ideal agents for maintenance therapy. The risk of adverse effects such as hypokalemia and dehydration is great because of their ability to remove large amounts of fluid from the body in a short time period. Loop diuretics are ototoxic, an effect more likely to occur in patients with renal insufficiency or when high doses are administered. Because of their greater toxicity, loop diuretics are sometimes reserved for patients with resistant HTN. Furosemide is the only loop diuretic in widespread use.

CONNECTION Checkpoint 37.1

Why must the thiazide diuretics be used with great caution in patients taking digoxin (Lanoxin)? *See Answer to Connection Checkpoint 37.1 on student resource website.*

TABLE 3 Drug Classes for Hypertension

Diuretics	Angiotensin II Receptor Blockers	Alpha₁ Blockers
Potassium-Sparing Type	candesartan (Atacand)	doxazosin (Cardura)
amiloride (Midamor)	eprosartan (Teveten)	prazosin (Minipress)
eplerenone (Inspra)	irbesartan (Avapro)	terazosin (Hytrin)
spironolactone (Aldactone)	losartan (Cozaar)	***Alpha₂-Adrenergic Agonists***
triamterene (Dyrenium)	olmesartan (Benicar)	clonidine (Catapres, Duraclon, Kapvay, Nexiclon XR)
Thiazide and Thiazide-Like	telmisartan (Micardis)	methyldopa (Aldomet)
chlorothiazide (Diuril)	valsartan (Diovan)	***Alpha and Beta Blockers (Centrally Acting)***
chlorthalidone (Hygroton)		carvedilol (Coreg)
hydrochlorothiazide (Microzide)	**Calcium Channel Blockers**	labetalol (Trandate, Normodyne)
indapamide (Lozol)	amlodipine (Norvasc)	***Adrenergic Neuron Blockers (Peripherally Acting)***
methyclothiazide (Enduron)	clevidipine (Cleviprex)	reserpine (Serpasil)
metolazone (Diulo, Mykrox, others)	diltiazem (Cardizem, Dilacor, others)	
Loop/High-Ceiling Type	felodipine (Plendil)	**Direct-Acting Vasodilators**
bumetanide (Bumex)	isradipine (DynaCirc)	hydralazine (Apresoline)
ethacrynic acid (Edecrin)	nicardipine (Cardene)	minoxidil (Loniten)
furosemide (Lasix)	nifedipine (Procardia, Adalat)	nitroprusside (Nitropress)
torsemide (Demadex)	nisoldipine (Nisocor, Sular)	
	verapamil (Calan, Isoptin, Verelan)	**Direct Renin Inhibitor**
ACE Inhibitors		aliskiren (Tekturna)
benazepril (Lotensin)	**Adrenergic Agents**	
captopril (Capoten)	***Beta Blockers***	
enalapril (Vasotec)	atenolol (Tenormin)	
fosinopril (Monopril)	betaxolol (Kerlone)	
lisinopril (Prinivil, Zestril)	bisoprolol (Zebeta)	
moexipril (Univasc)	metoprolol (Toprol, Lopressor)	
perindopril (Aceon)	nadolol (Corgard)	
quinapril (Accupril)	propranolol (Inderal)	
ramipril (Altace)	timolol (Betimol, others)	
trandolapril (Mavik)		

6 Calcium channel blockers have emerged as important drugs in the treatment of hypertension.

Calcium channel blockers (CCBs) are widely used in the treatment of HTN, angina pectoris, and dysrhythmias. The following section summarizes their application to the treatment of HTN.

CCBs exert beneficial effects on the heart and blood vessels by blocking calcium ion channels in cardiac and arteriolar smooth muscle. The flow of calcium ions into muscle cells is inhibited, limiting the degree of muscular contraction. At low doses, CCBs relax arterial smooth muscle, thus decreasing peripheral resistance and lowering blood pressure. Some CCBs such as nifedipine (Procardia) are selective for arterioles, whereas others such as verapamil (Calan) affect channels in both arterioles and the myocardium. CCBs vary in potency and in the frequency and types of adverse effects produced.

Due to their potent vasodilating effects, CCBs can cause reflex tachycardia, especially with those CCBs that are selective for arterioles. Because CCBs can slow myocardial conduction, they are contraindicated in patients with certain types of heart conditions such as sick sinus syndrome or third-degree AV block without the presence of a pacemaker. The CCBs that reduce myocardial contractility can worsen heart failure.

CCBs are usually not used as monotherapy for chronic HTN. They are, however, useful in combination therapy for treating certain populations such as older adults and African Americans who are sometimes less responsive to drugs in other antihypertensive classes.

CONNECTION Checkpoint 37.2

Verapamil and nifedipine are both calcium channel blockers used for HTN. Why would a beta blocker be used concurrently with nifedipine, but be contraindicated with verapamil? *See Answer to Connection Checkpoint 37.2 on student resource website.*

7 Blocking the renin-angiotensin-aldosterone system leads to a decrease in blood pressure.

The renin-angiotensin-aldosterone system (RAAS) is one of the primary homeostatic mechanisms controlling blood pressure and fluid balance. Drugs inhibiting the RAAS are widely used in the treatment of cardiovascular disease. Clinical research suggests ACE inhibitors are as effective as the diuretics in reducing HTN-related morbidity and mortality. The following section summarizes their applications to HTN pharmacotherapy.

Angiotensin-converting enzyme (ACE) inhibitors block the formation of angiotensin II, decreasing blood pressure through two mechanisms. First, ACE inhibitors block the intense vasoconstriction of arterioles caused by angiotensin II, which decreases blood pressure due to diminished peripheral resistance. Second, these drugs block the effects of angiotensin II on the secretion of aldosterone, which lowers blood pressure by decreasing blood volume. Through their inhibition of aldosterone secretion, ACE inhibitors enhance the effects of the thiazide diuretics; thus drugs from these two classes may be used concurrently in the management of HTN. Enalapril (Vasotec), lisinopril (Prinivil, Zestril), and captopril (Capoten) are three widely prescribed ACE inhibitors.

Adverse effects of ACE inhibitors are usually minor and include persistent cough and orthostatic hypotension, particularly following the first few doses of the drug. Hyperkalemia may occur, and can be a major concern for patients with diabetes, those with renal impairment, and patients taking potassium-sparing diuretics. Though rare, the most serious adverse effect of ACE inhibitors is the development of angioedema. When it does occur, angioedema most often develops within days after beginning ACE inhibitor therapy. Cough and angioedema arise more frequently in African Americans than in other ethnic groups.

The angiotensin II receptor blockers (ARBs) afford a second method for altering the RAAS pathway. ARBs such as losartan (Cozaar) block receptors for angiotensin II in arteriolar smooth muscle and in the adrenal gland, thus causing blood pressure to fall. Their actions are similar to those of the ACE inhibitors.

Angiotensin II receptor blockers have the lowest incidence of serious adverse effects of any of the antihypertensive classes. Most ARB adverse effects are related to hypotension. Unlike the ACE inhibitors, they do not cause cough, and angioedema is rare. Medications in this class are often combined with drugs from other classes in the management of HTN.

Aliskiren (Tekturna) was the first in a new class of antihypertensives called direct renin inhibitors approved in 2007. In 2008 the U.S. Food and Drug Administration (FDA) approved the combination of aliskiren with HCTZ (Tekturna ACT) for treating HTN. The most common adverse effects of aliskiren are diarrhea, cough, flulike symptoms, and rash.

8 Adrenergic antagonists are commonly used to treat hypertension.

The adrenergic antagonists, or blockers, are used for a wide variety of cardiovascular disorders, including HTN, angina pectoris, dysrhythmias, and MI prophylaxis. Blocking adrenergic receptors in the sympathetic nervous system has a number of beneficial effects on the heart and vessels. For example, by blocking the "fight-or-flight" responses, heart rate slows, blood pressure declines, and the bronchi dilate.

Adrenergic blockers affect the sympathetic division through a number of distinct mechanisms, although all have in common the effect of lowering blood pressure. These mechanisms include the following:

- Blockade of beta$_1$-adrenergic receptors
- Blockade of alpha$_1$-adrenergic receptors
- Nonselective blockade of both alpha$_1$- and beta-adrenergic receptors
- Stimulation of centrally acting alpha$_2$-adrenergic receptors in the brainstem
- Blockade of peripheral adrenergic neurons

The earliest drugs for HTN were nonselective agents that blocked nerve transmission at the ganglia or at both alpha- and beta-adrenergic receptors. Although the nonselective agents revolutionized the treatment of HTN, they caused significant adverse effects. These drugs are rarely used today because selective agents are more efficacious and better tolerated by patients. Of the five subclasses of adrenergic antagonists, only the beta-adrenergic antagonists are considered first-line drugs for the pharmacotherapy of HTN.

Beta-adrenergic antagonists: In this section, the discussion of beta-adrenergic antagonists is limited to their use in treating HTN. The student should be familiar with the basic pharmacology of this drug class. Other important therapeutic applications of the beta blockers include angina pectoris and MI, dysrhythmias, heart failure, and migraines.

Beta-adrenergic antagonists may be cardioselective (beta$_1$) or nonspecific (beta$_1$ and beta$_2$). Cardioselective beta blockers decrease heart rate, myocardial contractility, and cardiac conduction velocity. Nonspecific beta blockers produce the same effects, but also act on the respiratory system to cause bronchoconstriction. Decreasing the heart rate and contractility also reduces cardiac output and lowers systemic blood pressure. Some of their antihypertensive effect is also caused by the blockade of beta$_1$ receptors in the juxtaglomerular apparatus, which inhibits the secretion of renin and the formation of angiotensin II. The beta-adrenergic antagonists have been some of the most widely used drugs in the treatment of HTN.

At low doses, beta blockers are well tolerated and serious adverse events are uncommon. As the dosage is increased, however, adverse effects can become numerous and potentially serious in certain patients. Because nonselective beta blockers will slow the heart rate and cause bronchoconstriction, they should be used with caution in patients with asthma or heart failure. Heart rate and rhythm should be regularly monitored during beta-blocker therapy. Many patients report fatigue and activity intolerance at higher doses because the reduction in heart rate causes the heart to become less responsive to exertion. People with diabetes should be warned that symptoms of hypoglycemia (diaphoresis, nervousness, and palpitation) may become less observable while on beta-blocker therapy. Beta blockers have been reported to cause or worsen the symptoms of erectile dysfunction more than many other antihypertensive classes. Some drugs in this class are associated with clinical depression. When discontinuing a beta blocker, drug doses should be tapered over a several week period. Abrupt cessation of beta-blocker therapy can result in rebound HTN, angina, MI, and even death in patients with CAD.

CONNECTION Checkpoint 37.3

Should a hypertensive patient with asthma receive a selective beta$_1$ blocker or a nonselective beta blocker for HTN? *See Answer to Connection Checkpoint 37.3 on student resource website.*

Alpha$_1$-adrenergic antagonists:

The alpha$_1$-adrenergic antagonists have several clinical applications. In addition to their use in HTN, they are prescribed for benign prostatic hyperplasia (BPH) because their ability to relax smooth muscle in the prostate and bladder neck reduces urethral resistance.

The alpha$_1$-adrenergic antagonists lower blood pressure directly by blocking sympathetic receptors in arterioles, causing the vessels to dilate. They also dilate veins, which lowers blood pressure indirectly by decreasing venous return to the heart and reducing cardiac output. The alpha blockers are not first-line drugs for HTN. Although they are effective in reducing blood pressure, long-term clinical trials have shown them to be less effective at reducing the incidence of serious HTN-related cardiovascular events than diuretics. When used to treat HTN, the alpha blockers are used concurrently with other classes of antihypertensives, such as diuretics.

The alpha$_1$-adrenergic blockers may cause significant orthostatic hypotension. It is particularly serious with the initial doses of these medications and is referred to as the **first-dose phenomenon**, although orthostatic hypotension may persist throughout treatment. In severe cases, syncope can occur. Blood pressure should be assessed regularly during therapy to maintain patient safety. Other common adverse effects include weakness, dizziness, dry mouth, headache, and gastrointestinal (GI) complaints such as nausea and vomiting. The older adult is especially prone to orthostatic hypotension and to hypothermic effects related to vasodilation caused by these drugs. Less common, though sometimes a major cause for nonadherence, are adverse effects on male sexual function that include decreased libido and erectile dysfunction.

Nonselective alpha$_1$- and beta-adrenergic antagonists:

Carvedilol (Coreg) and labetalol (Normodyne) are unique in that they block both alpha$_1$- and beta-adrenergic receptors. These drugs act by a combination of effects: reducing cardiac output, inhibiting renin secretion, and blocking vasoconstriction of arterioles and veins. As expected, their adverse effects are a combination of alpha and beta blockade and include orthostatic hypotension, bradycardia, and bronchoconstriction.

Alpha$_2$-adrenergic agonists:

If an alpha antagonist such as prazosin (Minipress) lowers blood pressure, it might be predicted that the administration of an alpha$_2$-adrenergic agonist would raise blood pressure. This is not the case. The answer to this contradiction lies in the different locations of the two subtypes of alpha receptors. The alpha$_1$ receptors blocked by prazosin lie in the peripheral nervous system (PNS), at arterioles. The alpha$_2$ receptors reside in the central nervous system (CNS).

When alpha$_2$ receptors are activated, the outflow of sympathetic nerve impulses from the CNS to the heart and arterioles is inhibited. In effect, this produces the same responses as inhibition of the alpha$_1$ receptor: slowing the heart rate and conduction velocity, and dilating the arterioles. Thus, activating alpha$_2$ receptors (in the CNS) produces similar actions as inhibiting alpha$_1$ receptors (in the PNS).

Although the two drug classes have similar actions and are both used for HTN, the centrally acting alpha$_2$ agonists are used less frequently than the alpha$_1$ antagonists. The alpha$_2$ agonists have a tendency to cause excessive sedation, dizziness, and orthostatic hypotension, which can be especially troublesome in older adults. Extended use results in sodium and water retention, which increases blood volume and counteracts the antihypertensive action of these drugs. Alpha$_2$ agonists are usually reserved for treating resistant HTN that cannot be managed by safer medications. The two drugs in this class are methyldopa and clonidine.

Methyldopa is an older drug approved in 1962. Its only indication is HTN that has not responded adequately to safer antihypertensives. The drug is normally administered by the oral (PO) route, although an intravenous (IV) form known as methyldopate is available for hypertensive crises. Compared to other antihypertensives given by the IV route, methyldopa has a relatively slow onset of action because it must first be metabolized inside neurons to an active metabolite, methyl norepinephrine. Methyldopa is sometimes used for treating HTN occurring during pregnancy because it maintains stable blood flow to the uterus, and its safety to the fetus has been demonstrated in long-term studies.

Because methyldopa is a centrally acting agent, CNS effects such as drowsiness, depression, headache, sedation, and bizarre dreams are relatively common. Orthostatic hypotension may occur, but it is less severe than that produced by the alpha$_1$ antagonists. Peripheral edema due to sodium retention may occur, which can be managed by administration of a thiazide diuretic. A significant number of patients develop a positive Coombs' test, which detects antibodies against the patient's own red blood cells. In a small number of patients, the positive Coombs' test is associated with hemolytic anemia. The drug should be discontinued if signs of anemia develop. Because tolerance develops after 3 to 4 months of therapy, a dosage increase may be required to manage HTN. This drug is pregnancy category B.

Approved in 1974, clonidine (Catapres, Duraclon, Kapvay, Nexiclon XR) activates alpha$_2$-adrenergic receptors in the cardiovascular control centers in the brainstem. The reduced sympathetic outflow causes vasodilation and slows the heart rate. As an antihypertensive, it is available as regular oral tablets, extended release tablets or suspension (Nexiclon), or a transdermal patch that releases the drug at a constant rate over 7 days. A second approved indication for clonidine (Duraclon) is intractable pain in patients with cancer that is not relieved by opiates.

Pain control is achieved by a continuous epidural infusion of the drug. To assist in pain management, transdermal clonidine may be used to provide some degree of analgesia so that the dose of opiate can be reduced. In 2010, an extended-release form of clonidine (Kapvay) was approved to treat attention deficit/hyperactivity disorder.

Clonidine has many off-label indications. These include dysmenorrhea, menopausal flushing, migraine prophylaxis, smoking cessation, opiate and benzodiazepine withdrawal, and Tourette's syndrome.

The most common adverse effect of clonidine is dry mouth, which occurs in about 40% of the patients taking the drug. Like methyldopa, CNS adverse effects such as sedation, fatigue, drowsiness, and dizziness are common. Transdermal clonidine produces fewer serious adverse effects, although the patches can cause skin irritation and itching. The patient should be warned not to abruptly discontinue the drug, as severe rebound HTN, agitation, nervousness, and anxiety may result.

Adrenergic neuron–blocking agents: The adrenergic neuron-blocker class consists of two drugs that inhibit the synthesis or release of norepinephrine (NE) in sympathetic neurons. With less NE available to cross the synapse, sympathetic activity is diminished at both alpha- and beta-adrenergic receptors. In effect, the actions of these drugs are the same as the nonselective alpha$_1$- and beta-adrenergic antagonists: reduced heart rate and cardiac output (beta effects) combined with dilation of arterioles (alpha effect).

The adrenergic neuron–blocking agents have mostly historical interest, as they are rarely prescribed today due to the availability of safer medications. Reserpine (Serpalan), isolated from the shrub *Rauwolfia serpentina* in 1952, was one of the earliest drugs used for HTN. It is an ancient drug, used for centuries in India as an herbal tea to produce sedation and calm the nerves. Reserpine lowers blood pressure by irreversibly binding to NE storage vesicles, causing depletion of NE and other neurotransmitters in both the central and peripheral nervous systems. The drug may take 2 to 6 weeks to deplete NE and produce an optimal antihypertensive effect. Unfortunately, reserpine can cause profound depression and sedation, and cardiovascular adverse effects such as bradycardia and orthostatic hypotension can be severe. Effects are often prolonged because once depleted of NE, neurons may take several weeks to synthesize adequate amounts of the neurotransmitter. Reserpine is only prescribed when patients are unable to tolerate safer antihypertensives. Although it was once used to treat psychotic disorders, it is no longer used for this purpose because more effective drugs are available.

Guanethidine (Ismelin) is also an adrenergic neuron–blocking drug. It acts by preventing the storage and release of NE in nerve terminals. As with reserpine, depletion of NE causes the heart rate to slow, and blood pressure to fall. The limiting adverse effects of guanethidine are severe diarrhea and orthostatic hypotension, which occur frequently and can be serious enough to cause syncope. Guanethidine is rarely prescribed due to the potential for serious adverse effects. A third drug in this class, guanadrel (Hylorel), has similar actions and adverse effects to guanethidine, but its use has been discontinued in the United States.

9 Direct-acting vasodilators lower blood pressure by relaxing arteriolar smooth muscle.

The ability to cause vasodilation is a property shared by many different classes of drugs, as shown in Figure 1. Most vasodilators are used to treat HTN, and some are used for the pharmacotherapy of heart failure, angina pectoris, and MI. Some of the drugs presented in previous sections of this chapter produce vasodilation indirectly by affecting autonomic nerves or by influencing the renin-angiotensin-aldosterone pathway. The agents presented in this section affect the vascular smooth muscle itself; thus, they are called direct vasodilators.

Direct relaxation of arteriolar smooth muscle is an effective way to reduce blood pressure. Indeed, sodium nitroprusside (Nitropress) and diazoxide (Hyperstat IV) are used in hypertensive emergencies and can lower blood pressure almost instantaneously. Unfortunately, the medications in this class have the potential to produce serious adverse effects. This limits their applications in the pharmacotherapy of HTN to hypertensive emergencies and for HTN unresponsive to medications from safer drug classes.

All direct vasodilators cause **reflex tachycardia**, a compensatory increase in heart rate due to the sudden decrease in blood pressure. The baroreceptor reflex is an essential component of the normal physiological control of blood pressure. However, when reflex tachycardia occurs as the result of vasodilator agents, the heart is forced to work harder and the resultant blood pressure increase counteracts the effect of the antihypertensive drug. Patients with CAD may experience an acute angina attack due to the sudden increase in cardiac workload. Fortunately, reflex tachycardia can be prevented by administering a beta-adrenergic blocker, such as propranolol (Inderal). Beta blockers are often administered concurrently with direct vasodilators for this reason.

A second potentially serious adverse effect of direct vasodilator therapy is salt and water retention. The reduction in blood pressure from the vasodilator causes a compensatory increase in aldosterone secretion by the adrenal gland. The increased aldosterone level signals the kidney to retain more sodium and water. Blood volume increases, thus raising blood pressure and canceling the antihypertensive action of the vasodilator. A diuretic may be administered concurrently with a direct vasodilator in order to prevent fluid retention.

Other adverse effects are drug specific. Hydralazine can induce a lupus-like syndrome characterized by myalgia, arthralgia, fever, and the presence of antinuclear antibodies. Although rare, symptoms may persist for 6 months or longer and antinuclear antibodies may be present for 9 years. The occurrence of this lupus-like syndrome is more common in Caucasians who are slow acetylators. Antinuclear antibody titers should be determined prior to initiating therapy, and periodically thereafter to identify the development of this syndrome.

PROTOTYPE DRUG   Hydralazine (Apresoline)

Classification: **Therapeutic:** Antihypertensive
                Pharmacologic: Direct vasodilator

Therapeutic Effects and Uses: In 1952, hydralazine was one of the first oral antihypertensive medications marketed in the

United States. It is most commonly administered in tablet form for moderate to severe HTN, usually in combination with other antihypertensives. Apresazide is a fixed-dose combination of hydralazine with HCTZ. When given orally, hydralazine is administered 2 to 4 times per day, usually with food because this increases its bioavailability. Therapy is generally begun with low doses, which are gradually increased until the desired therapeutic response is obtained. After several months of therapy, tolerance to the drug develops and a dosage increase may be necessary. Although it produces an effective reduction in blood pressure, drugs in other antihypertensive classes have largely replaced hydralazine.

Hydralazine is also available by the intramuscular (IM) and IV routes for hypertensive emergencies, especially those associated with preeclampsia, although it is not a drug of choice for this indication. It is sometimes administered to patients with acute heart failure because the drug reduces the workload on the heart due to its antihypertensive action. ACE inhibitors have largely replaced the drug for patients with heart failure. A fixed-dose combination therapy of isosorbide dinitrate and hydralazine (BiDil) is available for the treatment of heart failure in African American patients.

Mechanism of Action: By causing peripheral vasodilation, hydralazine acts directly to relax arterial smooth muscle. The decreased peripheral resistance is accompanied by an increase in heart rate and cardiac output. The overall result is a reduction in afterload. Because the drug is selective for arterioles and does not cause dilation of veins, orthostatic hypotension is not a major adverse effect.

Pharmacokinetics:

Route(s)	PO, IM, IV
Absorption	Rapidly absorbed PO and well absorbed IM
Distribution	Widely distributed; crosses the placenta and is secreted in breast milk; 87% bound to plasma protein
Primary metabolism	GI mucosa and liver; extensive first-pass metabolism
Primary excretion	90% renal, 10% feces
Onset of action	PO: 20–30 min; IM: 10–30 min; IV: 5–20 min
Duration of action	2–6 h; half-life: 3–7 h

Adverse Effects: Hydralazine may cause several adverse events that have the potential to prompt discontinuation of therapy. Headache, tachycardia, palpitations, flushing, nausea, and diarrhea are common, but may resolve as therapy progresses. Orthostatic hypotension, fluid retention, and peripheral edema may also occur. Patients who are slow acetylators and those with renal impairment or who are receiving high doses of hydralazine are susceptible to experiencing a lupus-like syndrome. Symptoms may include rash, urticaria, myalgia, fever, chills, and fatigue. Blood dyscrasias such as agranulocytosis and leukopenia are rare, though potentially serious, adverse effects.

Contraindications/Precautions: Patients with lupus should not receive hydralazine, as the drug can worsen symptoms. The drug is contraindicated in patients with cerebrovascular disease or rheumatic heart disease. Patients should discontinue

hydralazine gradually because abrupt withdrawal may cause severe rebound HTN and anxiety. Because it is excreted primarily by the kidneys, the drug should be used with caution in patients with renal impairment. Caution must be used when administering hydralazine to patients who are known slow acetylators because plasma drug levels will be significantly higher in these patients. Caution should be used when treating patients with CAD, because hydralazine can precipitate angina attacks and an acute MI.

Drug Interactions: Administering hydralazine with other antihypertensives or monoamine oxidase inhibitors (MAOIs) may cause severe hypotension. This includes all drug classes used as antihypertensives. NSAIDs may decrease the antihypertensive action of hydralazine. Beta blockers are usually used concurrently with hydralazine to block reflex tachycardia, and heart rate should be carefully monitored to avoid bradycardia. Hydralazine may produce false-positive Coombs' tests. **Herbal/Food:** Hawthorn should be avoided because it may cause additive hypotensive effects.

Pregnancy: Category C.

Treatment of Overdose: Treatment includes gastric lavage, activated charcoal, and administration of a plasma volume expander to raise blood pressure. Tachycardia may require treatment with a beta blocker.

Nursing Responsibilities: Key nursing implications for patients receiving hydralazine are included in the Nursing Practice Application for Patients Receiving Direct Vasodilator Therapy.

Lifespan and Diversity Considerations:

- Use caution when administering the drug to the older adult who is at greater risk for hypotension, dizziness, and falls. Provide assistance with ambulation as needed.

- Because hydralazine is known to metabolize more slowly in some patients (slow acetylators) with resulting higher drug levels and because this cannot always be predicted, more frequent monitoring especially in the early stages of drug therapy is advised.

Patient and Family Education:

- Do not abruptly stop taking this drug because dangerously high blood pressure and anxiety could result.

- Headache and palpitations may occur within 2 to 4 hours after the first oral dose, but these symptoms usually subside.

- Avoid alcohol because alcohol intake could result in dizziness.

- Take the drug with a full glass of water.

- Do not breast-feed without approval of the health care provider.

Drugs Similar to Hydralazine (Apresoline)

Other direct vasodilators used for HTN include diazoxide, minoxidil, and nitroprusside. Nitroprusside is a drug of choice for hypertensive emergencies and is presented as a prototype drug in Section 10. Diazoxide (Hyperstat IV) is a rapid-acting vasodilator that is no longer marketed for blood pressure control. An oral form of diazoxide (Proglycem) is available to treat various hypoglycemic states, usually caused by the presence of excessive insulin (hyperinsulinism).

Minoxidil (Loniten): Minoxidil is a direct vasodilator with profound vasodilation activity that is selective for arterioles: It does not dilate veins. It is administered by the oral route for severe HTN that is unresponsive to drugs from other classes. Because of its efficacy and the potential for serious effects on the cardiovascular system, initial doses are very low, and the amount is increased gradually. It is a pregnancy category C drug.

Minoxidil is considerably more toxic than hydralazine. The most serious adverse effects are cardiovascular in nature, including reflex tachycardia and plasma volume expansion due to sodium and water retention. Beta blockers are usually administered concurrently to minimize tachycardia, and diuretics to prevent fluid retention. Although rare, pericardial effusion has been reported with minoxidil use. Minoxidil causes **hypertrichosis:** the elongation, thickening, and increased pigmentation of body hair. This is normal and will reverse when the drug is discontinued. The drug's effect on hair growth is used to the patient's advantage in Rogaine, a topical form of minoxidil used to stimulate hair growth in patients with male-pattern baldness. The topical form of the drug is not absorbed into the systemic circulation, thus Rogaine produces none of the serious cardiovascular effects observed with Loniten.

Management of Hypertensive Emergency

10 Hypertensive crisis is a medical emergency that is treated by the intravenous administration of antihypertensive medications.

A **hypertensive emergency (HTN-E)**, also called hypertensive crisis, is defined as a diastolic pressure of greater than 120 mmHg, with evidence of target-organ system damage. HTN-E requires aggressive treatment, usually within minutes to hours, to prevent further organ damage. A related condition, **hypertensive urgency**, is when a patient presents with severe HTN, but has no evidence of target-organ damage.

Target-organ damage from extreme HTN most often occurs in the cardiovascular system, the kidneys, or the CNS. In the cardiovascular system, the increased workload on the heart leads to acute left heart failure with pulmonary edema, sometimes accompanied by myocardial ischemia or infarction. Chest pain and dyspnea are the most common symptoms in patients with HTN-E. Renal function is diminished, as evidenced by oliguria, hematuria, and proteinuria. Acute renal failure may occur, or preexisting chronic renal failure may worsen. In the brain, thrombotic or hemorrhagic stroke may occur. The capillaries in the brain become leaky, producing hypertensive encephalopathy, with resulting headache, paralysis, seizures, or coma. In addition, retinal hemorrhages and edema of the retina (papilledema) are signs of severe HTN.

The most common cause of HTN-E is untreated or poorly controlled essential HTN. In some cases, the patient has abruptly discontinued use of the antihypertensive medication. There are, however, a large number of possible secondary causes of HTN-E, including the following conditions:

- Renovascular hypertension
- Pheochromocytoma
- Cocaine use
- Eclampsia or preeclampsia
- Head injuries
- Primary hyperaldosteronism
- Coarctation of the aorta
- Hyperthyroidism or thyroid storm

In the management of HTN-E, the therapeutic goal is to lower blood pressure quickly. Care must be taken, however, to not decrease blood pressure too quickly because rapid and intense vasodilation can result in serious hypoperfusion of the cerebral, coronary, or renal vascular capillaries. This can cause ischemia or infarction, worsening target-organ damage to the brain, heart, kidneys, or retina. It is recommended that the pretreatment blood pressure be progressively reduced by 20% to 25%, over 30 to 60 minutes. Additional, gradual reductions are made over a 12- to 48-hour period until blood pressure is reduced to a value within the normal range. Parenteral antihypertensives are preferred over PO medications due to their rapid onset of action and because infusions offer more precise control during the gradual pressure reduction.

In patients with hypertensive urgencies, target-organ damage has not yet developed. These patients are treated more conservatively by increasing the dose of their current antihypertensive drug, or by adding a second drug to the regimen. Oral medications are used to lower blood pressure because these drugs are less toxic than parenteral antihypertensives. Oral agents with a relatively rapid onset of action that may be used for hypertensive urgency include clonidine (Catapres), captopril (Capoten), or labetalol (Normodyne). The patient should be monitored for several hours, and doses may be repeated at frequent intervals, as needed, to lower pressure to acceptable levels. All patients with hypertensive urgency should receive follow-up assessments after 1 to 3 days on the new regimen.

PROTOTYPE DRUG	Nitroprusside Sodium (Nipride, Nitropress)

Classification: **Therapeutic:** Drug for hypertensive emergency
Pharmacologic: Direct vasodilator

Therapeutic Effects and Uses: Nitroprusside is a first-line drug for patients with aggressive, life-threatening HTN because it has the ability to lower blood pressure almost instantaneously upon IV administration. The drug has a short half-life, and the hypotensive effects disappear approximately 3 minutes after the infusion is discontinued. Unlike most direct vasodilators, nitroprusside causes very little reflex tachycardia. Although discovered in 1850, the drug was not approved by the FDA until 1974.

Patients must be continuously monitored while receiving nitroprusside to prevent hypotension due to overtreatment. Therapy is limited to 72 hours because the drug is metabolized to toxic thiocyanate and cyanide compounds. This is of special concern to patients with renal impairment who are unable to excrete the cyanide. If serum thiocyanate exceeds 12 mg/dL, the nitroprusside infusion should be discontinued. As a general rule, patients are switched from nitroprusside to an oral antihypertensive as soon as blood pressure has stabilized.

Mechanism of Action: Nitroprusside dilates both arteries and veins; therefore, the hypotensive action of nitroprusside is due to direct relaxation of arteriolar smooth muscle and to blood pooling in the veins. In most patients, heart rate is mildly increased, while cardiac output is decreased. In patients with severe left ventricular hypertrophy, however, cardiac output may increase.

Pharmacokinetics:

Route(s)	IV
Absorption	N/A
Distribution	Unknown
Primary metabolism	Metabolized to thiocyanates in erythrocytes and other tissues
Primary excretion	Renal
Onset of action	1–2 min
Duration of action	1–10 min

Adverse Effects: Signs and symptoms of vasodilation such as hypotension, headache, dizziness, and flushing of the skin are expected adverse effects. With extended therapy, thiocyanate toxicity may manifest. Thiocyanate poisoning is characterized by hypotension, lethargy, blurred vision, metabolic acidosis, faint heart sounds, and loss of consciousness. Irritation may occur at the infusion site. **Black Box Warning**: Nitroprusside requires dilution prior to infusion and is not suitable for direct injection. The drug can cause irreversible ischemic injury and death due to significant drops in blood pressure. Accumulation of cyanide ion may occur.

Contraindications/Precautions: Patients with inadequate cerebral circulation or who have compensatory HTN should not receive nitroprusside. Because the kidneys excrete the toxic thiocyanate metabolite of the drug, patients with serious renal impairment should be treated cautiously. Nitroprusside is contraindicated in patients with high intracranial pressure because the drug may worsen this condition.

Drug Interactions: Antihypertensive agents, ethanol, general anesthetics, and ganglionic blockers should be used with caution with nitroprusside because additive hypotension could result. Sympathomimetics such as epinephrine will block the antihypertensive actions of nitroprusside. Dobutamine (Dobutrex) and nitroprusside are sometimes administered concurrently because this interaction results in a beneficial synergistic increase in cardiac output and decrease in pulmonary capillary wedge pressure. **Herbal/Food**: Hawthorn may cause additive hypotensive effects.

Pregnancy: Category C.

Treatment of Overdose: Extreme hypotension may be treated with a vasopressor. Cyanide toxicity caused by the overdose may require the use of a cyanide antidote kit, which contains amyl nitrate, sodium nitrite, and sodium thiosulfate. The purpose of these drugs is to convert toxic cyanide into nontoxic thiocyanate.

Nursing Responsibilities: Key nursing implications for patients receiving nitroprusside are included in the Nursing Practice Application for Patients Receiving Direct Vasodilator Therapy.

Lifespan and Diversity Considerations:
- Use extreme caution when administering the drug to the older adult who is at greater risk for hypotension, dizziness, and falls. Provide assistance with ambulation as needed if ambulation is allowed.

Patient and Family Education:
- Be aware that therapy is short term and will be discontinued when blood pressure is controlled. The patient may need to remain in an intensive care setting during drug administration.

TABLE 4 Drugs for Hypertensive Emergency

Drug	Class	Applications
clevidipine (Cleviprex)	Calcium channel blocker	Newer drug with an onset of action of 2–4 min and a short duration, allowing for rapid blood pressure reduction
enalaprilat (Enalapril IV)	ACE inhibitor	Onset of action is 15–30 min; useful in HTN-E associated with heart failure or high plasma levels of angiotensin II
esmolol (Brevibloc)	Beta-adrenergic antagonist	Onset of action is 1–5 min; useful for patients with severe left ventricular dysfunction or with peripheral vascular disease
fenoldopam (Corlopam)	Dopamine agonist	Onset of action is 5 min; useful for patients with renal impairment, as the drug increases renal blood flow
hydralazine (Apresoline)	Direct vasodilator	Onset of action is 5–20 min; useful in HTN-E due to eclampsia and preeclampsia because it increases uterine blood flow
labetalol (Normodyne)	Alpha- and beta-adrenergic antagonist	Onset of action is 2–5 min; reduces incidences of MI and death
nicardipine (Cardene IV)	Calcium channel blocker	Onset of action is 1 min; rapid and effective for most HTN-E, with fewer adverse effects than some other HTN-E drugs
nitroprusside sodium (Nipride, Nitropress)	Direct vasodilator	Onset of action is 1 min; drug of choice for many HTN-E
phentolamine (Regitine)	Alpha-adrenergic antagonist	Onset of action is 1–5 min; rarely used due to high incidence of reflex tachycardia and myocardial ischemia; useful for HTN-E due to pheochromocytoma

Drugs Similar to Nitroprusside Sodium (Nipride, Nitropress)

Other vasodilators for HTN-E include clevidipine, enalaprilat, esmolol, fenoldopam, hydralazine, labetalol, nicardipine, and phentolamine. Table 4 summarizes their applications to the pharmacotherapy of hypertensive crisis.

PharmFact

Hypertensive crisis is a common condition, affecting 1% of the patients with primary HTN. The most common presentation, occurring in 25% of patients, is stroke. The 1-year survival rate for a patient presenting with a HTN crisis has improved from only 20% prior to 1950 to more than 90% with current medical treatment (Hopkins, 2011).

CONNECTIONS: NURSING PRACTICE APPLICATION

Patients Receiving Direct Vasodilator Therapy

Assessment	Potential Nursing Diagnoses
Baseline assessment prior to administration: • Understand the reason the drug has been prescribed in order to assess for therapeutic effects. • Obtain a complete health history: cardiovascular (including MI, heart failure), cerebrovascular and neurologic (including level of consciousness [LOC], history of stroke, head injury, increased intracranial pressure), respiratory, and the possibility of autoimmune diseases, especially systemic lupus erythematosus. Obtain a drug history including allergies, current prescription and over-the-counter drugs, and herbal preparations. Be alert to possible drug interactions. • Evaluate appropriate laboratory findings: electrolytes, especially sodium and potassium levels, hepatic and renal function studies, and lipid profiles. • Obtain baseline weight, vital signs, pulse oximetry, breath and heart sounds, and cardiac monitoring (e.g., ECG, cardiac output). Assess location and character of peripheral edema if present. • Assess the patient's ability to receive and understand instructions. Include family and caregivers as needed.	• *Decreased Cardiac Output* • *Deficient Knowledge* (Drug Therapy) • *Risk for Decreased Cardiac Tissue Perfusion* • *Risk for Imbalanced Fluid Volume* • *Risk for Injury* • *Risk for Impaired Skin Integrity*, related to adverse effects from intravenous infusion of medication
Assessment throughout administration: • Assess for desired therapeutic effects (e.g., lowered blood pressure within established limits). • Continue frequent and careful monitoring of vital signs, pulse oximetry, urinary and cardiac output, and daily weight, especially if IV administration is used. Blood pressure and pulse must be monitored every 5 min or as ordered while on IV infusion of the drug. (Invasive monitoring, such as arterial lines, is often used for this purpose.) • Continue periodic monitoring of electrolytes, especially potassium. • Continue frequent physical assessments, particularly neurologic, cardiac, and respiratory systems. • Assess for and promptly report adverse effects: excessive hypotension, dysrhythmias, reflex tachycardia (from too rapid decrease in blood pressure or significant hypotension), headache, decreased urinary output, peripheral edema, and priapism (prolonged erection in the absence of sexual stimulation). Severe hypotension, seizures, dysrhythmias, or palpitations may signal drug toxicity and are immediately reported.	

Planning: Patient Goals and Expected Outcomes

The patient will:

• Experience therapeutic effects dependent on the reason the drug is being given (e.g., decreased blood pressure).
• Be free from or experience minimal adverse effects.
• Verbalize an understanding of the drug's use, adverse effects, and required precautions.
• Demonstrate proper self-administration of the medication (e.g., dose, timing, and when to notify the provider).

Implementation

Interventions and (Rationales)	Patient-Centered Care
Ensuring therapeutic effects: • Continue frequent assessments as above for therapeutic effects. IV infusion of vasodilators may be titrated frequently to achieve desired effects. Vital signs, cardiac and urinary output, and daily weights should remain within the limits set by the health care provider. (Pulse, blood pressure, and respiratory rate should be within normal limits or acceptable parameters. An increase in weight of more than 1 kg [2.2 lb] per day may indicate excessive fluid gain, and may require judicious diuretic therapy.)	• To allay possible anxiety, teach the patient, family, or caregiver the rationale for all equipment used and the need for frequent monitoring. • Teach the patient, family, or caregiver how to monitor pulse and blood pressure as appropriate if the patient is on oral therapy at home. Ensure proper use and functioning of any home equipment obtained. • Have the patient weigh self daily along with blood pressure and pulse measurements. Report a weight gain or loss of more than 1 kg (2.2 lb) in a 24-h period.

(continued)

Minimizing adverse effects:

- Continue to monitor vital signs frequently. Be particularly cautious with older adults who are at increased risk for hypotension, patients with a preexisting history of cardiac or cerebrovascular ischemia, which may be worsened by decreased blood pressure, patients with dehydration, and patients with lupus erythematosus. Immediately notify the health care provider if the blood pressure or pulse decrease beyond established parameters or if hypotension is accompanied by reflex tachycardia. (Direct-acting vasodilators cause significant vasodilation, resulting in the potential for dramatically and rapidly lowered blood pressure accompanied by reflex tachycardia. Reflex tachycardia may require treatment with beta-blocking drugs.)

- Instruct the patient, family, or caregiver to report angina-like symptoms (e.g., chest, arm, back or neck pain), palpitations, faintness, dizziness, drowsiness, or headache.

- Continue cardiac monitoring (e.g., ECG) and invasive monitoring (e.g., cardiac output, arterial line pressures) as ordered in the hospitalized patient. (Monitoring devices assist in detecting early signs of adverse effects as well as monitoring for therapeutic effects.)

- To allay possible anxiety, teach the patient, family, or caregiver the rationale for all equipment used and the need for frequent monitoring.

- Continue frequent physical assessments, particularly neurologic, cardiac, and respiratory. Immediately report any changes in LOC, headache, or changes in heart or lung sounds. (Vasodilator therapy may worsen preexisting neurologic, cardiac, or respiratory conditions as blood pressure drops and perfusion to vital organs diminishes.)

- When on oral therapy at home, the patient, family, or caregiver should immediately report changes in mental status or LOC, palpitations, dizziness, dyspnea, increasing productive cough, especially if frothy sputum is present, and seek medical attention.

- Weigh the patient daily and report weight gain or loss of 1 kg (2.2 lb) or more in a 24-h period or significant peripheral edema. (Daily weight is an accurate measure of fluid status and takes into account intake, output, and insensible losses. Weight gain or edema may signal blood pressure has lowered too quickly, stimulating renin release, and may require judicious use of diuretic therapy to treat.)

- When on oral therapy at home, have the patient weigh self daily, ideally at the same time of day, and record weight along with blood pressure and pulse measurements. Have the patient report a weight gain or loss of more than 1 kg (2 lb) in a 24-h period, or peripheral edema, especially if increasing.

- Continue to monitor IV infusion sites frequently. (Direct-acting vasodilators may cause tissue damage if the drug extravasates.)

- Instruct the patient to report any burning or stinging pain, swelling, warmth, redness, or tenderness at the IV insertion site.

- Observe for signs and symptoms of lupus in patients taking vasodilators, particularly hydralazine. (Hydralazine has been linked to drug-induced/drug-related lupus. Other direct vasodilators are used with caution for this reason.)

- Instruct the patient to report symptoms such as a butterfly-shaped rash over the nose and cheeks, muscle aches, and fatigue when taking oral vasodilators, particularly hydralazine.

- Monitor for the development of priapism and notify the health care provider. (Priapism may result in tissue damage if unrelieved and is considered a medical emergency.)

- Instruct the patient to report a sustained erection that lasts more than 4 h if on vasodilator therapy at home and to seek immediate medical care.

- For oral drug therapy, give the first dose of the drug at bedtime. (A first-dose response may result in a greater initial drop in blood pressure than subsequent doses.)

- Instruct the patient to take the first dose of the medication at bedtime, immediately before going to bed, and to avoid driving or other substantial activities for 12 to 24 h after the first dose or when the dosage is increased until effects are known.

- Do not abruptly stop medication. (Rebound HTN and tachycardia may occur.)

- Teach the patient, family, or caregiver not to stop the medication abruptly and to call the health care provider if the patient is unable to take the medication for more than 1 day due to illness.

- Encourage appropriate lifestyle changes: lowered fat intake, gradual increase in exercise, limited alcohol intake, smoking cessation. Provide for dietitian consultation as needed. (Healthy lifestyle changes will support and minimize the need for drug therapy. Direct vasodilators decrease blood pressure substantially, and concurrent beta-blocker use may decrease heart rate. Given alone or together, this may lead to exercise intolerance. Activity levels should be increased gradually to patient tolerance. If dizziness or shortness of breath occur, decrease exercise levels to a comfortable level. Alcohol consumption may increase the risk of blood pressure–related adverse effects.)

- Encourage the patient, family, or caregivers to adopt a healthy lifestyle of low-fat food choices, reduced sodium intake, increased exercise, decreased alcohol consumption, and smoking cessation.
- Caution the patient about sudden increases in activity level. Report dizziness, palpitations, or shortness of breath that occurs while exercising.

Patient understanding of drug therapy:

- Use opportunities during administration of medications and during assessments to discuss the rationale for drug therapy, desired therapeutic outcomes, commonly observed adverse effects, parameters for when to call the health care provider, and any necessary monitoring or precautions. (Using time during nursing care helps to optimize and reinforce key teaching areas.)

- The patient, family, or caregiver should be able to state the reason for the drug, appropriate dose and scheduling, what adverse effects to observe for and when to report them, and the anticipated length of medication therapy.

Patient self-administration of drug therapy:

- When administering medications, instruct the patient, family, or caregiver in proper self-administration techniques. (Utilizing time during nurse-administration of these drugs helps to reinforce teaching.)

- Instruct the patient in proper administration techniques, followed by return demonstration.
- The patient, family, or caregiver is able to discuss appropriate dosing and administration needs.

Evaluation of Outcome Criteria

Evaluate the effectiveness of drug therapy by confirming that patient goals and expected outcomes have been met (see "Planning").

UNDERSTANDING THE CHAPTER

Key Concepts Summary

1 Hypertension is classified by stages, based on the degree of elevation of systolic and diastolic blood pressure.

2 Failure to properly manage hypertension can lead to stroke, heart failure, or myocardial infarction.

3 Therapeutic lifestyle changes can reduce blood pressure and lessen the need for antihypertensive medications.

4 The choice of antihypertensive medication is determined by the degree of hypertension and the presence of other medical conditions.

5 Diuretics are often drugs of first choice for treating mild to moderate hypertension.

6 Calcium channel blockers have emerged as important drugs in the treatment of hypertension.

7 Blocking the renin-angiotensin-aldosterone system leads to a decrease in blood pressure.

8 Adrenergic antagonists are commonly used to treat hypertension.

9 Direct-acting vasodilators lower blood pressure by relaxing arteriolar smooth muscle.

10 Hypertensive crisis is a medical emergency that is treated by the IV administration of antihypertensive medications.

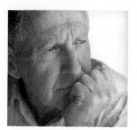

Making the PATIENT Connection

Remember the patient "Elmer Foley" at the beginning of the chapter? Now read the remainder of the case study. Based on the information presented within this chapter, respond to the critical thinking questions that follow.

Elmer Foley is a 72-year-old Caucasian male with a 10-month history of uncontrolled HTN. Initially, Elmer was prescribed the thiazide diuretic HCTZ (Microzide). However, after 1 week of therapy his blood pressure has remained at 168/102 mmHg. Next, Elmer's health care provider added an angiotensin-converting enzyme inhibitor, captopril (Capoten), to the regimen. Still, Elmer's blood pressure remained above normal limits. Lastly, the health care provider discontinued the captopril and started Elmer on hydralazine (Apresoline). With this visit, his blood pressure is 146/90 mmHg.

When Elmer was first told he had HTN, he began many of the suggested lifestyle changes encouraged by his health care provider. He has lost a total of 15 kg (33 lb) since starting his diet 10 months ago. Elmer started walking daily for exercise and can now walk up to 1 mile without fatigue. He avoids all salty foods and diligently checks food labels for fat and salt content. Elmer occasionally drinks a glass of wine, although never more than 1 to 2 glasses per month. Although it was difficult for Elmer to stop smoking totally, he proudly claims he has been smokeless for 8 months.

Critical Thinking Questions

1. How would you respond to Elmer's question, "What else can I do?" Is there anything else he can do to reduce his blood pressure?

2. Elmer wants to know why the previous therapies were unsuccessful. What would you say as his nurse?

3. As the nurse, how can you support Elmer before he leaves the clinic?

See Answers to Critical Thinking Questions on student resource website.

NCLEX-RN® Review

1 Methyldopa (Aldomet) is being initiated for a client with hypertension. Which health teaching would be most appropriate for this drug?

1. Avoid hot baths and showers, and prolonged standing in one position.
2. This drug may discolor the urine a pinkish-brown color.
3. You may experience bloating and weight gain.
4. The tablet should be taken only with food or milk.

2 A client is receiving hydralazine (Apresoline) for elevated blood pressure levels. The nurse would include in the care plan to monitor the client for which adverse effects?

1. Atelectasis
2. Crystalluria
3. Photosensitivity
4. Orthostatic hypotension

3. The nurse determines that the client understands an important principle in self-administration of hydralazine (Apresoline) when the client makes which statement?

1. "I should not drive until the response to drug therapy is determined."

2. "I can stop taking this medication once I begin to feel better."

3. "If I experience dizziness, I should take only half the dose."

4. "I should avoid air travel while taking this medication."

4. A client with hypertensive crisis is started on nitroprusside (Nipride) therapy. The nurse would perform what priority intervention during the course of this treatment?

1. Monitor for the presence or absence of bowel sounds

2. Obtain urine samples for specific gravity measurements and glucose levels

3. Observe skin pressure points for turgor and integrity

4. Titrate intravenous infusion rate according to the blood pressure response

5. Methyldopa (Aldomet) has been associated with the development of antibodies (positive Coombs' test) in a significant number of clients. To determine if a client is developing a further complication associated with these antibodies, what will the nurse also monitor?

1. Red blood cell count

2. Cardiac output

3. Development of urticaria

4. Plasma drug levels

6. A client is receiving nitroprusside (Nipride) and is being monitored in the intensive care unit. Because of toxic cyanide metabolites that develop, which of the following should the nurse evaluate in the client? Select all that apply.

1. Cardiac status and cardiac output

2. Renal function and creatinine levels

3. Past history of alcohol use

4. Level of consciousness

5. Skin color and turgor

Additional Case Study

Helen Edwards is a 44-year-old African American woman who presents to the emergency department with headache and shortness of breath. Helen has a long-standing history of HTN. She has never consistently adhered to any HTN management strategies and has been nonadherent with her medication regimen for the past 8 months. Upon arrival at the emergency department her blood pressure is 192/126 mmHg.

When you assess the patient, it is noted that she is approximately 1.7 m (5'6") in height and the self-reported weight is 107 kg (235 lb). She is slightly lethargic and reports having left arm numbness and tingling. Other physical assessment parameters are normal.

Helen is started on an infusion of nitroprusside (Nipride) 50 mg in 250 mL in D$_5$W. The dose will be titrated between 0.5 to 10 mcg/kg/min to maintain the patient's diastolic pressure at less than 100 mmHg.

1. Describe the mechanism of action related to nitroprusside (Nipride).

2. For what adverse effects should you monitor in patients receiving this drug therapy?

3. What factors does this patient have that predisposes her to hypertensive crises?

See Answers to Additional Case Study on student resource website.

Pearson Nursing Student Resources

Find additional review materials at nursing.pearsonhighered.com

Prepare for success with additional NCLEX®-style practice questions, interactive assignments and activities, web links, animations, videos, and more!

References

American Heart Association. (2011). *High blood pressure statistics*. Retrieved from http://www.americanheart.org/presenter .jhtml?identifier=4621

Centers for Disease Control and Prevention. (2011). *High blood pressure facts*. Retrieved from http://www.cdc.gov/bloodpressure/ facts.htm

Hopkins, C. H. (2011). Hypertensive emergencies. *Medscape Reference*. Retrieved from http://www.emedicine.com/emerg/ TOPIC267.HTM

National Center for Complementary and Alternative Medicine. (2010). *Herbs at a glance: Grape seed extract*. Retrieved from http://nccam.nih.gov/health/grapeseed/ ataglance.htm

National Institutes of Health, National Heart, Lung, and Blood Institute, National High Blood Pressure Education Program Coordinating Committee. (2003). *JNC-7 express: The seventh report of the Joint National Committee on Prevention, Detection Evaluation and Treatment of High Blood Pressure*. Bethesda, MD: Author. Retrieved from http://www.nhlbi.nih.gov/guidelines/ hypertension/express.pdf

Seguin, B., Hardy, B., Singer, P. A., & Daar, A. S. (2008). BiDil: Reconceptualizing the race debate. *The Pharmacogenomics Journal*, *8*(3), 169–173. doi:10.1038/sj.tpj.6500489

Tam, S. W., Sabolinski, M. L., Worcel, M., Packer, M., & Cohn, J. N. (2007). Lack of bioequivalence between different formulations of isosorbide dinitrate and hydralazine and the fixed-dose combination of isosorbide dinitrate/hydralazine: The V-HeFT paradox. *Clinical Pharmacokinetics*, *46*(10), 885–895. doi:10.2165/00003088-200746100-00006

University of Maryland Medical Center (2010). *Grape seed*. Retrieved from http://www .umm.edu/altmed/articles/grape-seed-000254.htm

Selected Bibliography

Clark, C. E., Smith, L. F., Taylor, R. S., & Campbell, J. L. (2010). Nurse led interventions to improve control of blood pressure in people with hypertension: Systematic review and meta-analysis. *British Medical Journal*, *341*, c3995. doi:10.1136/bmj .c3995

Colbert, B. J., & Mason, B. J. (2012). *Integrated cardiopulmonary pharmacology* (3rd ed.). Upper Saddle River, NJ: Pearson Prentice Hall.

Hill, M. N., Miller, N. H., & DeGeest, S. (2010). Adherence and persistence with taking medication to control high blood pressure. *Journal of the American Society of Hypertension*, *5*(1), 56–63. doi:10.1016/ j.jash.2011.01.001

Israili, Z. H., Hernandez-Hernandez, R., & Valasco, M. (2007). The future of antihypertensive treatment. *American Journal of Therapeutics*, *14*(2), 121–134. doi:10.1097/ 01.pap.0000249915.12185.58

Jayasinghe, J. (2009). Non-adherence in the hypertensive patient: Can nursing play a role in assessing and improving compliance? *Canadian Journal of Cardiovascular Nursing*, *19*(1), 7–12.

Kotchen, T. A. (2010). The search for strategies to control hypertension. *Circulation*, *122*, 1141–1143. doi:10.1161/ CIRCULATIONAHA.110.978759

McLean, D. L. (2007). Nurses managing high blood pressure in patients with diabetes in community pharmacies. *Canadian Journal of Cardiovascular Nursing*, *17*(2), 17–21.

Michel, T., & Hoffman, B. B. (2011). Treatment of myocardial ischemia and hypertension. In L. L. Brunton, B. A. Chabner, & B. C. Knollman (Eds.), *The pharmacological basis of therapeutics* (12th ed., pp. 745–788). New York, NY: McGraw-Hill.

Ong, K. L., Cheung, B. M. Y., Man, Y. B., Lau, C. P., & Lam, K. S. L. (2007). Prevalence, awareness, treatment, and control of hypertension among United States adults 1999–2004. *Hypertension*, *49*(12), 69–75.

Touyz, R. M. (2011). Advancement in hypertension pathogenesis: Some new concepts. *Current Opinion in Nephrology & Hypertension*, *20*(2), 105–106. doi:10.1097/ MNH.0b013e328343f526

Answers to NCLEX-RN® Review

1 Answer: 1 Rationale: Hot baths and showers, prolonged standing in one position, and strenuous exercise may enhance orthostatic hypotension. Options 2, 3, and 4 are incorrect. Methyldopa does not discolor the urine. Bloating and weight gain are not typical adverse effects of methyldopa, and methyldopa can be taken without food. Cognitive Level: Applying; Client Need: Physiological Integrity; Nursing Process: Implementation

2 Answer: 4 Rationale: Orthostatic hypotension is a common adverse effect of vasodilators such as hydralazine. Options 1, 2, and 3 are incorrect. Hydralazine does not typically cause atelectasis. Crystalluria is not an adverse effect of hydralazine and it does not cause photosensitivity. Cognitive Level: Applying; Client Need: Physiological Integrity; Nursing Process: Planning

3 Answer: 1 Rationale: Clients who have recently been prescribed hydralazine may experience dizziness initially and should be instructed not to engage in activities that may be hazardous. Options 2, 3, and 4 are incorrect. Clients should always consult their health care providers before discontinuing antihypertensive medications. Clients should report dizziness to the health care provider, and should not adjust the dosage until the etiology of the problem is determined. Clients on this drug have no restriction on air travel. Cognitive Level: Analyzing; Client Need: Health Promotion and Maintenance; Nursing Process: Evaluation

4 Answer: 4 Rationale: The nurse will titrate (adjust) the rate of infusion based on the client's blood pressure. Options 1, 2, and 3 are incorrect. Listening for bowel sounds in the client with hypertensive crisis is not a nursing priority. Urine specific gravity and glucose levels may be obtained but are not associated with hypertensive crisis or the administration of this drug. Observing skin pressure points is a nursing intervention that does not directly relate to hypertensive crisis or nitroprusside therapy. Cognitive Level: Applying; Client Need: Physiological Integrity; Nursing Process: Implementation

5 Answer: 1 Rationale: The RBC count should be monitored periodically. Antibodies created by methyldopa, as noted on a Coombs' test, work against the client's own RBCs and, in a significant number of clients, results in hemolytic anemia. Options 2, 3, and 4 are incorrect. Cardiac output, development of urticaria, or plasma drug level will not provide an indication that hemolytic anemia is occurring. Cognitive Level: Analyzing; Client Need: Physiological Integrity; Nursing Process: Evaluation

6 Answer: 1, 2, 4 Rationale: Thiocyanate poisoning may develop more quickly in clients with impaired renal function. Renal function and creatinine levels should be evaluated before starting the drug. Signs of thiocyanate poisoning include hypotension, lethargy, unconsciousness, and faint heart sounds. Options 3 and 5 are incorrect. Past alcohol use will not determine whether thiocyanate poisoning develops or influences its symptoms. While flushing of the skin may occur with nitroprusside administration, skin color and turgor are not reliable indicators of thiocyanate poisoning. Cognitive Level: Analyzing; Client Need: Physiological Integrity; Nursing Process: Evaluation

Pharmacotherapy of Angina Pectoris and Myocardial Infarction

From Chapter 38 of *Pharmacology: Connections to Nursing Practice*, Second Edition. Michael Patrick Adams, Carol Quam Urban. Copyright © 2013 by Pearson Education, Inc. All rights reserved.

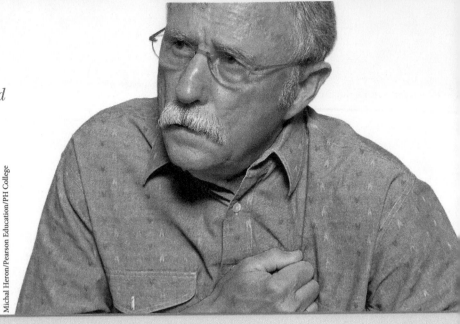

> *"I was simply sitting and reading the newspaper, when suddenly my chest felt tight, I felt weak, and I had difficulty breathing."*
>
> Patient "Michael Graff"

Michal Heron/Pearson Education/PH College

Pharmacotherapy of Angina Pectoris and Myocardial Infarction

Learning Outcomes

After reading this chapter, the student should be able to:

1. Describe factors that affect myocardial oxygen supply and demand.
2. Explain the relationship between atherosclerosis and coronary artery disease.
3. Explain the pathophysiology of angina pectoris and myocardial infarction.
4. Discuss the role of therapeutic lifestyle changes in the management of coronary artery disease.
5. Describe the pharmacologic management of the different types of angina.
6. Describe the pharmacologic management of myocardial infarction.
7. For each of the classes shown in the chapter outline, identify the prototype and representative drugs and explain the mechanism(s) of drug action, primary indications, contraindications, significant drug interactions, pregnancy category, and important adverse effects.
8. Apply the nursing process to care for patients receiving pharmacotherapy for angina and myocardial infarction.

Chapter Outline

Pathophysiology of Myocardial Ischemia

Etiology of Coronary Artery Disease

Pathophysiology of Angina Pectoris

Nonpharmacologic Therapy of Coronary Artery Disease

Pharmacologic Management of Angina Pectoris

Drug Classes for Angina Pectoris

Organic Nitrates

PROTOTYPE **Nitroglycerin (Nitrostat, Nitro-Bid, Nitro-Dur, Others)**

Beta-Adrenergic Blockers

PROTOTYPE **Atenolol (Tenormin)**

Calcium Channel Blockers

Pathophysiology of Myocardial Infarction

Pharmacologic Management of Myocardial Infarction

Thrombolytics and Adjunct Medications for Myocardial Infarction

The tissues of the body depend on a continuous supply of oxygen and vital nutrients to support life and health. The heart is particularly demanding of a steady source of oxygen. Insufficient arterial blood supply to cardiac muscle may result in angina pectoris, acute myocardial infarction (heart attack), and possibly death. This chapter focuses on the pharmacologic interventions related to angina pectoris and myocardial infarction (MI).

Pathophysiology of Myocardial Ischemia

1 Myocardial ischemia develops when there is inadequate blood supply to meet the metabolic demands of cardiac muscle.

Myocardial ischemia is a condition in which the heart is receiving an insufficient amount of oxygen to meet its metabolic demands. This occurs when there is an imbalance between oxygen supply and oxygen demand in myocardial cells. Knowledge of factors affecting myocardial oxygen supply and demand is necessary for understanding the pharmacotherapy of the diseases associated with myocardial ischemia.

Myocardial Oxygen Supply

The heart, from the moment it begins to function *in utero* until death, works to distribute oxygen and nutrients by means of its nonstop pumping action. It is the hardest working organ in the body, functioning continuously during both activity and rest. Because the heart is a muscle, it needs a steady supply of nourishment to sustain itself and maintain the systemic circulation in a balanced state of equilibrium. Any disturbance in blood flow to the myocardium—even for brief episodes—can result in life-threatening consequences.

As with other arteries in the body, the amount of blood flow through the coronary arteries is dependent on a number of hemodynamic factors. Of these, blood pressure is the most important. When systolic blood pressure falls, the quantity of blood flowing to the coronary arteries is diminished. If this occurs suddenly, such as in acute shock, it could be life threatening. Immediate restoration of blood pressure is required to reestablish an adequate oxygen supply to the myocardium, as well as to other vital tissues. Other important hemodynamic factors affecting the myocardial oxygen supply include changes in blood volume (e.g., hemorrhage) and disorders that reduce the oxygen content or carrying capacity of the blood (e.g., anemia).

The narrowing of a coronary artery resulting from atherosclerosis or coronary artery disease (CAD) deprives cells of needed oxygen and nutrients. If the narrowing develops over a long period of time, the heart compensates for its inadequate blood supply and the patient may be asymptomatic. Indeed, coronary arteries may be occluded as much as 50% or more and cause no symptoms.

Myocardial Oxygen Demand

As CAD progresses, cardiac muscle does not receive enough oxygen to meet the body's metabolic demands. The physiological demands on the heart are highly variable and depend on a large number of hemodynamic and lifestyle factors.

Basically, anything that increases the workload of the heart will increase myocardial oxygen demand. It is not difficult to think of the many daily activities that increase cardiac workload. Exercise, for example, will cause the heart to beat faster in order to pump more blood to muscles. This physical activity need not be extreme: Simply walking at a normal pace will increase cardiac workload over resting levels.

In some patients, the increased cardiac workload can be the result of mental, rather than physical, stressors. Think of the first time (or last time) you had to give a speech in front of a group, or became angry with a child, spouse, or coworker. These activities resulted in your heart pumping harder or faster, even though there was no physical activity involved. What factors do physical exercise and mental stress have in common that produced the increased cardiac workload?

The answer is simple. Anything that increases heart rate, contractility, or tension on the ventricular walls causes the heart to work harder. For example, if heart rate increases due to exercise or hyperthyroidism, it is easy to understand why the heart needs more oxygen because it must beat more times per minute. Similarly, the heart will need more oxygen if it beats more forcefully (increased contractility). A patient with heart failure (HF) has a thickened myocardium (increased tension) that will require more work to contract. The heart of a hypertensive patient will have to work harder to eject blood. It is important to remember that anything that makes the heart beat faster or contract with more force will increase myocardial oxygen demand. Drugs that diminish these factors are of value in the treatment of angina, MI, and HF.

Etiology of Coronary Artery Disease

2 Coronary artery disease is the major cause of myocardial ischemia.

Coronary artery disease (CAD) is one of the leading causes of mortality in the United States. The primary defining characteristic of CAD is narrowing or occlusion of one or more coronary arteries. Narrowing can result in symptoms of angina pectoris, whereas occlusion results in MI. The two disorders are closely related, as most patients who experience an MI have narrowing of the coronary vessels.

The most common etiology of CAD in adults is **atherosclerosis**, the presence of **plaque**—a fatty, fibrous material—within the walls of the coronary arteries. Plaque develops progressively over time, producing varying degrees of intravascular narrowing, a situation that results in partial or total blockage of the vessel. During periods of rest, demands on the

Key Terms

angina pectoris

atherosclerosis

coronary artery disease (CAD)

glycoprotein IIb/IIIa

myocardial infarctions (MIs)

myocardial ischemia

nitric oxide

partial fatty-acid oxidation inhibitors

plaque

silent angina

stable angina

unstable angina

vasospastic (Prinzmetal's) angina

229

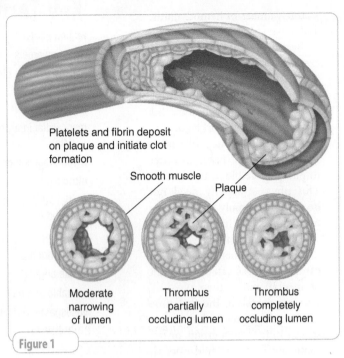

Platelets and fibrin deposit
on plaque and initiate clot
formation

Smooth muscle

Plaque

Moderate	Thrombus	Thrombus
narrowing	partially	completely
of lumen	occluding lumen	occluding lumen

Figure 1

Atherosclerosis in the coronary arteries.

heart are less and a partially occluded artery may be able to provide adequate oxygen. During exercise (or a pharmacology test), however, workload on the heart increases, the cardiac muscle distal to the obstruction receives insufficient oxygen supply, and ischemia results.

A healthy heart responds to stress by changing the diameter of the coronary arteries. Thus, when the oxygen demands of the heart increase, the vessels respond immediately by dilating to bring more oxygen to the myocardium. Plaque impairs normal elasticity, and the coronary vessels are unable to dilate properly when the myocardium demands additional oxygen. Myocardial ischemia occurs when cardiac demands exceed the amount of oxygen that can be supplied through the narrowed, inelastic vessels characteristic of CAD.

Plaque accumulation occurs gradually, over periods of 40 to 50 years in some individuals, but actually begins to accrue very early in life. The development of atherosclerosis is illustrated in Figure 1.

CONNECTION Checkpoint 38.1

Predict what would happen to the cardiac workload when plasma volume is increased by an infusion of normal saline. What effect might this have on a patient with CAD? *See Answer to Connection Checkpoint 38.1 on student resource website.*

Pathophysiology of Angina Pectoris

3 Angina pectoris is characterized by severe chest pain brought on by physical exertion or emotional stress.

Angina pectoris is acute chest pain caused by myocardial ischemia. The classic presentation of angina pectoris is steady, intense pain, sometimes with a crushing sensation in the anterior chest. Typically, the discomfort radiates to the left shoulder and proceeds down the left arm. It may also extend to the posterior thoracic region or move upward to the jaw, and in some patients the pain is experienced in the epigastrium or abdominal area. Accompanying the discomfort is severe emotional distress—a feeling of panic with fear of impending death. There is usually pallor, dyspnea with cyanosis, diaphoresis, tachycardia, and elevated blood pressure.

Anginal pain is usually precipitated by physical exertion or emotional excitement—events associated with increased myocardial oxygen demand. Angina pectoris episodes are of short duration. With physical rest and mental relaxation, the workload demands upon the heart diminish and the discomfort subsides within 5 to 10 minutes. Descriptions of the four basic types of angina follow.

When angina occurrences are fairly predictable in frequency, intensity, and duration, the condition is described as classic or **stable angina**. Rest usually relieves the pain associated with stable angina.

Vasospastic (Prinzmetal's) angina occurs when the decreased myocardial blood flow is caused by spasms of the coronary arteries. The vessels undergoing spasms may or may not contain atherosclerotic plaque. Thus, the primary cause of the narrowing and subsequent angina pain is vasoconstriction, rather than plaque buildup in the artery. Vasospastic angina pain occurs most often during periods of rest, although it may occur unpredictably, unrelated to rest or activity.

Although most people equate angina with chest pain, this is not always the case. When myocardial ischemia occurs in the absence of pain, it is called **silent angina**. Although one or more coronary arteries are partially occluded, the patient is asymptomatic. Some patients diagnosed with stable angina also experience silent angina. Although the mechanisms underlying silent angina are not completely understood, the condition is associated with a high risk for acute MI and sudden death.

Unstable angina occurs when episodes of angina occur suddenly, have added intensity, and occur during periods of rest. Unstable angina is a type of acute coronary syndrome in which an atherosclerotic plaque within a coronary artery ruptures. A thrombus quickly builds on the displaced plaque, and the artery becomes at serious risk of occlusion. This condition is a medical emergency requiring aggressive intervention because it is associated with an increased risk for MI.

Anginal pain often parallels the signs and symptomatology of MI. It is extremely important that the nurse be able to accurately identify the characteristics that differentiate the two conditions, since the pharmacologic interventions related to angina differ considerably from those of MI. Angina, while aggravating and uncomfortable, rarely leads to a fatal outcome and the chest pain is usually immediately relieved by nitroglycerin. MI, however, carries with it a high mortality rate if appropriate treatment is delayed (Section 9). In the event of MI, pharmacologic intervention must be initiated immediately and systematically maintained. When a patient presents with chest pain, the foremost objective for the health care provider is to quickly determine the cause of the pain so that proper, effective interventions can be delivered.

Nonpharmacologic Therapy of Coronary Artery Disease

4 Therapeutic lifestyle changes can decrease the frequency of anginal episodes and reduce the risk of coronary artery disease.

A combination of variables influences the development and progression of angina, including dietary patterns and lifestyle choices. The nurse is instrumental in teaching patients the means of preventing CAD, as well as how to lower the rate of recurrence of anginal episodes. Such support includes the formulation of a comprehensive plan of care that incorporates psychosocial support and an individualized teaching plan. The patient needs to understand the causes of angina, identify the conditions and situations that trigger it, and develop the motivation to modify behaviors associated with their disease.

Listing therapeutic lifestyle changes that modify the development and progression of cardiovascular disease (CVD) may seem repetitious, as these same factors have been included in chapters on hypertension (HTN) and heart disease. However, the importance of prevention and management of CVD through nonpharmacologic means cannot be overemphasized. Making healthy lifestyle choices can prevent CAD in many individuals, and slow the progression of the disease in those who have existing plaque. The following interventions have been shown to reduce the incidence of CAD:

- Limit alcohol consumption to small or moderate amounts.
- Eliminate foods high in cholesterol or saturated fats.
- Keep blood cholesterol and other lipid indicators within the normal ranges.
- Keep blood pressure within the normal range.
- Maintain blood glucose levels within the normal range.
- Exercise regularly and maintain optimum weight.
- Do not use tobacco.

When the patient is unable or unwilling to adopt healthy lifestyle choices, preventive drug therapy may be used to lower CAD risk factors. For example, antihypertensives are often used to manage blood pressure, statins to lower blood lipids, and insulin or oral hypoglycemics to keep blood glucose within the normal range. The nurse should teach patients that therapeutic lifestyle changes should be incorporated into their daily routine, even if medications are necessary to control major risk factors.

Pharmacologic Management of Angina Pectoris

5 The pharmacologic management of angina includes organic nitrates, beta-adrenergic blockers, and calcium channel blockers.

There are several desired therapeutic goals for a patient receiving pharmacotherapy for angina. A primary goal is to reduce the frequency and intensity of angina episodes. Additionally, successful pharmacotherapy should improve exercise tolerance and allow the patient to actively participate in activities of daily living. Long-term goals include extending the patient's life span by preventing the serious consequences of ischemic heart disease such as dysrhythmias, HF, and MI. Pharmacotherapy alone, however, cannot usually achieve these outcomes; the patient must be willing to implement therapeutic lifestyle changes that promote a healthy heart.

Medications for angina are sometimes placed into two categories: those that terminate an acute angina episode in progress, and those that decrease the frequency of angina episodes.

CONNECTIONS: Complementary and Alternative Therapies — Omega-3 Fatty Acids

Description: Omega-3 fatty acids are unsaturated fats found in fatty fish such as salmon, mackerel, and tuna; vegetable oils such as canola and soybean; and nuts, green leafy vegetables, and beans. Omega-3 fatty acids are essential to the body and necessary for regulating muscle function, blood clotting, digestion, cell growth, and other functions (National Center for Complementary and Alternative Medicine, 2010).

History and Claims: Omega-3 fatty acids have been claimed to reduce inflammation and prevent or treat conditions such as heart disease, high blood pressure, rheumatoid arthritis, lupus, asthma, inflammatory bowel disease, and cancer.

Standardization: There are different types of omega-3 fatty acids: alpha-linolenic acid (ALA), eicosapentaenoic acid (EPA), and docosahexaenoic acid (DHA). While a balance of omega-3 and omega-6 fatty acids in the diet is important, the average U.S. diet tends to contain as much as 10 to 25 times more omega-6 than omega-3, due in large part to the consumption of meats that are higher in omega-6. Doses of less than 3 g per day of omega-3 fatty acids are usually recommended to prevent GI side effects such as diarrhea. The American Heart Association has recommended up to 4 g for patients with high lipid levels and 1 g daily for patients with coronary artery disease (University of Maryland Medical Center, 2010).

Evidence: Research has shown that omega-3 fatty acids may reduce the incidence of cardiovascular disease. In some research studies, patients have shown improvement in lipid levels, and in inflammatory conditions such as rheumatoid arthritis or inflammatory bowel disease. Larger studies need to be conducted however, to determine the extent of such benefits. (Office of Dietary Supplements, National Institutes of Health n.d.). While obtaining omega-3 fatty acids through dietary means is highly recommended, concern about mercury levels in fatty fish has recently been raised, and the American Heart Association (2010) recommends that pregnant women and children avoid eating fish with the potential for high mercury levels, for example, tuna, shark, and swordfish.

The primary means by which antianginal medications act is by reducing the myocardial demand for oxygen. This may be accomplished by the following mechanisms:

- Slowing the heart rate
- Dilating veins so that the heart receives less blood (reduced preload)
- Causing the heart to contract with less force (reduced contractility)
- Lowering blood pressure (reduced afterload)

The pharmacotherapy of angina uses three primary classes of drugs: organic nitrates, beta-adrenergic blockers, and calcium channel blockers (CCBs). Rapid-acting organic nitrates are drugs of choice for *terminating* an acute angina episode. Beta-adrenergic blockers are first-line drugs for *prophylactic* treatment. CCBs are used when beta blockers are not tolerated well by a patient. Long-acting nitrates, given by the oral (PO) or transdermal routes, are alternatives for prophylaxis. Persistent angina requires drugs from two or more classes, such as a beta blocker combined with a long-acting nitrate or a CCB. Pharmacotherapy Illustrated 1

illustrates the mechanisms of action of medications used to prevent and treat CAD.

Approved in 2006, ranolazine (Ranexa) belongs to a class of drugs called **partial fatty-acid oxidation inhibitors**. Although its exact mechanism is not known, ranolazine is believed to act by shifting the metabolism of cardiac muscle cells so that they utilize glucose as the primary energy source rather than fatty acids. This decreases the metabolic rate and oxygen demands of myocardial cells. Thus, this is the only antianginal that acts through its metabolic effects, rather than hemodynamic effects. Effects on heart rate and blood pressure are minimal. The drug is only approved for chronic angina that has not responded to other agents. Another drug in this class, trimetazidine, is used in Europe to treat angina but has not received FDA approval in the United States.

CONNECTION Checkpoint 38.2

Many patients take HMG-CoA reductase inhibitors (statins) concurrently with antianginal medications. What is the rationale for prescribing drugs from this class for a patient with CAD? *See Answer to Connection Checkpoint 38.2 on student resource website.*

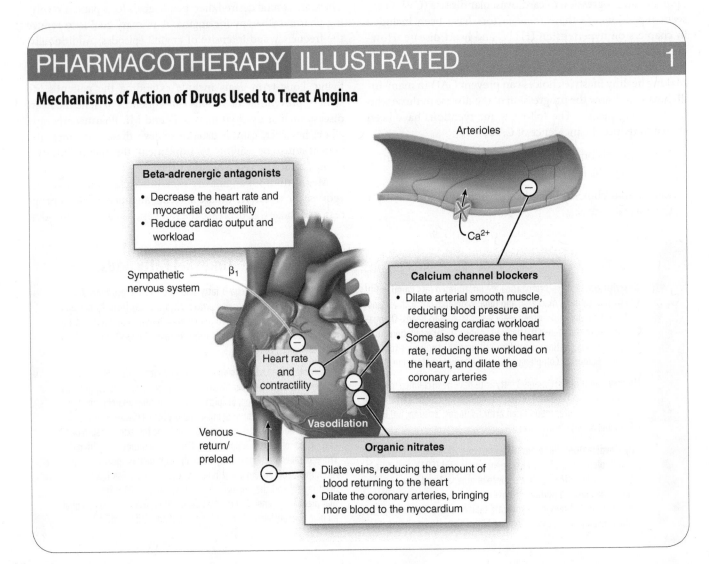

PHARMACOTHERAPY ILLUSTRATED   1

Mechanisms of Action of Drugs Used to Treat Angina

Arterioles

Beta-adrenergic antagonists

- Decrease the heart rate and myocardial contractility
- Reduce cardiac output and workload

Ca^{2+}

Sympathetic nervous system β_1

Calcium channel blockers

- Dilate arterial smooth muscle, reducing blood pressure and decreasing cardiac workload
- Some also decrease the heart rate, reducing the workload on the heart, and dilate the coronary arteries

Heart rate and contractility

Venous return/ preload

Vasodilation

Organic nitrates

- Dilate veins, reducing the amount of blood returning to the heart
- Dilate the coronary arteries, bringing more blood to the myocardium

Drug Classes for Angina Pectoris

6 Organic nitrates may be used to terminate or prevent angina episodes.

After their medicinal properties were discovered in 1857, the organic nitrates became the mainstay for the treatment of angina for the next 100 years. Their mechanism of action results from the formation of **nitric oxide** in vascular smooth muscle. Nitric oxide is an important cell-signaling molecule and a potent vasodilator, causing relaxation of both arterial and venous smooth muscle. Dilation of veins reduces the amount of blood returning to the heart (preload), and the chambers contain a smaller volume. With less blood for the ventricles to pump, cardiac output is reduced and the workload on the heart is decreased, thereby lowering myocardial oxygen demand. The therapeutic outcome is that chest pain is alleviated and episodes of angina become less frequent. The organic nitrates are listed in Table 1.

Organic nitrates also have the ability to dilate coronary arteries, which was once thought to be their primary mechanism of action. It seems logical that dilating a partially occluded coronary vessel would allow more oxygen to reach ischemic tissue. While this effect does indeed occur, it is no longer considered the primary mechanism of nitrate action in the treatment of stable angina. Coronary artery vasodilation, however, is crucial in treating vasospastic angina, in which the chest pain is caused by coronary artery spasm. The organic nitrates relax these spasms, allowing more oxygen to reach the myocardium, thereby terminating the pain.

Organic nitrates are classified by their onset and duration of action. The short-acting nitrates, such as nitroglycerin, may be taken sublingually or as an oral spray or buccal tablet to quickly terminate an acute anginal episode. Long-acting nitrates, such as isosorbide dinitrate (Isordil), are taken orally or are absorbed slowly through a transdermal patch to decrease the frequency and severity of angina episodes. Long-acting organic nitrates are occasionally used to treat symptoms of HF.

Tolerance is a common and potentially serious problem with the long-acting organic nitrates. The magnitude of the tolerance depends on the dosage and the frequency of drug administration. Although tolerance develops rapidly—as quickly as 24 hours after the initiation of therapy in some patients—it also disappears rapidly when the drug is withheld. Patients are often instructed to remove the transdermal patch for 6 to 12 hours each day or withhold a nighttime dose of the

TABLE 1 Administration of Organic Nitrates	
Route	**Administration**
Sublingual tablet	• Give 1 tablet. If pain is unrelieved, may give additional tablets at 5-min intervals up to 3 tablets in a 15-min period. • Moisture on sublingual tissue is necessary for the sublingual tablet to dissolve. A patient may be unresponsive to sublingual nitroglycerin, as the anxiety caused by chest pain typically leads to dry mouth.
Sustained-release buccal tablet	• Place 1 tablet between lip and gum above incisors or between cheek and gum. Allow to slowly dissolve over 3–5 h. • Avoid touching tongue to tablet or drinking hot fluids, as these can increase dissolving of the tablet, decrease duration of the medicinal effect, and lead to the onset of angina pain. • Avoid chewing, crushing, or swallowing the tablet.
Sustained-release tablet or capsule	• Give on an empty stomach with a full glass of water 1 h before, or 2 h after, meals. The tablet should be swallowed whole. • Note that the sustained-release form helps to prevent angina attacks but is not intended for immediate relief of angina. • Avoid chewing or crushing the tablet.
Translingual spray	• Avoid shaking medicine canister. Spray on or under the tongue. Never inhale spray. • Repeat spray every 5 minutes if needed for a maximum of 3 metered doses. • Teach the patient to avoid swallowing for at least 10 sec.
Transdermal ointment	• Avoid touching ointment with fingers. Squeeze the prescribed dosage onto the dose-determining applicator (paper application patch) in the medication package. Spread ointment in a thin, even layer to premarked 5.5- by 9-cm (2 1/4- by 3 1/2-in.) square. Place patch with ointment side down onto nonhairy skin surface such as the forearm, chest, abdomen, or anterior thigh. Cover with transparent wrap and secure with tape. • Rotate application sites to prevent skin inflammation and sensitization. Remove any residual ointment before reapplication. • Keep medication container closed and stored in a cool place. • Contact with water, such as in swimming or bathing, does not affect the transdermal patch.
Transdermal unit	• Apply transdermal patch at the same time each day to nonhairy or closely trimmed area without excessive movement. • Avoid application on irritated or scarred skin. • Rotate application site each time to prevent skin irritation and sensitization.
Intravenous (IV)	• Verify with health care provider the correct IV concentration, rate of infusion, and use the supplied IV tubing for administration. • Remove any existing transdermal or ointment in place on the patient before starting IV infusion to prevent overdosage. • Note that IV nitroglycerin can cause hypotension, so give with extreme caution to patients with preexisting hypotension or hypovolemia. • Monitor patient closely for any change in levels of consciousness and for dysrhythmias, because IV nitroglycerin contains a substantial amount of ethanol as a diluent. Ethanol intoxication with symptoms of nausea, vomiting, coma, lethargy, and alcohol breath can occur with high doses of IV nitroglycerin. Stop infusion if intoxication occurs. The patient should recover immediately when drug administration is discontinued.

oral medications in order to delay the development of tolerance. Because the oxygen demands of the heart during sleep are diminished, the patient with stable angina experiences few angina episodes during this drug-free interval.

Most adverse effects of the organic nitrates are extensions of their hypotensive action. Flushing of the face and headache are common effects, secondary to vasodilation. Orthostatic hypotension is a frequent adverse effect of this drug class, and patients should be advised to change positions gradually to prevent lightheadedness. Blood pressure should be carefully monitored, and the nurse should hold nitrates and remove topical forms if serious hypotension is discovered. Taking organic nitrates concurrently with alcohol may cause severe hypotension and even cardiovascular collapse.

An additional adverse effect that can be limiting in some patients is reflex tachycardia. When the organic nitrates dilate vessels and blood pressure falls, the baroreceptor reflex is triggered. Sympathetic stimulation of the heart increases heart rate and contractility, which are undesirable effects in a patient with angina. This adverse effect is often transient and asymptomatic. Patients who report significant palpitations may be administered a beta blocker, which will prevent the reflex cardiac stimulation.

PROTOTYPE DRUG | Nitroglycerin (Nitrostat, Nitro-Bid, Nitro-Dur, Others)

Classification: **Therapeutic:** Antianginal drug
Pharmacologic: Organic nitrate, vasodilator

Therapeutic Effects and Uses: Nitroglycerin, the oldest and most widely used organic nitrate, can be delivered by a number of different routes: sublingual, lingual spray, PO, intravenous (IV), transmucosal, transdermal, topical, and extended release forms. The rapid-acting forms may be taken while an acute angina episode is in progress or just prior to physical activity. When given sublingually, it reaches peak plasma levels within minutes, thus quickly terminating angina pain. Chest pain that does not respond within 10 to 15 minutes after two or three doses of sublingual nitroglycerin may indicate MI, and emergency medical services (EMS) should be contacted. The transdermal and oral sustained release forms are for prophylaxis only, since they have a relatively slow onset of action. The long-acting forms should be discontinued gradually because vasospasm may result if they are abruptly withheld.

There are indications for nitroglycerin other than angina. When administered by the IV route, the drug is approved for controlled hypotension induction during anesthesia, and the treatment of HF, acute pulmonary edema, acute MI, severe HTN, or hypertensive emergency. Off-label indications include use as a uterine relaxant to aid in the extraction of a retained placenta and for pain associated with anal fissures or hemorrhoids.

Mechanism of Action: Upon reaching vascular smooth muscle, nitroglycerin forms nitric oxide, which triggers a cascade resulting in the release of calcium ions in smooth muscle. Nitroglycerin relaxes both arterial and venous smooth muscle.

The venous dilation decreases the amount of blood returning to the heart, reducing preload. With less blood for the ventricles to pump, myocardial oxygen demand is decreased. In addition, direct vasodilation of coronary arteries enhances the blood supply to the myocardium, and is partially responsible for its therapeutic effects.

Pharmacokinetics:

Route(s)	PO: sublingual tablets, sublingual spray, buccal tablets; transdermal patch, topical ointment
Absorption	Rapid
Distribution	Widely distributed; 60% bound to plasma protein
Primary metabolism	Hepatic; extensive first-pass metabolism
Primary excretion	Renal
Onset of action	Sublingual: 1–3 min; buccal: 2–5 min; transdermal patch: 40–60 min; topical ointment: 20–60 min
Duration of action	Sublingual: 30–60 min; buccal: 2 h; transdermal patch: 18–24 h; topical ointment: 12 h

Adverse Effects: Most patients experience flushing of the face and a throbbing, transient headache, which result from the drug's vasodilation action. Orthostatic hypotension and syncope may occur. Stinging and rash may occur with ointments and transdermal patches. Methemoglobinemia is a rare adverse effect that can cause shock and coma. Anaphylaxis leading to circulatory collapse due to severe hypotension is rare. Tolerance develops with continuous therapy or large doses of the drug.

Contraindications/Precautions: Nitrates are contraindicated in patients with preexisting hypotension, shock, head injury with increased intracranial pressure, or head trauma because additive vasodilation would worsen these conditions. Drugs in this class are contraindicated in pericardial tamponade and constrictive pericarditis because the heart is unable to increase cardiac output to maintain blood pressure when the drug causes vasodilation. Sustained release forms of the medicine should not be given to patients with glaucoma because the drug may increase intraocular pressure. Nitroglycerin should be used cautiously in patients with severe liver or renal disease, as the drug could build to toxic levels. Dehydration or hypovolemia should be corrected before nitroglycerin is administered; otherwise serious hypotension may result.

Drug Interactions: Concurrent use with sildenafil (Viagra) or other phosphodiesterase-5 inhibitors may cause life-threatening hypotension and cardiovascular collapse. Nitrates should not be taken within 24 hours before or after taking these drugs. Concurrent use with ethanol, CCBs, antidepressants, phenothiazines, or antihypertensive drugs may cause additive hypotension. Sympathomimetics such as epinephrine will antagonize the vasodilation effects of nitroglycerin. **Herbal/Food:** Use with hawthorn may result in additive hypotension.

Pregnancy: Category C.

Treatment of Overdose: During overdose, hypotension may be reversed with the IV administration of normal saline. If methemoglobinemia is suspected, methylene blue may be administered.

Nursing Responsibilities: Key nursing implications for patients receiving nitroglycerin are included in the Nursing Practice Application for Patients Receiving Organic Nitrate Therapy for Angina.

Lifespan and Diversity Considerations:

- Use caution when administering the drug to the older adult who is at greater risk for hypotension, dizziness, and falls. Provide assistance with ambulation as needed.
- Due to differences in reporting pain, use subjective and objective data when evaluating pain relief from nitroglycerin in ethnically diverse and older adult patients.

Patient and Family Education:

- At the earliest sign of oncoming angina pain, sit or lie down and take the drug. Stop any activity that may have caused the onset of chest pain.
- Pain unrelieved by three sublingual tablets over a 15-minute period (one tablet every 5 minutes) may indicate a heart attack. Call the EMS within the community (911).
- Tablets can cause a sweet-tasting, tingling, or burning feeling under the tongue, which is normal.
- Do not breast-feed while taking this drug without approval of the health care provider.

Drugs Similar to Nitroglycerin
(Nitrostat, Nitro-Bid, Nitro-Dur, Others)

Other organic nitrates include isosorbide dinitrate and isosorbide mononitrate. Another older drug in this class, amyl nitrite, is given by the inhalation route but is rarely used for angina.

Isosorbide dinitrate (Dilatrate SR, Isordil): Approved in 1961, isosorbide dinitrate is an organic nitrate used to terminate anginal attacks (sublingual) and for the prophylaxis of angina (sustained release tablets). It is occasionally used to treat HF. The dosing schedule must allow for a drug-free period of at least 14 hours to prevent tolerance to the drug's effects. The PO forms of the drug should not be used to terminate angina attacks in progress because it takes as long as 60 minutes to reach therapeutic drug levels. Adverse effects are similar to those of nitroglycerin. A fixed-dose combination of isosorbide dinitrate with hydralazine (BiDil) was approved in 2005 to reduce morbidity and mortality associated with HF. This drug is pregnancy category C.

Isosorbide mononitrate (Imdur, Ismo, Monoket): Approved in 1991, isosorbide mononitrate is an active, long-acting metabolite of isosorbide dinitrate. The mononitrate is only used for prophylaxis: Its 30-60 minute onset of action makes it unacceptable for termination of acute anginal pain. The dosing schedule must allow for a drug-free period of at least 7 hours to prevent the development of tolerance to the drug's effects. It is available in tablet form only. Imdur is an extended release form of the drug that permits once-daily dosing. Adverse effects are the same as the other organic nitrates. This drug is pregnancy category C.

7 Beta-adrenergic blockers are sometimes drugs of choice for stable angina.

Beta-adrenergic antagonists or blockers decrease cardiac workload by lowering blood pressure, slowing heart rate, and reducing contractility. These actions on the heart are particularly beneficial during exercise. Beta blockers are as effective as the organic nitrates in decreasing the frequency and severity of anginal episodes caused by exertion. For the pharmacotherapy of CAD, cardioselective beta$_1$ antagonists are preferred over nonselective beta antagonists because they are less likely to cause bronchoconstriction (a beta$_2$ response). Beta-adrenergic antagonists are not effective for treating vasospastic angina and may, in fact, worsen this condition.

Beta-adrenergic blockers offer several advantages over the organic nitrates. Tolerance does not develop to the antianginal effects of the beta blockers during prolonged therapy. They possess antidysrhythmic properties, which help prevent cardiac conduction abnormalities that are common complications of patients with ischemic heart disease. Beta blockers are ideal for patients who have both HTN and CAD due to their antihypertensive action. They have also been shown to reduce the incidence of MI. Because of these cardioprotective actions, beta blockers are considered drugs of choice for the prophylaxis of chronic angina. The beta blockers used for angina are listed in Table 1. Beta blockers are widely used in medicine.

Beta-adrenergic antagonists are well tolerated by most patients. In some patients, fatigue, lethargy, and depression are reasons for discontinuation of beta-blocker therapy. At high doses, drugs in this class can cause shortness of breath and respiratory distress due to bronchoconstriction, and they should be used cautiously in patients with asthma or chronic obstructive pulmonary disease (COPD). Because beta blockers slow the heart rate and myocardial conduction velocity, they are contraindicated in patients with bradycardia and greater than first-degree heart block. Heart rate should be closely monitored so that it does not fall below 50 to 60 beats/minute at rest or 100 beats/minute during exercise. Beta blockers are also contraindicated in cardiogenic shock and overt cardiac failure.

Patients with diabetes who are prescribed beta blockers should be aware that the actions of beta blockers can obscure the initial symptoms of hypoglycemia (palpitations, diaphoresis, and nervousness). Because of this, blood glucose levels should be monitored more frequently, and insulin doses may need to be adjusted accordingly.

Beta-adrenergic antagonists should never be abruptly discontinued. With long-term beta blocker use, the heart becomes more sensitive to catecholamines, which are blocked by these medications. When withdrawn abruptly, adrenergic receptors are activated and rebound excitation occurs. In patients with CAD, this can exacerbate angina, precipitate tachycardia, or cause an MI.

CONNECTIONS: NURSING PRACTICE APPLICATION

Patients Receiving Organic Nitrate Therapy for Angina

Assessment	Potential Nursing Diagnoses
Baseline assessment prior to administration: • Understand the reason the drug has been prescribed in order to assess for therapeutic effects. • Obtain a complete health history: cardiovascular (including previous MI, HF, valvular disease), cerebrovascular and neurologic (including level of consciousness, history of stroke, head injury, increased intracranial pressure), renal or hepatic dysfunction, dysrhythmias, pregnancy, or lactation. Obtain a drug history including allergies, current prescription and over-the-counter (OTC) drugs, herbal preparations, and alcohol use. Be aware that use of erectile dysfunction drugs (e.g., sildenafil [Viagra], vardenafil [Levitra], or tadalafil [Cialis]) within the past 24 to 48 h may cause profound and prolonged hypotension when nitrates are administered. Be alert to possible drug interactions. • Obtain baseline weight, vital signs (especially blood pressure and pulse), and ECG. Assess for location and character of angina if currently present. • Evaluate appropriate laboratory findings, electrolytes, renal function studies, and lipid profiles. Troponin and/or CK-MB laboratory values may be ordered to rule out MI. • Assess the patient's ability to receive and understand instructions. Include family and caregivers as needed.	• *Decreased Cardiac Output* • *Acute Pain* • *Fatigue* • *Activity Intolerance* • *Deficient Knowledge* (Drug Therapy) • *Risk for Decreased Cardiac Tissue Perfusion*, related to adverse effects of drug therapy • *Risk for Falls*, related to adverse effects of drug therapy • *Risk for Injury*, related to adverse effects of drug therapy
Assessment throughout administration: • Assess for desired therapeutic effects (e.g., chest pain has subsided or has significantly lessened), heart rate and blood pressure remain within normal limits, ECG remains within normal limits without signs of ischemia or infarction. • Continue periodic monitoring of ECG for ischemia or infarct. • Continue frequent monitoring of blood pressure and pulse whenever IV nitrates are used or when giving rapid-acting (e.g., sublingual) nitrates. With sublingual nitrates, take blood pressure before and 5 min after giving dose and hold the drug if blood pressure is less than 90/60 mmHg, pulse over 100 beats/min, or parameters as ordered, and check with the health care provider before continuing to give the drug. • Assess for and promptly report adverse effects: severe hypotension, dysrhythmias, reflex tachycardia (from too rapid decrease in blood pressure or severe hypotension), headache that does not subside within 15–20 min, or when accompanied by neurologic changes or decreased urinary output. Immediately report severe hypotension, seizures, dysrhythmias, or palpitations. Chest pain remaining present after three sublingual nitroglycerin tablets given 5 min apart should be reported immediately, even if pain has lessened, as this may be a sign of impending ischemia or infarction.	

Planning: Patient Goals and Expected Outcomes

The patient will:

• Experience therapeutic effects dependent on the reason the drug is being given (e.g., angina subsides or substantially diminishes, heart rate and blood pressure remain within established parameters, and ECG within normal limits).
• Be free from or experience minimal adverse effects.
• Verbalize an understanding of the drug's use, adverse effects, and required precautions.
• Demonstrate proper self-administration of the medication (e.g., dose, timing, and when to notify the provider).

Implementation

Interventions and (Rationales)	Patient-Centered Care
Ensuring therapeutic effects: • Continue frequent assessments as above for therapeutic effects. (Because nitrates cause vasodilation, preload and afterload diminish, decreasing myocardial oxygenation needs, and chest pain diminishes.)	• Ask the patient to briefly describe the location and character of pain (use a pain rating scale for rapid assessment) prior to and after giving nitrates to assess for extent of relief. Correlate with objective assessment findings.
• Continue to monitor ECG, blood pressure, and pulse. (Nitrates cause vasodilation and possible hypotension. Blood pressure assessment aids in determining drug frequency and dose. ECG monitoring helps detect adverse effects such as reflex tachycardia, ischemia, or infarction.)	• Teach the patient, family, or caregiver how to monitor pulse and blood pressure. Ensure proper use and functioning of any home equipment obtained.

CONNECTIONS: NURSING PRACTICE APPLICATION (continued)

* Evaluate the need for adjunctive treatment with the health care provider for angina prevention and treatment (e.g., beta blockers, aspirin therapy) or further cardiac studies. (Patients with unstable angina may require adjunctive drug therapy or definitive cardiac studies to determine the need for other treatment options.)

* Encourage the patient to discuss any changes in character, severity, or frequency of angina episodes with the health care provider. Instruct the patient not to take routine (daily) aspirin without discussing with the provider first, because the drug may be contraindicated depending on other conditions or medications.

* For patients on transdermal nitroglycerin patches, remove patch for 6–12 h at night, or as directed by the health care provider. (Removing the transdermal patch at night helps prevent or delay the development of tolerance to nitrates. Removing the patch at night, when cardiac workload is lessened helps avoid possible anginal attacks during the daytime when workload is greater.)

* Instruct the patient on proper use of nitroglycerin and the rationale for removing transdermal patches. Also instruct patients on transdermal patches to always remove the old patch, cleanse the skin underneath gently, and to rotate sites before applying a new patch.

* Encourage appropriate lifestyle changes: lowered fat intake, restricted sodium or fluid intake if ordered, gradually increased levels of exercise, limited alcohol intake, and smoking cessation. Provide for dietitian consultation as needed. (Healthy lifestyle changes will support the benefits of drug therapy.)

* Encourage the patient, family, and caregivers to adopt a healthy lifestyle of low-fat food choices, increased exercise, decreased alcohol consumption, and smoking cessation. Provide educational materials on low-fat, low-sodium food choices.

Minimizing adverse effects:

* Continue to monitor vital signs frequently. Be particularly cautious with older adults who are at increased risk for hypotension, patients with a preexisting history of cardiac or cerebrovascular disease, or patients with a recent head injury, which may be worsened by vasodilation. Notify the health care provider immediately if angina remains unrelieved or if blood pressure or pulse decrease beyond established parameters, or if hypotension is accompanied by reflex tachycardia. (Nitrates may cause significant vasodilation, resulting in the potential for hypotension accompanied by reflex tachycardia. Reflex tachycardia increases myocardial oxygen demand, worsening angina.)

* Instruct the patient, family, or caregiver to report dizziness, faintness, palpitations, or headache unrelieved after taking nonnarcotic analgesics (e.g., acetaminophen).
* Instruct the patient on nitrates to rise from lying to sitting or standing slowly to avoid dizziness or falls, especially if taking sublingual nitrates, or until drug effects are known.

* Continue cardiac monitoring (e.g., ECG) as ordered if IV nitrates are administered. (Monitoring devices assist in detecting early signs of adverse effects of drug therapy, myocardial ischemia or infarction, as well as monitoring for therapeutic effects.)

* To allay possible anxiety, teach the patient, family, or caregiver the rationale for all equipment used and the need for frequent monitoring.

* Continue frequent physical assessments, particularly neurologic, cardiac, and respiratory. Immediately report any changes in level of consciousness, headache, or changes in heart or lung sounds. (Nitrate therapy may worsen preexisting neurologic, cardiac, or respiratory conditions as blood pressure drops and perfusion to vital organs diminishes. Lung congestion may signal impending HF.)

* When on PO therapy at home, the patient, family, or caregiver should immediately report changes in mental status or level of consciousness, palpitations, dizziness, dyspnea, and increasing productive cough, especially if frothy sputum is present, and seek medical attention.

* Review the medications taken by the patient before sending the patient home, and review all prescription as well as OTC medications with the patient. Current use of erectile dysfunction drugs, as noted on medication history, is contraindicated with nitrates. (Erectile dysfunction drugs lower blood pressure and when combined with nitrates, can result in severe and prolonged hypotension.)

* Instruct the patient to not take sildenafil (Viagra), vardenafil (Levitra), or tadalafil (Cialis) while taking nitrates and to discuss treatment options for erectile dysfunction with the health care provider.

Patient understanding of drug therapy:

* Use opportunities during administration of medications and during assessments to discuss the rationale for the drug therapy, desired therapeutic outcomes, commonly observed adverse effects, parameters for when to call the health care provider, and any necessary monitoring or precautions. (Using time during nursing care helps to optimize and reinforce key teaching areas.)

* The patient, family, or caregiver should be able to state the reason for the drug; appropriate dose and scheduling; what adverse effects to observe for and when to report them; equipment needed as appropriate and how to use that equipment; and the required length of medication therapy needed with any special instructions regarding renewing or continuing the prescription as appropriate.

Patient self-administration of drug therapy:

* When administering medications, instruct the patient, family, or caregiver in the proper self-administration of drugs and when to contact the provider. (Utilizing time during nurse-administration of these drugs helps to reinforce teaching.)

* The patient should be able to state how to use sublingual nitroglycerin at home:
  * Take one nitroglycerin tablet, under the tongue, for angina/chest pain. Remain seated or lie down to avoid dizziness or falls.
  * If chest pain continues, repeat one nitroglycerin tablet, under the tongue, in 5 min. Remain seated or lying down.
  * If chest pain continues, repeat nitroglycerin, under the tongue, in 5 min.
  * If chest pain continues, even if reduced, do not take further nitroglycerin unless specifically directed by the health care provider. Call EMS (e.g., 911) for assistance. Do *not* drive self, or have family drive the patient, to the emergency department.
* (If blood pressure monitoring equipment is available at home, have the patient, family, or caregiver take blood pressure prior to the second and third nitroglycerine doses. Hold the drug and contact EMS if blood pressure is less than 90/60 mmHg.

Evaluation of Outcome Criteria

Evaluate the effectiveness of drug therapy by confirming that patient goals and expected outcomes have been met (see "Planning").

PROTOTYPE DRUG	Atenolol (Tenormin)

Classification: **Therapeutic:** Antianginal agent
Pharmacologic: Beta-adrenergic antagonist

Therapeutic Effects and Uses: Atenolol is one of the most frequently prescribed drugs in the United States, due to its relative safety and effectiveness in treating a number of chronic disorders, including HF, HTN, stable angina, and acute MI. Approved in 1981, it is given by the PO route and has a long duration of action that allows for once-daily dosing. Off-label indications for atenolol include ethanol withdrawal, migraine prophylaxis, and unstable angina.

Mechanism of Action: Atenolol selectively blocks beta$_1$-adrenergic receptors in the heart. Its effectiveness in angina is attributed to its ability to slow the heart rate and reduce contractility, both of which lower myocardial oxygen demand.

Pharmacokinetics:

Route(s)	PO, IV
Absorption	50% absorbed from the gastrointestinal (GI) tract
Distribution	Distributed to most tissues including the placenta; secreted in breast milk; does not readily cross the blood–brain barrier; 5–15% bound to protein
Primary metabolism	Not metabolized
Primary excretion	Renal (50%) feces (50%)
Onset of action	PO: 1 h; IV: immediate
Duration of action	PO/IV: 24 h; half-life: 6–7 h

Adverse Effects: Oral atenolol is well tolerated by most patients. Beta-blocking effects can result in bradycardia and hypotension. Fatigue, weakness, and dizziness are other potential adverse effects. Nausea and vomiting occur in some patients. **Black Box Warning:** Abrupt discontinuation should be avoided in patients with ischemic heart disease; doses should be gradually reduced over a 1- to 2-week period. If angina worsens during the withdrawal period, the drug should be reinstituted, at least temporarily.

Contraindications/Precautions: Because atenolol slows heart rate, it should not be used by patients with severe bradycardia, advanced atrioventricular (AV) heart block, cardiogenic shock, or decompensated HF. Due to its vasodilation effects, it is contraindicated in patients with severe hypotension. Patients with severe renal impairment should receive reduced doses to prevent drug accumulation. Because atenolol reduces cardiac output, patients with stroke or low cerebrovascular blood flow should not receive this drug. Patients with major depression should not receive beta blockers because these drugs can worsen this condition.

Drug Interactions: Anticholinergics may decrease the absorption of atenolol from the GI tract. Use with digoxin or other antidysrhythmic agents that depress myocardial conduction may cause AV heart block. Concurrent use of atenolol with other antihypertensives may result in additive hypotension. Although CCBs are often used concurrently with beta block-

ers for their additive therapeutic actions, patients must be monitored carefully due to the possibility of excessive cardiac suppression. **Herbal/Food:** Use with hawthorn may result in additive hypotension.

Pregnancy: Category D.

Treatment of Overdose: The most serious symptoms of atenolol overdose are hypotension and bradycardia. Atropine or isoproterenol may be used to reverse bradycardia, or a cardiac pacemaker may be used to stabilize cardiac rhythm. Atenolol can be removed from the systemic circulation by hemodialysis.

Nursing Responsibilities: Key nursing implications for patients receiving atenolol are included in the Nursing Practice Application for Adrenergic Antagonists in the chapter "Adrenergic Antagonists."

Lifespan and Diversity Considerations:

- Monitor the older adult more frequently, especially during initiation and early use of drug therapy. Orthostatic hypotension may be more common in these patients and may increase the risk of falls.

- Monitor ethnically diverse patients for increased risk of hypotension. Research indicates differing responses to drugs with antihypertensive effects in ethnically diverse populations compared to non-Hispanic whites.

Patient and Family Education:

- If diabetic, remember that this drug suppresses signs of hypoglycemia such as increased pulse rate and changes in blood pressure. Monitor blood glucose frequently and report other possible signs of hypoglycemia such as sweating, fatigue, hunger, or lack of concentration.

- Do not breast-feed while taking this drug without approval of the health care provider.

- Do not discontinue this drug without consulting the health care provider.

Drugs Similar to Atenolol (Tenormin)

Atenolol, metoprolol, propranolol, and timolol are equally effective in treating chronic angina. The student should review general information on beta blockers.

8 Calcium channel blockers are effective at reducing myocardial oxygen demand and treating stable and vasospastic angina.

Blockade of calcium channels has a number of effects on the heart, most of which are similar to those of beta blockers. Although the first approved indication for CCBs was for the treatment of angina, these medications are also used for HTN and dysrhythmias. The actions of CCBs relevant to ischemic heart disease are discussed in this section. The CCBs used for angina are listed in Table 2.

CCBs have several actions on the cardiovascular system that benefit the patient with angina. Most importantly, CCBs relax arteriolar smooth muscle, thus reducing blood pressure. This reduction in afterload decreases myocardial oxygen demand. Some of the CCBs also slow cardiac conduction velocity through the AV node, thereby decreasing heart rate and contributing to the reduced cardiac workload. An additional effect of the CCBs is their ability to dilate the coronary arteries, bringing more oxygen to the myocardium. This vasodilation is especially important in patients with vasospastic angina. CCBs are considered drugs of choice for that condition. For stable, exertional angina, they may be used as monotherapy in patients unable to tolerate beta blockers. In patients with persistent symptoms, CCBs may be administered concurrently with organic nitrates or beta blockers.

Adverse effects of CCBs are generally not serious and are related to vasodilation: headache, dizziness, and edema of the ankles and feet. CCBs should be used with caution in patients taking other cardiovascular medications that slow conduction through the AV node, particularly digoxin or beta-adrenergic blockers. The combined effects of these drugs may cause partial or complete AV heart block, HF, or dysrhythmias. Some CCBs worsen HF by reducing myocardial contractility.

CONNECTION Checkpoint 38.3

For patients with asthma, calcium channel blockers are generally the preferred antianginal agents, rather than beta-adrenergic antagonists. Why would calcium channel blockers be preferred for patients with this comorbid condition? *See Answer to Connection Checkpoint 38.3 on student resource website.*

TABLE 2 Selected Drugs for Angina and Myocardial Infarction

Drug	Route and Adult Dose (maximum dose where indicated)	Adverse Effects
Organic Nitrates		
isosorbide dinitrate (Dilatrate SR, Isordil)	PO: 2.5–30 mg 4 times daily (max: 480 mg/day) Sustained release: 40 mg daily (max: 160 mg/day)	*Headache, orthostatic hypotension, flushing of the face, dizziness, rash (transdermal patch), tolerance*
isosorbide mononitrate (Imdur, Ismo, Monoket)	PO: 20 mg qid Ismo, Monoket: 20 mg bid (max: 40 mg/day) Imdur: 30–60 mg each morning (max: 240 mg/day)	<u>Anaphylaxis, circulatory collapse due to hypotension, syncope due to orthostatic hypotension</u>
nitroglycerin (Nitrostat, Nitro-Dur, Nitro-Bid, Others)	SL: 1 tablet (0.3–0.6 mg) or 1 spray (0.4–0.8 mg) every 3–5 min (max: 3 doses in 15 min)	
Beta-Adrenergic Antagonists		
atenolol (Tenormin)	PO: 25–50 mg daily (max: 100 mg/day)	*Fatigue, insomnia, drowsiness, impotence or decreased libido, bradycardia, and confusion*
metoprolol (Lopressor, Toprol XL)	PO: 100 mg bid (max: 400 mg/day)	
propranolol (Inderal, Inderal LA)	PO: 10–20 mg bid tid (max: 320 mg/day)	<u>Agranulocytosis, laryngospasm, Stevens–Johnson syndrome, anaphylaxis; if the drug is abruptly withdrawn, palpitations, rebound HTN, life-threatening dysrhythmias or myocardial ischemia may occur</u>
timolol (Betimol, Timoptic, Timoptic XE)	PO: 15–45 mg tid (max: 60 mg/day)	
Calcium Channel Blockers		
amlodipine (Norvasc)	PO: 5–10 mg daily (max: 10 mg/day)	*Flushed skin, headache, dizziness, peripheral edema, lightheadedness, nausea, diarrhea*
bepridil (Vascor)	PO: 200 mg daily (max: 400 mg/day)	
diltiazem (Cardizem, Cartia XT, Dilacor XR, Others)	PO regular release: 30 mg tid qid (max: 480 mg/day) Extended release: 20–240 mg bid (max: 540 mg/day)	<u>Hepatotoxicity, MI, HF, confusion, mood changes</u>
nicardipine (Cardene)	PO: 20–40 mg tid or 30–60 mg sustained release bid (max: 120 mg/day)	
nifedipine (Adalat, Procardia, Others)	PO: 10–20 mg tid (max: 180 mg/day) Extended release: 30–90 mg once daily	
verapamil (Calan, Covera-HS, Isoptin SR, Verelan)	PO: 80 mg 3–4 times daily (max: 480 mg/day)	
Other Agents		
ranolazine (Ranexa)	PO: 500–1,000 mg bid (max: 2,000 mg/day)	*Dizziness, constipation, headache, and nausea* <u>QT interval prolongation</u>

Note: *Italics* indicate common adverse effects. <u>Underline</u> indicates serious adverse effects.

Pathophysiology of Myocardial Infarction

9 The early diagnosis and pharmacotherapy of myocardial infarction increase chances of survival.

Myocardial infarctions (MIs), blood clots that block coronary arteries, are responsible for a substantial number of deaths each year. Many patients die before reaching a medical facility for treatment, or within 48 hours following the initial MI, due to complications of the disorder. Clearly, MI is a serious and frightening disease and one responsible for a large percentage of sudden deaths.

The primary cause of MI is advanced CAD: atherosclerotic plaque accumulation in the endothelial wall of one or more branches of the coronary arteries. Pieces of unstable plaque in a coronary artery can ulcerate or rupture and lodge in a small vessel serving a portion of the myocardium. Exposed plaque activates the clotting cascade, resulting in platelet aggregation. A new clot quickly builds on the existing plaque, making obstruction of the vessel imminent.

Deprived of adequate oxygen supply, the obstructed region of the myocardium becomes ischemic. The myocytes shift to anaerobic metabolism after only 8 to 10 seconds of oxygen loss. Anaerobic metabolism, however, is inefficient and cannot produce enough ATP to keep the heart beating efficiently for prolonged periods. Lactic acid accumulates, causing acidosis, which affects contractility and suppresses normal conduction across the myocardium. As contractility diminishes, the patient may experience HF. Myocytes will begin to die in about 20 minutes unless the blood supply is quickly restored. The necrosis of myocardial tissue, which may be irreversible, releases certain "marker" enzymes, such as creatine phosphokinase (CK) or cardiac-specific troponin (cTn), which can be measured in the blood to confirm the patient has experienced an MI.

Extreme chest pain is often the first symptom of MI, and the one that drives most patients to seek medical attention. An electrocardiogram (ECG) can give important clues as to the extent and location of the MI because the infarcted region of the myocardium is nonconducting, producing abnormalities of Q waves, T waves, and ST segments. Patients showing elevation of the ST segment on the ECG are at highest risk for death and require immediate treatment. Laboratory test results are used to aid in diagnosis and monitor progress after an MI. Table 3 describes some of these important laboratory values.

Early diagnosis and prompt pharmacotherapy of MI can significantly reduce the mortality and long-term disability associated with MI. The pharmacologic goals for treating a patient with an acute MI are as follows:

- If cardiac arrest has occurred, restart the heart and restore normal blood pressure with vasopressors.
- Restore blood supply (reperfusion) to the damaged myocardium as quickly as possible through the use of thrombolytics.
- Reduce myocardial oxygen demand with organic nitrates, beta blockers, or CCBs to lower the risk of additional infarctions.
- Control or prevent MI-associated dysrhythmias with amiodarone (Cordarone), beta blockers, or other antidysrhythmics.
- Reduce post-MI mortality with aspirin, beta blockers, and ACE inhibitors.
- Manage severe MI pain and associated anxiety with narcotic analgesics.

Pharmacologic Management of Myocardial Infarction

10 Thrombolytic agents can restore perfusion to ischemic regions of the myocardium if administered soon after a myocardial infarction.

Thrombolytic therapy is administered to dissolve clots obstructing the coronary arteries in order to restore circulation to the ischemic region of the myocardium. Clinical research has confirmed that quick restoration of coronary circulation reduces mortality following an acute MI. After the clot is successfully dissolved, anticoagulant or antiplatelet therapy is initiated to prevent additional clot formation.

TABLE 3 Changes in Blood Test Values with Acute Myocardial Infarction

Blood Test	Initial Elevation After MI	Peak Elevation After MI	Duration of Elevation	Normal Range
CK: Total creatine kinase (also called creatine phosphokinase)	3–8 h	12–24 h	2–4 days	Males: 5–35 mcg/L Females: 5–25 mcg/L
CK-MB	4–6 h	10–24 h	3–4 days	0–3% of CK
ESR (erythrocyte sedimentation rate)	2–3 days	4–5 days	Several weeks	Males: 15–20 mm/h Females: 20–30 mm/h
LDH: Total (lactate dehydrogenase)	12–24 h	2–5 days	6–12 days	70–250 units/L
Myoglobin	2–6 h	8–12 h	1–2 days	12–90 ng/mL
Troponin I	1–3 h	24–36 h	5–9 days	0.1–0.5 mcg/L
Troponin T	1–3 h	24–36 h	10–14 days	<0.2 mcg/L

Thrombolytics are most effective when administered from 20 minutes to 12 hours after the onset of MI symptoms. Ideally, the time from presentation in the emergency department to administration of the thrombolytic agent should be 30 minutes or less. Research has demonstrated little or no therapeutic benefit if the drugs are administered 24 hours or more after the MI onset. In addition, research suggests that patients over age 75 do not experience reduced mortality from these drugs. Because thrombolytic therapy is expensive and has the potential to produce serious adverse effects, it is important to identify circumstances that contribute to successful therapy. The development of clinical practice guidelines for thrombolytic therapy remains an area of active research. Pharmacotherapy Illustrated 2 illustrates this reperfusion process.

Thrombolytics exhibit a narrow margin of safety between dissolving clots and producing serious adverse effects. Although therapy is usually targeted to a single thrombus in a specific artery, once infused in the blood the drugs travel to all vessels and may cause adverse effects anywhere in the body. The primary risk of thrombolytics is excessive bleeding from interference with the clotting process. Vital signs must be monitored continuously and signs of bleeding call for discontinuation of therapy. Because these medications have a brief half-life and are rapidly destroyed in the blood, stopping the infusion normally results in the rapid termination of adverse effects. Physical and laboratory assessment for the possibility of abnormal bleeding should continue for 2 to 4 days after therapy is discontinued.

Thrombolytic therapy is contraindicated for many conditions, including recent trauma or surgery, internal bleeding (other than menses), active peptic ulcer, postpartum (within 10 days), history of intracranial hemorrhage, suspected ischemic stroke within the past 3 months, bleeding disorders, severe liver disease, or thrombocytopenia. Caution should be used when administering thrombolytics to patients taking anticoagulants or antiplatelet drugs.

11 Drugs are used to treat the symptoms and complications of acute myocardial infarction.

The most immediate needs of the patient with MI are to ensure that the heart continues functioning, and that permanent damage from the infarction is minimized. In addition to restoring perfusion to the myocardium with thrombolytic therapy, drugs from several other classes are administered soon after the onset of symptoms, to prevent reinfarction and to ultimately reduce mortality from the episode.

Aspirin

Unless contraindicated, 160 to 325 mg of aspirin is given as soon as an MI is suspected. Research has determined that aspirin use in the weeks following an acute MI dramatically reduces mortality. These effects from aspirin are believed to be due to several mechanisms. Clearly, aspirin has antiplatelet action that reduces platelet aggregation and thus the formation or enlargement of thrombi. Additionally, its anti-inflammatory properties decrease the formation of C-reactive protein, which is associated with an increased risk of MI.

CONNECTIONS

Evidence-Based Practice   Nitroglycerin and Chest Pain

Clinical Question
Does relief of chest pain by the administration of nitroglycerin indicate the presence of CAD with myocardial ischemia?

Evidence
Relief of chest pain following administration of nitroglycerin has been used as an indicator for CAD with myocardial ischemia since the late 1970s. More recent studies questioned the validity of that conclusion, and even complete relief of chest pain, experienced by only approximately 70% of patients, was not found to correlate directly with the presence or absence of CAD.

In a comprehensive review of clinical studies, the American Heart Association confirmed that relief of chest pain by nitroglycerin was not an adequate indicator of the presence or absence of CAD or cardiac pathologies and because it did not predict myocardial ischemia, it should not be used as the sole indicator (Amsterdam et al., 2010). Further diagnostic studies, including cardiac markers (e.g., troponin), ECG, and noninvasive or invasive studies such as echocardiography when appropriate, should be used to evaluate the presence of CAD with or without myocardial ischemia.

Implications
Nitroglycerin plays a key role in the treatment of myocardial ischemia and continues to be a part of the treatment plan. Health care providers should not rely on the presence or absence of chest pain following nitroglycerin use as an indicator of CAD, myocardial ischemia, or impending MI; other laboratory work and cardiac studies should also be used for diagnosis. The nurse can help patients understand that the provider should be notified if nitroglycerin is taken for chest pain, particularly if frequent or escalating use is required. The nurse can also teach the patient, family, or caregiver that the relief of chest pain after nitroglycerin use is not the only indicator that MI is not occurring or impending. Other symptoms such as fatigue, chest pressure, dizziness, sweating, or abdominal discomfort should be considered as possible symptoms of myocardial ischemia and the patient should seek emergency assistance if the symptoms continue to exist after taking nitroglycerin for chest pain.

Critical Thinking Questions
In addition to angina, what are other signs and symptoms of myocardial ischemia? What should the nurse teach the patient if sublingual nitroglycerin is prescribed?

See Answers to Critical Thinking Questions on student resource website.

PHARMACOTHERAPY ILLUSTRATED

2

Thrombolytic Pharmacotherapy

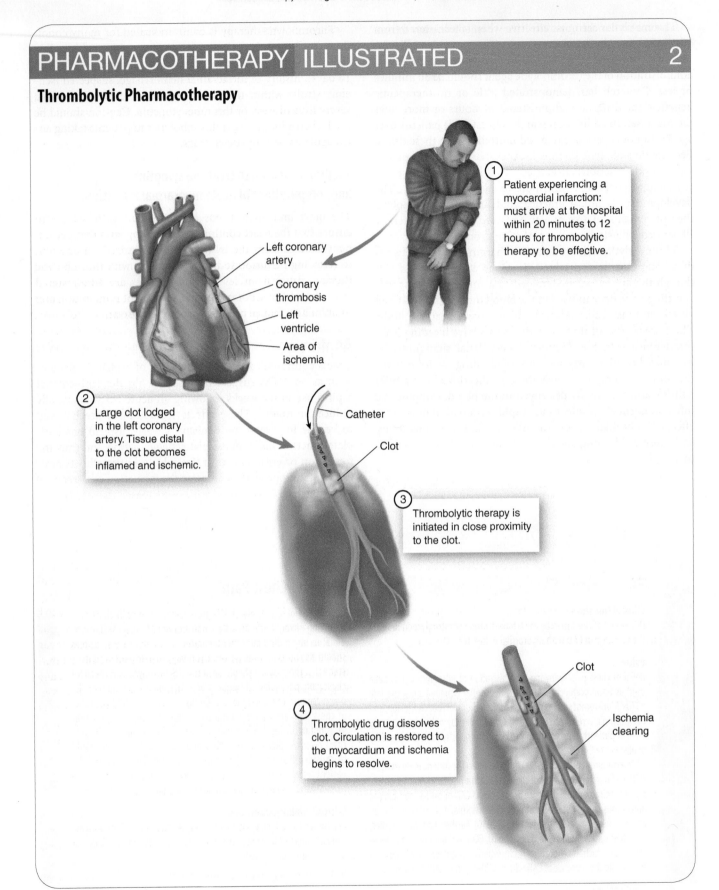

① Patient experiencing a myocardial infarction: must arrive at the hospital within 20 minutes to 12 hours for thrombolytic therapy to be effective.

Left coronary artery

Coronary thrombosis

Left ventricle

Area of ischemia

② Large clot lodged in the left coronary artery. Tissue distal to the clot becomes inflamed and ischemic.

Catheter

Clot

③ Thrombolytic therapy is initiated in close proximity to the clot.

④ Thrombolytic drug dissolves clot. Circulation is restored to the myocardium and ischemia begins to resolve.

Clot

Ischemia clearing

The major concern over aspirin use is its tendency to promote GI bleeding in some patients. This could be a serious adverse effect, given that some post-MI patients receive anticoagulants. However the benefits of taking aspirin following an acute MI generally outweigh the risks for most patients. Aspirin maintenance therapy can cut the risk of death due to a subsequent MI by as much as 50% in some populations. Furthermore, the low doses used in maintenance therapy (75–150 mg/day) rarely cause GI bleeding.

ADP Receptor Blockers

Clopidogrel (Plavix) and ticlopidine (Ticlid) are effective antiplatelet agents that are approved for the prevention of thrombotic stroke and MI. Research has demonstrated that these agents reduce mortality associated with thromboembolic events. Because they are more expensive than aspirin, they are usually considered for antiplatelet therapy for patients allergic to aspirin or who are at high risk for GI bleeding from aspirin. Some protocols call for combination therapy with clopidogrel and aspirin. Clopidogrel is the more frequently used of the two drugs in the class.

Glycoprotein IIb/IIIa Inhibitors

Glycoprotein IIb/IIIa is a receptor found on the surface of platelets. Drugs that occupy the glycoprotein IIb/IIIa receptor inhibit thrombus formation by a mechanism of action distinct from that of aspirin.

Glycoprotein IIb/IIIa inhibitors are sometimes indicated for unstable angina or MI, or for those undergoing percutaneous coronary intervention (PCI) procedures such as angioplasty. The most common drug in this class, abciximab (ReoPro), is infused at the time of PCI, and continued for 12 hours after the procedure is completed to prevent reinfarction.

As with other drugs having an anticoagulant effect, glycoprotein IIb/IIIa inhibitors are contraindicated in the presence of active bleeding, recent surgery, or trauma. They may be used in combination therapy with aspirin and heparin, thus increasing the need for careful monitoring for bleeding.

Anticoagulants

Upon diagnosis of MI in the emergency department, patients may be placed on the anticoagulant heparin to prevent additional thrombi from forming. Unfractionated heparin therapy is sometimes continued for 48 hours, or until PCI is completed, at which time the patients are switched to warfarin (Coumadin) or clopidogrel (Plavix). An alternative is to administer a low-molecular-weight heparin, such as enoxaparin (Lovenox).

Some patients may remain on anticoagulant therapy on a chronic basis after hospital discharge. These include patients at high risk for thromboembolic disease and those with chronic atrial fibrillation. Research has not shown that the use of warfarin lowers mortality in post-MI patients; however, it does increase the risk of bleeding. For most patients, anticoagulation with aspirin or clopidogrel is sufficient for protection from thromboembolic events. The long-term use of heparin in post-MI patients is limited unless other conditions are present that warrant the use of the drug.

Nitrates

The value of nitrates in treating myocardial ischemia was presented in Section 6. Nitrates have additional uses in the patient with a suspected MI. At the initial onset of chest pain, sublingual nitroglycerin is administered to assist in the diagnosis, and three doses may be taken 5 minutes apart. Pain that persists 5 to 10 minutes after the initial dose may indicate an MI, and the patient should seek medical assistance. Thus, nitrates serve a diagnostic role for MI patients.

Patients with persistent pain, HF, or severe HTN may receive IV nitroglycerin for 24 hours following the onset of pain. The arterial and venous dilation produced by the drug reduces myocardial oxygen demand. Organic nitrates also relieve coronary artery vasospasm, which may be present during the acute stage of MI. Upon discharge from the hospital, organic nitrates are discontinued, unless the patient needs them for relief of stable anginal pain.

Beta-Adrenergic Blockers

Beta blockers have the ability to slow heart rate, decrease contractility, and reduce blood pressure. These three factors reduce myocardial oxygen demand, which is critical for patients experiencing a recent MI. In addition, they slow impulse conduction through the heart, suppressing dysrhythmias, which are serious and sometimes fatal complications following an MI. Research has clearly demonstrated that beta blockers can reduce MI-associated mortality if administered within 8 hours of MI onset. These drugs may be initially administered IV, and then switched to oral dosing for chronic therapy. Unless contraindicated, beta-blocker therapy continues for the remainder of the patient's life. For patients unable to tolerate beta blockers, CCBs are an alternative. The beta blockers most often used for MI are listed in Table 1.

Angiotensin-Converting Enzyme Inhibitors

Clinical research has demonstrated increased survival for patients administered the angiotensin-converting enzyme (ACE) inhibitors captopril (Capoten) or lisinopril (Prinivil, Zestoretic) following an acute MI. These drugs are most effective when therapy is started within 24 hours after the onset of symptoms. Oral doses are normally begun after thrombolytic therapy is completed and the patient's condition has stabilized. IV therapy may be used during the early stages of MI pharmacotherapy.

The benefit of ACE inhibitors is believed to be due to their ability to prevent cardiac remodeling, and their ability to suppress dysrhythmias. Unless otherwise contraindicated, post-MI patients should receive an ACE inhibitor indefinitely to prevent HF and future ischemic development.

Pain Management

The pain associated with an MI can be debilitating and stressful, creating an increased workload for the myocardium. Pain control is essential in order to ensure patient comfort and to reduce stress. Narcotic analgesics such as morphine sulfate or meperidine (Demerol) are given to ease extreme pain and to sedate the anxious patient.

PharmFACT

About 1.5 million Americans experience a new or recurrent MI each year. About one third of the patients experiencing an MI will die from it (Zafari, 2011).

12 Vasopressors are used following cardiopulmonary arrest to reestablish coronary and cerebral blood flow.

Cardiopulmonary arrest is a complete stoppage of heart and lungs activity, usually resulting from a dysrhythmia such as ventricular fibrillation or pulseless ventricular tachycardia. Most patients who experience cardiopulmonary arrest have underlying CAD.

Cardiopulmonary resuscitation (CPR) must be initiated as quickly as possible to restore ventilation and blood circulation to avoid hypoxic injury to the tissues. Electrical defibrillation is used to restore normal cardiac rhythm.

Pharmacotherapy is an important component of CPR. The primary drugs used in the initial phase of resuscitation are sympathomimetics, and epinephrine is the drug of choice. Sympathomimetics cause vasoconstriction, immediately raising cerebral, coronary, and systemic blood pressure. Vasopressin, also called antidiuretic hormone, is an alternative therapy.

Following restoration of cardiac function and ventilation, it is critical that the heart maintain normal conduction in order to prevent the recurrence of ventricular fibrillation or the establishment of other serious dysrhythmias. Historically, lidocaine has been the agent of choice for ventricular dysrhythmias associated with MI. Clinical research, however, has shown that the administration of amiodarone (Cordarone) results in improved patient survival. If the risk of dysrhythmia is high, a loading dose of amiodarone is given by infusion, and the patient is switched to oral forms after a therapeutic plasma level of the drug has been achieved.

UNDERSTANDING THE CHAPTER

Key Concepts Summary

1 Myocardial ischemia develops when there is inadequate blood supply to meet the metabolic demands of cardiac muscle.

2 Coronary artery disease is the major cause of myocardial ischemia.

3 Angina pectoris is characterized by severe chest pain brought on by physical exertion or emotional stress.

4 Therapeutic lifestyle changes can decrease the frequency of anginal episodes and reduce the risk of coronary artery disease.

5 The pharmacologic management of angina includes organic nitrates, beta-adrenergic blockers, and calcium channel blockers.

6 Organic nitrates may be used to terminate or prevent angina episodes.

7 Beta-adrenergic blockers are sometimes drugs of choice for stable angina.

8 Calcium channel blockers are effective at reducing myocardial oxygen demand and treating stable and vasospastic angina.

9 The early diagnosis and pharmacotherapy of myocardial infarction increase chances of survival.

10 Thrombolytic agents can restore perfusion to ischemic regions of the myocardium if administered soon after a myocardial infarction.

11 Drugs are used to treat the symptoms and complications of acute myocardial infarction.

12 Vasopressors are used following cardiopulmonary arrest to reestablish coronary and cerebral blood flow.

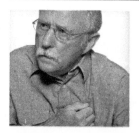

Making the PATIENT Connection

Remember the patient "Michael Graff" at the beginning of the chapter? Now read the remainder of the case study. Based on the information presented within this chapter, respond to the critical thinking questions that follow.

Early one morning, 60-year-old Michael Graff began to feel severe anterior crushing chest pain that lasted for 35 minutes. He experienced dizziness, cold sweats, and nausea. Although he considered driving to the local emergency department, his family insisted on calling an ambulance for emergency transport to the hospital.

Michael, a general contractor, is a 2-pack-per-day smoker and consumes alcohol (beer) two to three times per week. He has a family history of coronary artery disease, diabetes mellitus, and hyperlipidemia. It has been at least 10 years since his last physical examination.

Upon arrival at the emergency department, he presents with symptoms of anxiety, moderate chest pain, and cold extremities. Auscultation of the thorax revealed tachycardia and clear lung fields. Blood pressure was slightly above normal at 156/90 mmHg. He had no neck venous distention. His white blood cell count was 7,600/mm^3, hematocrit 43.8%, platelets 256,000/mm^3, creatine phosphokinase (CPK) 87 international units/L, and troponin-I < 4.1 mcg/L. An ECG showed ST-segment elevation.

Once stabilized, Michael is transported to the coronary care unit with the admission diagnosis of unstable angina and to rule out MI. In the coronary care unit, he receives IV nitroglycerin 50 mg in D$_5$W 25 mL. The nurse begins the infusion at 10 mcg/min and titrates the rate based on his report of chest pain every 5 to 10 min (5–10 mcg/min).

Critical Thinking Questions

1. Michael and his family ask you to explain what is occurring with his heart. How would you describe the pathophysiology of Michael's condition to them?

2. Discuss the reason Michael is receiving nitroglycerin.

3. What adverse effects should the nurse monitor with patients receiving IV nitroglycerin?

4. How do nitroglycerin infusions differ from other IV infusions?

See Answers to Critical Thinking Questions on student resource website.

NCLEX-RN® Review

1. Nitroglycerin topical ointment is being initiated for a client with angina. Which health teaching would be most appropriate?

1. Keep the medication in the refrigerator.
2. Only take this medication when chest pain is severe.
3. Remove the old paste before applying the next dose.
4. Apply the ointment on the chest wall only.

2. A client with chest pain is receiving sublingual nitroglycerin. The nurse would include in the care plan to monitor the client for which adverse effect?

1. Photosensitivity
2. Elevated blood pressure
3. Vomiting and diarrhea
4. Decreased blood pressure

3. The client states, "I always put my nitroglycerin patch in the same place so I do not forget to take it off." The nurse's response would be based on which of the following physiological concepts?

1. Clients are more likely to remember to apply the patch if the same site is used daily.
2. Repeated use of the same application site will enhance medication absorption.
3. Rebound phenomenon is likely to occur when the same site is used more than once.
4. Skin irritation due to the nitroglycerin ointment can occur if the same site is used repeatedly.

4. The nurse is caring for a client with chronic angina pectoris. The client is receiving isosorbide dinitrate (Isordil) oral tablets. Which client manifestations would the nurse conclude are common adverse effects of this medication?

1. Flushing and headache
2. Tremors and anxiety
3. Lightheadedness and dizziness
4. Sleepiness and lethargy

5. The client asks how atenolol (Tenormin) helps angina. The response provided by the nurse is based on which concept? This medication:

1. Slows the heart rate and reduces contractility.
2. Increases the heart rate and diminishes contractility.
3. Blocks sodium channels and elevates depolarization.
4. Decreases blood pressure and blocks the alpha$_2$ receptors.

6. Which of the following assessment findings, if discovered in a client receiving verapamil (Calan) for angina, would be cause for the nurse to withhold the medication? Select all that apply.

1. Bradycardia: heart rate of 40 beats/minute
2. Tachycardia: heart rate of 126 beats/minute
3. Hypotension: blood pressure 76/46 mmHg
4. Tinnitus with hearing loss
5. Hypertension: blood pressure 156/92 mmHg

Additional Case Study

Bill Shackley, a 52-year-old man, is prescribed a daily nitroglycerin transdermal patch. While discussing his medications, Bill shares several of his concerns. How would you respond to the following questions?

1. "I heard that I can become 'tolerant' to this drug. What does this mean? How can it be avoided?"

2. "Sometimes, after applying the nitroglycerin patch, I get a throbbing headache. Is there anything I can do about this?"

3. "I was told to report episodes of dizziness when I stand up plus rapid heart rates. How does nitroglycerin cause these?"

See Answers to Additional Case Study on student resource website.

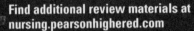

Pearson Nursing Student Resources

Find additional review materials at
nursing.pearsonhighered.com

Prepare for success with additional NCLEX®-style practice questions, interactive assignments and activities, web links, animations, videos, and more!

References

Alaeddini, J. (2010). Angina pectoris. *Medscape Reference.* Retrieved from http://emedicine.medscape.com/article/150215-overview

American Heart Association. (2010). *Fish and omega-3 fatty acids.* Retrieved from http://www.heart.org/HEARTORG/GettingHealthy/NutritionCenter/HealthyDietGoals/Fish-and-Omega-3-Fatty-Acids_UCM_303248_Article.jsp

Amsterdam, E. A., Kirk, J. D., Bluemke, D. A., Diercks, D., Farkouh, M. E., Garvey, J. L., et al. (2010). Testing of low-risk patients presenting to the emergency department with chest pain: A scientific statement from the American Heart Association. *Circulation, 122*(17), 1756–1776. doi:10.1161/CIR.0b013e3181ec61df

National Center for Complementary and Alternative Medicine. (2010). *Omega-3 supplements.* Retrieved from http://nccam.nih.gov/health/omega3/introduction.htm

Office of Dietary Supplements, National Institutes of Health. (n.d.). *Omega-3 fatty acids and health.* Retrieved from http://ods.od.nih.gov/factsheets/omega3fattyacidsandhealth

University of Maryland Medical Center. (2010). *Omega-3 fatty acids.* Retrieved from http://www.umm.edu/altmed/articles/omega-3-000316.htm

Zafari, A. M. (2011). *Myocardial infarction.* Retrieved from http://emedicine.medscape.com/article/155919-overview

Selected Bibliography

Aronow, W. S., Frishman, W. H., & Cheng-Lai, A. (2007). Cardiovascular drug therapy in the elderly. *Cardiology in Review, 15*(4), 195–215.

Bhat, D. L. (2010). Acute coronary syndrome update for hospitalists. *Journal of Hospital Medicine, 5*(Suppl 4), S15–S21. doi:10.1002/jhm.830

Gehi, A. K., Ali, S., Na, B., & Whooley, M. A. (2007). Self-reported medication adherence and cardiovascular events in patients with stable coronary heart disease: The heart and soul study. *Archives of Internal Medicine, 167*(16), 1798–1803. doi:10.1001/archinte.167.16.1798

Jackevicius, C. A., Li, P., & Tu, J. V. (2008). Prevalence, predictors, and outcomes of primary nonadherence after acute myocardial infarction. *Circulation, 117*(2), 1028–1036. doi:10.1161/CIRCULATIONAHA.107.706820

Jayasekara, R. (2010). Effect of early treatment with antihypertensive drugs on short- and long-term mortality in patients with an acute cardiovascular event. *International Journal of Evidence-Based Healthcare, 8*(1), 41. doi:10.1111/j.1744-1609.2010.00155.x

Kee, J. L. (2010). *Laboratory and diagnostic tests with nursing implications* (8th ed.). Upper Saddle River, NJ: Pearson Education.

Manfredini, R., Salmi, R., & Manfredini, F. (2008). Survival patterns with in-hospital cardiac arrest. *Journal of the American Medical Association, 299*(22), 2625–2626. doi:10.1001/jama.299.22.2625-a

Maron, B. A., & Rocco, T. P. (2011). Pharmacotherapy of heart failure. In L. L. Brunton, B. A. Chabner, & B. C. Knollman (Eds.), *The pharmacological basis of therapeutics* (12th ed., pp. 789–814). New York, NY: McGraw-Hill.

Norton, C., Georgiopoulou, V., Kalogeropoulos, A., & Butler, J. (2011). Chronic stable angina: Pathophysiology and innovations in treatment. *Journal of Cardiovascular Medicine, 12*(3), 218–219. doi:10.2459/JCM.0b013e328343e974

Rasmussen, J. N., Chong, A., & Alter, D. A. (2007). Relationship between adherence to evidence-based pharmacotherapy and long-term mortality after acute myocardial infarction. *Journal of the American Medical Association, 297*(2), 177–186. doi:10.1001/jama.297.2.177

Wright, R. S., Anderson, J. L., Adams, C. D., Bridges, C. R., Casey, D. E., Ettinger, S. M., et al. (2011). ACCF/AHA focused update of the guidelines for the management of patients with unstable angina/non–ST-elevation myocardial infarction (updating the 2007 guideline): A report of the American College of Cardiology Foundation/American Heart Association Task Force on Practice Guidelines. *Journal of the American College of Cardiology, 57,* 1929–1959. doi:10.1016/j.jacc.2011.02.009

Answers to NCLEX-RN® Review

1 Answer: 3 Rationale: Clients should be taught to remove the old ointment before applying the next dose. Options 1, 2, and 4 are incorrect. Nitroglycerin should be kept at room temperature, not in the refrigerator. Clients should take the medication before chest pain becomes severe. Nitroglycerin can be applied to any skin surface. However, absorption is decreased when applied to hairy areas, soles of feet, and palms. Cognitive Level: Applying; Client Need: Health Promotion and Maintenance; Nursing Process: Implementation

2 Answer: 4 Rationale: A decline in blood pressure is an expected adverse effect. The nurse should always assess the blood pressure prior to and 5 min after administering nitroglycerin. Options 1, 2, and 3 are incorrect. Photosensitivity, vomiting, and diarrhea are not expected adverse effects. Nitroglycerin will cause a decline in blood pressure not an increase. Cognitive Level: Applying; Client Need: Physiological Integrity; Nursing Process: Planning

3 Answer: 4 Rationale: Skin irritation due to the nitroglycerin ointment can occur if the same site is used repeatedly. Options 1, 2, and 3 are incorrect. Clients should be instructed to rotate the site of application when using nitroglycerin ointment. Repeated use of the same application site may actually decrease absorption. Rebound phenomenon is not an expected occurrence with nitroglycerin. Cognitive Level: Applying; Client Need: Health Promotion and Maintenance; Nursing Process: Implementation

4 Answer: 3 Rationale: Clients may experience light-headedness or dizziness as a result of the hypotensive effects of isosorbide. Options 1, 2,

and 4 are incorrect. Because the oral form of isosorbide has a slower onset than sublingual forms, a flushing sensation and headache are not usually experienced as they are with nitroglycerin sublingual. Tremors and anxiety are not associated adverse effects with this drug. Isosorbide does not usually cause sleepiness or lethargy, and if these occur they should be evaluated. Cognitive Level: Analyzing; Client Need: Physiological Integrity; Nursing Process: Evaluation

5 Answer: 1 Rationale: Atenolol increases blood flow to the myocardium, thereby increasing oxygen supply by reducing the heart rate and decreasing the contractility. Options 2, 3 and 4 are incorrect. Atenolol is a beta-adrenergic antagonist, which decreases heart rate. This drug does not affect the sodium channels. Although this drug reduces blood pressure, the mechanism of action is not by blocking the alpha$_2$ receptors. Cognitive Level: Applying; Client Need: Physiological Integrity; Nursing Process: Implementation

6 Answer: 1, 3 Rationale: Verapamil decreases blood pressure and heart rate. The administration of this drug may cause significant hypotension and bradycardia in some clients. Options 2, 4, and 5 are incorrect. Verapamil may be used to treat fast heart rates and HTN in addition to angina. Tinnitus and hearing loss are not adverse effects associated with verapamil. Cognitive Level: Analyzing; Client Need: Physiological Integrity; Nursing Process: Evaluation

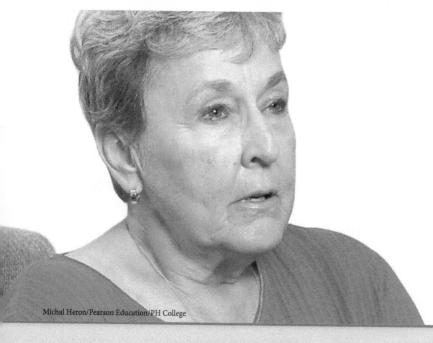

"It seems that over the past 2 weeks, I have become more short of breath just walking around my apartment. Walking up stairs and unloading my groceries have become impossible."

Patient "Thelma Walters"

Pharmacotherapy of Heart Failure

Chapter Outline

Learning Outcomes

After reading this chapter, the student should be able to:

1. Identify the major diseases associated with heart failure.
2. Relate how the symptoms associated with heart failure may be caused by a weakened heart muscle and diminished cardiac output.
3. Identify compensatory mechanisms used by the body to maintain cardiac output in patients with heart failure.
4. Describe how heart failure is classified.
5. Describe the nurse's role in the pharmacologic management of heart failure.
6. For each of the classes shown in the chapter outline, identify the prototype and representative drugs and explain the mechanism(s) of drug action, primary indications, contraindications, significant drug interactions, pregnancy category, and important adverse effects.
7. Apply the nursing process to care for patients receiving pharmacotherapy for heart failure.

From Chapter 39 of *Pharmacology: Connections to Nursing Practice*, Second Edition. Michael Patrick Adams, Carol Quam Urban. Copyright © 2013 by Pearson Education, Inc. All rights reserved.

Key Terms

cardiac remodeling

digitalization

diuretic resistance

heart failure (HF)

natriuretic peptides

phosphodiesterase III

reverse remodeling

Heart failure is one of the most common and fatal of the cardiovascular diseases, and its incidence is increasing as the population ages. Although improved treatment of myocardial infarction and hypertension has led to declines in mortality due to heart failure, approximately one in five patients still dies within a year of diagnosis of heart failure, and 50% die within 5 years. Historically, this condition was called *congestive heart failure*; however, because not all incidences of this disease are associated with congestion, the more appropriate name is *heart failure*.

PharmFACT

Each year, about 550,000 new cases of heart failure are diagnosed and over 300,000 deaths are attributed to HF in the United States. Although the incidence is equal in men and women, females develop HF later in life and survive longer with the disease (Dumitru, 2011).

Etiology of Heart Failure

1 Heart failure is closely associated with disorders such as chronic hypertension, coronary artery disease, and diabetes.

Heart failure (HF) is the inability of the heart to pump enough blood to meet the metabolic demands of the body. HF can be caused by any disorder that affects the heart's ability to receive or eject blood. While weakening of cardiac muscle is a natural consequence of aging, the process can be caused or accelerated by the following:

- Coronary artery disease (CAD)
- Mitral stenosis
- Myocardial infarction (MI)
- Chronic hypertension (HTN)
- Diabetes mellitus

The student should detect a common theme throughout the chapters on cardiovascular pharmacology. That theme is the ability to prevent major causes of morbidity and mortality through control of healthy lifestyle choices. Controlling lipid levels, implementing a regular exercise program, maintaining optimum body weight, and keeping blood pressure within normal limits reduce the incidences of CAD and MI. Maintaining blood glucose within the normal range reduces the consequences of uncontrolled diabetes. Thus, for many patients, HF is a preventable condition; controlling associated diseases will greatly reduce the risk of development and progression of HF.

Since there is no cure for HF, the treatment goals are to prevent, treat, or remove the underlying causes whenever possible and treat its symptoms, so that the patient's quality of life can be improved. Advances in understanding the pathophysiology of HF during the past two decades have led to a change in pharmacotherapeutic goals. No longer is therapy of HF focused on end stages of the disorder. Pharmacotherapy is now targeted at prevention and slowing the progression of HF. This change in emphasis has led to significant improvements in survival and quality of life in patients with HF.

Pathophysiology of Heart Failure

2 The body attempts to compensate for heart failure by increasing cardiac output.

HF is a general term used to describe several different types of cardiac dysfunction. The dysfunction may occur on the left side, the right side, or on both sides of the heart.

Left-sided HF is called congestive heart failure (CHF) because it is characterized by an accumulation of fluid causing congestion in the pulmonary capillary beds. Although left-sided HF is more common, the right side of the heart can also become weak, either simultaneously with the left side or independently from the left side. In right-sided HF, the blood pools in the veins resulting in peripheral edema and engorgement of organs such as the liver.

Left-sided HF is further subdivided into two types. Systolic HF occurs when cardiac output (CO) is diminished due to decreased contractility of the myocardium. Approximately 60% to 80% of left-sided HF is the systolic type. Diastolic HF occurs when the lungs become congested even though cardiac output is normal. Diastolic HF is caused by a restriction in ventricular filling, resulting in higher-than-normal pressure in the ventricle. Although cardiac output is normal, the increased pressure in the ventricle creates higher pressure in the pulmonary capillaries, resulting in pulmonary edema. A patient may have both systolic and diastolic HF. Pharmacotherapy of the two types differs somewhat. For example, inotropic drugs that increase contractility are more successful with systolic HF than diastolic HF.

HF may progress slowly over many years, or it may have an acute onset. Once HF reaches the stage where cardiac output is affected, tissues receive inadequate perfusion and organ failure is possible. The body has developed a complex series of actions to compensate for HF. Knowledge of these compensatory mechanisms is important to understanding the pharmacotherapy of HF. Prior to continuing in this chapter, factors affecting cardiac output, stroke volume, afterload, and preload, should be reviewed. The pathophysiology of HF is illustrated in Figure 1.

Ventricular Hypertrophy

In left HF, the left ventricle is forced to work harder due to the increased preload or afterload. Over time, the wall of the left ventricle thickens and enlarges (ventricular hypertrophy) in an attempt to compensate for the increased workload. Changes in the size, shape, and structure of the myocardial cells (myocytes) occur. These compensatory changes in structure benefit the heart by allowing it to better maintain adequate stroke volume and cardiac output. The term **cardiac remodeling** is sometimes used to describe these changes to myocyte structure and function.

The benefits of cardiac remodeling as a compensatory mechanism, however, are limited. Myocytes continually die, likely due to workload injury, and fibrotic tissue fills the spaces

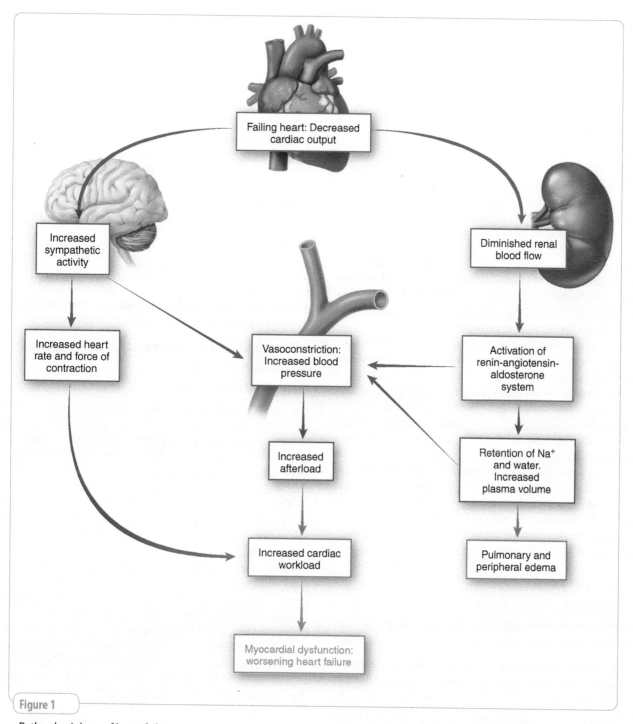

Figure 1

Pathophysiology of heart failure.

between them. These tissue changes stiffen the myocardium, causing diminished contractility and reduced cardiac output. The heart responds with even more remodeling, continuing the destructive cycle. Without intervention, the abnormal structural changes can result in irreversible cardiac impairment.

Activation of the Sympathetic Nervous System

One of the fastest homeostatic responses to diminished cardiac output is activation of the sympathetic nervous system (SNS). The increased heart rate resulting from sympathetic

activation is a normal compensatory mechanism that serves to increase cardiac output.

The SNS, however, also constricts arteries and activates the renin-angiotensin-aldosterone system (RAAS). Higher angiotensin II levels raise blood pressure and afterload, causing the heart to work harder. The stressed myocardium, which already has reduced contractility and is having difficulty maintaining cardiac output, is faced with even greater challenges by this additional workload. The diminished cardiac output caused by the high afterload produces an ongoing activation of the SNS. Patients with preexisting CAD may experience an anginal attack from the increased SNS activity. Again, although there are certain compensatory benefits to activating the SNS to maintain cardiac output, a destructive cycle is created that can lead to or worsen HF.

CONNECTION Checkpoint 39.1

Propranolol (Inderal) is an example of a negative inotropic agent. Explain why this type of drug should be administered with caution to a patient with heart failure who also has asthma. *See Answer to Connection Checkpoint 39.1 on student resource website.*

Increased Plasma Volume and Preload

When cardiac output in a patient with HF is diminished, blood flow to the kidneys is reduced. The kidneys respond to the decreased perfusion by secreting renin and activating the RAAS. As a result of the action of angiotensin II, aldosterone secretion is increased, and the body retains sodium and water. This has the beneficial effects of increasing preload, stretching the myocardial fibers, and increasing contractility, thus returning cardiac output to normal levels. This is an important compensatory mechanism in normal hearts.

However, the heart has a limited ability to increase contractility. In a diseased heart, the increased preload leads to volume overload and pulmonary congestion. In addition, the increased plasma volume increases blood pressure, which further adds to afterload and to the burden of an already weak heart.

Research has discovered additional detrimental effects related to activation of the RAAS. Angiotensin II has been found to promote ventricular hypertrophy, myocyte death, and fibrosis formation in the myocardium. Aldosterone also has direct effects on the myocardium, promoting fibrosis and stiffening of the ventricular wall. Angiotensin-converting enzymes (ACE) inhibitors have become preferred drugs for HF, in part, because they are able to block these detrimental effects of angiotensin II and aldosterone on cardiac remodeling.

Natriuretic Peptides and Neurohumoral Factors

Natriuretic peptides are substances secreted in response to increased pressure in the heart. Three types have been identified:

1. Atrial natriuretic peptide (ANP) is secreted by the atria.
2. B-type natriuretic peptide (BNP) is secreted by the ventricles.
3. C-type natriuretic peptide (CNP) is secreted by the brain.

The physiological functions of ANP and BNP are to cause diuresis, vasodilation, and decreased aldosterone secretion, thus balancing the effects of the SNS and RAAS activation. Nesiritide (Natrecor), a drug structurally identical to BNP, has a limited role in the treatment of HF, as discussed in Section 8.

Research has identified several other substances as potential mediators in the progression of HF. Two proinflammatory substances, tumor necrosis factor (TNF) and interleukin, are found in high levels in patients with HF, and are associated with a poor prognosis. The hormone endothelin is a vasoconstrictor that also is associated with a poor prognosis in HF patients. Vasopressin (antidiuretic hormone), which is elevated in HF patients, causes fluid retention and worsens this condition. It

TABLE 1 Drugs That May Worsen Heart Failure	
Mechanism	**Example Drugs and Classes**
Negative inotropic effect: slow heart rate or reduce contractility	Antidysrhythmics Beta-adrenergic blockers Calcium channel blockers Itraconazole
Cardiotoxicity: damage to the myocardium	Cyclophosphamide Daunomycin Doxorubicin
Increase blood volume: cause sodium and water retention and fluid overload	Androgens Estrogens Glucocorticoids NSAIDs Rosiglitazone and pioglitazone

is likely that research will identify additional mediators of HF, along with potential novel therapies for the disease.

3 Symptoms of heart failure occur when compensatory mechanisms fail to maintain adequate cardiac output.

The classic symptoms of HF are dyspnea on exertion, fatigue, pulmonary congestion, and peripheral edema. Lung congestion causes a cough and orthopnea (difficulty breathing when recumbent). If pulmonary edema occurs, the patient feels as if he or she is suffocating and extreme anxiety may result. The condition often worsens at night.

Through pharmacotherapy and lifestyle modifications, many patients with HF can be maintained in a symptom-free, compensated state for years. The most common reason patients experience decompensation is fluid overload due to nonadherence to sodium and water restrictions. The second most common reason is nonadherence to the pharmacotherapeutic regimen. The nurse must stress to patients the importance of sodium restriction and treatment adherence to maintain a properly functioning heart. Cardiac events such as myocardial ischemia, MI, or dysrhythmias can also precipitate acute HF. Certain medications can worsen HF, and the nurse should use these drugs with caution. A list of selected drugs that may worsen HF is shown in Table 1.

Pharmacologic Management of Heart Failure

4 The specific therapy for heart failure depends on the clinical stage of the disease.

Several models are available to guide the pharmacologic management of HF. The New York Heart Association (NYHA) classification has been widely used in clinical practice for the staging of HF. This model classifies symptomatic HF into four functional classes:

- I: Patients with cardiac disease but with no symptoms during physical activity

Evidence-Based Practice   Diabetes and Heart Failure

Clinical Question
Does maintaining glucose control in diabetes decrease the incidence of heart failure?

Evidence
Diabetics have a higher incidence of CAD and an increased risk of heart disease and HF. Studies of the incidence of HF often include multiple risk factors including smoking, physical inactivity, and lipid levels that make determining the impact of diabetes alone difficult to assess. Van Melle et al. (2010) analyzed data collected in the 2003 Heart and Soul Study of depression and quality-of-life indicators in patients with heart failure. Regression analyses demonstrated that for patients with diabetes, serum control as measured by the A1C level was an independent risk factor for the development of HF in patients with stable CAD. This finding was also noted by Dungan et al. (2010), and further studies were suggested to support or refute the findings. When teaching patients, nurses can emphasize the need for stable glucose control (A1C levels) over time as an important means to decrease the risk of

HF in patients with diabetes who also have CAD, even if no symptoms are present currently.

Implications
Maintaining glucose control is an important part of a diabetes regimen. People with diabetes have a higher incidence of CAD, which may progress to heart disease, MI, and HF. Recent studies suggest that poor glucose control is linked to the development of HF in people with diabetes. Nurses teaching the patient with diabetes should include a discussion of the risks for heart disease and HF, and emphasize the need to maintain stable glucose levels as measured by the A1C level.

Critical Thinking Question
A patient is evaluated by a cardiologist for mild chest pain. The patient has type 2 diabetes managed with both oral medication and insulin therapy. What teaching would the nurse need to give this patient?

See Answers to Critical Thinking Questions on student resource website.

- II: Patients with cardiac disease who have slight limitations on physical activity, with symptoms such as fatigue, palpitations, dyspnea, or angina
- III: Patients with cardiac disease who have marked limitations during physical activity
- IV: Patients with cardiac disease who are unable to perform physical activity, and who have symptoms at rest

A more recent model, proposed by the American College of Cardiology (ACC) and the American Heart Association (AHA), categorizes HF into four stages, as listed in Table 2. Although similar to the NYHA model, the ACC/AHA model better illustrates the progressive nature of the disease and the role of risk factor modification.

Drugs for Heart Failure

Pharmacotherapy of HF focuses on three primary goals:

1. Reduction of preload
2. Reduction of systemic vascular resistance (afterload reduction)
3. Inhibition of both the RAAS and vasoconstrictor mechanisms of the sympathetic nervous system.

The first two goals provide symptomatic relief but do not reverse the progression of the disease. In addition to reducing symptoms, inhibition of the RAAS and vasoconstriction by the sympathetic nervous system also result in a significant reduction in morbidity and mortality from HF. These mechanisms are illustrated in Pharmacotherapy Illustrated 1.

TABLE 2 Stages for Treating Heart Failure

Stage	Description	Treatment Examples
A	Patients are at high risk of developing HF.	Make lifestyle modifications. Treat and control associated conditions: HTN, dyslipidemia, and diabetes. If hypertensive, use ACE inhibitor.
B	Patients have structural evidence of heart disease, such as a previous MI or valvular disease, but no symptoms of HF. (Includes NYHA Class I patients.)	Continue treatments for Stage A. Treat with ACE inhibitor (or an angiotensin II receptor blocker [ARB] if patient is intolerant to ACE inhibitors). Beta blockers are added for those with prior HF symptoms. Diuretics and salt restriction are added for patients with fluid retention.
C	Patients have structural evidence of heart disease with symptoms of HF such as fatigue, fluid retention, or dyspnea. (Includes NYHA Class II and III patients.)	Treat with ACE inhibitor (or ARB) and beta blocker. Add digoxin and spironolactone if needed to control symptoms. If symptoms do not improve, add a loop or thiazide diuretic, and a combination nitrate with hydralazine.
D	Patients have symptoms at rest, despite optimal medical therapy; decompensated HF. (Includes NYHA Class IV patients.)	Treatment may include intravenous (IV) diuretics, dopamine, dobutamine, IV nitroglycerin, nesiritide, or phosphodiesterase inhibitors.

Source: From "2009 Focused Update: ACCF/AHA Guidelines for the Diagnosis and Management of Heart Failure in Adults. A Report of the American College of Cardiology Foundation/American Heart Association Task Force on Practice Guidelines Developed in Collaboration with the International Society for Heart and Lung Transplantation," 2009, *Journal of the American College of Cardiology, 53,* pp. 1343–1382.

PHARMACOTHERAPY ILLUSTRATED 1

Mechanisms of Action of Drugs Used for Heart Failure

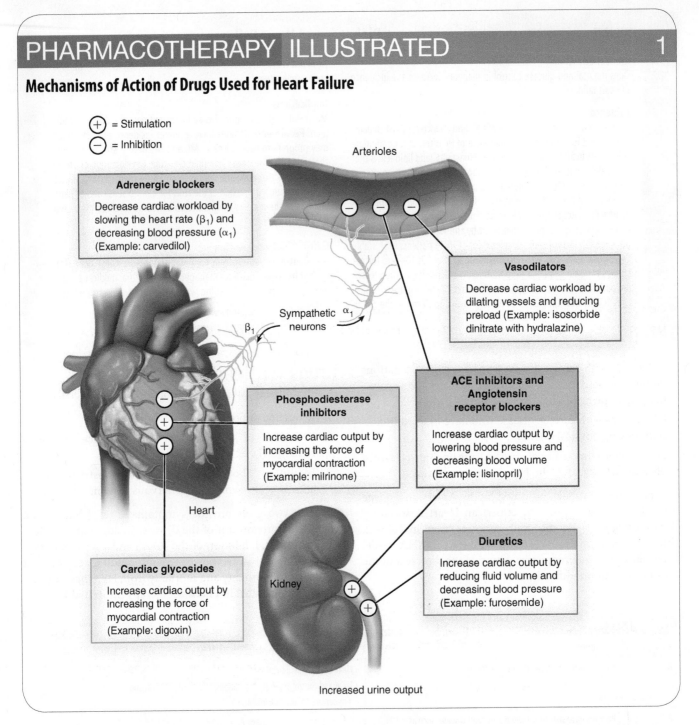

$\oplus$ = Stimulation
$\ominus$ = Inhibition

Arterioles

Adrenergic blockers

Decrease cardiac workload by slowing the heart rate (β_1) and decreasing blood pressure (α_1) (Example: carvedilol)

Sympathetic neurons α_1

β_1

Vasodilators

Decrease cardiac workload by dilating vessels and reducing preload (Example: isosorbide dinitrate with hydralazine)

Phosphodiesterase inhibitors

Increase cardiac output by increasing the force of myocardial contraction (Example: milrinone)

ACE inhibitors and Angiotensin receptor blockers

Increase cardiac output by lowering blood pressure and decreasing blood volume (Example: lisinopril)

Heart

Cardiac glycosides

Increase cardiac output by increasing the force of myocardial contraction (Example: digoxin)

Kidney

Diuretics

Increase cardiac output by reducing fluid volume and decreasing blood pressure (Example: furosemide)

Increased urine output

5 Angiotensin-converting enzyme inhibitors are drugs of choice for heart failure.

Due to their effectiveness and relative safety, the ACE inhibitors have replaced digoxin as first-line drugs for the treatment of chronic HF. Indeed, unless specifically contraindicated, all patients with HF and many patients at high risk of HF should receive an ACE inhibitor. The following section focuses on the benefits of these drugs for patients with HF.

Clinical research has clearly demonstrated that ACE inhibitors slow the progression of HF and reduce mortality

from this disease. Although this is probably true for all ACE inhibitors, the largest body of research has been conducted using captopril (Capoten) and lisinopril (Prinivil, Zestril). Doses for the ACE inhibitors indicated for HF are listed in Table 3.

The two primary actions of the ACE inhibitors are to lower peripheral resistance through the inhibition of angiotensin II formation, and to reduce blood volume through inhibition of aldosterone secretion. The resultant reduction of arterial blood pressure diminishes afterload, and increases cardiac output. An additional effect of the ACE inhibitors is dilation of veins. This action, which is probably not directly related to their inhibition of angiotensin, lowers preload and reduces pulmonary

TABLE 3 Drugs for Early and Moderate Heart Failure

Drug	Route and Adult Dose (maximum dose where indicated)	Adverse Effects
ACE Inhibitors and Angiotensin Receptor Blockers (ARBs)		
candesartan (Atacand)	PO: start at 4 mg/day and increase gradually (max: 32 mg/day)	*Headache, dizziness, orthostatic hypotension, cough* Severe hypotension (first-dose phenomenon), syncope, angioedema, blood dyscrasias, fetal toxicity
captopril (Capoten)	PO: 6.25–12.5 mg tid (max: 450 mg/day)	
enalapril (Vasotec)	PO: 2.5 mg qid–bid (max: 40 mg/day)	
fosinopril (Monopril)	PO: 5–40 mg/day (max: 40 mg/day)	
lisinopril (Prinivil, Zestril)	PO: 10 mg/day (max: 80 mg/day)	
quinapril (Accupril)	PO: 10–20 mg/day (max: 40 mg/day)	
ramipril (Altace)	PO: 2.5–5 mg bid (max: 10 mg/day)	
valsartan (Diovan)	PO: 80 mg/day (max: 320 mg/day)	
Diuretics		
Loop or High Ceiling		
bumetanide (Bumex)	PO: 0.5–2 mg/day (max: 10 mg/day)	Loop and thiazides: *Electrolyte imbalances, fatigue, orthostatic hypotension* Severe hypotension, dehydration, serious hypokalemia, hyponatremia, hyperglycemia (thiazides), ototoxicity (loop diuretics)
furosemide (Lasix)	PO: 20–80 mg in one or more divided doses (max: 600 mg/day)	
torsemide (Demadex)	PO/IV: 10–20 mg/day (max: 200 mg/day)	
Thiazide and Thiazide-Like		
hydrochlorothiazide (Microzide)	PO: 25–200 mg in one to three divided doses (max: 200 mg/day)	Potassium-sparing: *Hyperkalemia, gynecomastia in males, fatigue* Dysrhythmias due to hyperkalemia
Potassium-Sparing (Aldosterone Antagonist)		
eplerenone (Inspra)	PO: 25–50 mg once daily (max: 100 mg/day)	
spironolactone (Aldactone)	PO: 5–200 mg in divided doses	
Beta-Adrenergic Blockers		
carvedilol (Coreg)	PO: 3.125 mg bid for 2 weeks (max: 25 mg bid if less than 85 kg or 50 mg bid if more than 85 kg) Sustained release: 10 mg/day (max: 80 mg/day)	*Fatigue, insomnia, drowsiness, impotence or decreased libido, bradycardia, confusion* Agranulocytosis, laryngospasm, Stevens–Johnson syndrome, anaphylaxis; if the drug is abruptly withdrawn, palpitations, rebound HTN, life-threatening dysrhythmias, or myocardial ischemia may occur
metoprolol extended release (Toprol-XL)	PO: 25 mg/day for 2 weeks; 12.5 mg/day for severe cases (max: 200 mg/day)	
Vasodilator		
isosorbide dinitrate with hydralazine (BiDil)	PO: 1 tablet tid (max: 2 tablets tid); each tablet contains 20 mg of isosorbide dinitrate and 37.5 mg of hydralazine	*Headache, flushing of face, orthostatic hypotension, dizziness, reflex tachycardia* Fainting, severe headache, severe hypotension with overdose, lupus-like reaction (hydralazine)
Cardiac Glycoside		
digoxin (Lanoxin, Lanoxicaps)	PO: 0.125–0.5 mg/day	*Nausea, vomiting, headache, and visual disturbances such as seeing halos, a yellow or green tinge, or blurring* Dysrhythmias, AV block

Note: Italics indicate common adverse effects. <u>Underline</u> indicates serious adverse effects.

congestion and peripheral edema. The combined reductions in preload, afterload, and blood volume from the ACE inhibitors substantially decrease the workload on the heart and allow it to work more efficiently for patients with cardiac impairment. Patients taking ACE inhibitors experience fewer HF-related symptoms, hospitalizations, and treatment failures. Exercise tolerance is improved.

Research has also demonstrated that several ACE inhibitors are effective in preventing HF following an acute MI. Furthermore, post-MI therapy with ACE inhibitors reduces mortality and decreases reinfarction rates. Although these effects are most prominent when therapy is initiated within 36 hours after the onset of the MI, benefits are also obtained when therapy is begun later and continued for several years.

Therapy with ACE inhibitors is generally begun at low doses, and the amount is gradually increased until the desired therapeutic level is reached. Clinical research has not shown a significant difference in mortality between patients receiving low versus high doses. Because higher doses reduce HF symptoms more effectively, however, patients often receive doses in the higher range, as long as significant adverse effects do not interfere with therapy. Symptomatic relief from HF symptoms occurs within days of initiating therapy, but maximum benefits may take several weeks.

The ACE inhibitors are well tolerated by most patients with HF. Hypotension is the most common adverse effect, and the risk is increased when the patient is receiving other drugs that lower blood pressure such as diuretics and beta blockers. Hypotension is generally worse at the beginning of therapy or when dosage is increased. Multidrug therapy is common in these patients and the nurse serves a key role in teaching patients how to space drug administration times to minimize hypotensive adverse effects.

An additional concern during ACE inhibitor therapy is functional renal insufficiency. Patients with severe HF have high circulating levels of angiotensin II, which helps to maintain renal blood flow by constricting efferent arterioles in the kidney. When ACE inhibitors are administered, the level of angiotensin II declines rapidly, leading to reduced blood flow through the kidneys. During therapy with ACE inhibitors, renal insufficiency may also result from sodium depletion, often secondary to the concurrent use of diuretics. To avoid this potentially serious adverse effect, serum creatinine, serum electrolytes, and blood urea nitrogen (BUN) should be monitored during therapy. Should an assessment discover signs of renal impairment, the dose should be immediately decreased or the drug discontinued.

Other adverse effects of ACE inhibitors are angioedema, cough, and hyperkalemia.

Another mechanism that blocks the effects of angiotensin II is the use of angiotensin receptor blockers (ARBs). Pharmacologically, the effects of the ARBs are very similar to those of the ACE inhibitors, as would be expected because drugs from both classes inhibit the actions of angiotensin II. In patients with HF, ARBs show equivalent efficacy to the ACE inhibitors. Clinical research, however, has suggested that combining ARBs with ACE inhibitors does not improve patient survival but does increase the risk of adverse effects. Because they show no clear advantage over other HF medications, the use of ARBs in the treatment of HF is usually reserved for patients who are unable to tolerate the adverse effects of ACE inhibitors.

6 Diuretics relieve symptoms of heart failure by reducing fluid overload and decreasing blood pressure.

Diuretics are common medications for the treatment of patients with HF, since they are effective at reducing peripheral edema and pulmonary congestion and produce few adverse effects. By reducing blood volume and lowering blood pressure, the workload on the heart is reduced, and cardiac output increases. Diuretics are rarely used alone for HF, but are frequently prescribed in combination with ACE inhibitors, beta blockers, and other HF medications. Doses for selected diuretics are listed in Table 3.

Although diuretics are effective at relieving HF symptoms, clinical research has not demonstrated their effectiveness in slowing the progression of HF or in decreasing the mortality rate associated with the disease. Indeed, some of the actions of the diuretics, particularly effects on potassium balance, may increase the risk of adverse effects from other HF drugs. Because of this, diuretics are only indicated when there is evidence of fluid retention. In patients presenting with fluid retention, especially with symptoms of severe pulmonary congestion or peripheral edema, diuretics are essential medications.

Of the diuretic classes, the loop diuretics are most commonly prescribed for HF, due to their effectiveness in removing fluid from the body. Loop diuretics are also able to function in patients with renal impairment, an advantage for many patients with decompensated HF. Another major advantage in treating acute HF is that loop diuretics act quickly, within minutes for IV formulations. For chronic HF, therapy is begun with low doses of furosemide (Lasix), bumetanide (Bumex), or torsemide (Demadex), and gradually increased until the desired volume reduction is obtained.

As therapy continues with loop diuretics, some patients become less responsive, a phenomenon known as **diuretic resistance**. The loop diuretics exhibit a ceiling effect; once the "ceiling dose" is reached, increases in dosage will not produce additional diuresis. To obtain additional diuresis and volume reduction, the loop diuretic may be administered more frequently, or a diuretic from a different class may be added to the regimen.

Thiazide diuretics are also used in the pharmacotherapy of HF, sometimes combined with loop diuretics to achieve a more effective diuresis in patients with acute HF. Because they are less effective than the loop diuretics, thiazides are generally reserved for patients with mild-to-moderate HF.

In addition to being a potassium-sparing diuretic, spironolactone is also classified as an aldosterone antagonist. As a diuretic, spironolactone has a limited role in HF, due to its low efficacy. Clinical research, however, has demonstrated that the drug is able to block the deleterious effects of aldosterone on the heart. High levels of aldosterone promote cardiac remodeling and the deposition of fibrotic tissue in the myocardium of patients with HF. By blocking these cardiac effects, spironolactone decreases mortality due to sudden death, as well as progression to advanced HF.

At the low doses used for HF patients (25 mg daily), spironolactone produces few adverse effects. The most common adverse effect at this dose is gynecomastia in male patients. More serious, however, is the risk of hyperkalemia. Caution must be used when administering spironolactone concurrently with ACE inhibitors due to the possibility of additive hyperkalemia. Care must be taken to educate patients to limit potassium-rich foods in the diet and eliminate potassium supplements.

Diuretic use in HF patients should be carefully monitored to avoid dehydration or electrolyte imbalances. These adverse effects are more likely to occur in HF patients who have comorbid renal impairment. During maintenance therapy, patients are urged to weigh themselves frequently, and report significant changes to their health care provider. Frequent laboratory tests for blood electrolyte levels are obtained to prevent the development of hypokalemia during loop or thiazide diuretic therapy. This is especially important in patients who are also taking digoxin (Lanoxin), because hypokalemia may induce fatal dysrhythmias.

CONNECTION Checkpoint 39.2

Conn's syndrome is characterized by excess secretion of aldosterone. What effect would you predict this syndrome would have on the heart, and what medication might be a drug of choice? *See Answer to Connection Checkpoint 39.2 on student resource website.*

7 Beta-adrenergic antagonists can dramatically reduce hospitalizations and increase the survival of patients with heart failure.

Cardiac glycosides, beta-adrenergic agonists, and other medications that produce a positive inotropic effect serve important roles in reversing the diminished contractility that is the hallmark of HF. It may seem somewhat surprising, then, to find beta-adrenergic blockers—drugs that exhibit a negative inotropic effect—prescribed for this disease. Even though this class of drugs has the potential to worsen HF, beta-adrenergic blockers are standard therapy for many patients with this chronic disorder. Why is this the case?

In patients with HF, high levels of endogenous norepinephrine and other catecholamines cause excessive activation of the sympathetic nervous system, and are associated with cardiac remodeling and progression of the disease. Beta-adrenergic antagonists block the actions of these catecholamines, slowing the heart rate and reducing blood pressure, thus decreasing the cardiac workload. After several months of therapy, heart size, shape, and function return to normal in some patients, in essence producing a **reverse remodeling** of the heart. Extensive clinical research has demonstrated that the careful use of beta-adrenergic antagonists can dramatically reduce the number of HF-associated hospitalizations and deaths. They are effective in all stages of symptomatic HF. Doses for selected beta-adrenergic antagonists are listed in Table 3.

To benefit patients with HF, however, beta-adrenergic antagonists must be administered in a very specific manner. Initial doses must be 1/10 to 1/20 of the target dose. Doses are doubled every 2 weeks until the target dose is reached. If therapy is begun with the target dose, or the dose is increased too rapidly, beta blockers can worsen HF. Carvedilol and metoprolol are the two beta-adrenergic antagonists approved for HF, although bisoprolol has also been shown to be effective. When treating HF, beta blockers are almost always combined with other agents, especially the ACE inhibitors.

Adherence to beta-blocker therapy can be a major clinical challenge for some patients. The patient may not report symptomatic improvement with the drug and, in fact, may feel worse at the initiation of therapy. To achieve maximum patient adherence, the nurse must teach the patient the important long-term benefits of beta blockers.

Beta-adrenergic antagonists are contraindicated in patients with chronic obstructive pulmonary disease (COPD), severe bradycardia, or heart block. These medications should be used with caution in patients with diabetes, peripheral vascular disease, and hepatic impairment. Caution is needed with older adults because these patients often require a reduced dose. Hepatic function tests should be performed periodically, and the prescriber notified if signs or symptoms of liver toxicity become apparent.

8 Vasodilators reduce symptoms of heart failure by reducing preload or afterload.

Vasodilators relax blood vessels and lower blood pressure, creating less workload on the heart. They serve a limited role in the pharmacotherapy of HF.

Hydralazine with isosorbide dinitrate (BiDil): Hydralazine and isosorbide dinitrate were used off-label for many years in patients who did not respond well to drugs from other classes. In 2005, the fixed-dose combination of the two (BiDil) was approved as an adjunct to standard therapy for HF. The drug was shown to be particularly effective in treating African American patients, who are sometimes resistant to therapy for hypertension and heart failure.

Hydralazine acts on arterioles to decrease peripheral resistance, reduce afterload, and increase cardiac output. It is an effective antihypertensive drug, although it is not a drug of first choice for this indication because hypotension and reflex tachycardia are common, and may limit therapy. The drug must be taken three to four times daily, which places an extensive pill burden on HF patients, who often are taking multiple drugs.

Isosorbide dinitrate (Isordil) is a long-acting organic nitrate that reduces preload by directly dilating veins. The drug is not very effective as monotherapy, and tolerance develops to its actions with continued use. Isosorbide dinitrate is usually combined with hydralazine (BiDil) because the two drugs act synergistically when used in HF patients. The high incidence of adverse effects in some patients such as reflex tachycardia and orthostatic hypotension limits their use.

Nesiritide (Natrecor): A third vasodilator used for HF is very different from hydralazine or isosorbide dinitrate. Approved in 2001, nesiritide (Natrecor) is a small-peptide hormone, produced through recombinant DNA technology, that is structurally identical to human beta-type natriuretic peptide (hBNP). When heart failure occurs, the ventricles begin to secrete hBNP

TABLE 4 Drugs for Advanced Heart Failure

Drug	Route and Adult Dose (maximum dose where indicated)	Adverse Effects
Beta-Adrenergic Agonists		
dobutamine (Dobutrex)	IV: Infused at a rate of 2.5–40 mcg/kg/min for a max of 72 h	*Headache, palpitations, nausea, vomiting, changes in blood pressure (hypo- or hypertension)*
dopamine (Dopastat, Intropin)	IV: 2–5 mcg/kg/min initial dose; may be increased to 20–50 mcg/kg/min (max: 50 mcg/kg/min)	
epinephrine (Adrenalin)	Subcutaneous: 0.1–0.5 mL of 1:1,000 every 10–15 min prn IV: 0.1–0.25 mL of 1:1,000 every 10–15 min	<u>Dysrhythmias, gangrene, severe HTN</u>
isoproterenol (Isuprel)	IV infusion: 0.5–5 mcg/min	
norepinephrine (Levophed)	IV: Initially, 0.5–1 mcg/min until pressure stabilizes, then 2–4 mcg/min for maintenance (max: 30 mcg/min)	
Phosphodiesterase Inhibitors		
inamrinone (Inocor)	IV: 0.75 mg/kg bolus given slowly over 2–3 min; then 5–10 mcg/kg/min (max: 10 mg/kg/day)	*Headache, hypotension*
milrinone (Primacor)	IV: 50 mcg/kg over 10 min; then 0.375–0.75 mcg/kg/min	<u>Dysrhythmias</u>
Vasodilators		
nesiritide (Natrecor)	IV: 2 mcg/kg bolus followed by continuous infusion at 0.1 mcg/kg/min	*Hypotension, increased serum creatinine* <u>Dysrhythmias</u>

Note: Italics indicate common adverse effects. <u>Underline</u> indicates serious adverse effects.

in response to the increased stretch on the ventricular walls. hBNP enhances diuresis and renal excretion of sodium.

In therapeutic doses, nesiritide causes vasodilation, which contributes to reduced preload. By reducing preload and afterload, the drug compensates for diminished cardiac function. The use of nesiritide is very limited because it can rapidly cause severe hypotension, which can persist several hours after the infusion is discontinued. The drug is given by IV infusion, and patients require continuous monitoring. It is approved only for patients with acutely decompensated heart failure. The dosage for nesiritide is shown in Table 4. Nesiritide is pregnancy category C.

CONNECTION Checkpoint 39.3

Isosorbide dinitrate is also used for angina. Why is nitroglycerin a preferred drug for acute angina, rather than isosorbide dinitrate? *See Answer to Connection Checkpoint 39.3 on student resource website.*

9 Cardiac glycosides increase the force of myocardial contraction and were once drugs of choice for heart failure.

Once used as arrow poisons by African tribes and as medicines by the ancient Egyptians and Romans, the value of the cardiac glycosides in treating heart disorders has been known for over 2,000 years. Originally extracted from the beautiful flowering plants, *Digitalis purpura* (purple foxglove) and *Digitalis lanata* (white foxglove), the cardiac glycosides were the mainstay of HF treatment until the discovery of the ACE inhibitors. During the past 20 years, the role of the cardiac glycosides in the pharmacotherapy of HF has become more limited. The two primary cardiac glycosides, digoxin and digitoxin, are quite similar in efficacy; the primary difference is that the latter has a more prolonged half-life. Digitoxin is no longer available in the United States. The dose for digoxin is listed in Table 3.

Because of its long historical use, the effectiveness of digitalis in the pharmacotherapy of HF remained unquestioned until the late 1980s, when a controlled study of 6,800 patients with HF revealed no significant difference in mortality between patients who took digoxin and those who received a placebo. The drug did, however, produce symptomatic benefit in patients. Based on this study, and the development of safer and more effective drug classes, cardiac glycosides are now limited to late-stage HF, in combination with other agents. Digoxin remains an important therapy in HF patients with supraventricular tachyarrhythmias, because the drug has antidysrhythmic activity that can stabilize these types of cardiac conduction abnormalities.

The margin of safety between a therapeutic dose and a toxic dose of cardiac glycosides is very narrow, and severe adverse effects may result from poorly managed therapy. **Digitalization** refers to the procedure by which the dose of digoxin is gradually increased until tissues become saturated with the medication, and the symptoms of HF diminish. If the patient is critically ill, digitalization can be done rapidly with IV doses in a controlled clinical environment, where adverse effects may be carefully monitored. As an outpatient, digitalization may be completed over a period of 7 days, using oral (PO) dosing. In either case, the goal is to determine the proper dose of medication to be administered, without undue adverse effects.

PROTOTYPE DRUG	Digoxin (Lanoxin, Lanoxicaps)

Classification: **Therapeutic:** Drug for heart failure
Pharmacologic: Cardiac glycoside, inotropic agent

Therapeutic Effects and Uses: The primary benefit of digoxin is its ability to increase the strength of myocardial contraction, a positive inotropic action. By increasing myocardial contractility, digoxin directly increases cardiac output, which alleviates symptoms of HF and improves exercise tolerance. The higher cardiac output increases urine production and results in a desirable reduction in blood volume, relieving the distressing symptoms of pulmonary congestion and peripheral edema. In current clinical practice, digoxin use is usually limited to patients who are not responding adequately to ACE inhibitor therapy or to HF patients with atrial fibrillation.

In addition to its positive inotropic effect, digoxin also affects the speed of myocardial conduction. Through a mechanism not fully understood, digoxin decreases SNS activity and increases parasympathetic activity. This helps attenuate the excessive sympathetic activation that causes tachycardia and worsens HF (Section 2). Digoxin has the ability to suppress the sinoatrial node and slow electrical conduction through the atrioventricular node. The heart rate decreases, allowing greater diastolic filling of the ventricles. Because the heart rate may decline too much, health care providers establish parameters for each patient. As a general rule, if the apical pulse falls below 60 beats per minute, the medication is withheld and the health care provider notified.

Digoxin is available by the PO or IV route. The capsule formulation (Lanoxicaps) has a more predictable bioavailability than the tablet form, but it is more expensive. Because differences in bioavailability of digoxin formulations can potentially affect drug action and the potential for adverse effects, it is advisable to continue with the same brand name, unless otherwise changed by the prescriber.

Mechanism of Action: Digoxin inhibits Na^+-K^+-ATPase, the critical enzyme responsible for pumping sodium ions out of the myocardial cells in exchange for potassium ions. As sodium ions accumulate in myocytes, calcium ions are released from their storage areas in the cell to activate contractile elements. The release of calcium ions produces a more forceful contraction of myocardial fibers.

Pharmacokinetics:

Route(s)	PO, IV
Absorption	70–90% absorbed from the gastrointestinal (GI) tract
Distribution	Widely distributed; crosses the placenta; secreted in breast milk; 20–25% bound to protein
Primary metabolism	Hepatic, 14%
Primary excretion	Renal
Onset of action	PO: 30–90 min; IV: 5–30 min
Duration of action	Half-life: 3–4 days

Adverse Effects: Adverse effects of digoxin involve multiple body systems and can be severe. The most dangerous adverse effect is its ability to cause ventricular dysrhythmias, which may result in sudden cardiac death. The most common cause of digoxin-induced dysrhythmias is hypokalemia due to diuretic use. Other factors placing patients at risk for digoxin-induced dysrhythmias include hypomagnesemia, hypercalcemia, and impaired renal function. Additional serious adverse cardiac effects include atrioventricular (AV) block, atrial dysrhythmias, and sinus bradycardia. Frequent electrocardiograms (ECGs) should be obtained to assess for cardiotoxicity.

Noncardiac adverse effects include general malaise, dizziness, headache, anorexia, nausea, and vomiting. The drug may produce unusual visual effects such as halos, changes in color perception, and photophobia.

Frequent serum digoxin levels should be obtained during therapy, and the dosage adjusted based on the laboratory results and the patient's clinical response. Clinical research suggests that digoxin levels from 0.5 to 2 ng/mL give the most therapeutic benefit, with an acceptable risk of adverse effects for most patients. Raising the dose does not increase the therapeutic effect, but it does increase the risk of serious digoxin toxicity. For each patient, the health care provider should establish acceptable parameters for serum digoxin levels, and the drug should be discontinued should the level rise above the maximum. Digoxin levels greater than 2.0 ng/mL are considered toxic. However, the nurse should remember that toxicity should be based on patient symptoms rather than serum level. Levels should be taken 6 to 12 hours after a dose, because digoxin has a prolonged distribution time.

Contraindications/Precautions: Patients with AV block or ventricular dysrhythmias unrelated to HF should not receive digoxin, because the drug may worsen these conditions. Digoxin should be administered with caution to older adults because these patients experience a higher incidence of adverse effects. Patients with renal impairment should receive lower doses of digoxin, because the drug is excreted by this route. The drug should be used with caution in patients with MI, cor pulmonale, or hypothyroidism.

Drug Interactions: Digoxin interacts with many drugs. Concurrent use of digoxin with diuretics must be carefully monitored, since diuretics can cause hypokalemia and increase the risk of dysrhythmias. Use with ACE inhibitors, spironolactone, or potassium supplements can lead to hyperkalemia and reduce the therapeutic action of digoxin. Administration of digoxin with other positive inotropic agents can cause additive effects on myocardial contractility. Concurrent use with beta blockers may result in additive bradycardia. Antacids and cholesterol-lowering drugs can decrease the absorption of digoxin. If calcium is administered intravenously together with digoxin, it can increase the risk of dysrhythmias. Quinidine, verapamil, amiodarone, and alprazolam will decrease the distribution and excretion of digoxin, thus increasing the risk of digoxin toxicity. **Herbal/Food:** The drug should be used with caution with ginseng, which may increase the risk of digoxin toxicity.

Pregnancy: Category A.

Treatment of Overdose: Digoxin overdose can be fatal and the nurse should be prepared to administer digoxin immune Fab (Digibind). Digoxin immune Fab consists of digoxin-specific antibodies, which form a complex with digoxin that prevents the drug from reaching the tissues, and is removed through renal excretion. Reversal of adverse effects occurs quickly: 90% of patients respond within an hour after IV administration. As digoxin is removed from the body, the inotropic effects of the drug will diminish, and the patient may be at risk of HF. The patient must be monitored continuously during the infusion.

Nursing Responsibilities: Key nursing implications for patients receiving digoxin are included in the Nursing Practice

Application for Patients Receiving Pharmacotherapy for Heart Failure.

Lifespan and Diversity Considerations:

- Digoxin is included in the Beers list of potentially inappropriate drugs for the older adult and warrants careful monitoring. Because of decreased excretion related to renal changes associated with aging, closely monitor for adverse effects.
- Use extreme caution in measuring liquid doses for infants and children to ensure proper dosing.

Patient and Family Education:

- Take digoxin precisely as prescribed. Do not skip or double a dose or change dose intervals, and take it at the same time each day.
- Do not switch brands of digoxin originally prescribed, unless directed by the prescriber.
- Do not breast-feed while taking this drug without approval of the health care provider.

Drugs Similar to Digoxin (Lanoxin, Lanoxicaps)

Digoxin is the only cardiac glycoside available in the United States.

CONNECTION Checkpoint 39.4

Cholestyramine reduces the bioavailability of digoxin, thus potentially decreasing the actions of the cardiac glycoside. What is the primary indication for cholestyramine and what is the likely reason this drug causes a decrease in digoxin bioavailability? *See Answer to Connection Checkpoint 39.4 on student resource website A.*

10 Phosphodiesterase III inhibitors and other positive inotropic agents are used for acute decompensated heart failure.

Advanced or decompensated HF can be a medical emergency, and prompt, effective treatment is necessary to avoid organ failure or death. In addition to high doses of loop diuretics, positive inotropic drugs are often necessary. The two primary classes of inotropic agents used for decompensated HF are beta-adrenergic agonists and phosphodiesterase inhibitors. Doses for these agents are listed in Table 4.

Beta-Adrenergic Agonists (Sympathomimetics)

Beta-adrenergic agonists used for HF include isoproterenol (Isuprel), epinephrine, norepinephrine, dopamine (Dopastat, Intropin), and dobutamine (Dobutrex). Dobutamine has been a traditional drug of choice in this class because it has the ability to rapidly increase myocardial contractility, with minimal changes to heart rate or blood pressure. This is important because increases in heart rate or blood pressure will create greater oxygen demands on the heart and possibly worsen HF. Therapy with dobutamine is usually limited to 72 hours, as continuous infusion of the drug causes the heart to become tolerant to beta adrenergic activation, making the drug less effective. The two most common adverse effects with beta-agonists are tachycardia and dysrhythmias.

Patients who have both HF and hypotension benefit from dopamine, which not only increases myocardial contractility but also activates alpha-adrenergic receptors to increase blood pressure. However, tachycardia is more prominent with dopamine than with dobutamine. Patients who have been receiving a beta-adrenergic antagonist for their HF may require a higher initial dose of beta-agonist.

Phosphodiesterase III Inhibitors

In the 1980s, two medications became available that block the enzyme **phosphodiesterase III** in cardiac and smooth muscle, which leads to increases in the amount of calcium available for myocardial contraction. The enzyme inhibition results in two main actions that benefit patients with HF: a positive inotropic

---

Complementary and Alternative Therapies   Carnitine (L-Carnitine)

Description: Carnitine is a natural substance that is structurally similar to amino acids. Its primary function in metabolism is to move fatty acids from the bloodstream into cells, where it assists in the breakdown of lipids in the mitochondria. This breakdown produces energy and increases the availability of oxygen, particularly in muscle cells. A congenital deficiency of carnitine leads to severe brain, liver, and heart damage. The best food sources of carnitine are organ meats, fish, muscle meats, and milk products.

History and Claims: Carnitine has been claimed to enhance energy and sports performance, heart health, memory, immune function, and male fertility. It is also being marketed as a "fat burner" for weight reduction.

Standardization: Carnitine is available as a supplement in several forms, including L-carnitine, D-carnitine, and L-acetylcarnitine. D-carnitine is associated with potential adverse effects, and should be avoided. Doses range from 2 to 6 g/day.

Evidence: Carnitine has been well studied but large, controlled research trials are still needed to explore the effects for certain conditions. There is solid evidence to support supplementation in patients who are deficient in carnitine (Flanagan, Simmons, Vehige, Wilcox, & Garrett, 2010). Although a normal diet supplies 300 mg per day, certain patients may need additional amounts. Vegans are at risk for carnitine depletion, since plant protein supplies little or no carnitine.

Carnitine supplementation has been shown to improve exercise tolerance in patients with angina. The use of carnitine may prevent the occurrence of dysrhythmias in the early stages of heart disease. Carnitine has also been shown to decrease triglyceride levels while increasing HDL serum levels, thus helping to minimize one of the major risk factors associated with heart disease.

Research has not shown carnitine supplementation to be of significant benefit in enhancing sports performance, improving brain function in patients with Alzheimer's disease, or weight loss (University of Maryland Medical Center, 2009).

action and vasodilation. Cardiac output is increased due to the increase in contractility and the decrease in left ventricular afterload. There is little effect on heart rate. Arterial pressure is either decreased or, in some patients, it remains unchanged.

Although the actions of the phosphodiesterase III inhibitors are very similar to dobutamine, they have a much longer half-life. This makes it more difficult to make rapid changes in dose when controlling acute HF. In addition, if adverse effects do occur, they are more prolonged than with dobutamine.

Phosphodiesterase inhibitors have serious toxicity that limits their use to patients with resistant HF who have not responded to ACE inhibitors, digoxin, or other therapies. Therapy is limited to 2 to 3 days and the patient is continuously monitored for ventricular dysrhythmias, including ectopic beats, supraventricular dysrhythmias, premature ventricular contractions, ventricular tachycardia, and ventricular fibrillation. If the patient presents with hypokalemia, this should be corrected before administering phosphodiesterase III inhibitors because this can increase the likelihood of dysrhythmias. These medications can cause hypotension. When using inamrinone, frequent laboratory blood tests should be conducted to assess for thrombocytopenia.

PROTOTYPE DRUG	Milrinone (Primacor)

Classification: **Therapeutic:** Drug for heart failure
Pharmacologic: Phosphodiesterase inhibitor; inotropic agent

Therapeutic Effects and Uses: Approved in 1987, milrinone is indicated for the short-term treatment of patients with acute decompensated heart failure. Although inamrinone was the first drug in this class to be marketed, milrinone is generally preferred because it has a shorter half-life and fewer adverse effects. It is only given intravenously, and peak effects occur in 2 minutes. Immediate effects of milrinone include an increased force of contraction (positive inotropic effect) and a resulting increase in cardiac output. Research has not yet demonstrated any decrease in mortality or morbidity with the use of milrinone infusions. In patients with Class II or IV HF, drug therapy with milrinone is generally limited to 48 hours.

Mechanism of Action: Milrinone inhibits phosphodiesterase III, the enzyme responsible for the breakdown of cAMP to AMP, in cardiac and vascular smooth muscle. The rise in cAMP levels increases intracellular calcium, resulting in greater contractility. Cardiac output is increased and pulmonary capillary wedge pressure is decreased.

Pharmacokinetics:

Route(s)	IV
Absorption	N/A
Distribution	Unknown; 70% bound to plasma protein
Primary metabolism	Unknown; 83% is excreted unchanged
Primary excretion	Renal
Onset of action	2–10 min
Duration of action	Half-life: 3–6 h

Adverse Effects: The most serious adverse effect of milrinone is ventricular dysrhythmia, which can occur in more than 10% of patients taking the drug. The ECG is monitored continuously during the infusion of the drug to prevent serious dysrhythmias, especially ventricular dysrhythmias. Blood pressure is also continuously monitored during the infusion to avoid hypotension. Patients with Class IV HF are at high risk for life-threatening cardiovascular reactions. Less serious adverse effects include headache, nausea, and vomiting.

Contraindications/Precautions: Milrinone is contraindicated in patients with severe obstructive valvular heart disease. The drug should be used with caution in patients with preexisting dysrhythmias. Hypovolemia or electrolyte imbalances should be corrected before starting the infusion, and the dose should be reduced in patients with renal impairment.

Drug Interactions: Caution should be used when administering milrinone with digoxin, dobutamine, or other inotropic drugs, since their cardiac effects may be additive. Use with antihypertensive agents may cause additive hypotension. **Food/Herbal:** Ginger may contribute to the cardiac actions of milrinone.

Pregnancy: Category C.

Treatment of Overdose: Overdose of milrinone causes hypotension, which may be treated with the administration of normal saline or a vasopressor.

Nursing Responsibilities: Key nursing implications for patients receiving milrinone are included in the Nursing Practice Application for Patients Receiving Pharmacotherapy for Heart Failure.

Lifespan and Diversity Considerations:
- Because of decreased excretion related to renal changes associated with aging, closely monitor for adverse effects in the older adult.

Patient and Family Education:
- Immediately report chest pain (angina) to the health care provider should it occur during the infusion.
- This drug may cause a headache, which can be treated with analgesics.

Drugs Similar to Milrinone (Primacor)

The only other drug in the phosphodiesterase inhibitor class is inamrinone.

Inamrinone (Inocor): Approved in 1984, inamrinone has similar indications and inotropic actions as milrinone. Its only approved use is for the short-term therapy of serious or decompensated HF. Like milrinone, it is administered by IV infusion with continuous monitoring to detect the possibility of dysrhythmias and to avoid hypotension. One difference is that inamrinone causes a higher incidence of thrombocytopenia. The nurse should assess for signs and symptoms of bleeding during therapy. Because the liver metabolizes inamrinone, caution must be used when treating patients with hepatic impairment. Prior to 2000, inamrinone was called amrinone. The name was changed to avoid medication errors. The name amrinone looked and sounded too similar to amiodarone, an antidysrhythmic drug. This drug is pregnancy category C.

CONNECTIONS: NURSING PRACTICE APPLICATION

Patients Receiving Pharmacotherapy for Heart Failure

Assessment	Potential Nursing Diagnoses
Baseline assessment prior to administration: • Understand the reason the drug has been prescribed in order to assess for therapeutic effects. • Obtain a complete health history: cardiovascular (including previous MI, HF, valvular disease, dysrhythmias [especially heart block] renal dysfunction, pregnancy, or lactation. Obtain a drug history including allergies, current prescription and over-the-counter (OTC) drugs, herbal preparations, and alcohol use. Be alert to possible drug interactions. • Obtain baseline weight, vital signs (especially pulse and blood pressure), breath sounds, and ECG. Assess for location and character of edema if present. • Evaluate appropriate laboratory findings, electrolytes, especially potassium level, renal function studies, and lipid profiles. • Assess the patient's ability to receive and understand instructions. Include family and caregivers as needed.	• *Decreased Cardiac Output* • *Fatigue* • *Activity Intolerance* • *Excess Fluid Volume* • *Deficient Knowledge* (Drug Therapy) • *Risk for Reduced Cardiac Tissue Perfusion* • *Risk for Falls*, related to adverse drug effects • *Risk for Injury*, related to adverse drug effects
Assessment throughout administration: • Assess for desired therapeutic effects (e.g., heart rate and blood pressure return to, or remain within, normal limits; urine output returns to, or is within, normal limits; respiratory congestion (if present) is improved; peripheral edema (if present) is improved; level of consciousness, skin color, capillary refill, and other signs of adequate perfusion are within normal limits; fatigue lessens). • Continue periodic monitoring of electrolytes, especially potassium, renal function, and drug levels. • Assess for adverse effects: hypotension, fatigue, dizziness, or drowsiness. Bradycardia, nausea, vomiting, anorexia, visual changes (e.g., halos around lights, yellow or yellowish-green tint to colors) may also occur with digoxin. A pulse rate below 60 or above 100 beats/min, palpitations, significant dizziness or syncope, dyspnea, persistent anorexia or vomiting, or visual changes should be reported to the provider immediately. • Exercise extra caution when giving the drug to older adults, pediatric patients, or patients with renal insufficiency. Immature renal function or declines in renal function make these populations more susceptible to adverse effects.	

Planning: Patient Goals and Expected Outcomes

The patient will:

• Experience therapeutic effects dependent on the reason the drug is being given (e.g., heart rate and blood pressure remain within established parameters, urine output increases to normal, fatigue lessens, lung sounds clear, peripheral edema decreases).

• Be free from or experience minimal adverse effects.

• Verbalize an understanding of the drug's use, adverse effects, and required precautions.

• Demonstrate proper self-administration of the medication (e.g., dose, timing, and when to notify the provider).

Implementation

Interventions and (Rationales)	Patient-Centered Care
Ensuring therapeutic effects: • Continue frequent assessments as above for therapeutic effects. (As the heart contracts more forcefully, blood pressure and pulse should return to within normal limits or within the parameters set by the health care provider; urine output returns to within normal limits, peripheral edema decreases, and lung sounds clear.)	• Teach the patient, family, or caregiver how to monitor the pulse and blood pressure. Ensure proper use and functioning of any home equipment obtained.
• Encourage appropriate lifestyle changes: lowered fat intake, restricted sodium or fluid intake if ordered, gradually increased levels of exercise, limited alcohol intake, and smoking cessation. Provide for dietitian consultation as needed. (Healthy lifestyle changes will support the benefits of drug therapy.)	• Encourage the patient, family, or caregiver to adopt a healthy lifestyle of low-fat food choices, increased exercise, decreased alcohol consumption, and smoking cessation. Provide educational materials on low-fat, low-sodium food choices.

CONNECTIONS: NURSING PRACTICE APPLICATION (continued)

Minimizing adverse effects:

- Continue to monitor vital signs. Take an apical pulse for 1 full minute before giving the drug. Hold the drug and notify the health care provider if heart rate is below 60 or above 100 beats/min and contact the provider. Monitor ECG during infusion of milrinone (Primacor) and during the digitalization period for dysrhythmias or bradycardia. (Drugs that are positive inotropes increase myocardial contractility but may affect cardiac conduction. Milrinone is associated with serious and potentially life-threatening dysrhythmias. Digoxin slows the heart rate and may cause bradycardia.)

- Teach the patient, family, or caregiver how to take a peripheral pulse for 1 full minute before taking the drug. Assist the patient to find the most convenient and easily felt pulse area. Record daily pulse rates and bring the record to each health care visit. Instruct the patient to not take the drug if pulse is below 60 or above 100 beats/min, and to contact the provider for further direction. If the patient, family, or caregiver chooses to buy a stethoscope to take pulse, ensure proper understanding of heart sounds (i.e., lub-dub of heartbeat is *ONE* heartbeat) and appropriate stethoscope placement. Have the patient, family, or caregiver return demonstrate. (With easier accessibility to OTC medical equipment such as stethoscopes, patients, family, or caregivers may try to emulate the health care provider. Ensure proper use before the patient goes home.)

- Continue to monitor electrolyte levels periodically, especially potassium, renal function laboratory values, drug levels, and ECG. (Hypokalemia increases the risk of dysrhythmias from drugs used to treat HF.)

- Instruct the patient on the need to return periodically for laboratory work.
- Advise the patient to carry a wallet identification card or wear medical identification jewelry indicating drug therapy for HF.

- Weigh the patient daily and report a weight gain or loss of 1 kg (2.2 lb) or more in a 24-h period. (Daily weight is an accurate measure of fluid status and takes into account intake, output, and insensible losses. Weight gain or edema may signal impending HF with reduced organ perfusion, stimulating renin release.)

- Have the patient weigh self daily, ideally at the same time of day, and record weight along with pulse measurements. Instruct the patient to report a weight loss or gain of more than 1 kg (2.2 lb) in a 24-h period.

- Monitor for signs of worsening HF (e.g., increasing dyspnea or postural nocturnal dyspnea, rales or crackles in lungs, frothy pink-tinged sputum) and report immediately. (Positive inotropic drugs such as digoxin or phosphodiesterase inhibitors are usually reserved for patients with more advanced stages of HF. If signs and symptoms worsen, other treatment options may need to be considered.)

- Instruct the patient to immediately report any severe shortness of breath, frothy sputum, profound fatigue, or swelling of extremities as possible signs of HF.

- For patients taking digoxin, report signs of possible toxicity immediately to the provider and obtain a drug level. (Digoxin levels should remain less than 1.8 mg/mL. Signs and symptoms such as bradycardia, nausea and vomiting, anorexia, visual changes, depression, changes in level of consciousness, fatigue, dizziness, or syncope should be reported.)

- Instruct the patient, family, or caregiver on signs to report to the health care provider. Encourage the patient to report any significant change in overall health or mental activity promptly.

- Use extra caution when measuring the precise dose of medication ordered and use extreme caution when measuring liquid doses, especially for pediatric patients. (For drugs such as digoxin with a long half-life and duration, toxic levels may result with only small amounts of additional drug.)

- Caution the patient on taking the precise dose of medication ordered, not doubling the dose if a dose is missed, and to use extreme caution when measuring liquid doses, especially for pediatric patients.

Patient understanding of drug therapy:

- Use opportunities during administration of medications and during assessments to discuss the rationale for the drug therapy, desired therapeutic outcomes, commonly observed adverse effects, parameters for when to call the health care provider, and any necessary monitoring or precautions. (Using time during nursing care helps to optimize and reinforce key teaching areas.)

- The patient, family, or caregiver should be able to state the reason for the drug, appropriate dose and scheduling, what adverse effects to observe for and when to report them, and the anticipated length of medication therapy.

Patient self-administration of drug therapy:

- When administering medications, instruct the patient, family, or caregiver in the proper self-administration techniques. (Utilizing time during nurse-administration of these drugs helps to reinforce teaching.)

- Instruct the patient in proper administration techniques, followed by return demonstration.
- The patient, family, or caregiver is able to discuss appropriate dosing and administration needs.

Evaluation of Outcome Criteria

Evaluate the effectiveness of drug therapy by confirming that patient goals and expected outcomes have been met (see "Planning").

UNDERSTANDING THE CHAPTER

Key Concepts Summary

1 Heart failure is closely associated with disorders such as chronic hypertension, coronary artery disease, and diabetes.

2 The body attempts to compensate for heart failure by increasing cardiac output.

3 Symptoms of heart failure occur when compensatory mechanisms fail to maintain adequate cardiac output.

4 The specific therapy for heart failure depends on the clinical stage of the disease.

5 Angiotensin-converting enzyme inhibitors are drugs of choice for heart failure.

6 Diuretics relieve symptoms of heart failure by reducing fluid overload and decreasing blood pressure.

7 Beta-adrenergic antagonists can dramatically reduce hospitalizations and increase the survival of patients with heart failure.

8 Vasodilators reduce symptoms of heart failure by reducing preload or afterload.

9 Cardiac glycosides increase the force of myocardial contraction and were once drugs of choice for heart failure.

10 Phosphodiesterase III inhibitors and other positive inotropic agents are used for acute decompensated heart failure.

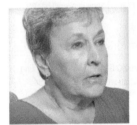

Making the PATIENT Connection

Remember the patient "Thelma Walters" at the beginning of the chapter? Now read the remainder of the case study. Based on the information presented within this chapter, respond to the critical thinking questions that follow.

Thelma Walters is a 77-year-old woman who arrives via EMS at the emergency department after experiencing increasing dyspnea for the past 2 days. She has also noticed swelling in her feet and ankles. Due to her onset of shortness of breath, she has had to sleep in a recliner and is unable to lay flat in bed at night. Her past medical history includes a myocardial infarction 3 years ago and an episode of heart failure 1 year ago. The heart failure was treated with captopril (Capoten) and furosemide (Lasix), which she has been taking since that time. Her surgical history includes a hysterectomy 20 years ago. She has never used tobacco or alcohol.

As the nurse performs the initial physical assessment the following relevant findings are discovered. The patient is 1.7 m (5'6") tall and weighs 82 kg (180 lb). The patient's blood pressure is 162/92 mmHg, her heart rate is 148 beats/min and irregular, and her respiratory rate is 38 breaths/min and labored. The neck veins of the patient are distended when she is placed at a 45-degree incline. She is orthopneic and cannot tolerate the head of

the bed being lowered below 45 degrees. The nurse notes scattered crackles bilaterally throughout the lung fields. The patient has a productive cough with frothy, pink-tinged sputum. 4+ pitting edema of both hands and legs is noted with the nail beds moderately cyanotic. Circumoral cyanosis is also noted.

Immediately upon arrival at the emergency department, the patient received oxygen therapy and an IV line was started. Blood is collected for initial laboratory data with the following results: serum sodium 136 mEq/L (normal 135–147 mEq/L), serum potassium 3.1 mEq/L (normal 3.5–5.2 mEq/L), and arterial blood gases on room air: pH 7.32, PaO_2 54, $PaCO_2$ 48, SaO_2 68%, indicating overall hypoxemia. Thelma is in acute distress and admitted to the intensive care unit (ICU) with a diagnosis of heart failure. She is given a dose of furosemide (Lasix) 20 mg intravenously and she will receive milrinone (Primacor) by IV infusion after admission to the ICU.

Critical Thinking Questions

1. Describe how milrinone (Primacor) aids in treating heart failure.

2. During the infusion of milrinone (Primacor), Thelma's ECG and blood pressure will be monitored closely. What adverse effects does milrinone have on the heart rhythm and blood pressure?

3. Because Thelma has been taking furosemide (Lasix) at home and has received another dose in the emergency department, what will the nurse assess prior to starting the milrinone (Primacor)? What electrolyte imbalance must be corrected before Thelma receives the milrinone (Primacor)?

See Answers to Critical Thinking Questions on student resource website.

NCLEX-RN® Review

1 A client newly diagnosed with heart failure following an acute myocardial infarction has a prescription for enalapril (Vasotec). This drug class is frequently used in early heart failure because of what clinical improvement?

1. It strengthens the force of myocardial contraction to improve cardiac output.
2. It decreases peripheral resistance, increasing cardiac output.
3. It slows the heart rate, improving filling time and increasing cardiac output.
4. It has diuretic effects, decreasing peripheral edema and pulmonary congestion.

2 In providing the client with heart failure information prior to discharge, the nurse will discuss digoxin (Lanoxin) therapy. Which point would the nurse include in the client's teaching?

1. Take the drug in the morning before rising.
2. Monitor the pulse daily prior to taking the drug.
3. Discontinue the drug if the pulse rate is 70 beats per minute.
4. Eat a diet high in bran fiber and calcium.

3 The nurse is evaluating the therapeutic effects of milrinone (Primacor). The nurse knows that this drug is given to:

1. Increase the force of cardiac contractions and improve cardiac output.
2. Decrease the volume of the cardiac output to reduce hypertension.
3. Relax the myocardial muscle, decreasing myocardial oxygen requirements.
4. Inhibit cardiac irregularities, decreasing the sensation of palpitations.

4 The client is receiving hydralazine with isosorbide (BiDil) for heart failure. The nurse should monitor this client for:

1. Confusion and agitation.
2. Bleeding.
3. Tingling or cramping in the legs.
4. Dizziness and rapid heart rate.

5 A client will begin taking carvedilol (Coreg) for heart failure. Before teaching the client about this drug, the nurse will discuss the strategy for drug dosage with the health care provider because of which recommended routine for beta-adrenergic blockers in heart failure?

1. Significantly lower dosages are used first and gradually increased to a target dose.
2. A loading dose that is higher than the subsequent daily dose must be given.
3. The beta-adrenergic blocker dosage must be lowered if the client is also on ACE inhibitors.
4. Beta-adrenergic blockers are almost never used in HF and the order must be confirmed.

6 When planning client education, the nurse knows that client adherence to beta-adrenergic blocker therapy in heart failure may be difficult to achieve despite the usefulness of these drugs. What will the nurse need to address in the teaching plan? Select all that apply.

1. The dosage must be gradually adjusted over time to a beneficial dose.
2. The client may not notice significant improvement during early therapy.
3. The drug may require changes to many other medications the client is taking.
4. The drug has significant benefit in reducing mortality from heart failure.
5. The drug will require extensive lifestyle changes.

Additional Case Study

Jim Mabry, a 77-year-old man, currently takes the following medications daily: digoxin (Lanoxin) 0.125 mg; furosemide (Lasix) 20 mg daily; and potassium supplementation (K-Dur) 20 mEq. As his nurse, you will be discussing Jim's medication regimen and his next health care provider office visit after discharge from the hospital.

1. Discuss the relationship among the three medications.
2. Jim will have a digoxin serum level collected during the health care provider office visit. What does he need to know about this procedure?
3. Jim asked you to compile a list of foods that are rich in potassium. Prepare the list.

See Answers to Additional Case Study on student resource website.

Pearson Nursing Student Resources

Find additional review materials at
nursing.pearsonhighered.com
Prepare for success with additional NCLEX®-style practice
questions, interactive assignments and activities, web links,
animations, videos, and more!

References

American College of Cardiology/American Heart Association Task Force on Practice Guidelines. (2009). 2009 focused update *ACCF/AHA guidelines for the diagnosis and management of heart failure in adults.* A report of the American College of Cardiology Foundation/American Heart Association Task Force on Practice Guidelines Developed in collaboration with the International Society for Heart and Lung Transplantation. *Journal of the American College of Cardiology, 53,* 1343–1382. doi:10.1016/j.jacc.2008.11.009

Dumitru, I. (2011). Heart failure. *Medscape Reference.* Retrieved from http://emedicine.medscape.com/article/163062-overview

Dungan, K. M., Osei, K., Nagaraja, H. N., Schuster, D. P., & Binkley, P. (2010). Relationship between glycemic control and readmission rates in patients hospitalized with congestive heart failure during implementation of hospital-wide initiatives. *Endocrine Practice, 16*(6), 945–951. doi:10.4158/EP10093.OR

Flanagan, J. L., Simmons, P. A., Vehige, J., Wilcox, M., & Garrett, Q. (2010). Role of carnitine in disease. *Nutrition and Metabolism, 7,* 30. doi:10.1186/1743-7075-7-30

University of Maryland Medical Center. (2009). *Carnitine (L-carnitine).* Retrieved from http://www.umm.edu/altmed/articles/carnitine-l-000291.htm

van Melle, J. P., Bot, M., de Jonge, P., de Boer, R. A., van Veldhuisen, D. K., & Whooley, M. A. (2010). Diabetes, glycemic control, and new-onset heart failure in patients with stable coronary artery disease. *Diabetes Care, 33*(9), 2084–2089. doi:10.2337/dc10-0286

Selected Bibliography

Albert, N. M., Yancy, C. W., Li Liang, X. Z., Hernandez, A. F., Peterson, A. D., Cannon, C. P., & Fonarow, G. G. (2009). Use of aldosterone antagonists in heart failure. *Journal of the American Medical Association, 302*(15), 1658–1665. doi:10.1001/jama.2009.1493

Al-Mohammad, A., & Mant, J. T. (2011). The diagnosis and management of chronic heart failure: Review following the publication of the NICE guidelines. *Heart, 97*(5), 411–416. doi:10.1136/hrt.2010.214999

Case, R., Haynes, D., Holaday, B., & Parker, V. G. (2010). Evidence-based nursing: The role of the advanced practice registered nurse in the management of heart failure patients in the outpatient setting. *Dimensions of Critical Care Nursing, 29*(2), 57–62. doi:10.1097/DCC.0b013e3181c92efb

DeFelice, P., Masucci, M., McLoughlin, J., Salvatore, S., Shane, M., & Wong, D. (2010). Congestive heart failure: Redefining health care and nursing. *Journal of Continuing Education in Nursing, 41*(9), 390–391. doi:10.3928/00220124-20100825-03

Dupree, C. S. (2010). Primary prevention of heart failure: An update. *Current Opinion in Cardiology, 25*(5), 478–483. doi:10.1097/HCO.0b013e32833cd550

Gislason, G. H., Rasmussen, J. N., Abildstrom, S. Z., Schramm, T. K., Hansen, M. L., Buch, P., et al. (2007). Persistent use of evidence-based pharmacotherapy in heart failure is associated with improved outcomes. *Circulation, 116*(10), 734–744.

Jugdutt, B. I. (2010). Aging and heart failure: Changing demographics and implications for therapy in the elderly. *Heart Failure Reviews, 15*(5), 401–405. doi:10.1007/s10741-010-9164-8

Kee, J. L. (2010). *Laboratory and diagnostic tests with nursing implications* (8th ed.). Upper Saddle River, NJ: Pearson Education.

Maron, B. A., & Rocco, T. P. (2011). Pharmacotherapy of congestive heart failure. In L. L. Brunton, B. A. Chabner, & B. C. Knollman (Eds.), *The pharmacological basis of therapeutics* (12th ed., pp. 789–814). New York, NY: McGraw-Hill.

Answers to NCLEX-RN® Review

1 Answer: 2 Rationale: ACE inhibitors such as enalapril lower peripheral resistance through the inhibition of angiotensin II formation, and reduce blood volume through inhibition of aldosterone secretion. This reduces arterial blood pressure, decreasing afterload and increasing cardiac output. Options 1, 3, and 4 are incorrect. Enalapril is not a positive inotropic agent and does not strengthen the force of myocardial contraction. It does not slow heart rate (negative chronotropic and dromotropic effects) and it does not have diuretic effects. Cognitive Level: Analyzing; Client Need: Physiological Integrity; Nursing Process: Evaluation

2 Answer: 2 Rationale: The client will be taught to take the pulse daily and to contact the prescriber if the pulse rate is less than 60 or greater than 100 beats per min. Options 1, 3, and 4 are incorrect. The medication should be taken at the same time each day, but preferably after the client has been active for a period of time (midmorning). Typically, the pulse rate will be lower in the morning before the client rises. Digoxin should be withheld if the pulse rate is below 60 beats per min. A high-fiber diet may decrease the absorption of digoxin, and the drug should not be taken along with meals high in fiber. Furthermore, foods high in calcium may create hypercalcemia, which will potentiate the possibility of digoxin toxicity. Cognitive Level: Applying; Client Need: Health Promotion and Maintenance; Nursing Process: Implementation

3 Answer: 1 Rationale: Milrinone is a positive inotropic drug and is given to increase the force of the contraction of the heart, which improves cardiac output. Options 2, 3, and 4 are incorrect. Inotropic effects increase the volume of the cardiac output rather than decrease it, and do not relax the myocardial muscle. Milrinone may cause cardiac dysrhythmias as an adverse effect. Cognitive Level: Analyzing; Client Need: Physiological Integrity; Nursing Process: Evaluation

4 Answer: 4 Rationale: Hydralazine with isosorbide may cause hypotension with reflex tachycardia, resulting in dizziness and rapid heart rate. Options 1, 2, and 3 are incorrect. Hydralazine with isosorbide does not cause confusion, agitation, bleeding, or tingling of the extremities. If these occur, other causes should be investigated. Cognitive Level: Analyzing; Client Need: Physiological Integrity; Nursing Process: Evaluation

5 Answer: 1 Rationale: Beta-adrenergic blockers such as carvedilol must be started at 1/10 to 1/20 of a usual dose and gradually increased to a target dosage. Options 2, 3, and 4 are incorrect. Because lower dosages are required, a higher loading dose will not be given, and beta-adrenergic blockers are often combined with ACE inhibitors, although dosage will not be directly related to the ACE inhibitor. While caution is required if beta-adrenergic blockers are used to treat HF, they are an important drug group used to treat heart failure. Cognitive Level: Applying; Client Need: Physiological Integrity; Nursing Process: Implementation

6 Answer: 1, 2, 4 Rationale: Beta-adrenergic blockers require gradual increases in dosage amount approximately every 2 weeks to a target dosage. Significant improvement may not be noticed in early therapy and the client may feel worse during initiation of therapy. Overall, however, the therapy has been proven to reduce the number of HF-related hospitalizations and mortalities. Options 3 and 5 are incorrect. Beta-adrenergic blocker therapy may require alterations in dosage for other cardiac drugs but not all drugs will be affected. Lifestyle changes may be advisable in HF but are not necessarily directly related to beta-adrenergic blocker use. Cognitive Level: Applying; Client Need: Health Promotion and Maintenance; Nursing Process: Planning

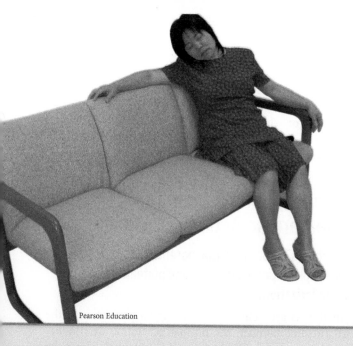

"I will never forget the fear that overwhelmed me as I woke up in the emergency department. I had no idea what had happened. I only remember a strange sensation in my chest. It was like my heart was fluttering. Then I must have passed out."

Patient "Jada Chinn Nguyen"

Pharmacotherapy of Dysrhythmias

Chapter Outline

Etiology of Dysrhythmias

Phases and Measurement of the Cardiac Action Potential

Classification of Dysrhythmias

General Principles of Dysrhythmia Management

Drugs for Dysrhythmias

Sodium Channel Blockers: Class I

PROTOTYPE **Procainamide**

Beta-Adrenergic Antagonists: Class II

Potassium Channel Blockers: Class III

PROTOTYPE **Amiodarone (Cordarone, Pacerone)**

Calcium Channel Blockers: Class IV

Miscellaneous Antidysrhythmics

Learning Outcomes

After reading this chapter, the student should be able to:

1. Identify disorders associated with an increased risk of dysrhythmias.

2. Explain how rhythm abnormalities can affect cardiac function.

3. Sketch a typical cardiac action potential and label the flow of potassium, sodium, and calcium ions during each phase.

4. Design a table that indicates the classification of dysrhythmias and the types of drugs used to treat them.

5. Describe general principles guiding the management of dysrhythmias.

6. Identify the primary mechanisms of action of antidysrhythmic drugs.

7. For each of the classes shown in the chapter outline, identify the prototype and representative drugs and explain the mechanism(s) of drug action, primary indications, contraindications, significant drug interactions, pregnancy category, and important adverse effects.

8. Apply the nursing process to care for patients receiving pharmacotherapy for dysrhythmias.

From Chapter 40 of *Pharmacology: Connections to Nursing Practice*, Second Edition. Michael Patrick Adams, Carol Quam Urban. Copyright © 2013 by Pearson Education, Inc. All rights reserved.

Dysrhythmias are disorders of cardiac rhythm characterized by abnormal heart rate or irregular contractions. Also called arrhythmias, they encompass a number of different disorders that range from harmless to life threatening. Diagnosis is difficult and patients often must be connected to an electrocardiogram (ECG) and must be experiencing symptoms in order to determine the exact type of rhythm disorder. Proper diagnosis and optimum pharmacotherapy can significantly affect the frequency of dysrhythmias and their consequences.

Etiology of Dysrhythmias

1 Some dysrhythmias produce no patient symptoms, while others may be life threatening.

Some dysrhythmias are asymptomatic and have no effect on cardiac function, while others require immediate treatment. Typical symptoms of dysrhythmias include dizziness, weakness, fatigue, decreased exercise tolerance, palpitations, dyspnea, and syncope. It is difficult to estimate the frequency of the disease, although it is likely that dysrhythmias are quite common in the population. Patients often wait until these symptoms occur more frequently or become acute before seeking medical intervention.

Dysrhythmias occur in all age groups, and in both healthy and diseased hearts. While the actual cause of most dysrhythmias is elusive, the majority are closely associated with certain conditions, primarily heart disease and myocardial infarction (MI): 90% of patients experiencing an MI will develop a dysrhythmia. Persistent dysrhythmias are associated with increased risk of stroke and heart failure (HF), and severe dysrhythmias may result in sudden death. Conditions that promote the formation of cardiac rhythm abnormalities are called **prodysrhythmics**. Following are some of the diseases and conditions associated with dysrhythmias:

- Hypertension (HTN)
- Cardiac valve disease such as mitral stenosis
- Coronary artery disease (CAD)
- Low or high potassium levels in the blood
- Myocardial infarction (MI)
- Stroke
- Diabetes mellitus
- Heart failure

In addition to the preceding list, a number of medications have been found to cause new dysrhythmias or worsen existing ones. Caution must be used when administering prodysrhythmic drugs to patients with preexisting cardiac impairment or who may have any of the above conditions. Table 1 lists selected drugs known to have prodysrhythmic properties.

Phases and Measurement of the Cardiac Action Potential

2 The phases of cardiac action potential include rapid depolarization, a long plateau, and repolarization.

Dysrhythmias are defects in the electrical properties of the heart. In some manner, the normal generation or conduction of the electrical impulse, or action potential, across the myocardium has been altered. Because antidysrhythmic drugs act by correcting or modifying impulse conduction, a firm grasp of cardiac electrical properties is essential for understanding drug mechanisms. Before proceeding, the student should review the normal pathway of impulse conduction in the heart.

Action potentials occur in neurons and cardiac muscle cells due to the changes in the concentration of specific ions found inside and outside the cell. Under resting conditions, sodium ions (Na^+) and calcium ions (Ca^{2+}) are in higher concentrations outside of myocardial cells, while potassium ions (K^+) are found in higher concentration inside these cells. These imbalances are, in part, responsible for the inside of a myocardial cell membrane having a slightly negative charge (80–90 mV), relative to the outside of the membrane. A cell having this negative membrane potential is **polarized**.

An action potential illustrating the steps in electrical conduction is shown in Figure 1. The changes in ions, or fluxes, occurring during an action potential may be grouped into five phases.

Phase 4: It is easiest to begin with phase 4 because this is the period during which the cell is "resting" and the action potential has not yet occurred. Note in Figure 1, however, that during phase 4 the membrane potential is slowly increasing toward a potential that will trigger an action potential: the

TABLE 1 Selected Prodysrhythmic Drugs	
Class of Medication	Example Drugs
Antidysrhythmic drugs	amiodarone, disopyramide, dofetilide, flecainide, ibutilide, procainamide, propafenone, quinidine, sotalol
Autonomic agents	atenolol, clonidine, methyldopa, nadolol, propranolol
Calcium channel blockers	diltiazem, nifedipine, verapamil
Cardiac glycosides	digoxin
Miscellaneous agents	amitriptyline, chloroquine, cimetidine, haloperidol, lithium carbonate, phenothiazines

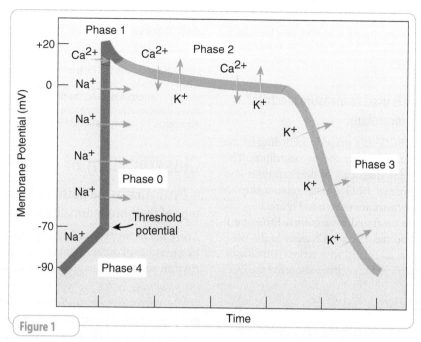

Figure 1

Phases of the myocardial action potential. Ion movements during each phase are shown.

threshold potential. Sodium is slowly "leaking" into the cell during this period, causing the change in potential, which gives certain regions such as the sinoatrial (SA) node the property of automaticity, the ability to depolarize spontaneously, without input from the nervous system.

Phase 0: An action potential begins when the threshold potential is reached and gated sodium ion channels located in the plasma membrane become activated and open. Sodium ions rush into the cell producing a rapid **depolarization**, or loss of membrane potential. Because they open and close rapidly, these sodium channels are sometimes referred to as "fast" channels. During this period, Ca^{2+} also enters the cell through calcium ion channels, although the influx is slower than that of sodium. In cells located in the SA and atrioventricular (AV) nodes, it is the influx of Ca^{2+}, rather than Na^+, which generates the rapid depolarization of the membrane.

Phase 1: During depolarization, the inside of the plasma membrane temporarily reverses its charge, becoming positive. This is a brief, transient phase.

Phase 2: During phase 2, a plateau is reached in which depolarization is maintained. The entry of Ca^{2+} into the cells signals the release of additional calcium ions that had been held in storage inside the sarcoplasmic reticula. This large and sudden increase in intracellular Ca^{2+} is responsible for the contraction of cardiac muscle. Gated potassium ion channels open, causing an efflux of K^+ from the cells. The plateau is maintained as long as the positive calcium ions entering the cell are balanced by the positive potassium ions leaving the cell. Action potentials in skeletal muscle lack this plateau phase.

Phase 3: During phase 3, the calcium channels close and additional potassium channels open, thus causing a net loss of positive ions from the cell. This **repolarization** returns the negative resting membrane potential to the cell.

The synchronized pumping action of the heart requires alternating periods of contraction and relaxation. There is a brief period of time following depolarization and most of repolarization during which the cell cannot initiate a subsequent action potential. This **refractory period** ensures that the myocardial cell finishes contracting before a second action potential begins.

Although learning about the different ions involved in an action potential may seem complicated, they are very important to cardiac pharmacology. Blocking potassium, sodium, or calcium ion channels is a pharmacologic strategy used to terminate or prevent dysrhythmias. In addition, the therapeutic effect of some antidysrhythmic agents is due to their prolongation of the refractory period. It is not possible to understand drug mechanisms without adequate knowledge of the normal electrical conduction properties of the heart. In general, most cardiac drugs:

- Increase impulse formation or automaticity.
- Increase conduction velocity.
- Increase both impulse formation or automaticity and conduction velocity.

   OR

- Decrease impulse formation or automaticity.
- Decrease conduction velocity.
- Decrease both impulse formation or automaticity and conduction.

CONNECTION Checkpoint 40.1

What are the three types of calcium channels? Which type is blocked by calcium channel blocker medications? *See Answer to Connection Checkpoint 40.1 on student resource website.*

3 The electrocardiogram is used to measure electrical conduction across the myocardium.

The **electrocardiogram (ECG)** is a graphic recording of the wave of electrical conduction across the myocardium. The ECG is a primary tool in the diagnosis of dysrhythmias and other heart diseases. A normal ECG and its relationship to impulse conduction in the heart are shown in Figure 2.

Three distinct waves are produced by a normal ECG: the P wave, the QRS complex, and the T wave. Changes to the wave patterns or in their timing are associated with certain pathologies. The different classes of antidysrhythmic drugs also affect the ECG

in characteristic manners. A summary of the different waves and their importance to cardiac physiology is given in Table 2.

PharmFACT

Long QT syndrome (LQTS) is a hereditary dysrhythmia that causes about 4,000 deaths in children and young adults each year. The condition is usually asymptomatic and the first sign may be syncope followed by sudden cardiac death. Most people with known LQTS are treated with beta-adrenergic blockers (National Heart, Lung, and Blood Institute, 2009).

Classification of Dysrhythmias

4 Dysrhythmias are classified by the impulse origin and type of rhythm abnormality produced.

There are many types of dysrhythmias and they are classified by a number of different methods. The two broad categories of rhythm abnormalities are those that affect impulse formation

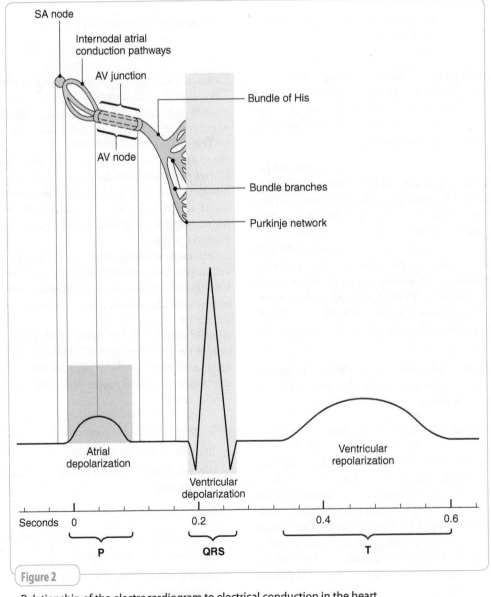

Figure 2

Relationship of the electrocardiogram to electrical conduction in the heart.

TABLE 2 ECG Waves and Intervals

Wave or Interval	Physiological Significance	Importance
P wave	Represents atrial depolarization.	A large P wave (voltage greater than 2.5 mm or 2 ½ small boxes on the readout) suggests the atria may be enlarged.
PQ segment	Represents the delay at the AV node; sometimes referred to as the PR segment.	This delay is vital so the ventricles can fill with blood. Prolonged PQ segments suggest slow or nonconducting fibrotic areas in the myocardium.
PQ interval	Represents all electrical activity prior to the impulse reaching the ventricles and contains the P wave and the PQ segment; sometimes referred to as the PR interval.	Normal measurements range between 0.12 and 0.20 sec. Slightly prolonged PQ intervals are common and considered harmless. More prolonged PQ intervals suggest a first-degree heart block.
QRS complex	Represents ventricular depolarization.	An exaggerated R wave suggests enlargement of the ventricles. The QRS should not be longer than 0.11 sec. Patients experiencing an MI may show QRS complexes that are abnormally high or that have extended durations.
T wave	Represents ventricular repolarization.	A flat T wave suggests ischemia to the myocardium.
ST segment	Represents the plateau phase of the action potential when the ventricles are depolarized.	Elevated ST segments are used to guide the pharmacotherapy of MI.
QT interval	Represents the time from the start of ventricular depolarization to the completion of ventricular repolarization.	Drugs that lengthen the QT interval have been linked to cardiac dysrhythmias, cardiac arrest, and sudden death. At the same time, prolongation of the action potential duration is a primary antidysrhythmic mechanism.

and those that affect impulse conduction. Although a correct diagnosis of the type of dysrhythmia is sometimes difficult, it is essential for effective treatment.

Bradydysrhythmias are disorders characterized by a heart rate of less than 60 beats/minute. Bradydysrhythmias are very common in older adults because the number of cells in the SA node declines progressively such that by age 75 about 90% of the cells are nonfunctional. Similar age-related changes occur in the AV node, where normal cells progressively die and are replaced by fibrotic tissue. Bradydysrhythmias are the major indication for pacemaker implantation. Common bradydysrhythmias include the following:

- **Sinus bradycardia.** The most common slow heart rhythm. Sinus bradycardia generally does not require treatment unless the patient is experiencing syncope or dizziness due to lack of sufficient blood flow to the brain, or if the heart rate fails to increase during periods of exertion.

- **Sinoatrial node dysfunction (sick sinus syndrome).** The SA node fails to generate or transmit sufficient electrical impulses. Patients with this condition may experience severe bradycardia (less than 40 beats/minute resting), failure of the heart rate to increase with exercise, or significant sinus "pauses." Severe episodes of bradycardia may alternate with periods of abnormally rapid heart rates.

- **Atrioventricular conduction block.** The AV node fails to conduct impulses to the rest of the myocardium. AV blocks are classified by degree. In first-degree AV block, the AV node conducts the impulse slowly, and conduction is delayed but not prevented. In second-degree AV block, some, but not all, impulses are prevented (blocked) from leaving the AV node. Second-degree AV block results in nonconducted P waves. A third-degree AV block results in total stoppage of impulses through the AV node. None of the impulses originating in the atria can make their way

through the block into the ventricles. Second- and third-degree blocks require pharmacotherapy or the insertion of a temporary or permanent pacemaker. Some AV blocks are temporary in origin, and can be due to cardiac drug toxicity. Any drug that slows AV conduction can cause a temporary form of AV block.

Tachydysrhythmias are disorders exhibiting a heart rate greater than 100 beats/minute. The incidence of tachydysrhythmias increases in older adults and in patients with preexisting cardiovascular disease. The simplest method for categorizing tachydysrhythmias is according to the type of rhythm abnormality produced and its location. Dysrhythmias that originate in the atria are sometimes referred to as supraventricular. Those that originate in the ventricles are generally more serious because they are more likely to interfere with the normal function of the heart.

- **Atrial tachycardia.** May be caused by a rapidly firing SA node or by an ectopic focus in the atria that suppresses the SA node and establishes a rapid heart rate, often between 160 and 200 beats/minute. When these episodes alternate with periods of normal rhythm, it is called paroxysmal atrial tachycardia (PAT), or **paroxysmal supraventricular tachycardia (PSVT)**.

- **Atrial flutter.** A rapid, regular heartbeat in which the atria may beat 250 to 350 times per minute. During atrial flutter, the job of the AV node is to selectively block some of the impulses coming from the atria, so the ventricular rate (pulse) is 125 to 175 beats/minute (usually two, three, or four atrial beats for each ventricular beat).

- **Atrial fibrillation.** A complete disorganization of rhythm, this is the most common type of dysrhythmia. It is caused by multiple sites of impulse formation in the atria, all firing in a chaotic fashion. The atrial rate can range from 300 to 600 beats/minute, causing an irregular ventricular rate ranging from 50 to 200 beats/minute. The rapid atrial rate causes a loss of organized atrial contraction, and results in quivering (fibrillation). This lack of contraction causes blood to lie dormant in parts of the atria and may give rise to clots. Because of the potential for clot formation, atrial fibrillation is a leading risk factor for stroke.

- **Ventricular tachycardia.** Usually recognized by regular, rapid, wide beats with a ventricular rate of 100 to 200 beats/minute. Patients with sustained or symptomatic ventricular tachycardia must be treated immediately because this condition is associated with a high risk of sudden death. **Torsades de pointes** is a specific type of ventricular tachycardia that is characterized by rates between 200 and 250 beats/minute and "twisting of the points" of the QRS complex on the ECG.

- **Ventricular fibrillation.** A complete disorganization of rhythm in which the ventricles pump little or no blood, quickly starving the tissues of oxygen. Ventricular fibrillation is now considered cardiac arrest.

General Principles of Dysrhythmia Management

5 Antidysrhythmic drugs are only used when there is a clear benefit to the patient.

Some antidysrhythmic drugs have the potential to produce serious adverse effects. The very drugs used to treat dysrhythmias may actually worsen or create new dysrhythmias. Furthermore, research suggests that mortality may actually increase when some of these drugs are used to treat or prevent dysrhythmias. The following guidelines are used in the management of the patient with dysrhythmias.

Asymptomatic dysrhythmias: Research has shown little or no benefit to the patient in treating asymptomatic dysrhythmias with medications. Antidysrhythmic drugs are normally reserved for patients experiencing overt symptoms or for those whose condition cannot be controlled by other means.

Acute dysrhythmias: Some types of dysrhythmias are serious and may be life threatening. In these cases, pharmacotherapy or cardioversion is warranted. For example, ventricular dysrhythmias often interfere with cardiac output and have greater potential for harm than atrial dysrhythmias. Dysrhythmias that are sustained may worsen and affect cardiac function. Several antidysrhythmics available by the intravenous (IV) route have an immediate onset of action to terminate life-threatening dysrhythmias.

Prophylaxis of dysrhythmias: Patients who are afflicted with recurring dysrhythmias or who have a comorbid condition, such as preexisting heart disease, may benefit from prophylactic therapy with antidysrhythmics. These patients should be monitored regularly to assess for prodysrhythmic effects from the drugs. Drug combinations that have the potential to prolong the QT interval are avoided and doses are kept as low

To the Community
Dysrhythmias and Diet

Patients with dysrhythmias may benefit from education about certain foods that may increase cardiac problems. The patient should avoid foods and beverages that trigger an irregular heartbeat and should eat a healthy low-salt, low-fat diet. Alcohol, including beer, wine, or hard liquor, may trigger dysrhythmias in some patients; for example, atrial fibrillation can occur after an alcohol binge. Because food and drinks with caffeine may also trigger dysrhythmias, the nurse should advise the patient to avoid coffee, tea, and some soft beverages, as well as chocolate. Another caution comes with herbal remedies, especially substances used to improve sports performance. Maintaining a healthy, well-balanced diet while avoiding food triggers may help to decrease dysrhythmias.

as possible to minimize risk. Prophylactic therapy should only be initiated for high-risk patients.

Nonpharmacologic treatment: Serious types of dysrhythmias are corrected through electrical shock of the heart, a treatment called **cardioversion** or **defibrillation**. The electrical shock momentarily stops all electrical impulses in the heart, both normal and abnormal. Under ideal conditions, the temporary cessation of electrical activity will allow the SA node to automatically return conduction to a normal sinus rhythm.

Other types of nonpharmacologic treatment include identification and destruction of the myocardial cells responsible for the abnormal conduction through a surgical procedure called catheter ablation. Cardiac pacemakers are sometimes inserted to correct the types of dysrhythmias that cause the heart to beat too slowly. Implantable cardioverter defibrillators (ICDs) are placed in a patient to restore normal rhythm by either pacing the heart or giving it an electric shock when dysrhythmias occur. In addition, the ICD is capable of storing information regarding the heart rhythm for the health care provider to evaluate.

Drugs for Dysrhythmias

6 Antidysrhythmic drugs are classified by their mechanism of action.

The therapeutic goals of antidysrhythmic pharmacotherapy are to terminate existing dysrhythmias or to prevent abnormal rhythms for the purpose of reducing the risks of sudden death, stroke, or other complications resulting from the disease. Antidysrhythmic drugs act by altering specific electrophysiologic properties of the heart. They do this through two basic mechanisms: blocking flow through ion channels (conduction) or altering autonomic activity (automaticity).

The most common method of classifying antidysrhythmic drugs is called the Vaughan Williams classification, which was begun in 1985. This classification scheme groups drugs as Classes I, II, III, and IV based on the stage at which they affect the action potential. A fifth group includes miscellaneous drugs

TABLE 3 Classification of Antidysrhythmics

Class	Actions	Primary Indications
I: Sodium Channel Blockers		
IA	Delays repolarization; slows conduction velocity; increases duration of the action potential	Atrial fibrillation, premature atrial contractions, premature ventricular contractions, tachycardia
IB	Accelerates repolarization; slows conduction velocity; decreases duration of action potential	Severe ventricular dysrhythmias
IC	No significant effect on repolarization; slows conduction velocity	Severe ventricular dysrhythmias
II: Beta-Adrenergic Blockers	Slows conduction velocity; decreases automaticity; prolongs refractory period	Atrial flutter and fibrillation, tachydysrhythmias, ventricular dysrhythmias
III: Drugs That Slow Repolarization	Slows repolarization; increases duration of action potential; prolongs refractory period	Severe atrial and ventricular dysrhythmias
IV: Calcium Channel Blockers	Slows conduction velocity; decreases contractility; prolongs refractory period	Paroxysmal supraventricular tachycardia, supraventricular tachydysrhythmias

not acting by one of the first four mechanisms. Although widely used, the Vaughan Williams classification method is simplistic because some of these drugs act by more than one mechanism and the drugs within each class have unique properties that distinguish them from each other. For example, the Class I drugs have three subclasses. The categories of antidysrhythmics and their mechanisms are shown in Table 3.

The use of antidysrhythmic drugs has significantly declined in recent years. The reason for this decline is that research studies determined that the use of antidysrhythmic medications for prophylaxis can actually increase patient mortality. Drugs affecting cardiac electrophysiology have a narrow margin of safety between a therapeutic effect and a toxic effect. They have the ability not only to correct dysrhythmias, but also to worsen or even create new dysrhythmias. These prodysrhythmic effects have resulted in less use of drugs in Class I; however, drugs in Class II and Class III (specifically amiodarone) have increased in usage.

Another reason for the decline in antidysrhythmic drug use is the success of nonpharmacologic techniques. Catheter ablation and implantable defibrillators are more successful in managing many types of dysrhythmias than is the prophylactic use of medications.

Sodium Channel Blockers: Class I

7 Class I antidysrhythmics act by blocking ion channels in myocardial cells.

Sodium channel blockers, the Class I drugs, are the largest group of antidysrhythmics. They are further divided into three subgroups (IA, IB, and IC) based on subtle differences in their mechanisms of action. Because initiation of the action potential is dependent on the opening of gated sodium ion channels, a blockade of these channels will prevent depolarization of the myocardium. The spread of the action potential will slow, and areas of ectopic pacemaker activity will be suppressed. The sodium channel blockers are shown in Table 4 and Figure 3.

The sodium channel blockers are similar in structure and action to local anesthetics. In fact, the Class I antidysrhythmic lidocaine is a prototype local anesthetic. This anesthetic-like action slows impulse conduction across the heart. Some, such as quinidine and procainamide, are effective against many types of dysrhythmias. The remaining Class I drugs are more specific, and indicated only for life-threatening ventricular dysrhythmias.

The adverse effects of the sodium blockers vary with each individual drug. All these agents can cause new dysrhythmias or worsen existing ones. The slowing of the heart rate can cause hypotension, dizziness, and fainting. During pharmacotherapy, the ECG should be monitored for signs of cardiotoxicity, such as increases in the PR and QT intervals and widening of the QRS complex. Some Class I drugs have significant anticholinergic adverse effects such as dry mouth, constipation, and urinary retention. Special precautions should be taken with older adults, because anticholinergic adverse effects may worsen urinary hesitancy in men with prostate enlargement.

Class IA: The class IA antidysrhythmics include quinidine, disopyramide (Norpace), and procainamide. Although quinidine is the oldest and best known Class IA drug, procainamide is the prototype because it has been more widely used than quinidine in recent decades. All are available by the oral (PO) route and act by blocking sodium ion channels during phase 0 of the action potential.

The primary action responsible for the antidysrhythmic effects of the Class IA drugs is a slowing of conduction velocity. These agents also inhibit potassium channels, which delays repolarization and increases the refractory period. Subsequent action potentials must wait slightly longer before triggering the next electrical impulse. These actions allow the Class IA drugs to inhibit the formation of ectopic foci in both the atria and ventricles.

The effects of the Class IA agents can be recognized on the ECG. The QRS complex widens, owing to the slowed depolarization of the ventricles. The QT interval is increased due to the delay in repolarization of the ventricles.

TABLE 4 Antidysrhythmic Drugs

Drug	Route and Adult Dose (maximum dose where indicated)	Adverse Effects
Class IA: Sodium Channel Blockers		
disopyramide (Norpace)	PO: 100–200 mg qid (max: 1,200–1,600 mg/day)	*Nausea, vomiting, diarrhea, dry mouth, urinary retention, cinchonism (quinidine), anorexia, rash, photosensitivity*
procainamide	PO: 1 g loading dose followed by 250–500 mg every 3 h	
quinidine gluconate	PO: 200–600 mg tid qid (max: 3–4 g/day) IV: 0.25 mg/kg/min (max: 5–10 mg/kg)	May produce new dysrhythmias or worsen existing ones; hypotension, torsades de pointes, blood dyscrasias, hepatotoxicity (quinidine), lupus (procainamide)
quinidine sulfate	PO: 200–400 mg tid qid (max: 3–4 g/day); therapeutic serum drug level is 2–5 mcg/mL	
Class IB: Sodium Channel Blockers		
lidocaine (Xylocaine)	IV: 1–4 mg/min infusion (max: 3 mg/kg per 5–10 min)	*Nausea, vomiting, drowsiness, dizziness, lethargy, confusion (phenytoin)*
mexiletine (Mexitil)	PO: 200–300 mg tid (max: 1,200 mg/day)	May produce new dysrhythmias or worsen existing ones; hypotension, bradycardia, CNS toxicity (lidocaine), malignant hyperthermia (lidocaine), cardiac arrest (lidocaine), status epilepticus if abruptly withdrawn (phenytoin), blood dyscrasias (phenytoin)
phenytoin (Dilantin, Phenytek)	IV: 50–100 mg every 10–15 min until dysrhythmia is terminated (max: 1 g/day) PO: 100–200 mg tid (max: 625 mg/day)	
Class IC: Sodium Channel Blockers		
flecainide (Tambocor)	PO: 100 mg bid; increase by 50 mg bid every 4 days (max: 400 mg/day)	*Nausea, vomiting, fatigue, dizziness, headache, visual disturbances (flecainide)*
propafenone (Rythmol)	PO: 150–300 mg tid (max: 900 mg/day)	May produce new dysrhythmias or worsen existing ones; hypotension, bradycardia, cardiac arrest (flecainide), blood dyscrasias, lupus (propafenone), HF (propafenone), acute liver injury (propafenone)
Class II: Beta-Adrenergic Antagonists		
acebutolol (Sectral)	PO: 200–600 mg bid tid (max: 1,200 mg/day)	*Fatigue, insomnia, drowsiness, impotence, decreased libido, dizziness, bradycardia, confusion*
esmolol (Brevibloc)	IV: 500 mcg/kg/min loading dose; maintenance dose 50–300 mcg/kg/min (maintenance max: 200 mcg/kg/min)	Agranulocytosis, HF, bronchospasm, hypotension, Stevens–Johnson syndrome, anaphylaxis; if the drug is abruptly withdrawn, palpitations, rebound HTN, life-threatening dysrhythmias, or myocardial ischemia may occur
propranolol (Inderal)	PO: 10–30 mg 3–4 times daily (max: 480 mg/day) IV: 0.5–3.1 mg every 4 h or prn	
Class III: Potassium Channel Blockers		
amiodarone (Cordarone, Pacerone)	PO: 400–600 mg/day in 1–2 divided doses (max: 1,600 mg/day as loading dose)	*Blurred vision (amiodarone), photosensitivity, nausea, vomiting, anorexia*
dofetilide (Tikosyn)	PO: 125–500 mcg bid based on creatinine clearance	May produce new dysrhythmias or worsen existing ones; hypotension, HF, heart block, bradycardia, pneumonia-like syndrome (amiodarone), angioedema (dofetilide), CNS toxicity (ibutilide)
dronedarone (Multaq)	PO: 400 mg bid	
ibutilide (Corvert)	IV: 1 mg infused over 10 min (for patients over 60 kg); 0.01 mg/kg (for patients under 60 kg); (max: 2 mg infused over at least 20 min)	
sotalol* (Betapace, Betapace AF, Sorine)	PO: 80 mg bid (max: 320 mg/day)	
Class IV: Calcium Channel Blockers		
diltiazem (Cardizem, Dilacor, Taztia XR, Tiazac)	IV: 5–10 mg/h continuous infusion for a maximum of 24 h (max: 15 mg/h)	*Flushed skin, headache, dizziness, peripheral edema, lightheadedness, nausea, diarrhea, syncope*
verapamil (Calan, Isoptin, Verelan)	PO: 240–480 mg/day in divided doses; 5–10 mg IV direct over 2 min, may repeat in 15–30 min	Hepatotoxicity, MI, CHF, confusion, mood changes, hypotension
Miscellaneous Antidysrhythmics		
adenosine (Adenocard, Adenoscan)	IV: 6–12 mg given as a bolus injection every 1–2 min as needed (max: 12 mg/dose)	*Facial flushing, dyspnea, headache* May produce new dysrhythmias or worsen existing ones, AV block
digoxin (Lanoxin, Lanoxicaps)	PO: 0.125–0.5 mg 4 times daily Therapeutic serum drug level: 0.8–2 ng/mL	*Nausea, vomiting, headache, diarrhea, visual disturbances* May produce new dysrhythmias or worsen existing ones

Note: *Italics* indicate common adverse effects. Underline indicates serious adverse effects.
*Sotalol is a beta blocker, but because its cardiac effects are more similar to amiodarone, it is in Class III. Adverse effects are those of Class II and Class III.

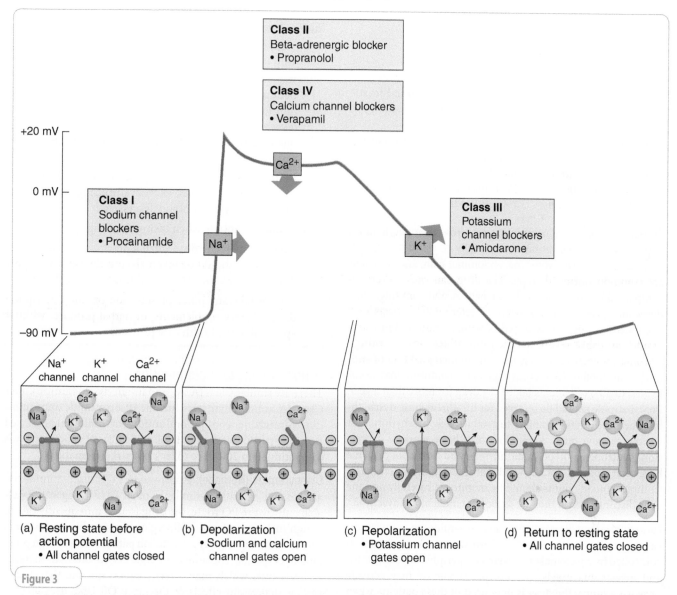

Figure 3

Ion channels in myocardial cells: (a) resting state before action potential (all channel gates closed); (b) depolarization (sodium and calcium channel gates open); (c) repolarization (potassium channel gates open); (d) return to resting state (all channel gates closed).

PROTOTYPE DRUG	Procainamide

Classification: **Therapeutic:** Antidysrhythmic, Class IA
Pharmacologic: Sodium channel blocker

Therapeutic Effects and Uses: Approved in 1950, procainamide is a broad-spectrum antidysrhythmic chemically related to the local anesthetic procaine that has the ability to correct many different types of atrial and ventricular dysrhythmias. Indications include ventricular tachycardia during cardiopulmonary resuscitation (CPR); refractory ventricular fibrillation or pulseless ventricular tachycardia during CPR; conversion to sinus rhythm in patients with paroxysmal atrial tachycardia, atrial flutter, or atrial fibrillation; and treatment or prophylaxis of PSVT. Procainamide is now considered a drug of last choice for advanced cardiac life support due to its toxicity; it is used when other drugs have failed to reverse a severe dysrhythmia. The major hepatic metabolite of the drug, N-acetyl procainamide, also has antidysrhythmic activity. Because the rate of acetylation to the active metabolite is genetically determined, "slow acetylators" and "fast acetylators" will require adjustments in dosages to obtain optimum therapeutic results.

Procainamide is available in IV and intramuscular (IM) formulations: PO forms of procainamide have been discontinued. Dosage is guided by periodic serum drug levels, which are maintained between 4 and 8 mcg/mL. The supine position should be used during IV administration because severe hypotension may occur during the infusion. Use of procainamide must be terminated if the QRS widens more that 50% of its original width.

Mechanism of Action: Procainamide blocks sodium ion channels in myocardial cells, thus reducing automaticity and slowing the velocity of the action potential across the myocardium. This slight delay in conduction velocity prolongs the refractory period and can suppress dysrhythmias.

277

Pharmacokinetics:

Route(s)	IV, IM
Absorption	Readily absorbed
Distribution	Widely distributed; crosses the placenta; secreted in breast milk; 15% bound to plasma protein
Primary metabolism	Hepatic; metabolized to active metabolite
Primary excretion	Renal, 50–70% unchanged
Onset of action	IV: immediate; IM: 10–30 min
Duration of action	IM/IV: 3–4 h

Adverse Effects: Procainamide has a narrow therapeutic index and dosage must be monitored carefully to avoid serious adverse effects. Nausea, vomiting, abdominal pain, and headache are common during therapy. The drug can cause fever, accompanied by anorexia, weakness, nausea, and vomiting. High doses may produce central nervous system (CNS) effects such as confusion or psychosis. Rapid IV administration of procainamide can cause severe hypotension. **Black Box Warnings:** Chronic administration may result in an increased titer of antinuclear antibodies (ANAs). A lupus-like syndrome may occur in 30% to 50% of patients taking the drug for more than a year. Procainamide should be reserved for life-threatening dysrhythmias because it has the ability to produce new dysrhythmias or worsen existing ones. Agranulocytosis, bone marrow depression, neutropenia, hypoplastic anemia, and thrombocytopenia have been reported, usually within the first 3 months of therapy. Complete blood counts should be monitored carefully and the drug discontinued at the first sign of potential blood dyscrasia.

Contraindications/Precautions: Procainamide is contraindicated in patients with second- or third-degree AV block (unless controlled by a pacemaker), severe HF, peripheral neuropathy, and myasthenia gravis. Because procainamide may activate or worsen lupus, the drug is only used in these patients when there is no safer alternative. Doses must be lowered in patients with renal impairment due to possible accumulation of the drug. Patients in shock or with severe hypotension should not receive this drug due to additive hypotension. Procainamide may worsen blood dyscrasias; thus, it should be used with caution in patients with preexisting bone marrow suppression.

Drug Interactions: Additive cardiac depressant effects may occur if procainamide is administered with other antidysrhythmics. Additive anticholinergic adverse effects will occur if procainamide is used concurrently with anticholinergic agents. Procainamide may increase plasma levels of amiodarone or quinidine. Use with antihypertensives may result in hypotension. **Herbal/Food:** Although no interactions have been well documented, the use of all herbal products or supplements should be avoided unless approved by the health care provider due to the toxicity of the drug.

Pregnancy: Category C.

Treatment of Overdose: No specific therapy is available for overdose. Supportive treatment is targeted to reversing hypotension with vasopressors and preventing or treating procainamide-induced dysrhythmias.

Nursing Responsibilities: Key nursing implications for patients receiving procainamide are included in the Nursing Practice Application for Patients Receiving Antidysrhythmic Therapy.

Lifespan and Diversity Considerations:

- Because of differences in metabolism rates and acetylation to procainamide's active form, monitor ethnically diverse populations more frequently to ensure optimal therapeutic effects and minimize adverse effects.

Patient and Family Education:

- Immediately report wheezing, fever, mouth soreness or sore throat, infections, excessive bruising, or bleeding. The drug may cause blood dyscrasias.

- Avoid alcohol use when taking this drug.

- Do not double the dose when a previous dose is missed. Medication should be taken around the clock in evenly spaced doses.

- Do not take any other prescription or nonprescription drugs, dietary supplements, or herbal products without approval of the health care provider.

Drugs Similar to Procainamide

There are similar Class IA, IB, and IC antidysrhythmics. Other Class IA antidysrhythmics include disopyramide and quinidine. Moricizine, a unique oral antidysrhythmic that possessed some properties attributed to all three Class I subclasses, was discontinued in 2007 due to lack of market demand.

Disopyramide (Norpace): Approved in 1977, disopyramide has actions and indications similar to other Class IA agents. Available only by the PO route, the drug is used infrequently due to a high incidence of anticholinergic effects such as xerostomia (dry mouth) and urinary retention in patients with benign prostatic hyperplasia. The anticholinergic effects cause an increase in heart rate, which may directly cancel out the therapeutic cardiac depressant effects of the drug. Off-label uses include maintenance of, or conversion to, sinus rhythm in patients with atrial flutter or atrial fibrillation. Disopyramide has a black box warning that the drug should be restricted to patients with life-threatening dysrhythmias. This drug is pregnancy category C.

Quinidine: Approved in 1938, quinidine is the oldest antidysrhythmic drug, originally obtained as a natural substance from the bark of the South American Cinchona tree. Like procainamide, quinidine is a broad-spectrum drug having the ability to correct many different types of atrial and ventricular dysrhythmias. The two salts of quinidine are sulfate, which is given PO, and gluconate, which is given PO and IV. Like other drugs in this class, quinidine blocks sodium ion channels in myocardial cells, thus reducing automaticity and slowing the velocity of the action potential across the myocardium. In addition to dysrhythmias, quinidine gluconate may be used to treat malaria and persistent hiccups. The most common adverse effect of quinidine is diarrhea, which occurs in approximately one third of patients, and may be intense. The drug can induce various types of dysrhythmias when serum levels rise above normal. High doses result in a syndrome called **cinchonism** with symptoms such as tinnitus, headache, blurred vision, hearing loss, and dysrhythmias. These symptoms are reversible once the drug is discontinued. Quinidine is contraindicated in patients with incomplete AV block because it can induce total blockage of conduction. Quinidine carries a black box warning that the drug has resulted in increased mortality when used for non-life-threatening dysrhythmias. This drug is pregnancy category C.

Class IB: The class IB antidysrhythmics include lidocaine, mexiletine, and phenytoin. Like other Class I drugs, these agents act by blocking gated sodium ion channels in cardiac muscle cells. Unlike the Class IA drugs, the Class IB agents shorten the refractory period and have little effect on conduction velocity. The Class IB drugs have minimal effects on the ECG and their primary indication is ventricular dysrhythmias. A fourth drug in this class, tocainide, was discontinued in 2003 due to a high incidence of adverse effects.

Lidocaine (Xylocaine): Lidocaine is the most frequently prescribed Class IB antidysrhythmic. It is an important treatment for life-threatening ventricular dysrhythmia, although amiodarone is considered a preferred drug for this indication. It is not effective in preventing or treating atrial dysrhythmias. Lidocaine decreases the refractory period of the action potential, especially in ischemic myocardial tissue. For acute conditions, lidocaine is administered by IV bolus or infusion; it is rarely given by the IM or subcutaneous routes. Serum lidocaine levels may be monitored and should be between 2 and 6 mcg/mL. The first signs of lidocaine toxicity usually involve the CNS and include confusion, anxiety, tremors, and paresthesias. As doses increase, the patient may become comatose and experience seizures or respiratory arrest. The correct lidocaine formulation must be used for IV infusions: Local anesthetic lidocaine preparations may contain preservatives and epinephrine. This drug is pregnancy category B.

Mexiletine (Mexitil): Approved in 1985, mexiletine is chemically similar to lidocaine, has local anesthetic properties, and is used only for serious ventricular dysrhythmias. Mexiletine, however, is well absorbed orally. An off-label indication is for the treatment of neuropathic pain. The most common adverse effects are nausea and vomiting. CNS effects such as dizziness, tremor, and ataxia are common. Less common, though potentially serious adverse effects include blood dyscrasias, pulmonary fibrosis, and worsening of HF. A black box warning has been issued regarding the possibility of acute liver damage in patients taking mexiletine. The target range for serum mexiletine concentration is 0.5 to 2 mcg/mL. This drug is pregnancy category C.

Phenytoin (Dilantin): The primary use for phenytoin is to treat seizures. As an antidysrhythmic, phenytoin may be administered by the oral or IV routes. IV phenytoin must be pushed extremely slowly: 100 mg over 5 minutes. Phenytoin is rarely used for its antidysrhythmic properties and is not approved by the U.S. Food and Drug Administration (FDA) for this purpose. Historically, it has been used to treat dysrhythmias secondary to digoxin (Lanoxin) toxicity. If used for dysrhythmias, serum phenytoin levels should be carefully monitored to be 10 to 20 mcg/mL because the drug can have multiple serious adverse effects, including seizures, ataxia, coma, blood dyscrasias, and hepatotoxicity. This drug is pregnancy category D.

Class IC: The Class IC antidysrhythmics include two drugs: flecainide and propafenone. Like other Class agents, these drugs block gated sodium ion channels in cardiac muscle cells. The Class IC antidysrhythmics profoundly decrease conduction velocity. Thus the PR, QRS, and QT intervals are often prolonged. The refractory period may be shortened slightly, but is mostly unchanged by the Class IC drugs. Their primary indication is for life-threatening atrial dysrhythmias, although they can also prevent ventricular dysrhythmias. Research has shown these drugs to have a pronounced prodysrhythmic effect that has the potential to increase mortality in patients who have experienced a recent MI.

Flecainide (Tambocor): Flecainide is an oral drug used primarily to treat or prevent paroxysmal atrial fibrillation or atrial flutter due to its ability to markedly decrease conduction velocity. It is indicated for the prophylaxis of life-threatening ventricular dysrhythmias, although it is rarely used for this purpose. The FDA has issued several black box warnings regarding flecainide. The prodysrhythmic effects of the drug may generate new ventricular dysrhythmias in about 10% of the patients. Due to an excessive mortality rate, the drug is contraindicated in patients with left ventricular dysfunction who have experienced a recent MI. Serum flecainide levels should be monitored, especially in patients with renal or hepatic impairment, and maintained between 0.2 and 1 mcg/mL. Pulmonary fibrosis and bone marrow suppression are potentially serious adverse effects. Other adverse effects include dizziness, headache, asthenia, tremor, and malaise. This drug is pregnancy category C.

Propafenone (Rythmol): Approved in 1989, propafenone is an oral drug similar to flecainide that is used primarily for atrial fibrillation and the prophylaxis of PSVT. Its prodysrhythmic activity limits its use in treating ventricular dysrhythmias. Unlike flecainide, propafenone exhibits clinically significant beta-adrenergic antagonist activity. This beta-blocker action may cause a negative inotropic effect that can worsen symptoms of CHF. Furthermore, the beta-blocking actions may cause bronchospasm in patients with asthma or chronic obstructive pulmonary disease (COPD). An extended release formulation (Rythmol SR) allows for twice-daily dosing. Propafenone is metabolized to active metabolites, which account for much of the drug's effects. In addition to exacerbating or creating new dysrhythmias, propafenone may cause dizziness and dysgeusia (altered sense of taste). This drug is pregnancy category C.

Beta-Adrenergic Antagonists: Class II

8 Beta-adrenergic antagonists reduce automaticity as well as slow conduction velocity in the heart.

Beta-adrenergic antagonists, or blockers, are used to treat HTN, MI, HF, and dysrhythmias. Only the actions of these drugs that relate to dysrhythmias are discussed in this section.

As expected from their effects on the autonomic nervous system, beta-adrenergic antagonists slow the heart rate (negative chronotropic effect) and decrease conduction velocity. These effects are primarily caused by the blockade of calcium ion channels in the SA and AV nodes, although these drugs also block gated sodium ion channels in the atria and ventricles. The reduction in myocardial automaticity stabilizes many types of dysrhythmias. The main value of beta blockers as antidysrhythmic agents is to treat atrial dysrhythmias associated with HF. When administered to post-MI patients, beta blockers decrease the likelihood of sudden death due to fatal dysrhythmias. Tachydysrhythmias respond well to beta blockers, including those that are induced by exercise.

Only a few beta blockers are approved for dysrhythmias, due to potential adverse effects, and these are listed in Table 4. Unless a functioning pacemaker is present, these drugs are contraindicated in patients with severe bradycardia, sick sinus syndrome, or advanced AV block because they depress conduction through the AV node. Blockade of beta-adrenergic receptors in the heart causes bradycardia, which may not be well tolerated in patients with preexisting cardiac disease, and hypotension may cause dizziness and possible fainting. Nonselective beta blockers may affect beta$_2$ receptors in the lung, causing bronchospasm in patients with asthma or COPD. Higher doses may produce depression, as well as hallucinations and psychosis, especially in older adults. Abrupt discontinuation of beta blockers can lead to dysrhythmias and HTN.

Acebutolol (Sectral): Approved in 1984, acebutolol is a cardioselective beta$_1$-adrenergic antagonist available only by the oral route. Like other beta blockers, acebutolol reduces sympathetic activity to the heart, thus lowering heart rate. It also has a negative inotropic effect. As an antidysrhythmic, it is used to treat premature ventricular contractions and reduce exercise-induced tachycardia. Other indications include chronic, stable angina, and HTN. Adverse effects such as hypotension and bradycardia are extensions of its beta-blocking action. At high doses, the selectivity for beta$_1$ receptors diminishes and the drug may cause bronchoconstriction (beta$_2$ receptors). Because the negative inotropic effects of the drug may worsen symptoms of HF, it is usually contraindicated in patients with HF. This drug is pregnancy category B.

Esmolol (Brevibloc): Approved in 1986, esmolol differs from the other antidysrhythmic beta blockers in that it is has a very short half-life of 9 minutes and is only given by IV infusion. As an antidysrhythmic, esmolol is used for the immediate termination of atrial tachyarrhythmias and noncompensatory sinus tachycardia, and to control ventricular rate in patients with atrial flutter or fibrillation. When a loading dose is administered, peak plasma levels can be reached after only 5 minutes. Off-label indications include treatment of hypertensive emergencies, acute MI, and unstable angina. Hypotension and bradycardia are common adverse effects but they quickly resolve once the infusion

is discontinued. At therapeutic doses, the drug is selective for beta$_1$-adrenergic receptors. This drug is pregnancy category C.

Propranolol (Inderal): Propranolol is a nonselective beta-adrenergic antagonist. Because it slows automaticity, propranolol is indicated for many types of dysrhythmias including suppression of exercise-induced tachycardia, atrial dysrhythmias, ventricular dysrhythmias, premature ventricular contractions, and digoxin-induced tachydysrhythmias. Propranolol exhibits few serious adverse effects at therapeutic doses. At high doses, patients may experience bradycardia, hypotension, HF, and bronchospasm. This drug is pregnancy category C.

CONNECTION Checkpoint 40.2

Both alpha$_1$ blockers and beta$_1$ blockers are used to treat HTN but only the beta$_1$ blockers are antidysrhythmics. Explain why the selective alpha blockers are not used to treat dysrhythmias. *See Answer to Connection Checkpoint 40.2 on student resource website.*

Potassium Channel Blockers: Class III

9 Potassium channel blockers prolong the refractory period of the heart.

The potassium channel blockers are a small but diverse class of drugs that have very important applications to the treatment of dysrhythmias. After the action potential has passed and the myocardial cell is in a depolarized state, repolarization depends on removal of potassium from the cell. The drugs in Class III exert their actions by blocking potassium ion channels in myocardial cells. Although there are significant differences among the drugs, all have in common the ability to delay repolarization and prolong the refractory period. This action is reflected by an increase in the QT interval on the ECG. Automaticity is also reduced.

Most drugs in this class have multiple actions on the heart and also affect adrenergic receptors or sodium channels. For example, in addition to blocking potassium channels, sotalol

(Betapace) is considered a beta-adrenergic blocker. The potassium channel blockers are listed in Table 4.

Drugs in this class have limited uses due to potentially serious toxicity. Like other antidysrhythmics, potassium channel blockers slow the heart rate, resulting in bradycardia and possible hypotension in a significant percentage of patients. These agents can create or worsen dysrhythmias, especially during the first few doses. Older adults with preexisting HF must be carefully monitored because these patients are at higher risk for the cardiac adverse effects of potassium channel blockers.

PROTOTYPE DRUG | Amiodarone (Cordarone, Pacerone)

Classification: **Therapeutic:** Antidysrhythmic, Class III
Pharmacologic: Potassium channel blocker

Therapeutic Effects and Uses: Approved in 1985, amiodarone is the most frequently prescribed Class III antidysrhythmic. It is considered a broad-spectrum antidysrhythmic because it is effective in terminating both atrial and ventricular dysrhythmias. It is approved for the treatment of resistant ventricular tachycardia and recurrent fibrillation that may prove life threatening, and it has become a medication of choice for the treatment of atrial dysrhythmias in patients with HF.

Amiodarone is available as PO tablets and as an IV infusion. IV infusions are limited to short-term therapy, normally only 2 to 4 days. Although its onset of action may take several weeks when the medication is given PO, its effects can last 4 to 8 weeks after the drug is discontinued because it has an extended half-life that may exceed 100 days. Amiodarone is a structural analog of thyroid hormone. The therapeutic serum level for amiodarone is 1 to 2.5 mcg/mL.

Mechanism of Action: Amiodarone exerts multiple, complex actions on the heart, and its exact mechanism of action is not completely known. In addition to blocking potassium ion channels, some of this drug's actions relate to its blockade of sodium ion channels and inhibiting sympathetic activity to the heart. Repolarization is delayed, the refractory period prolonged, and automaticity reduced. In addition to prolonging the QT interval, amiodarone increases the PR interval and widens the QRS complex on the ECG.

Pharmacokinetics:

Route(s)	PO, IV
Absorption	Completely absorbed by the gastrointestinal (GI) tract
Distribution	Widely distributed; crosses the placenta; secreted in breast milk; concentrated in the lung, kidneys, spleen, and adipose tissue
Primary metabolism	Hepatic; some enterohepatic recirculation occurs
Primary excretion	Primarily biliary; some feces
Onset of action	PO: 2–3 days; IV: 2 h
Duration of action	PO/IV; 10–150 days

Adverse Effects: Potentially serious adverse effects limit the use of amiodarone. Amiodarone may cause nausea, vomiting, anorexia, fatigue, dizziness, and hypotension. Visual disturbances are common in patients taking this drug for extended periods and include blurred vision due to cornea deposits, photophobia, xerostomia, cataracts, and macular degeneration. Rashes, photosensitivity, and other skin reactions occur in 10% to 15% of patients taking the drug. Certain tissues concentrate this medication; thus, adverse effects may be slow to resolve, persisting long after the drug has been discontinued. **Black Box Warning (oral form only):** Amiodarone causes a pneumonia-like syndrome in the lungs. Because the pulmonary toxicity may be fatal, baseline and periodic assessment of lung function is essential. Amiodarone has prodysrhythmic action and may cause bradycardia, cardiogenic shock, or AV block. Mild liver injury is frequent with amiodarone.

Contraindications/Precautions: Amiodarone is contraindicated in patients with severe bradycardia, cardiogenic shock, sick sinus syndrome, severe sinus node dysfunction, or third-degree AV block. Because amiodarone contains iodine in its chemical structure, patients who have hypersensitivity to this element should not receive the drug. It should be used with caution in patients with HF because it has a negative inotropic effect that can worsen symptoms. Electrolyte imbalances, especially hypokalemia and hypomagnesemia, should be corrected before administering amiodarone because these conditions predispose the patient to the development of dysrhythmias. Due to the drug's pulmonary toxicity, it is contraindicated in patients with COPD or respiratory insufficiency. Breast-feeding during amiodarone therapy may cause infant hypothyroidism; thus, the drug is contraindicated during lactation.

Drug Interactions: Amiodarone is metabolized by the cytochrome P450 enzymes and markedly inhibits the metabolism of many other drugs. This can raise the serum levels of these drugs and cause toxicity. For example, amiodarone can increase serum digoxin levels by as much as 70%. Amiodarone greatly enhances the actions of anticoagulants, thus the dose of warfarin must be cut by as much as half. Use with beta-adrenergic blockers or calcium channel blockers (CCBs) may potentiate sinus bradycardia, sinus arrest, or AV block. Amiodarone may increase phenytoin levels two- to threefold. Caution must be used during therapy with loop diuretics because hypokalemia can enhance the prodysrhythmic properties of amiodarone. Because of the large number of potential drug interactions, the nurse should regularly check current reference sources when patients are taking amiodarone concurrently with other medications. **Herbal/Food:** Use with echinacea may increase the risk of hepatotoxicity. Aloe may cause an increased effect of amiodarone. When the drug is administered PO, grapefruit juice can increase serum amiodarone levels by over 80%.

Pregnancy: Category D.

Treatment of Overdose: Overdose will cause bradycardia, hypotension, and life-threatening dysrhythmias. Supportive treatment is targeted to reversing hypotension with vasopressors and bradycardia with atropine or isoproterenol.

Nursing Responsibilities: Key nursing implications for patients receiving amiodarone are included in the Nursing Practice Application for Patients Receiving Antidysrhythmic Therapy.

Lifespan and Diversity Considerations:

- Monitor pulmonary function more frequently with the older adult, because normal physiological changes related to aging may increase the risk for pulmonary toxicity.

- Monitor potassium and magnesium levels frequently in the older adult who is at greater risk for the development of hypokalemia and hypomagnesemia while on these drugs.

- Because amiodarone is metabolized through one of the P450 system pathways, monitor ethnically diverse populations and older adults more frequently to ensure optimal therapeutic effects and minimize the risk of adverse effects.

Patient and Family Education:

- Do not take any other prescription or nonprescription drugs, dietary supplements, grapefruit or grapefruit juice, or herbal products without approval of the health care provider.

- Assess for history of iodine allergy, and withhold the drug until the provider is notified.

- Immediately notify the health care provider of any known or suspected pregnancy.

Drugs Similar to Amiodarone (Cordarone, Pacerone)

Other Class III antidysrhythmics include dofetilide, dronedarone, ibutilide, and sotalol. A fifth drug in this class, bretylium, was discontinued in the United States due to the availability of safer and more effective antidysrhythmic drugs.

Dofetilide (Tikosyn): Approved in 1999, dofetilide is an oral drug indicated for conversion of symptomatic atrial flutter or fibrillation to normal sinus rhythm. Like other potassium channel blockers, dofetilide prolongs the refractory period and action potential duration, thus increasing the QT interval. Dofetilide does not exhibit a negative inotropic effect, as do amiodarone and sotalol. The drug has no effect on the PR interval and it does not widen the QRS complex. Dofetilide has many potentially serious adverse effects, and a black box warning states that therapy should begin in a clinical setting under continuous monitoring for a minimum of 3 days. The drug exhibits significant dose-related prodysrhythmic effects, including heart block, ventricular tachycardia, and torsades de pointes. The risk for drug-induced dysrhythmias is increased when dofetilide is administered concurrently with other medications that prolong the QT interval, including Class I and Class III antidysrhythmics. Dofetilide may accumulate to toxic levels in patients with renal impairment. Therefore, serum creatinine levels are monitored frequently during therapy. Electrolyte imbalances, especially hypokalemia or hypomagnesemia, should be corrected before administering dofetilide because these conditions predispose the patient to developing dysrhythmias. This drug is pregnancy category C.

Dronedarone (Multaq): Approved in 2009, dronedarone is a newer antidysrhythmic. Given by the oral route, the drug is indicated to reduce the risk of hospitalization in patients with atrial dysrhythmias and associated cardiovascular risk factors such as HTN, diabetes, or previous stroke. The drug has a black box warning that it is contraindicated in patients with advanced HF with recent decompensation. It is also contraindicated in patients with bradycardia (less than 50 bpm), prolonged QT interval, and severe hepatic impairment. The most common adverse effects are diarrhea, nausea, abdominal pain, vomiting, and asthenia. Dronendarone inhibits CYP enzymes and can participate in multiple drug–drug interactions with other cardiovascular medications. Dronedarone is a category X drug and should not be taken during pregnancy or lactation.

Ibutilide (Corvert): Approved in 1995, ibutilide is only administered as an IV infusion. Continuous ECG monitoring should be conducted for at least 4 hours following the infusion to identify the potential development of new or worsening dysrhythmias. Administered over 10 minutes, ibutilide is a drug of choice for rapidly converting atrial flutter or fibrillation to normal sinus rhythm. The drug prolongs the duration of the cardiac action potential without affecting the PR interval or QRS complex. The infusion is stopped as soon as the dysrhythmia is terminated. Ibutilide is generally well tolerated, although it does have prodysrhythmic effects, including induction of ventricular tachycardia and torsades de pointes. Like other Class III agents, precautions must be taken when administering this drug concurrently with other medications that prolong the QT interval or if given to patients with hypokalemia or hypomagnesemia, as these conditions increase the risk of dysrhythmias. This drug is pregnancy category C.

Sotalol (Betapace, Betapace AF, Sorine): Approved in 1992, sotalol is unique in that the drug has both Class II and Class III antidysrhythmic properties. As a Class II agent, it is a nonselective beta blocker that slows conduction through the AV node. Its Class III actions delay repolarization and prolong the refractory period, thus widening the QT interval. Its mixed mechanisms are reflected in the diversity of indications for the drug.

Betapace and its generic equivalents are indicated for sustained ventricular fibrillation that is deemed to be life threatening. Betapace AF converts atrial fibrillation to normal sinus rhythm and is indicated for highly symptomatic atrial dysrhythmias. The drugs contain a black box warning stating that they are not interchangeable.

Because of its prodysrhythmic activity, the first 3 days of therapy with sotalol are usually conducted in a controlled clinical setting with continuous monitoring. The drug should be used with caution when taken concurrently with other medications that prolong the QT interval or if given to patients with hypokalemia or hypomagnesemia, as these conditions increase the risk of dysrhythmias. This drug is pregnancy category B.

Calcium Channel Blockers: Class IV

10 Calcium channel blockers are used to treat atrial dysrhythmias.

Although about 10 CCBs are available to treat cardiovascular disease, only a limited number are approved for dysrhythmias. Only actions relevant to dysrhythmias are discussed in this section. The antidysrhythmic CCBs are listed in Table 4.

Blockade of calcium ion channels has a number of effects on the heart, which are very similar to those of beta-adrenergic blockers. Effects include reduced automaticity in the SA node and slowed impulse conduction through the AV node. These effects are predictable, because nodal tissues are more dependent on calcium channels than other areas of the myocardium. This slows the heart rate and prolongs the refractory period. On an ECG, the most prominent effect of CCBs is prolongation of the PR interval. Indications include the control of ventricular rate in cases of atrial flutter or fibrillation, and prophylaxis of PSVT. CCBs are only effective against atrial dysrhythmias.

CCBs are safe medications that are well tolerated by most patients. As with many other antidysrhythmics, patients should be carefully monitored for bradycardia and hypotension. Because their cardiac effects are almost identical to those of beta-adrenergic blockers, patients concurrently taking drugs from both classes are especially at risk for bradycardia and possible HF. Because older adults often have multiple cardiovascular disorders, such as HTN, HF, and dysrhythmias, it is not unusual to find elderly patients taking drugs from multiple classes.

CONNECTION Checkpoint 40.3

Nifedipine (Procardia) is a prototype CCB. Why is this drug (and other dihydropyridines) not effective in treating dysrhythmias? *See Answer to Connection Checkpoint 40.3 on student resource website.*

Diltiazem (Cardizem, Dilacor, Taztia XR, Tiazac): Like other CCBs, diltiazem inhibits the transport of calcium into myocardial cells. The actions and indications for diltiazem are the same as those of verapamil. The IV form of the drug is indicated for the management of acute atrial dysrhythmias, including paroxysmal supraventricular tachycardia. In addition to its use in treating and preventing atrial dysrhythmias, the oral forms are indicated for HTN, as well as stable and vasospastic angina. Adverse effects of diltiazem are generally not serious and are related to vasodilation: headache, dizziness, and edema of the ankles and feet. Because of its profound depressant effects on nodal tissue, diltiazem is contraindicated in patients with severe bradycardia, AV block, or sick sinus syndrome. Concurrent use of diltiazem with digoxin or beta-adrenergic blockers may cause partial or complete heart block, HF, or dysrhythmias.

Verapamil (Calan, Isoptin, Verelan): Verapamil was the first CCB approved by the FDA. In the heart, verapamil slows conduction velocity and stabilizes dysrhythmias. The IV form of the drug is indicated for the rapid control of acute atrial dysrhythmias. Because verapamil can cause bradycardia and AV block, patients with HF should be carefully monitored. Because the drug may produce profound bradycardia, patients should notify their health care provider if their heart rate falls below 60 beats/minute or if systolic blood pressure falls below 90 mmHg. The therapeutic serum level is 0.08 to 0.3 mcg/mL.

PharmFACT

Sudden cardiac arrest (SCA), also called sudden cardiac death, is usually caused by ventricular defibrillation (VF). VF is commonly the first expression of coronary artery disease and is responsible for about 50% of deaths from CAD, often within the first hour after the onset of an acute myocardial infarction. The mortality rate is as high as 95% (Zevitz, 2010).

Miscellaneous Antidysrhythmics

11 Adenosine and digoxin are used for specific dysrhythmias.

Two other medications, adenosine and digoxin, are occasionally used to treat specific dysrhythmias, but they do not act by the mechanisms described above. Doses for these miscellaneous agents are listed in Table 4.

Adenosine (Adenocard, Adenoscan): Adenosine is a naturally occurring nucleoside that activates potassium channels in the SA and AV nodes, causing the potassium to leave cardiac muscle cells. When given as a rapid 1- to 2-second IV bolus, adenosine blocks reentry pathways in the AV node and terminates the tachycardia. It is usually followed by a 1- to 5-second period of asystole. Patients should be laid supine prior to adenosine use, and warned that they may feel faint. The IV site used to give adenosine should be antecubital or above, and an 18-gauge angio catheter or larger should be used. If the tachycardia has not been eliminated in 1 to 2 minutes, a second rapid bolus may be given. The primary indication for adenosine is PSVT, for which it is a drug of choice. It is also used to assist in the diagnosis of coronary artery disease of dysrhythmias in patients who are unable to undergo a cardiac exercise stress test. It is not effective in treating ventricular dysrhythmias. Although the drug has prodysrhythmic effects and dyspnea is common, adverse effects are generally self-limiting because of its 10-second half-life. This drug is pregnancy category C.

Digoxin (Lanoxin, Lanoxicaps): Although digoxin is primarily used to treat HF, it is also prescribed for atrial flutter or fibrillation and PSVT because of its ability to decrease automaticity of the SA node and slow conduction through the AV node. The drug is not effective against ventricular dysrhythmias. Because excessive levels of digoxin can produce serious dysrhythmias, and interactions with other medications are common, patients must be carefully monitored during therapy.

CONNECTIONS: NURSING PRACTICE APPLICATION

Patients Receiving Antidysrhythmic Pharmacotherapy

Assessment	Potential Nursing Diagnoses
Baseline assessment prior to administration: • Understand the reason the drug has been prescribed in order to assess for therapeutic effects (e.g., atrial, ventricular dysrhythmias). • Obtain a complete health history including cardiovascular (including previous dysrhythmias, HTN, MI, HF), and the possibility of pregnancy. Obtain a drug history including allergies, current prescription and over-the-counter (OTC) drugs, herbal preparations, and alcohol use. Be alert to possible drug interactions. • Obtain baseline weight, vital signs (especially blood pressure and pulse), ECG (rate and rhythm), cardiac monitoring (such as cardiac output if appropriate), and breath sounds. Assess for location, character, and amount of edema, if present. • Evaluate appropriate laboratory findings: electrolytes, especially potassium and magnesium levels, renal and liver function studies, and lipid profiles. • Assess the patient's ability to receive and understand instructions. Include the family and caregivers as needed.	• *Decreased Cardiac Output* • *Anxiety* • *Fatigue* • *Activity Intolerance* • *Sexual Dysfunction* • *Deficient Knowledge* (Drug Therapy) • *Risk for Decreased Cardiac Tissue Perfusion* • *Risk for Injury*, related to hypotension or dizziness associated with dysrhythmias or to adverse effects of drug therapy • *Risk for Falls*, related to hypotension or dizziness associated with dysrhythmias or to adverse effects of drug therapy
Assessment throughout administration: • Assess for desired therapeutic effects (e.g., control or elimination of dysrhythmia, blood pressure and pulse within established limits). • Continue frequent monitoring of ECG (continuous if hospitalized). Check pulse quality, volume, and regularity, along with ECG. Assess for complaints of palpitations and correlate symptoms with ECG findings. • Continue periodic monitoring of electrolytes, especially potassium and magnesium. • Assess for adverse effects: lightheadedness or dizziness, hypotension, nausea, vomiting, headache, fatigue or weakness, flushing, sexual dysfunction, or impotence. Immediately report bradycardia, tachycardia, or new or different dysrhythmias to the health care provider.	

Planning: Patient Goals and Expected Outcomes

The patient will:

• Experience therapeutic effects dependent on the reason the drug is being given (e.g., decreased dysrhythmias, blood pressure and pulse within normal limits).
• Be free from or experience minimal adverse effects.
• Verbalize an understanding of the drug's use, adverse effects, and required precautions.
• Demonstrate proper self-administration of the medication (e.g., dose, timing, and when to notify the provider).

Implementation

Interventions and (Rationales)	Patient-Centered Care
Ensuring therapeutic effects: • Continue frequent assessments as above for therapeutic effects. (Dysrhythmias have diminished or are eliminated. Blood pressure and pulse should be within normal limits or within parameters set by the health care provider.)	• To allay possible anxiety, teach the patient, family, or caregiver the rationale for all equipment used and the need for frequent monitoring.
• Encourage appropriate lifestyle changes: lowered fat intake, increased exercise, limited alcohol intake, limited caffeine intake, and smoking cessation. Provide for dietitian consultation as needed. (Healthy lifestyle changes will support and minimize the need for drug therapy.)	• Encourage the patient and family to adopt a healthy lifestyle of low-fat food choices, increased exercise, decreased alcohol consumption, and smoking cessation.
Minimizing adverse effects: • Continue to monitor ECG and pulse for quality and volume. Take the pulse for 1 full minute to assess for regularity. Continue to assess for complaints of palpitations and correlate palpitations or pulse irregularities with the ECG. (Not all dysrhythmias are symptomatic. Correlating symptoms with an ECG may help determine the need for further symptom management.)	• Teach the patient, family, or caregiver how to take a peripheral pulse for 1 full minute before taking the drug. Assist the patient to find the pulse area most convenient and easily felt. Record daily pulse rates and regularity, and bring the record to each health care visit. Instruct the patient to notify the provider if the pulse is below 60 or above 100 beats/min, there is a noticeable change in regularity from previously felt pulse rate, or if palpitations develop or worsen.

CONNECTIONS: NURSING PRACTICE APPLICATION (continued)

• Take the blood pressure lying, sitting, and standing to detect orthostatic hypotension. Be particularly cautious with the first few doses of the drug and with the elderly who are at increased risk for hypotension. (Antidysrhythmic drugs may cause hypotension. A first-dose effect may occur with a significant drop in blood pressure with the first few doses. Orthostatic hypotension may increase the risk of falls and injury.)	• Teach the patient to rise from lying or sitting to standing slowly to avoid dizziness or falls. • Instruct the patient to take the first dose of the new prescription in the evening before bed if possible, and to be cautious during the next few doses until the drug effects are known. • Teach the patient, family, or caregiver how to monitor blood pressure if required. Ensure proper use and functioning of any home equipment obtained. • Instruct the patient to notify the health care provider if blood pressure is 90/60 mmHg or below, or below the parameters set by the health care provider.
• Continue to monitor periodic electrolyte levels, especially potassium and magnesium, renal function laboratory values, and drug levels as needed. (Hypokalemia and hypomagnesemia increase the risk of dysrhythmias. Inadequate or high levels of antidysrhythmic drugs may lead to increased or more lethal dysrhythmias.)	• Instruct the patient on the need to return periodically for laboratory work. • Advise the patient to carry a wallet identification card or wear medical identification jewelry indicating antidysrhythmic therapy.
• Weigh the patient daily and report weight gain or loss of 1 kg (2.2 lb) or more in a 24-h period. Continue to assess for edema, noting location and character. (Daily weight is an accurate measure of fluid status and takes into account intake, output, and insensible losses. Weight gain or edema may indicate adverse drug effects or worsening cardiovascular disease processes.)	• Have the patient weigh self daily, ideally at the same time of day, and record weight along with pulse measurements. Have the patient report weight loss or gain of more than 1 kg (2.2 lb) in a 24-h period.
• Monitor for breath sounds and heart sounds (e.g., increasing dyspnea or postural nocturnal dyspnea, rales or crackles in lungs, frothy pink-tinged sputum, murmurs, or extra heart sounds) and report immediately. (Increasing lung congestion or new or worsening heart murmurs may indicate impending HF. Potassium channel blockers are associated with pulmonary toxicity.)	• Instruct the patient to immediately report any severe shortness of breath, frothy sputum, profound fatigue, or swelling of extremities as possible signs of HF or pulmonary toxicity.
• Report any visual changes, skin rashes, or unusual sunburn to the health care provider. (Potassium channel blockers may cause photosensitivity, skin rashes, and blurred vision.)	• Teach the patient to report any visual changes promptly and to maintain regular eye examinations. • Teach the patient about the importance of wearing protective clothing and applying sunscreen regularly during periods of sun exposure.
Patient understanding of drug therapy: • Use opportunities during administration of medications and during assessments to discuss the rationale for the drug therapy, desired therapeutic outcomes, commonly observed adverse effects, parameters for when to call the health care provider, and any necessary monitoring or precautions. (Using time during nursing care helps to optimize and reinforce key teaching areas.)	• The patient, family, or caregiver should be able to state the reason for the drug, appropriate dose and scheduling, what adverse effects to observe for and when to report them, equipment needed as appropriate and how to use that equipment, and the required length of medication therapy needed, with any special instructions regarding renewing or continuing the prescription as appropriate.
Patient self-administration of drug therapy: • When administering medications, instruct the patient, family, or caregiver in proper self-administration techniques. (Utilizing time during nurse-administration of these drugs helps to reinforce teaching.)	• Teach the patient to take drugs as evenly spaced apart as possible, and not to double dose if a dose is missed. • Teach the patient, family, or caregiver not to stop the medication abruptly, and to call the health care provider if the patient is unable to take the medication for more than one day due to illness.

Evaluation of Outcome Criteria

Evaluate the effectiveness of drug therapy by confirming that patient goals and expected outcomes have been met (see "Planning").

UNDERSTANDING THE CHAPTER

Key Concepts Summary

1 Some dysrhythmias produce no patient symptoms, while others may be life threatening.

2 The phases of cardiac action potential include rapid depolarization, a long plateau, and repolarization.

3 The electrocardiogram is used to measure electrical conduction across the myocardium.

4 Dysrhythmias are classified by the impulse origin and type of rhythm abnormality produced.

5 Antidysrhythmic drugs are only used when there is a clear benefit to the patient.

6 Antidysrhythmic drugs are classified by their mechanism of action.

7 Class I antidysrhythmics act by blocking sodium ion channels in myocardial cells.

8 Beta-adrenergic antagonists reduce automaticity as well as slow conduction velocity in the heart.

9 Potassium channel blockers prolong the refractory period of the heart.

10 Calcium channel blockers are used to treat atrial dysrhythmias.

11 Adenosine and digoxin are used for specific dysrhythmias.

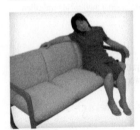

Making the PATIENT Connection

Remember the patient "Jada Chinn Nguyen" at the beginning of the chapter? Now read the remainder of the case study. Based on the information presented within this chapter, respond to the critical thinking questions that follow.

The day had been busy as Jada prepared for her daughter's upcoming wedding. There were so many arrangements to be made, and Jada felt overwhelmed. During the day she experienced heaviness in her chest, but she attributed it to the stress of the wedding and perhaps a touch of bronchitis. Nonetheless, she knew there was no time to stop and rest; there was too much to do.

Later that afternoon, she realized that she had to take it easy. Then she experienced that strange sensation once again. As she sat in a chair, Jada suddenly felt dizzy with extreme weakness and difficulty breathing. Her family members report that she became pale and unexpectedly collapsed.

Emergency personnel were called to the scene, and Jada was taken to the nearest hospital.

In the emergency department, Jada's physical examination revealed the following findings: weak, middle-aged Asian female; vital signs: blood pressure 102/68 mmHg, heart rate 116 beats/min, respiratory rate 18 breaths/min, afebrile; weight 53 kg (116 lb). She has clear bilateral breath sounds and active bowel sounds heard in all four quadrants. Her ECG reveals atrial fibrillation with a ventricular rate of 116 beats/min. She is admitted to the coronary care unit for further testing and observation.

Critical Thinking Questions

1. Jada's ECG shows atrial fibrillation. Trace the electrical conduction system through the heart. What part of the ECG complex would be most affected with this patient's medical diagnosis?

2. While in the coronary care unit, Jada will receive amiodarone (Cordarone) IV infusion. She wants to know how long she will need to receive the IV medication and how it works. How would you respond to this patient's questions?

3. The patient is being discharged on amiodarone 400 mg twice daily. What instructions should this patient receive?

4. List any drug–food interaction concerns you should discuss with Jada.

See Answers to Critical Thinking Questions on student resource website.

NCLEX-RN® Review

1 A health care provider has ordered procainamide for each of four clients. A nurse should question the order for a client with which condition?
   1. Ventricular tachycardia
   2. Paroxysmal atrial tachycardia
   3. Atrial fibrillation
   4. Severe heart failure

2 A client is receiving intravenous lidocaine for ventricular dysrhythmias. Which nursing intervention is appropriate for this therapy?
   1. Monitor the client for decreased platelet levels
   2. Place the client in a supine position during administration
   3. Monitor for paresthesias, drowsiness, or confusion
   4. Encourage coughing and deep breathing to remove secretions

3 The client with a rapid atrial dysrhythmia is being treated with verapamil (Calan). The nurse would monitor for therapeutic effectiveness by noting which of the following?
   1. Change in the blood pressure
   2. Increase in the serum potassium level
   3. Changes in the cardiac rhythm
   4. Reduction in the urine output

4 A client is to receive adenosine (Adenocard) for rapid supraventricular tachycardia. This drug must be administered:
   1. Over a 24-hour period by IV drip.
   2. Along with potassium chloride to prevent electrolyte imbalance.
   3. Over 20 to 30 minutes IV.
   4. By a rapid IV bolus injection over 1 to 2 seconds.

5 The client is prescribed propranolol (Inderal) for the treatment of atrial dysrhythmias associated with heart failure. The nurse knows this drug is used cautiously in patients with heart failure because of which effect?

1. It causes sodium retention, worsening congestion.
2. Its adverse effects include hypertension, worsening heart failure.
3. It is a negative inotropic agent and will decrease myocardial contractility and cardiac output.
4. It may cause bronchoconstriction.

6 A client is being discharged with a diagnosis of dysrhythmias. The nurse is teaching the client about amiodarone (Cordarone). What client teaching is needed related to this medication?

1. Avoid crowds while taking this medication.
2. Avoid birth control pills and use an alternate form of birth control.
3. Wear protective clothing and adequate sunscreen.
4. Use an electric razor to shave.

Additional Case Study

Malcolm Hibbert is a 56-year-old man who was diagnosed with a rapid atrial dysrhythmia and placed on diltiazem (Cardizem) to control the condition. He has been surfing the Internet to find out more about his condition and drug therapy. When he returns to the clinic, he has multiple questions to ask you. How would you respond to each of the following?

1. "My neighbor had a fast heartbeat and now he's on something called digoxin. Why didn't they use that for me?"
2. "If I'm on a calcium channel blocker, does that mean my bones might get weak?"
3. "Might any of my medications cause an increase in dysrhythmias?"

See Answers to Additional Case Study on student resource website.

Pearson Nursing Student Resources

Find additional review materials at nursing.pearsonhighered.com

Prepare for success with additional NCLEX®-style practice questions, interactive assignments and activities, web links, animations, videos, and more!

References

National Heart, Lung, and Blood Institute. (2009). *Long QT syndrome*. Retrieved from http://www.nhlbi.nih.gov/health/dci/Diseases/qt/qt_whatis.html

Zevitz, M. E. (2010). Ventricular fibrillation. *Medscape Reference*. Retrieved from http://emedicine.medscape.com/article/158712-overview

Selected Bibliography

Antzelevitch, C., & Burashnikov, A. (2011). Overview of basic mechanisms of cardiac arrhythmia. *Cardiac Electrophysiology Clinics*, 3(1), 23–45. doi:10.1016/j.ccep.2010.10.012

Ball, J. W., & Bindler, R. C. (2010). *Child health nursing: Partnering with children and families* (2nd ed.). Upper Saddle River, NJ: Pearson Education.

Marrouche, N. F., McMullan, L. L., & Gaston, V. (2010). Atrial fibrillation in the failing heart—A clinical review. *US Cardiology*, 7(1), 52–56.

National Heart, Lung, and Blood Institute. (2011). *Sudden cardiac arrest*. Retrieved from http://www.nhlbi.nih.gov/health/dci/Diseases/scda/scda_whatis.html

Rivero, A., & Curtis, A. B. (2010). Sex differences in arrhythmias. *Current Opinion in Cardiology*, 25(1), 8–15. doi:10.1097/HCO.0b013e328333f95f

Sampson, K. J., & Kaas, R. S. (2011). Antiarrhythmic drugs. In L. L. Brunton, B. A. Chabner, & B. C. Knollman (Eds.), *The pharmacological basis of therapeutics* (12th ed., pp. 815–848). New York, NY: McGraw-Hill.

Tsiperfall, A., Ottoboni, L. K., Beheiry, S., Al-Ahmad, A., Natale, A., & Wang, P. (2011). *Cardiac arrhythmia management: A practical guide for nurses and allied professionals*. Ames, IA: Wiley-Blackwell.

Zipes, D. P., Camm, A. J., Borggrefe, M., Buxton, A. E., Chaitman, B., Fromer, M., et al. (2006). ACC/AHA/ESC 2006 guidelines for management of patients with ventricular arrhythmias and the prevention of sudden cardiac death—Executive summary. *Journal of the American College of Cardiology*, 48, 1064–1108. doi:10.1016/j.jacc.2006.07.008

Answers to NCLEX-RN® Review

1 Answer: 4   Rationale: Procainamide should be avoided in clients suffering from severe HF since this drug can worsen the condition. Options 1, 2, and 3 are incorrect. Ventricular tachycardia, paroxysmal atrial tachycardia, and atrial fibrillation are indications for the use of procainamide. Cognitive Level: Applying; Client Need: Physiological Integrity; Nursing Process: Implementation

2 Answer: 3   Rationale: Early signs of lidocaine toxicity include CNS effects such as paresthesias, drowsiness, confusion, anxiety, or tremors. Options 1, 2, and 4 are incorrect. Decreased platelet levels are not related to the administration of lidocaine. Unless the client experiences hypotension, there is no need to routinely keep the client supine. Although coughing and deep breathing are effective nursing strategies to maintain pulmonary function, they are not pertinent for the administration of IV lidocaine. Cognitive Level: Applying; Client Need: Physiological Integrity; Nursing Process: Implementation

3 Answer: 3   Rationale: The therapeutic goal of verapamil is to stabilize the dysrhythmia by slowing the conduction. While the atrial dysrhythmia may continue, the rate should return to a normal range (e.g., 60–100 in an adult). Options 1, 2, and 4 are incorrect. Verapamil may cause hypotension, but as an adverse rather than a therapeutic effect. It should not cause increases in potassium levels or reduction in urine output. Cognitive Level: Analyzing; Client Need: Physiological Integrity; Nursing Process: Evaluation

4 Answer: 4   Rationale: Adenosine has an extremely short half-life and must be administered by rapid IV push, over 1 to 2 seconds. Options 1, 2, and 3 are incorrect. Adenosine is not given by IV infusion or slowly. While potassium is an important electrolyte to monitor in clients with dysrhythmias, adenosine does not cause hypo- or hyperkalemia. Cognitive Level: Applying; Client Need: Physiological Integrity; Nursing Process: Implementation

5 Answer: 3   Rationale: Beta blockers such as propranolol are negative inotropic agents and reduce myocardial contractility. In clients with existing HF, this may result in less cardiac output and worsening of symptoms. Options 1, 2, and 4 are incorrect. Propranolol does not cause sodium retention and its adverse effects include hypotension rather than HTN. It may cause bronchoconstriction because it is a nonselective beta-adrenergic antagonist (blocker), but this effect does not worsen HF. It warrants caution or is contraindicated in clients with COPD and other respiratory conditions. Cognitive Level: Analyzing; Client Need: Physiological Integrity; Nursing Process: Evaluation

6 Answer: 3   Rationale: An adverse effect associated with amiodarone is photosensitivity. The client should be instructed to avoid direct sunlight, wear protective clothing, and use adequate sunscreen lotions of SPF 15 or higher. Options 1, 2, and 4 are incorrect. Amiodarone is not known to cause immunosuppression or to interact with oral contraceptives. Increased bleeding tendencies are not an adverse effect of amiodarone. Cognitive Level: Applying; Client Need: Health Promotion and Maintenance; Nursing Process: Implementation

Pharmacotherapy of Asthma
and Other Pulmonary Disorders

From Chapter 47 of *Pharmacology: Connections to Nursing Practice*, Second Edition. Michael Patrick Adams, Carol Quam Urban. Copyright ©
2013 by Pearson Education, Inc. All rights reserved.

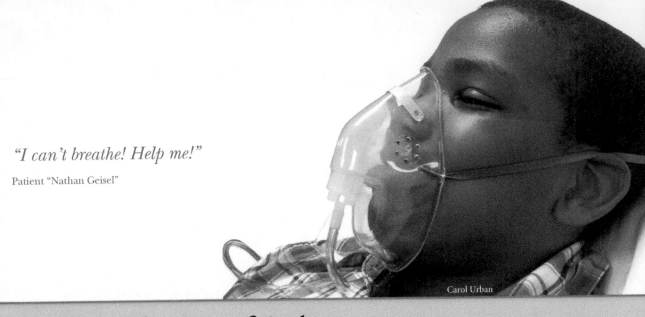

"I can't breathe! Help me!"

Patient "Nathan Geisel"

Carol Urban

Pharmacotherapy of Asthma and Other Pulmonary Disorders

Learning Outcomes

After reading this chapter, the student should be able to:

1. Identify the anatomic structures associated with the lower respiratory tract and their functions.

2. Explain how the autonomic nervous system regulates airway diameter.

3. Explain the role of inflammation and bronchospasm in the pathogenesis of asthma.

4. Compare the advantages and disadvantages of using the inhalation route of drug administration for pulmonary drugs.

5. Describe the types of devices used to deliver aerosol therapies via the inhalation route.

6. Explain the three basic principles of asthma management recommended by the National Asthma Education and Prevention Program.

7. Compare and contrast the indications for pharmacotherapy with the short- versus long-acting beta-adrenergic agonists.

8. Describe the nurse's role in the pharmacologic management of lower respiratory tract disorders.

9. For each of the classes shown in the chapter outline, identify the prototype and representative drugs and explain the mechanism(s) of drug action, primary indications, contraindications, significant drug interactions, pregnancy category, and important adverse effects.

10. Apply the nursing process to care for patients receiving pharmacotherapy for lower respiratory tract disorders.

Chapter Outline

Physiology of the Lower Respiratory Tract

Pathophysiology of Asthma

Administration of Pulmonary Drugs via Inhalation

Principles of Asthma Pharmacotherapy

Beta₂-Adrenergic Agonists

PROTOTYPE **Albuterol (Proventil, Ventolin, VoSpire)**

Anticholinergics

PROTOTYPE **Ipratropium (Atrovent)**

Corticosteroids

PROTOTYPE **Beclomethasone (Beconase AQ, Qvar)**

Mast Cell Stabilizers

PROTOTYPE **Cromolyn (Intal)**

Leukotriene Modifiers

PROTOTYPE **Zafirlukast (Accolate)**

Methylxanthines

PROTOTYPE **Theophylline (Theo-Dur, Others)**

Monoclonal Antibodies

Chronic Obstructive Pulmonary Disease

The flow of oxygen, carbon dioxide, and other gases in and out of the human body is in constant flux. Minute-by-minute control of the airways is necessary to bring an adequate supply of oxygen to the pulmonary capillaries and to rid the body of some of its most toxic waste products. Any restriction in this dynamic flow, even for brief periods, may result in serious consequences. This chapter examines drugs used in the pharmacotherapy of two primary pulmonary disorders: asthma and chronic obstructive pulmonary disease (COPD).

Physiology of the Lower Respiratory Tract

1 The physiology of the respiratory system involves two main processes: perfusion and ventilation.

The primary function of the respiratory system is to bring oxygen into the body and to remove carbon dioxide. The process by which these gases are exchanged is called respiration. The basic structures of the lower respiratory tract are shown in Figure 1.

Blood flow through the lung is called **pulmonary perfusion**. The bronchial tree ends in microscopic sacs called alveoli, which have no smooth muscle and inflate like balloons during inspiration. The alveoli are abundantly rich in capillaries. An extremely thin membrane in the alveoli separates the inspired air from the pulmonary capillaries, allowing gases to readily move between the internal environment of the blood and the inspired air. As oxygen crosses this membrane to enter the bloodstream, it is exchanged for carbon dioxide, which is a cellular waste product that leaves the bloodstream to enter the alveoli. The process of gas exchange is illustrated in Figure 1.

Ventilation is the process of moving air into and out of the lungs. As the diaphragm contracts and lowers in position, it creates a negative pressure that draws air into the lungs and inspiration occurs. During expiration the diaphragm relaxes and air leaves the lungs passively. Ventilation is a purely mechanical process that occurs approximately 12 to 18 times per minute in adults, which is a rate determined by neurons in the brainstem. This rate may be modified by a number of factors, including emotions, fever, stress, and the pH of the blood.

One of the most important factors that affect ventilation is the size of the thousands of tubes or passageways leading from the outside to the alveoli, collectively known as the airways. The nervous system controls ventilation by changing the diameter of the airways, specifically the very small and abundant bronchioles.

Bronchioles are muscular, elastic, tubular structures whose diameter, or lumen, varies with the contraction or relaxation of bronchiolar smooth muscle. Bronchodilation allows air to enter the alveoli more freely, thus increasing the supply of oxygen to the body's tissues during periods of exercise.

Key Terms

aerosol

asthma

bronchospasm

chronic bronchitis

chronic obstructive pulmonary disease (COPD)

dry powder inhaler (DPI)

emphysema

leukotrienes

metered-dose inhaler (MDI)

methylxanthines

mucolytics

nebulizer

pulmonary perfusion

small volume nebulizer

status asthmaticus

ventilation

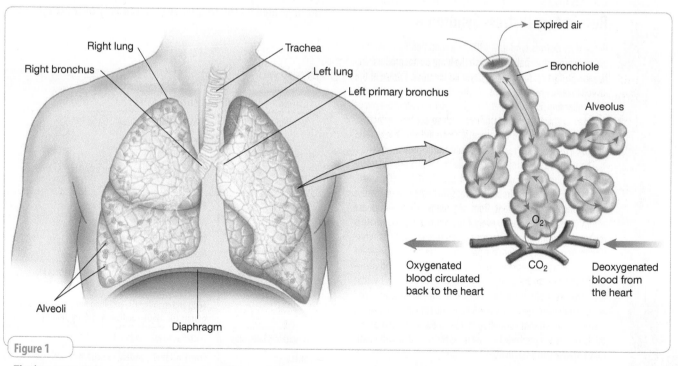

Figure 1

The lower respiratory tract and the process of gas exchange.

Bronchoconstriction increases airway resistance, resulting in less airflow. Bronchodilation and bronchoconstriction are largely regulated by the two branches of the autonomic nervous system:

- The sympathetic branch activates beta$_2$-adrenergic receptors, which causes bronchiolar smooth muscle to relax, the airway diameter to increase, and bronchodilation to occur.
- The parasympathetic branch causes bronchiolar smooth muscle to contract, the airway diameter to narrow, and bronchoconstriction to occur.

In practical terms, drugs that enhance bronchodilation will cause the patient to breathe easier. On the other hand, drugs that cause bronchoconstriction will cause breathing to become labored and the patient to become short of breath.

Bronchoconstriction is a common indication for pharmacotherapy. Bronchoconstriction may occur through several mechanisms, and the choice of pharmacotherapy will differ depending on the mechanism. The airways may narrow due to **bronchospasm**, a sudden contraction of the smooth muscle of the airways that causes acute dyspnea. Drug treatment for bronchospasm is targeted at immediately relaxing the smooth muscle spasm. A second mechanism of bronchoconstriction is the production of thick, viscous secretions that plug up the airways. Depending on the cause, treatment may involve antibiotics for an infection or drugs that break up viscous secretions (mucolytics). A third mechanism of bronchoconstriction is edema that is caused by engorgement of the pulmonary blood vessels. Treatment may include diuretics and drugs to enhance cardiac function.

Pathophysiology of Asthma

2 Asthma is a chronic disease that has both inflammatory and bronchospasm components.

Asthma is one of the most common chronic conditions in the United States, and it is increasing at an alarming rate. Asthma currently affects about 24 million Americans. The prevalence of asthma is three times greater among African Americans compared to European Americans, and women account for about 65% of all asthma patients. Although often considered a condition of childhood, asthma can occur at any age.

Asthma is characterized by chronic inflammation that occurs when potent mediators of the immune and inflammatory responses are released by mast cells lining the bronchial passageways. These mediators include histamine, leukotrienes, prostaglandins, and interleukins. The result of inflammation is an increase in airway edema coupled with increased mucus secretion, which narrows the airways, compromises the process of respiration, and contributes to airway obstruction. This is illustrated in Figure 2.

The second component in the pathogenesis of asthma is bronchospasm. The inflammatory conditions in the airway make the smooth muscle hyperresponsive to a variety of stimuli. Stimuli such as breathing smoke, pollutants, or cold air may trigger acute bronchospasm. Specific triggers are listed in Table 1. Some patients experience bronchospasm on exertion, a condition called exercise-induced asthma. Gastroesophageal reflux can trigger an asthma event when acid in the esophagus induces reflex bronchoconstriction.

The patient with asthma may present with a variety of symptoms, including evening cough, shortness of breath, chest tightness, and wheezing. Intervals between symptoms may vary from days to weeks to months. The severity of asthma is often graded by the frequency and intensity of acute episodes,

Treating the Diverse Patient
Respiratory Distress Syndrome

Respiratory distress syndrome (RDS) is a condition that primarily occurs in premature babies in which the lungs do not produce surfactant. Surfactant forms a thin layer on the inner surface of the alveoli to raise the surface tension, thereby preventing the alveoli from collapsing during expiration. If birth occurs before the pneumocytes in the lung are mature enough to secrete surfactant, the alveoli collapse and RDS results. There are also known and unknown genetic links to the lack of surfactant-producing cells.

The natural surfactant agents available for RDS are calfactant (Infasurf), beractant (Survanta), and poractant alfa (Curosurf). Calfactant is harvested from calf lungs, beractant from mature cattle lungs, and poractant from pig lungs. These drugs are administered intratracheally every 4 to 6 hours and the neonate is repositioned from side to side, prone, and supine during administration. Recent research into the possibility of nebulized surfactant has demonstrated positive outcomes. Shah (2011) found nebulized surfactant to be an effective administration strategy that would reduce or eliminate the adverse outcomes of intubation and administration-related adverse effects of the current intratracheal method. Randomized controlled studies are still needed before this becomes accepted practice, but it has the potential to dramatically improve outcomes in RDS.

TABLE 1 Common Triggers of Asthma	
Cause	Sources
Air pollutants	Tobacco smoke
	Ozone
	Nitrous and sulfur oxides
	Fumes from cleaning fluids or solvents
	Burning leaves
Allergens	Pollen from trees, grasses, and weeds
	Animal dander
	Household dust
	Mold
Chemicals and food	Drugs, including aspirin, ibuprofen, and beta blockers
	Sulfite preservatives
	Food and condiments, including nuts, monosodium glutamate (MSG), shellfish, and dairy products
Respiratory infections	Bacterial, fungal, and viral
Stress	Emotional stress, anxiety, exercise in dry, cold climates

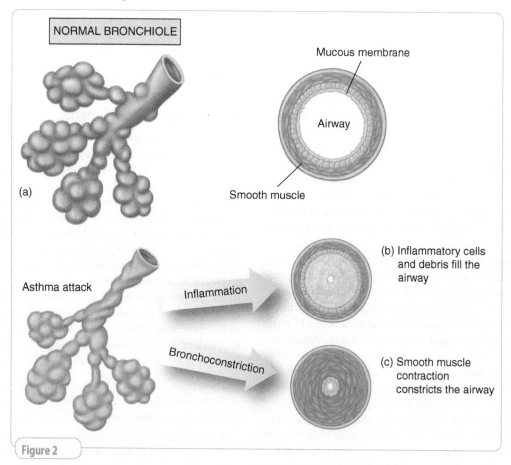

NORMAL BRONCHIOLE

Mucous membrane

Airway

(a)

Smooth muscle

Asthma attack

Inflammation

(b) Inflammatory cells and debris fill the airway

Bronchoconstriction

(c) Smooth muscle contraction constricts the airway

Figure 2

Changes in the bronchioles during an asthma attack: (a) Normal bronchiole. (b) The inflammatory component plugs the airway. (c) Bronchoconstriction narrows the airway.

as given in Table 2. **Status asthmaticus**, an emergency situation in which asthma is unresponsive to drug treatment, may lead to respiratory failure. Drugs may be given to prevent asthmatic attacks or to terminate attacks in progress.

PharmFACT

According to the Asthma and Allergy Foundation of America (n.d.), each day in the United States:

- 40,000 people miss school or work due to asthma.
- 30,000 people have an asthma attack.
- 5,000 people visit the emergency department for asthma treatment.
- 11 people die from asthma.

Administration of Pulmonary Drugs via Inhalation

3 Inhalation is a common route of administration for pulmonary drugs because it delivers drugs directly to their sites of action.

Many drugs that are used to treat asthma are available for administration by the inhalation route. Inhalation offers a rapid and efficient mechanism for delivering drugs directly to their site of action in the lungs. The enormous surface area of the bronchioles and alveoli and the rich blood supply to these

TABLE 2 Assessment of Asthma

Level	Frequency of Symptoms	Nocturnal Attacks	Activity
Intermittent	Less than 2 times/week	Less than 2 times/month	Not limited
Mild persistent	3–6 days/week	More than 2 times/month	Attacks may limit activity
Moderate persistent	Daily	More than 1 time/week	Attacks affect activity
Severe persistent	Continual	Frequent	Attacks limit physical activity

Source: From COLBERT, BRUCE J; KENNEDY, BARBARA J., INTEGRATED CARDIOPULMONARY PHARMACOLOGY, 2nd Ed., © 2008. Reprinted and Electronically reproduced by permission of Pearson Education, Inc., Upper Saddle River, New Jersey.

areas result in an almost instantaneous onset of action for inhaled substances.

Medications are delivered to the respiratory system by aerosol therapy. An **aerosol** is a suspension of minute liquid droplets or fine solid particles suspended in a gas. The major advantage of aerosol therapy is that it delivers the drugs directly to the site of action. Not only does this dramatically decrease the onset of action, but it also allows for much smaller doses of a drug. The small doses of drug given by the inhalation route minimize any systemic effects that might result from absorption across pulmonary capillaries when compared to PO medications. Several devices are used to deliver drugs via the inhalation route. The most common are metered-dose inhalers, dry power inhalers, and nebulizers.

The **metered-dose inhaler (MDI)**, often simply called an inhaler, is the most common type of aerosol delivery device. It consists of a canister that holds the medicine and a mouthpiece. To use an MDI, the patient presses the canister toward the mouthpiece to deliver a measured dose or "puff" of medication. By inhaling during drug delivery, the patient helps to ensure that the drug reaches the site of action in the lungs. Even when MDIs are used properly, however, the majority of the aerosolized drug never reaches the lungs. There are two primary reasons for this problem. One is that heavier aerosolized particles fall out by gravity and are deposited in the oropharynx. The other reason is that proper coordination of drug delivery with inhalation can be difficult for some patients. To decrease oropharyngeal deposition and to enhance drug delivery to the lungs, many health care providers recommend that patients use a spacer with their MDI. A spacer is a special tube that attaches to the mouthpiece that is designed to hold the cloud of aerosolized medication. This serves two primary purposes. First, the spacer holds drops that fall out of the aerosol so that less medication is deposited on the oropharynx and in the mouth. Second, because the spacer holds the medication, the patient does not have to precisely coordinate inhalation with activation, so that more drug reaches the site of action.

A **dry powder inhaler (DPI)** delivers the medication as a fine dry powder. Whereas the MDI is activated by pressing the canister, the DPI is automatically activated when the patient inhales through the mouthpiece. Because the timing of drug delivery and inhalation does not have to be coordinated, more medication is delivered to the lung with a DPI. The DPI has no propellants in the canister (propellants can be harmful to some patients with lung problems).

A **nebulizer** (or **small volume nebulizer**) is a machine that delivers medication as a fine mist. When using a nebulizer, the medication to be delivered is poured into a receptacle. The machine then vaporizes the liquid medication into a mist that is inhaled by using a face mask or other handheld device. These "breathing treatments" may take up to 30 minutes to administer the drug so it may not work as quickly as a drug taken from an MDI or DPI; however, medication delivered in this fashion is often more effective because it is delivered over many inhalations that occur during the period of medication delivery.

Principles of Asthma Pharmacotherapy

4 The goals of asthma pharmacotherapy are to terminate acute bronchospasms and to reduce the frequency of asthma attacks.

The choice of medications for asthma is determined by evidence-based guidelines coupled with the patient's response to therapy and adjusted according to the patient's individual situation. Evidence-based guidelines have been developed by experts in asthma management and are based on research findings. In the United States, the National Asthma Education and Prevention Program (NAEPP) issued guidelines for asthma treatment in 1991, which were updated in 1997, 2002, and 2007. The NAEPP guidelines (2007) recommend a stepwise approach to asthma control based on the frequency and severity of symptoms, as shown in Figure 3. As patient symptoms worsen, the pharmacotherapy is adjusted accordingly by going to the next step. This provides for a rational, evidence-based approach to asthma management. The three general strategies for asthma management from the NAEPP are as follows:

- Incorporate four components of care: medications, patient education, environmental control measures, and management of comorbidities.
- Initiate therapy based on asthma severity. For patients not taking long-term control therapy, select the treatment step based on severity. Patients who have persistent asthma require daily long-term control medication.
- Adjust the therapy based on asthma control. Once therapy is initiated, monitor the level of asthma control and adjust the therapy accordingly: step up if necessary and step down if possible to identify the minimum amount of medication required to maintain asthma control.

The goals of asthma pharmacotherapy are twofold: to terminate acute bronchospasms and to prevent or reduce the frequency of asthma attacks. Different medications are needed to achieve each of these goals. The NAEPP categorizes asthma drugs into two simple classes: quick-relief medications and long-term control medications. A summary of the different classes used for asthma management is given in Table 3.

PharmFACT

More than 7 million children have asthma in the United States. Children from poor households are more likely to have asthma than those from nonpoor households (Bloom, Cohen, & Freeman, 2010).

5 Beta₂-adrenergic agonists are the most effective drugs for relieving acute bronchospasm.

Beta-adrenergic agonists are some of the most frequently prescribed drugs for treating pulmonary disorders. Beta agonists are drugs that activate the sympathetic nervous system, which relaxes bronchial smooth muscle, resulting in bronchodilation. They are the drugs of choice in the treatment of bronchoconstriction.

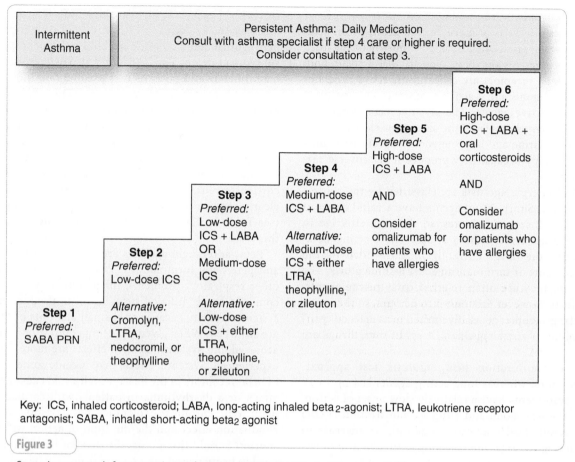

Key: ICS, inhaled corticosteroid; LABA, long-acting inhaled beta₂-agonist; LTRA, leukotriene receptor antagonist; SABA, inhaled short-acting beta₂ agonist

Figure 3

Stepwise approach for managing asthma in adults and patients 12 years and older.
Source: From *Expert Panel Report 3 (EPR3): Guidelines for the Diagnosis and Management of Asthma* (p. 343), by the National Asthma Education Prevention Program, coordinated by the National Heart, Lung, and Blood Institute of the National Institutes of Health, 2007. Retrieved from http://www.nhlbi.nih.gov/guidelines/asthma/asthgdln.htm

TABLE 3 Overview of Drug Classes for Asthma Management

Class	Mechanism	Use
Quick-Relief Medications		
Short-acting beta₂-adrenergic agonists (SABAs)	Bronchodilators	Preferred drugs for relief of acute symptoms.
Anticholinergics	Bronchodilators	Alternate drugs for those who cannot tolerate SABAs.
Corticosteroids: systemic	Anti-inflammatory	Although not rapid acting, these oral agents are used for short periods to reduce the frequency of acute exacerbations.
Long-Acting Medications		
Corticosteroids: inhaled	Anti-inflammatory	Preferred drugs for long-term asthma management. Oral doses may be required for severe, persistent asthma.
Mast cell stabilizers	Anti-inflammatory	Alternative drugs to control mild, persistent asthma or exercise-induced asthma.
Leukotriene modifiers	Anti-inflammatory	Alternative drugs to control mild, persistent asthma or as adjunctive therapy with inhaled corticosteroids.
Long-acting beta₂-adrenergic agonists (LABAs)	Bronchodilators	Used in combination with inhaled corticosteroids for prophylaxis of moderate to severe persistent asthma.
Methylxanthines	Bronchodilators	Used in combination with inhaled corticosteroids for prophylaxis of mild to moderate persistent asthma.
Immunomodulators	Monoclonal antibody	Used as adjunctive therapy for patients who have allergies and severe, persistent asthma.

Source: From *Expert Panel Report 3 (EPR3): Guidelines for the Diagnosis and Management of Asthma,* by the National Asthma Education and Prevention Program Coordinating Committee, coordinated by the National Heart, Lung, and Blood Institute of the National Institutes of Health, 2007. Retrieved from http://www.nhlbi.nih.gov/guidelines/asthma/asthgdln.htm

Beta-agonist medications may act on either beta$_1$ receptors, which are located primarily in the heart, or on beta$_2$ receptors, which are located in smooth muscle of the lung, uterus, and other organs. Beta agonists that activate both beta$_1$ and beta$_2$ receptors are called nonselective bronchodilators. Beta agonists that activate only the beta$_2$ receptors are called selective agents. The selective beta$_2$-adrenergic agonists have largely replaced the older, nonselective agents such as epinephrine and isoproterenol (Isuprel) for asthma pharmacotherapy because they produce fewer adverse cardiac effects.

Beta$_2$-adrenergic agonists are classified by their duration of action. Short-acting agents have a rapid onset of action, usually several minutes, so they are effective in terminating an acute asthma attack. Short-acting beta$_2$ agonists are the drugs currently recommended by the NAEPP to abort or terminate an acute asthma attack. For this reason, they are often referred to as rescue agents. Their effects, however, last only 2 to 6 hours, so the use of short-acting agents is generally limited to as-needed (prn) management of acute episodes. Doses of these drugs are listed in Table 4.

Intermediate-duration beta$_2$ agonists last approximately 8 hours, whereas long-acting agents last up to 12 hours. These agents have a relatively slow onset of action. In 2005, the U.S. Food and Drug Administration (FDA) issued a public health advisory regarding an increase in deaths among persons who take long-acting beta$_2$ agonists (LABAs). Because LABAs are not indicated to abort an asthma attack, taking a LABA instead of a short-acting beta agonist could result in unrelieved bronchospasm and subsequent death. The LABAs are also delivered via handheld inhalers and patients may assume that they have the same actions as the short-acting agents. Patients must be alerted to the dangers inherent in taking these during an acute episode. Although the risk of asthma-related death is small, LABAs should only be used as additional therapy for patients who are not adequately controlled on other asthma-controller medications, such as inhaled corticosteroids, or for patients with severe asthma who clearly require two medications for disease management (see Table 2). They are not to be used as monotherapy for this disease.

Beta$_2$-adrenergic agonists are available in PO, inhaled, and parenteral formulations. When taken for asthma and other respiratory problems, inhalation is by far the most common route. Inhaled beta$_2$ agonists produce minimal systemic toxicity because only small amounts of the drugs are absorbed. When given PO a longer duration of action is achieved, but systemic adverse effects are more frequently experienced. Systemic effects may include some activation of beta$_1$ receptors in the heart, which could cause an angina attack or a dysrhythmia in patients with cardiac impairment. With chronic use tolerance may develop to the bronchodilation effect and the duration of action will become shorter. Should this occur, the dose of beta$_2$ agonist may need to be increased, or a second drug may be added to the therapeutic regimen.

Evidence-Based Practice   Asthma Management

Clinical Question
What role do elementary school teachers play in the management of asthma?

Evidence
Multiple risk factors for asthma have been determined including family history, low socioeconomic status, lack of insurance coverage, obesity, and environmental and allergen exposures. Research into best practices for drug management have recently suggested that the combination of a long-acting beta agonist (LABA) paired with an inhaled corticosteroid (ICS) works well in preventing and controlling asthma symptoms for many patients, especially for those whose asthma is not controlled by ICS alone (Lemanske & Busse, 2010; O'Connor, Patrick, Parasuraman, Martin, & Goldman, 2010). Despite current knowledge into the risks, etiology, and treatment of asthma, childhood asthmatic attacks still cause lost school days and learning, lost parent productivity as days off from work are required to care for the child, and increasing medical expenses.

Teachers are with children up to one third of their waking hours during the week and as such, are in a key position to proactively assist the child and family to manage asthma. Bruzzese et al. (2010) found that despite experience with asthmatic children in the classroom, elementary school teachers were not always well prepared in asthma management. Overall, the majority of teachers had experience with children with asthma and could recognize common asthma triggers. While many could identify steps to prevent asthma attacks such as trigger avoidance and activity limitation, few identified actually taking more than one step. Fewer teachers identified steps to manage asthma symptoms, with most identifying "contacting the nurse" as the usual step taken. And while the teachers communicated about the child's asthma with both the parents and the school nurse, more teachers discussed asthma-related information with the parents than with the nurse.

Implications
Teachers must manage multiple academic responsibilities as well as health-related concerns such as asthma. The school nurse may be the most important person in assisting elementary teachers to proactively manage childhood asthma rather than reactively seeking assistance when an attack occurs. Working together as a team, nurses can help teachers become more knowledgeable about asthma triggers, symptoms, and treatment, and teachers can become more skilled in symptom recognition and prevention measures.

Critical Thinking Question
Discuss approaches that a school nurse could use to increase teachers' knowledge about asthma management. What are some strategies that could encourage students, parents, and their families to participate in a schoolwide effort to increase asthma knowledge?

See Answers to Critical Thinking Questions on student resource website.

CONNECTIONS

TABLE 4 Bronchodilators for Asthma

Drug	Route and Adult Dose (maximum dose where indicated)	Adverse Effects
Beta Agonists/Sympathomimetics		
albuterol (Proventil, Ventolin, VoSpire)	MDI: 2 inhalations every 4–6 h as needed (max: 12 inhalations/day) Nebulizer: 1.25–5 mg every 4–8 h as needed PO: 2–4 mg tid-qid (max: 32 mg/day); extended release tabs: 8 mg every 12 h (max: 32 mg/day divided)	*Headache, dizziness, tremor, nervousness, throat irritation, drug tolerance* Tachycardia, dysrhythmia, hypokalemia, hyperglycemia, paradoxical bronchoconstriction, hypomagnesemia, maternal heart problems during pregnancy (terbutaline), increased risk for asthma-related death
arformoterol (Brovana)	Nebulizer: 15 mcg twice daily (max: 30 mcg/day)	
formoterol (Foradil, Perforomist)	DPI: 12 mcg inhalation capsule every 12 h (max : 24 mcg/day) Nebulizer: 20 mcg bid (max: 40 mcg/day)	
indacaterol (Arcapta neohaler)	Inhalation: one 75 mcg capsule/day using the Neohaler	
levalbuterol HCl (Xopenex)	Nebulizer: 0.63 mg tid-qid MDI: 2 inhalations every 4–6 h	
pirbuterol (Maxair)	MDI: 2 inhalations qid (max: 12 puffs/day)	
salmeterol (Serevent)	DPI: 2 aerosol inhalations bid or 1 powder diskus bid	
terbutaline sulfate (Brethine)	PO: 2.5–5 mg tid (max: 15 mg/day) Subcutaneous: 0.25 mg, followed by an additional 0.25 mg if no response is noted in 30 min	
Anticholinergics		
ipratropium (Atrovent)	MDI: 2 inhalations (50 mcg) qid (max: 12 inhalations/day) Nebulizer: 500 mcg every 6–8 h as needed	*Headache, bad taste, cough, dry mouth, blurred vision* Pharyngitis
tiotropium (Spiriva)	DPI: 1 capsule inhaled/day	
Methylxanthines		
aminophylline (Truphylline)	PO: 380 mg/day in divided doses every 6–8 h (max: 928 mg/day) IV: 0.1–0.5 mg/kg/h (rate dependent on certain patient parameters)	*Nervousness, tremors, dizziness, headache, nausea, vomiting, anorexia* Tachycardia, dysrhythmias, hypotension, seizures, circulatory failure, respiratory arrest
dyphylline (Lufylline)	PO: 15 mg every 6 h	
theophylline (Theo-Dur, Others)	PO: 300–600 mg/day in divided doses (max: 900 mg/day) IV: 0.39–0.79 mg/kg/h (rate dependent on certain patient parameters)	

Note: *Italics* indicate common adverse effects. Underline indicates serious adverse effects.

PROTOTYPE DRUG | Albuterol (Proventil, Ventolin, VoSpire)

Classification: **Therapeutic:** Bronchodilator
Pharmacologic: Beta$_2$-adrenergic agonist

Therapeutic Effects and Uses: Approved in 1981, albuterol is a short-acting, beta$_2$-adrenergic agonist that is used to relieve and prevent the bronchospasm that is a characteristic pathophysiological feature of asthma. Its rapid onset and excellent safety profile have made inhaled albuterol a drug of choice for the termination of acute bronchospasm. In addition to relieving bronchospasm, the drug facilitates mucus drainage and can inhibit the release of inflammatory chemicals from mast cells. When inhaled 15 to 30 minutes prior to physical activity, it can prevent exercise-induced bronchospasm for 2 to 3 hours. Inhaled albuterol is considered safe for use during pregnancy.

Oral forms of albuterol include immediate release and extended release tablets (VoSpire) and an oral solution. The PO forms have a longer onset of action and are not suitable for terminating acute asthma attacks. The NAEPP does not recommend the use of short-acting beta$_2$ agonists for the management of asthma prophylaxis.

Mechanism of Action: Albuterol acts by selectively binding to beta$_2$-adrenergic receptors in bronchial smooth muscle to cause bronchodilation.

Pharmacokinetics:

Route(s)	Inhalation, PO
Absorption	Slow by the inhalation route. Some of the inhaled drug is swallowed and absorbed by the gastrointestinal (GI) tract. Rapid when given PO
Distribution	Delivered directly to the lungs (site of action); crosses the blood–brain barrier; may cross the placenta; unknown if secreted in breast milk
Primary metabolism	Hepatic (CYP450)
Primary excretion	Renal (less than 10% feces)
Onset of action	Inhalation: 5–15 min; PO: 30 min; peak effect: 0.5–2 h
Duration of action	Inhalation: 2–6 h; PO, sustained release: 8–12 h

Adverse Effects: Serious adverse effects from inhaled albuterol are uncommon when taken as directed; PO forms cause more sympathomimetic adverse effects. Some patients experience palpitations, headaches, throat irritation, tremor, nervousness, restlessness, and tachycardia. Less common adverse reactions include insomnia and dry mouth. Uncommon adverse effects include chest pain, paradoxical bronchospasm, and allergic reactions.

Contraindications/Precautions: Albuterol use is contraindicated if the patient has hypersensitivity to the drug. Because albuterol may exhibit cardiovascular effects in some patients, caution is required when administering these agents to persons with a history of tachyarrhythmias, prolongation of the QT interval, coronary artery disease, or hypertension (HTN).

Drug Interactions: Concurrent use with beta blockers will inhibit the bronchodilation effect of albuterol and may induce bronchospasm in patients with asthma. To prevent hypertensive crisis, patients should also avoid monoamine oxidase inhibitors (MAOIs) within 14 days of beginning therapy. Concurrent use with thyroid hormone may produce additive stimulatory effects on the cardiovascular system. **Herbal/Food:** Products containing caffeine such as coffee and tea may cause nervousness, tremor, or palpitations.

Pregnancy: Category C.

Treatment of Overdose:
Overdose results in an exaggerated sympathetic activation, causing dysrhythmias, hypokalemia, and hyperglycemia. Cardiac arrest and death have been reported. In severe cases, administration of a beta antagonist may be necessary.

Nursing Responsibilities: Key nursing implications for patients receiving albuterol are included in the Nursing Practice Application for Patients Receiving Pharmacotherapy for Asthma and Chronic Obstructive Pulmonary Disease.

Lifespan and Diversity Considerations:
- Monitor cardiac status in the older adult receiving albuterol. Undetected cardiac disease may increase the likelihood of adverse effects related to the drug.
- Supervise young children over the age of 2 to ensure appropriate use of the inhaler.

Patient and Family Education:
- Clean the mouthpiece at least weekly by removing the drug canister and running warm water through the top and bottom, shaking out excess water, and allowing to air dry. This will help to ensure there is no medication buildup with resulting improper drug delivery.
- Do not breast-feed while taking this drug without approval of the health care provider.
- Immediately notify the health care provider of any known or suspected pregnancy.

Drugs Similar to Albuterol (Proventil, Ventolin, VoSpire)

Other short-acting beta agonists include levalbuterol and pirbuterol. Long-acting beta agonists include arformoterol, formoterol, indacaterol, salmeterol, and terbutaline. Bitolterol mesylate is a drug in this class that has been discontinued in the United States. Adverse effects are the same as those of other beta₂ agonists and include tachycardia, nervousness, angina, and headache.

Arformoterol (Brovana): Arformoterol is one of the newer drugs in the class that was approved in 2007 for the treatment of COPD, including chronic bronchitis and emphysema. This drug is an isomer of formoterol and is the first LABA available by inhalation via nebulizer. Formoterol and salmeterol use DPIs. Arformoterol may be administered twice daily. Although it begins to relax bronchi within about 7 minutes, its maximum effects take 1 to 3 hours. Thus this drug is not suitable for terminating acute asthma attacks. Arformoterol is well tolerated and exhibits few serious adverse effects in most patients. The drug has a black box warning that it (and other LABAs) have been shown to increase the risk of asthma-related death; thus it should only be prescribed when short- and intermediate-acting drugs are unable to control symptoms. A combination drug (Dulera) containing arformoterol and mometasone was approved in 2010. Arformoterol is pregnancy category C.

Formoterol (Foradil, Perforomist): Approved in 2001, formoterol is a long-acting, selective beta₂ agonist that is administered using a DPI. Because the drug takes 1 to 3 hours for maximum effect, it is not suitable for terminating acute bronchospasm. Due to its long duration of action, formoterol is indicated for asthma prophylaxis, including the prevention of nocturnal symptoms and exercise-induced asthma. It is also approved by the FDA for the relief of bronchospasm due to COPD. This drug is well tolerated and has the same adverse effect profile as that of other drugs in this class. Formoterol has a black box warning that it (and other LABAs) have been shown to increase the risk of asthma-related death; thus it should only be prescribed when short- and intermediate-acting drugs are unable to control symptoms. This drug is pregnancy category C.

Indacaterol (Arcapta Neohaler): One of the newest drugs in this class, indacaterol was approved in 2011 as a maintenance bronchodilator for patients with COPD, including chronic bronchitis and emphysema. The drug comes as a capsule that is inserted into the neohaler device for inhalation. Its once daily dosing schedule offers an advantage over other LABAs. Indacaterol is not indicated for the termination of acute bronchospasm. Like other LABAs, indacaterol carries a black box warning that it should not be used for long-term asthma control due to the possibility of an increased risk of asthma-related death. This drug is pregnancy category C.

Levalbuterol (Xopenex): Approved in 1999, levalbuterol is an isomer of albuterol and has almost identical indications, actions, and adverse effects. This drug is administered via nebulized or aerosolized oral inhalation. It is indicated for the relief of acute bronchospasm symptoms and can be administered three to four times daily. Regular, daily use of levalbuterol is not recommended by the NAEPP as a means to prevent bronchospasm. Like other drugs in this class, levalbuterol has few serious adverse effects, with nervousness and tremor being the most frequently reported. This drug is pregnancy category C.

Pirbuterol (Maxair): Approved in 1986, pirbuterol is a short-acting, selective beta$_2$ agonist that has a structure very similar to that of albuterol. Its rapid, 5-minute onset of action makes it suitable for the termination of acute bronchospasm symptoms. Doses may be repeated every 4 to 6 hours, as needed. Like the other short-acting beta$_2$ agonists, this drug must not be used on a regular, daily basis to prevent asthmatic attacks. It is also FDA approved for the relief of bronchospasm due to COPD and may be prescribed off-label to prevent exercise-induced bronchospasm. It is available only by the inhalation route. Adverse effects are uncommon and include tachycardia and palpitation. This drug is pregnancy category C.

Salmeterol (Serevent): Approved in 1994, salmeterol is a LABA that is prescribed for asthma prophylaxis and the long-term therapy of bronchospasm associated with COPD. The LABAs salmeterol and formoterol are considered less effective at preventing asthma attacks than the inhaled corticosteroids. Salmeterol has a slow onset of action and should not be used to terminate acute bronchospasm. The aerosol form of salmeterol has been discontinued in the United States, although the DPI route is still available. Overall, the drug is well tolerated, and few serious adverse effects are reported. Pharyngitis and upper respiratory tract infections occur in patients who are taking the drug, and headache is a common adverse effect. Salmeterol has a black box warning that it (and other LABAs) have been shown to increase the risk of asthma-related death; thus it should only be prescribed when short- and intermediate-acting drugs are unable to control symptoms. This drug is pregnancy category C.

Terbutaline (Brethine): An older drug approved in 1974, terbutaline is indicated for the treatment of bronchospasm. Terbutaline is given by the PO route and may take 30 minutes or longer to act; thus it is too slow to be used for acute conditions. A subcutaneous form of terbutaline can relieve bronchospasm within 15 minutes. PO terbutaline has a shorter duration of action than albuterol or salmeterol and it must be administered three times daily. An inhalation form of the drug (Brethaire) was removed from the U.S. market in 1999. Terbutaline is moderately selective for beta$_2$ receptors but may produce some activation of beta$_1$ receptors in the heart. Adverse effects are similar to those observed with other drugs in this class. Terbutaline has been used off-label to delay premature labor contractions due to its effects on beta$_2$ receptors in the uterus that cause smooth muscle relaxation. However, in 2011 the FDA issued a black box warning that *oral* terbutaline should not be used to prevent or treat preterm labor because it has not been shown to be effective and there is a potential for serious maternal heart problems and death. In very serious conditions, the *injectable* form of the drug may still be used but treatment is limited to no longer than 48 to 72 hours to delay preterm labor. This drug is pregnancy category B.

CONNECTION Checkpoint 47.1

The agents for asthma are selective for beta$_2$-adrenergic receptors. What are the primary indications for the drugs selective for beta$_1$-adrenergic receptors? *See Answer to Connection Checkpoint 47.1 on student resource website.*

6 The inhaled anticholinergics are used for preventing bronchospasm.

Although short-acting beta agonists are the drugs of choice for treating acute bronchospasm, anticholinergics (cholinergic blockers or antagonists) are alternative bronchodilators. Although anticholinergics such as atropine have been available for many decades, the adverse effect profile of these agents made most anticholinergics poorly suited for the management of asthma. With the delivery of the anticholinergics by inhalation, however, they have become important drugs in the arsenal of asthma pharmacotherapy. Two inhalation anticholinergic agents are available for the treatment of bronchospasm: ipratropium (Atrovent) and tiotropium (Spiriva).

Anticholinergics block the parasympathetic nervous system. Blocking the parasympathetic nervous system results in actions similar to those of stimulating the sympathetic nervous system. It is predictable then that anticholinergic drugs would cause bronchodilation and have potential applications in the pharmacotherapy of asthma and COPD. Ipratropium is rapid acting and can be used to relieve acute bronchospasm, whereas tiotropium is better suited for maintenance therapy due to its longer onset of action.

Anticholinergics have actions that are similar to those of beta-adrenergic agonists and drugs from the two classes may be combined to produce a greater and more prolonged bronchodilation than either drug used separately. This additive effect is particularly useful for patients with persistent bronchospasm for whom either agent alone is inadequate to alleviate bronchoconstriction. Taking advantage of this increased effect, the pharmaceutical companies have developed inhalants that combine both an anticholinergic and a beta agonist into a single canister.

Anticholinergics are available in PO, inhaled, and injection formulations; however, when used for asthma and other respiratory conditions, the inhaled forms are typically prescribed. The inhaled anticholinergics are relatively safe medications. The wide range of anticholinergic adverse effects that is observed when drugs in this class are administered systemically rarely occurs when administered by inhalation.

PROTOTYPE DRUG | Ipratropium (Atrovent)

Classification: Therapeutic: Bronchodilator
Pharmacologic: Anticholinergic

Therapeutic Effects and Uses: Approved by the FDA in 1986, ipratropium is an anticholinergic agent that is delivered by the inhalation and intranasal routes. The inhalation form is approved to relieve and prevent the bronchospasm that is characteristic of asthma and COPD. It is a drug of choice for treating bronchospasms due to COPD (e.g., bronchitis and emphysema). Although it has not received FDA approval for the treatment of asthma, it is nevertheless prescribed off-label for the disorder. NAEPP guidelines state that the role of ipratropium in asthma management is as an alternative to short-acting beta agonists and for patients experiencing severe asthma exacerbations. It is sometimes combined with beta agonists or corticosteroids to provide additive bronchodilation. Ipratropium is much less effective than the beta$_2$ agonists at preventing exercise-induced bronchospasm. Combivent is a fixed dose combination of ipratropium and albuterol indicated for COPD.

When administered via inhalation, ipratropium can relieve acute bronchospasm within minutes of administration, although peak effects may take 1 to 2 hours. Bronchodilation action may continue for up to 6 hours.

The nasal spray formulation of ipratropium was approved in 1995 for the symptomatic relief of rhinorrhea associated with the common cold and perennial rhinitis. The drug inhibits nasal secretions but does not have decongestant action. Treatment is limited to 3 weeks.

Mechanism of Action: Ipratropium causes bronchodilation by blocking cholinergic receptors in bronchial smooth muscle. Intranasal administration blocks parasympathetic receptors, thus reducing nasal hypersecretion characteristic of the common cold.

Pharmacokinetics:

Route(s)	Inhalation, intranasal
Absorption	Minimal systemic absorption; some of the inhaled drug is swallowed but is not absorbed by the GI tract
Distribution	Small amount is secreted in breast milk; minimally bound to plasma protein
Primary metabolism	Hepatic (CYP450)
Primary excretion	Renal and feces
Onset of action	5–15 min; peak effect: 1.5–2 h
Duration of action	3–6 h; half-life: 1.5–2 h

Adverse Effects: Because it is not readily absorbed from the lungs, ipratropium produces few systemic adverse effects. Though rare it can worsen glaucoma with sufficient systemic absorption. Typical anticholinergic adverse effects such as dry mouth, nausea, and GI distress are among the most common adverse effects but occur in less than 3% of patients. Irritation of the upper respiratory tract may result in cough, drying of the nasal mucosa, or hoarseness. Paradoxical acute bronchospasm is a rare adverse effect that may be life threatening. This drug produces a bitter taste that some patients find problematic. Intranasal administration may cause epistaxis and excessive drying of the nasal mucosa.

Contraindications/Precautions: Ipratropium is contraindicated in patients with hypersensitivity to soya lecithin or related food products such as soybean and peanut. Soya lecithin is used as a propellant in the inhaler. Ipratropium is contraindicated in persons who have demonstrated a hypersensitivity to ipratropium. All anticholinergics should be used with caution in patients with closed-angle glaucoma or urinary tract obstruction because they may worsen these conditions.

Drug Interactions: Because it has little systemic absorption, ipratropium interacts with very few drugs. Use with other anticholinergics such as atropine may lead to additive anticholinergic adverse effects. **Herbal/Food:** Unknown.

Pregnancy: Category B.

Treatment of Overdose: Overdose with ipratropium is unlikely because very little of the drug is absorbed.

Nursing Responsibilities: Key nursing implications for patients receiving ipratropium are included in the Nursing Practice Application for Patients Receiving Pharmacotherapy for Asthma and Chronic Obstructive Pulmonary Disease.

Lifespan and Diversity Considerations:
- Monitor cardiac status in the older adult receiving albuterol. Undetected cardiac disease may increase the likelihood of adverse effects related to the drug.
- Monitor the older adult for urinary retention, dry mouth, and other anticholinergic effects.

Patient and Family Education:
- Clean the mouthpiece at least weekly by removing the drug canister and running warm water through the top and bottom, shaking out excess water, and allowing to air dry. This will help to ensure there is no medication buildup with resulting improper drug delivery.
- Do not give this drug to children without a prescription. Ipratropium is not recommended for children younger than 12 years of age.
- Do not breast-feed while taking this drug without approval of the health care provider.
- Immediately notify the health care provider of any known or suspected pregnancy.

Drugs Similar to Ipratropium (Atrovent)

The only other anticholinergic currently approved in the United States for inhalation is tiotropium.

Tiotropium (Spiriva): Approved in 2004, tiotropium is closely related to ipratropium and is indicated for the long-term maintenance treatment and prophylaxis of bronchospasm in patients with COPD, including chronic bronchitis and emphysema. It is not to be used to terminate acute bronchospasm; short-acting adrenergic agonists are indicated for this condition. An advantage of tiotropium is its long duration of action. Unlike ipratropium, which must be taken four or more times a day, tiotropium only needs to be taken once a day so patients are less likely to miss doses. Another difference between the two agents is that ipratropium is administered by MDI, whereas tiotropium is administered by DPI (HandiHaler device). For patients with COPD who have difficulty using an MDI device, tiotropium can be a viable alternative. Adverse effects are the same as those of ipratropium. This drug is pregnancy category C.

7 Inhaled corticosteroids are the most effective drugs for the long-term control of asthma.

Corticosteroids are the most potent natural anti-inflammatory substances known. Because asthma has a major inflammatory component, it should not be surprising that drugs in this class play a major role in the management of this disorder. *Inhaled corticosteroids are the drugs of choice for the prevention of*

TABLE 5 Anti-Inflammatory Drugs for Asthma and Chronic Obstructive Pulmonary Disease

Drug	Route and Adult Dose (maximum dose where indicated)	Adverse Effects
Inhaled Corticosteroids*		
beclomethasone (Beconase AQ, Qvar)	MDI: 1–2 inhalations tid-qid (max: 20 inhalations/day)	*Hoarseness, dry mouth, cough, sore throat* Oropharyngeal candidiasis, hypercorticism, hypersensitivity reactions
budesonide (Pulmicort)	DPI: 1–2 inhalations (200 mcg/inhalation) qid (max: 800 mcg/day)	
ciclesonide (Alvesco)	Intranasal: 2 sprays per nostril (200 mcg) once daily Inhalation: 2 inhalations (160–320 mcg/inhalation) daily	
flunisolide (AeroBid)	MDI: 2–3 inhalations bid-tid (max: 12 inhalations/day)	
fluticasone (Flovent)	MDI (44 mcg): 2 inhalations bid (max: 10 inhalations/day)	
mometasone (Asmanex)	DPI: 1 inhalation daily (max: 2 inhalations daily)	
triamcinolone (Azmacort)	MDI: 2 inhalations tid-qid (max: 16 inhalations/day)	
Mast Cell Stabilizers		
cromolyn (Intal)	MDI: 1 inhalation qid	*Nausea, sneezing, nasal stinging, throat irritation, unpleasant taste* Anaphylaxis, angioedema, bronchospasm
nedocromil (Tilade)	MDI: 2 inhalations qid	
Leukotriene Modifiers and Miscellaneous Drugs		
montelukast (Singulair)	PO: 10 mg/day in evening	*Headache, nausea, diarrhea, throat pain, weight loss (romflumilast)* Increased aspartate aminotransferase (AST), hepatotoxicity, psychiatric events including suicidality (roflumilast)
roflumilast (Daliresp)	PO: 500 mcg once daily	
zafirlukast (Accolate)	PO: 20 mg bid 1 h before or 2 h after meals	
zileuton (Zyflo CR)	PO: 1,200 mg bid (max: 2,400 mg/day)	

*For doses of systemic corticosteroids, refer to the chapter "Corticosteroids and Drugs Affecting the Adrenal Cortex."
Note: *Italics* indicate common adverse effects. <u>Underline</u> indicates serious adverse effects.

asthmatic attacks and for the management of chronic asthma. *Oral* corticosteroids are used for the short-term management of acute asthma attacks. The therapeutic actions of the corticosteroids have resulted in their widespread use in the pharmacotherapy of allergic rhinitis and other inflammatory disorders. Doses for the inhaled corticosteroids are given in Table 5.

Corticosteroids decrease inflammation of the airways by inhibiting the synthesis and release of inflammatory mediators, including histamine, leukotriene, cytokines, and prostaglandins. They also inhibit the number of circulating leukocytes and decrease vascular permeability. This results in diminished mucus production and edema, thus reducing airway obstruction. Although corticosteroids are not bronchodilators, they sensitize the bronchial smooth muscle to be more responsive to beta-agonist stimulation. In addition, they reduce the bronchial hyperresponsiveness to allergens, which is responsible for triggering many asthma attacks.

When inhaled on a daily schedule, corticosteroids suppress inflammation without producing major adverse effects. Although symptoms will improve in the first 1 to 2 weeks of therapy, 4 to 8 weeks may be required for maximum benefit. Because of the dangerous adverse effects of long-term therapy, systemic corticosteroids are generally reserved for short-term management of acute asthma exacerbations. For outpatient management in these instances, PO corticosteroids such as prednisone are given for the shortest length of time possible, usually 5 to 7 days. In the hospital setting, intravenous (IV)

corticosteroids may be given. Regardless, at the end of the brief treatment period, patients are usually switched to inhaled corticosteroids for long-term management.

When taken long term, both PO and inhaled formulations of corticosteroids have the potential to affect bone physiology in adults and children. Adults who are at risk for osteoporosis should receive periodic bone mineral density tests and possibly pharmacotherapy with bisphosphonates to prevent fractures. In children, small decreases in linear bone growth have been documented. Although these effects are usually temporary, growth should be monitored and the prescriber should weigh the risks of growth suppression against the benefits of corticosteroid use. In all cases, effects on bone growth are dose and frequency dependent; thus patients should be administered the lowest doses possible to maintain adequate asthma control.

PROTOTYPE DRUG | Beclomethasone (Beconase AQ, Qvar)

Classification: **Therapeutic:** Anti-inflammatory
Pharmacologic: Corticosteroid

Therapeutic Effects and Uses: Approved in 1976, beclomethasone is a corticosteroid that is available for administration by aerosol inhalation for asthma (Qvar) or as a nasal spray (Beconase AQ) for allergic rhinitis. Guidelines from the NAEPP place beclomethasone and other drugs in this class as preferred drugs for the long-term management of persistent asthma in both children and adults. Two inhalations, two to three times per day, usually provide adequate prophylaxis, although 3 to 4 weeks of therapy may be necessary before optimum benefits are achieved. In 2000, a double strength formulation (Qvar) was developed with smaller drug particles. It is able to deliver half the usual dose and achieve the same therapeutic effect. Beclomethasone is not a bronchodilator and should not be used to terminate asthma attacks in progress.

The intranasal formulation is effective at reducing the symptoms of allergic rhinitis. Therapeutic effects may take as long as 2 weeks to be fully apparent. Intranasal beclomethasone is also approved to prevent recurrence of nasal polyps following surgical removal. Very little of this drug is absorbed in the systemic circulation when it is administered by this route.

Mechanism of Action: Beclomethasone acts by reducing inflammation and immune responses, thus decreasing the frequency of asthma attacks.

Pharmacokinetics:

Route(s)	Inhalation
Absorption	Minimal systemic absorption
Distribution	Delivered directly to the lungs (site of action); small amount is secreted in breast milk
Primary metabolism	Liver (CYP450: 3A substrate) and lung
Primary excretion	Feces (less than 10% in urine)
Onset of action	Approximately 7 days
Duration of action	Half-life: 15 h

Adverse Effects: Inhaled beclomethasone produces few systemic adverse effects. Because small amounts may be swallowed with each dose, the patient should be observed for signs of corticosteroid toxicity (hypercorticism) when taking this drug for prolonged periods. Local effects may include hoarseness, dry mouth, and changes in taste. Inhaled corticosteroid use has been associated with the development of cataracts in adults. Some studies have shown that long-term intranasal or inhaled corticosteroids may cause growth inhibition in children.

Like all corticosteroids, the anti-inflammatory properties of beclomethasone can mask signs of infections and the drug is contraindicated if active infection is present. A large percentage of patients taking beclomethasone on a long-term basis will develop oropharyngeal candidiasis, a fungal infection in the throat, due to the constant deposits of drug in the oral cavity. Children who have not been vaccinated for varicella should receive the vaccine because of the potential for developing serious disseminated varicella infections during treatment with corticosteroids.

Contraindications/Precautions: The only contraindication to using beclomethasone is hypersensitivity to the drug.

Drug Interactions: Because very little of the drug is absorbed, no clinically significant drug interactions occur. **Herbal/Food:** None known.

Pregnancy: Category C.

Treatment of Overdose: Overdose does not occur when taken by the inhalation route.

Nursing Responsibilities: Key nursing implications for patients receiving beclomethasone are included in the Nursing Practice Application for Patients Receiving Pharmacotherapy for Asthma and Chronic Obstructive Pulmonary Disease.

Lifespan and Diversity Considerations:
- Monitor for vision changes in the older adult receiving beclomethasone. Encourage yearly eye exams to detect cataract formation.
- Monitor height in children with each office visit.
- Assess for previous history of varicella vaccination before therapy with beclomethasone is initiated.
- Supervise young children over 2 years of age to ensure the appropriate use of the inhaler.

Patient and Family Education:
- Clean the mouthpiece at least weekly by removing the drug canister and running warm water through the top and bottom, shaking out excess water, and allowing to air dry. This will help to ensure there is no medication buildup with resulting improper drug delivery.
- Watch for signs and symptoms of infections, particularly in the mouth. Report any mouth soreness or white patches in the mouth.
- Do not breast-feed while taking this drug without approval of the health care provider.
- Immediately notify the health care provider of any known or suspected pregnancy.

Drugs Similar to Beclomethasone (Beconase AQ, Qvar)

Other corticosteroids for inhalation include budesonide, ciclesonide, flunisolide, fluticasone, mometasone, and triamcinolone.

Budesonide (Pulmicort): Budesonide is a corticosteroid that is available by the intranasal route for allergic rhinitis (Rhinocort), oral inhalation, nebulizer for asthma prophylaxis (Pulmicort), or PO capsules for Crohn's disease (Entocort). The most common adverse effects with the inhaled use of budesonide include respiratory infections, rhinitis, cough, and otitis media. Visual impairment may occur. Growth effects should be monitored in pediatric patients. This drug is pregnancy category B.

Ciclesonide (Alvesco): Approved in 2006, ciclesonide is a corticosteroid available by the oral inhalation (Alvesco) route for asthma maintenance and prophylaxis in patients over 12 years of age or by the intranasal (Omnaris) route for allergic rhinitis. Ciclesonide is a prodrug that is converted to an active metabolite following administration. Like other drugs in this class, ciclesonide is not a bronchodilator and should not be used to treat acute bronchospasm. Actions and adverse effects are the same as other corticosteroids administered by inhalation. This drug is pregnancy category C.

Flunisolide (AeroBid): Flunisolide is a corticosteroid that is available by the intranasal route for allergic rhinitis (Nasarel) or by oral inhalation for asthma prophylaxis (AeroBid). The most common adverse effects with inhaled use include upper respiratory infections, dry mouth, hoarseness, nausea, vomiting, and taste changes. Like other drugs in this class, visual impairment may occur and growth effects should be monitored in pediatric patients. This drug is pregnancy category C.

Fluticasone (Flovent): Fluticasone is a corticosteroid that is available by the intranasal route for allergic rhinitis (Flonase); oral inhalation for asthma prophylaxis or COPD (Flovent); or topical cream or ointment for dermatitis, eczema, and other skin conditions (Cutivate). The most common adverse effects with the inhaled use of fluticasone include headache, throat irritation, and upper respiratory tract infections. Visual impairment may occur. Growth effects should be monitored in pediatric patients. Like other inhaled corticosteroids, fluticasone is not indicated for the relief of acute bronchospasm. This drug is pregnancy category C.

Mometasone (Asmanex): Mometasone is an inhaled corticosteroid that is available for the prevention of acute asthmatic attacks. When inhaled it may take an hour or longer to produce its effects; therefore it is not indicated for the relief of acute bronchospasm. Actions and adverse effects are the same as those of other inhaled corticosteroids. An intranasal form is available for allergic rhinitis (Nasonex), and a topical preparation (Elocon) is used to treat various inflammatory skin conditions. This drug is pregnancy category C.

Triamcinolone (Azmacort): Triamcinolone is available in a wide variety of formulations: oral inhalation for asthma (Azmacort), intranasal for allergic rhinitis (Nasacort), ophthalmic for ocular inflammation (Triesence), and various topical formulations for inflammatory skin conditions. Parenteral formulations (Kenalog) are available for a large number of allergic and inflammatory disorders. When inhaled, the adverse effects are the same as those of other corticosteroids, such as throat irritation, dry mouth, hoarseness, visual changes, possible growth retardation in children, and upper respiratory tract infections. This drug is pregnancy category C.

CONNECTION Checkpoint 47.2

Describe strategies that could be used to limit the incidence of serious adverse effects when corticosteroids must be taken PO for prolonged periods. *See Answer to Connection Checkpoint 47.2 on student resource website.*

8 Mast cell stabilizers are used for the prophylaxis of asthma and act by preventing the release of histamine.

Mast cell stabilizers serve limited, though important, roles in the prophylaxis of asthma. Mast cells are large cells that contain inflammatory granules, such as histamine, that mediate inflammatory and allergic reactions. When these cells are sensitized, they degranulate and release the inflammatory substances into the body where they initiate an inflammatory response. Mast cell stabilizers are helpful in managing asthma and COPD because they prevent degranulation of the mast cell, preventing the release of histamine and other inflammatory mediators in the airways. There are two currently approved mast cell stabilizers: cromolyn (Intal) and nedocromil (Tilade). Doses of these agents are listed in Table 5. Mast cell stabilizers are administered by inhalation via an MDI or a nebulizer. An intranasal form is available for management of allergic rhinitis.

| PROTOTYPE DRUG | Cromolyn (Intal) |

Classification: Therapeutic: Anti-inflammatory
Pharmacologic: Mast cell stabilizer

Therapeutic Effects and Uses: An older drug that was approved by the FDA in 1973, cromolyn prevents the inflammation that is a characteristic pathophysiological feature of asthma and COPD. Because it has no effect on previously released inflammatory mediators from mast cell degranulation, the effects will not be noted immediately. The NAEPP guidelines place cromolyn as an alternate drug for the treatment of mild to moderate asthma when corticosteroids are contraindicated or have not proven effective. This drug should not be used to terminate acute asthma attacks.

For asthma therapy the drug is administered via oral inhalation. An intranasal over-the-counter (OTC) formulation (Nasal-Crom) is available for allergic rhinitis. An ophthalmic solution (Crolom) is used to treat various allergic disorders of the conjunctiva. Gastrocrom is a PO dosage form of cromolyn that is the only FDA-approved drug to treat systemic mastocytosis, which is a rare condition in which the patient has an excessive number of mast cells. Gastrocrom is also used off-label to treat ulcerative colitis and to prevent symptoms associated with food allergies.

Mechanism of Action: By stabilizing mast cells, cromolyn helps to prevent the inflammatory response that occurs when mast cells degranulate.

Pharmacokinetics:

Route(s)	Inhalation
Absorption	Minimal systemic absorption (less than 1%)
Distribution	Delivered directly to the lungs (site of action); small amount crosses the placenta; small amount is secreted in breast milk
Primary metabolism	Hepatic
Primary excretion	Bile (and, subsequently, feces) and renal
Onset of action	Adequate effect may not be noted until 2–4 weeks of use
Duration of action	Unknown

Adverse Effects: Adverse effects are uncommon when the drug is administered by oral inhalation. The most common effects are bronchospasm, cough, and pharyngeal irritation. Intranasal and ophthalmic administration may cause local burning and stinging.

Contraindications/Precautions: As with any drug, persons who have demonstrated a hypersensitivity to this drug should not take it. It should be discontinued if the patient develops pulmonary eosinophilia.

Drug Interactions: No significant interactions are known. **Herbal/Food:** Unknown.

Pregnancy: Category B.

Treatment of Overdose: There are no noted problems associated with overdosage. Toxicity is unlikely.

Nursing Responsibilities: Key nursing implications for patients receiving cromolyn are included in the Nursing Practice Application for Patients Receiving Pharmacotherapy for Asthma and Chronic Obstructive Pulmonary Disease.

Lifespan and Diversity Considerations:
- Supervise young children over 5 years of age to ensure the appropriate use of the inhaler.

Patient and Family Education:
- Clean the mouthpiece at least weekly by removing the drug canister and running warm water through the top and bottom, shaking out excess water, and allowing to air dry. This will help to ensure there is no medication buildup with resulting improper drug delivery.
- If a bronchodilator aerosol spray such as albuterol (Proventil) is used in addition to cromolyn, the bronchodilator should be used first, and 5 minutes should elapse before the cromolyn is used.
- Do not breast-feed while taking this drug without approval of the health care provider.
- Immediately notify the health care provider of any known or suspected pregnancy.

Drugs Similar to Cromolyn (Intal)

Nedocromil is the only other mast cell stabilizer.

Nedocromil (Tilade): Approved in 1992, the profile for this agent is similar to that of cromolyn with the exception of a very bitter taste that causes some people to discontinue it. This is a particularly important consideration for children who will be less willing to taking distasteful medication. Like cromolyn, nedocromil is to be used only for asthma prophylaxis and not to terminate acute asthma attacks. The drug may require a week of therapy before benefits are obtained, and it must be taken on a continuous basis for asthma prophylaxis. An ophthalmic form (Alocril) is available to treat allergic conjunctivitis. This drug is pregnancy category B.

9 The leukotriene modifiers, which are primarily used for asthma prophylaxis, act by reducing the inflammatory component of asthma.

Leukotriene modifiers are one of the newest drug classes added to the arsenal of asthma management. They are able to ease bronchoconstriction by reducing inflammation. Because of their delayed onset, leukotriene modifiers are ineffective at terminating acute asthma attacks. The NAEPP guidelines list the leukotriene modifiers as alternative drugs to be considered when inhaled corticosteroids and short-acting beta agonists are unable to control asthma symptoms. Doses for these drugs are listed in Table 5.

Leukotrienes are mediators of the immune and inflammatory responses that are involved in allergic and asthmatic reactions. Leukotrienes are synthesized by mast cells as well as neutrophils, basophils, and eosinophils. When released in the airway,

they promote edema, inflammation, and bronchoconstriction. Leukotriene modifiers reduce inflammation by either blocking the enzyme that controls leukotriene synthesis or by blocking leukotriene receptors. They are not considered bronchodilators, although they do reduce bronchoconstriction indirectly. The leukotriene modifiers are only available by the PO route.

PROTOTYPE DRUG | **Zafirlukast (Accolate)**

Classification: **Therapeutic:** Agent for asthma prophylaxis, anti-inflammatory
Pharmacologic: Leukotriene modifier

Therapeutic Effects and Uses: Zafirlukast, the first leukotriene modifier, which was approved in 1996, is used for the prophylaxis of persistent, chronic asthma. This drug prevents the inflammation that is a characteristic pathophysiological feature of asthma and COPD. It is less effective than inhaled corticosteroids. Off-label uses include allergic rhinitis and prevention of exercise-induced bronchospasm.

Zafirlukast is given by the PO route. Its relatively long onset of action makes it unsuitable for the termination of acute bronchospasm.

Mechanism of Action: Zafirlukast prevents airway edema and inflammation by blocking leukotriene receptors in the airways.

Pharmacokinetics:

Route(s)	PO
Absorption	Rapidly absorbed, but decreased in presence of food
Distribution	Secreted in breast milk; more than 99% bound to plasma protein
Primary metabolism	Extensive hepatic metabolism (CYP2C9, CYP 3A4)
Primary excretion	Mostly bile; 10% renal
Onset of action	1 week
Duration of action	Unknown; half-life: 10 h

Adverse Effects: Zafirlukast produces few serious adverse effects. Headache is the most common complaint. Rhinitis, nausea, vomiting, and diarrhea are reported by some patients.

Contraindications/Precautions: The only absolute contraindication is hypersensitivity to this drug. Because a few rare cases of fatal hepatic failure have been reported, patients with preexisting hepatic impairment should be treated with caution. This drug should be avoided when breast-feeding.

Drug Interactions: Zafirlukast is metabolized by CYP450 enzymes and has the potential to interact with substrates of the inhibitors of this enzyme. Use with warfarin may significantly increase prothrombin time (PT). Erythromycin and theophylline may decrease the serum levels of zafirlukast. Concurrent use with aspirin can significantly increase zafirlukast levels. **Herbal/Food:** Food can reduce the bioavailability; thus the drug should be taken on an empty stomach.

Pregnancy: Category B.

Treatment of Overdose: Symptoms of overdose include headache, nausea, and vomiting. Treatment is supportive.

Nursing Responsibilities: Key nursing implications for patients receiving zafirlukast are included in the Nursing Practice Application for Patients Receiving Pharmacotherapy for Asthma and Chronic Obstructive Pulmonary Disease.

Lifespan and Diversity Considerations:

• Monitor hepatic function laboratory values more frequently in the older adult because normal physiological changes related to aging may affect the drug's metabolism.

• Monitor the older adult for signs or symptoms of infection. People older than age 55 may experience an increased frequency of infections while taking the drug.

Patient and Family Education:

• Do not breast-feed while taking this drug without approval of the health care provider.

• Immediately notify the health care provider of any known or suspected pregnancy.

Drugs Similar to Zafirlukast (Accolate)

Montelukast and zileuton are other leukotriene modifiers.

Montelukast (Singulair): Given by the PO route, montelukast acts by blocking leukotriene receptors in the airways. Montelukast is the only agent in this category that is approved for very young children, 12 months or older. For pediatric use it is available as chewable tablets and oral granules that may be sprinkled on soft food. The drug is approved for the prophylaxis of persistent, chronic asthma, allergic rhinitis, and exercise-induced bronchospasm. Like other drugs in this class, montelukast should not be used to treat acute asthma attacks. Adverse effects are generally mild. Headache is the most frequently reported adverse effect. This is a pregnancy category B drug.

Zileuton (Zyflo CR): Approved in 1996, zileuton is a PO drug that acts by inhibiting the lipoxygenase, which is the first enzyme in the pathway of leukotriene synthesis. Like other drugs in this class, zileuton is considered an alternate drug in the prophylaxis of persistent, chronic asthma. In 2007 an extended release formulation (Zyflo CR) was approved that allows for twice-daily dosing. Like other drugs in this class, zileuton should not be used to treat acute asthma attacks. This drug is generally well tolerated, with sinusitis, nausea, and throat pain being the most common adverse effects. The most serious concern with zileuton is the potential for liver damage. Zileuton raises liver enzymes (alanine aminotransferase), and cases of jaundice and severe hepatic injury have been reported. This drug is contraindicated in patients with hepatic impairment, and liver function tests should be conducted on a regular basis during therapy. Because zileuton can increase serum warfarin levels, PT should be regularly monitored. This is a pregnancy category C drug.

10 Methylxanthines were once the mainstay of asthma pharmacotherapy but are now rarely prescribed for that disorder.

The methylxanthines were considered the drugs of choice for treating asthma 30 years ago. Now they are primarily reserved for the long-term management of persistent asthma that is unresponsive to beta agonists or inhaled corticosteroids. One reason for the lessened use of methylxanthines is that their narrow therapeutic index increases the risk of toxicity, especially with prolonged use. These drugs also have significant interactions with numerous other drugs. Doses for these agents are listed in Table 4.

The methylxanthines are modest bronchodilators. They are chemically related to caffeine and share caffeine's stimulant effect. Methylxanthines are available in forms for PO, parenteral, and rectal administration. Because they are not available for inhalation, patients do not benefit from the smaller doses and direct effects that are provided by drugs that can be administered by the inhalation route. Interestingly, theobromine, an ingredient in chocolate, is also a methylxanthine.

PROTOTYPE DRUG	Theophylline (Theo-Dur, Others)

Classification: Therapeutic: Bronchodilator
Pharmacologic: Methylxanthine

Therapeutic Effects and Uses: Approved by the FDA in 1940, theophylline is a natural substance found in small amounts in tea. Theophylline relaxes bronchial smooth muscle and may exert some anti-inflammatory action that is beneficial to patients with asthma. It is considered an alternate drug by the NAEPP guidelines, to be considered for asthma prophylaxis when more effective drugs fail to bring symptomatic relief. It may be used in combination with a corticosteroid for persistent asthma. Although FDA-approved for treating acute bronchospasm, theophylline is not recommended by the NAEPP guidelines because the short-acting beta$_2$-adrenergic agonists (SABAs) are more effective.

Theophylline has several off-label indications. As a respiratory stimulant, theophylline and caffeine may be used to treat sleep apnea in neonates and in adults with chronic heart failure. Given IV, theophylline has been found to reduce neurotoxicity resulting from the drug methotrexate.

Mechanism of Action: Theophylline works by two mechanisms. It relaxes bronchial smooth muscle, which promotes bronchodilation, and it suppresses airway responsiveness to stimuli that promote bronchospasm.

Pharmacokinetics:

Route(s)	PO, parenteral, suppository
Absorption	Rapid absorption
Distribution	About 40% protein bound; remainder is distributed well in fluids and less well in body lipids
Primary metabolism	Hepatic (CYP1A2, CYP2E1, CYP3A3)
Primary excretion	Renal
Onset of action	Peak: approximately 60 min (highly variable)
Duration of action	Half-life: 6–10 h (highly variable)

Adverse Effects: Theophylline has a very narrow therapeutic index. Therapeutic levels are 10 to 15 mcg/mL and the toxic level is anything above 20 mcg/mL. Serum theophylline levels should be obtained during therapy. Common adverse effects include nausea, vomiting, headache, irritability, and insomnia. More serious reactions include dysrhythmias, hypotension, and seizures.

Contraindications/Precautions: Theophylline should be used with great caution in patients who have seizure disorders, heart failure, or cardiac dysrhythmias. Theophylline has also been shown to increase the production of gastric acid so use in patients with active peptic ulcer disease is not recommended. Because of the extensive hepatic metabolism, theophylline should be closely monitored in patients with a history of liver disease. As with any drug, this drug is contraindicated in persons who have demonstrated a hypersensitivity to it.

Drug Interactions: Because theophylline is highly metabolized by the CYP450 enzyme system, there are numerous drug interactions, including many common antibiotics (ciprofloxacin, clarithromycin, erythromycin) and antianxiety agents (diazepam, flurazepam, lorazepam, midazolam). When treating a patient who is receiving multiple drugs concurrently with theophylline, the nurse should consult current sources for potential drug interactions. There are also a number of IV incompatibilities, including emergency medications such as epinephrine, norepinephrine, and isoproterenol. Compatibility of any medication should be checked prior to initiating infusions in the same line. **Herbal/Food:** Foods and beverages containing caffeine will cause additive central nervous system (CNS) stimulation. St. John's wort may decrease the effectiveness of theophylline.

Pregnancy: Category C.

Treatment of Overdose: There is no specific antidote to theophylline. Gastric lavage is indicated in the event of an overdose of PO medications. Seizures and other CNS effects may respond to barbiturates or benzodiazepines. Supportive measures need to be provided for hypotension, shock, dysrhythmias, and other toxic effects. Serum levels should be monitored periodically until they are within normal limits.

Nursing Responsibilities: Key nursing implications for patients receiving theophylline are included in the Nursing Practice Application for Patients Receiving Pharmacotherapy for Asthma and Chronic Obstructive Pulmonary Disease.

Lifespan and Diversity Considerations:

- Monitor hepatic function laboratory values more frequently in the older adult because normal physiological changes related to aging may affect the drug's metabolism.
- Because theophylline is metabolized through one of the P450 system pathways, monitor ethnically diverse populations frequently to ensure optimal therapeutic effects and minimize adverse effects.

Patient and Family Education:

- Limit or eliminate tobacco use, because smoking increases the rate of drug clearance from the body, which may diminish the effectiveness of the drug.
- Do not breast-feed while taking this drug without approval of the health care provider.

Drugs Similar to Theophylline (Theo-Dur, Others)

Aminophylline and dyphylline are other methylxanthines. Oxtriphylline (Choledyl) is a drug in this class that has been discontinued in the United States.

Aminophylline: Approved in 1975, aminophylline is a theophylline salt that has enhanced water solubility. It is approved to treat symptoms of asthma and COPD. It has the same actions and adverse effects as theophylline. Aminophylline is shorter acting than theophylline and is available in PO, rectal, and IV forms. This drug is pregnancy category C.

Dyphylline (Lufyllin): Dyphylline is not a theophylline salt but it has similar actions. It is approved to treat acute bronchospasms associated with asthma and COPD. Approved in 1951, it is available in PO form and has a short half-life of only 2 hours, so it is usually given four times a day. It is 90% less potent than theophylline. but exerts fewer adverse effects. The intramuscular (IM) form of the drug has been discontinued in the United States. Indications are the same as those of theophylline. This drug is pregnancy category C.

11 Monoclonal antibodies are a newer form of therapy for the prevention of asthma symptoms.

Approved in 2003, omalizumab (Xolair) was the first biologic therapy used to treat asthma, offering a new approach to the management of the disease. This drug is approved for treating allergic rhinitis and moderate to severe, persistent asthma that cannot be controlled satisfactorily with inhaled corticosteroids. To receive omalizumab, the patient must have tested positive for an airborne allergen such as mold, pollen, or animal dander. Although it is only available by the subcutaneous route, injections are scheduled every 2 to 4 weeks, depending on the patient's response to therapy. It is approved for asthma prophylaxis in patients 12 years of age or older.

Omalizumab is a monoclonal antibody. Monoclonal antibodies are designed to attach to a specific receptor on a target cell or molecule. Most monoclonal antibodies are designed to attack cancer cells. However, omalizumab is designed to attach to a receptor on immunoglobulin E (IgE). The normal function of IgE is to react to antigens and cause the release of inflammatory chemical mediators from mast cells and basophils. By binding to IgE, omalizumab prevents inflammation and dampens the body's response to allergens that sometimes trigger asthma.

Omalizumab is reserved for patients with persistent asthma because of its expense, potential adverse effects, and the need for regular parenteral injections. Although adverse effects are uncommon, they may be serious and include anaphylaxis, bleeding-related events, or severe dysmenorrhea. Less serious adverse effects include rash, headache, and viral infections.

CONNECTION Checkpoint 47.3

Most monoclonal antibodies are classified as immunosuppressants. Explain methods by which these drugs can be used to suppress the immune system. *See Answer to Connection Checkpoint 47.3 on student resource website.*

CONNECTIONS: NURSING PRACTICE APPLICATION

Patients Receiving Pharmacotherapy for Asthma and Chronic Obstructive Pulmonary Disease

Assessment	Potential Nursing Diagnoses
Baseline assessment prior to administration:	• *Impaired Gas Exchange*
• Understand the reason the drug has been prescribed in order to assess for therapeutic effects.	• *Anxiety*
• Obtain a complete health history including previous history of symptoms and association with seasons, foods, or environmental exposures, existing cardiovascular, respiratory, hepatic, renal, or neurologic disease, glaucoma, prostatic hypertrophy, difficulty with urination, presence of fever or active infections, pregnancy or breast-feeding, alcohol use, or smoking. Obtain a drug history, noting the type of adverse reaction experienced to any medications.	• *Disturbed Sleep Pattern*, related to adverse drug effects
	• *Activity Intolerance*, related to disease processes or ineffective drug therapy
	• *Deficient Knowledge* (Drug Therapy)
	• *Risk for Ineffective Cardiac Tissue Perfusion*
• If asthma symptoms are of new onset, particularly in infants and young children, assess for any recent changes in diet, soaps including laundry detergent, laundry softener, cosmetics, lotions, and environmental factors (e.g., pets, travel, or recent carpet-cleaning) that may correlate with the onset of symptoms.	
• Obtain baseline vital signs, noting respiratory rate and depth.	
• Assess pulmonary function with pulse oximeter, peak expiratory flow meter, and/or arterial blood gases to establish baseline levels.	
• Evaluate appropriate laboratory findings (e.g., CBC, hepatic, and renal tests).	
• Assess symptom-related effects on eating, sleep, and activity level.	
• Assess the patient's ability to receive and understand instructions. Include the family and caregivers as needed.	
Assessment throughout administration:	
• Assess for desired therapeutic effects (e.g., increased ease of breathing, improvement in pulmonary function studies, improved signs of peripheral oxygenation and increased activity levels, maintenance of normal eating and sleep periods).	
• Continue periodic monitoring of pulmonary function with pulse oximeter, peak expiratory flow meter, and/or arterial blood gases as appropriate.	
• Assess vital signs, especially respiratory rate and depth. Assess breath sounds, noting the presence of adventitious sounds, and any mucus production.	
• Assess for adverse effects: dizziness, tachycardia, palpitations, blurred vision, or headache. Immediately report fever, confusion, tachycardia, palpitations, hypotension, syncope, dyspnea, or increasing pulmonary congestion.	

Planning: Patient Goals and Expected Outcomes

The patient will:

• Experience therapeutic effects dependent on the reason the drug is being given (e.g., increased ease of breathing, improvement in pulmonary function studies, able to experience normal sleep and eating periods, and able to carry out activities of daily living (ADLs) to a level appropriate for the condition).

• Be free from or experience minimal adverse effects.

• Verbalize an understanding of the drug's use, adverse effects, and required precautions.

• Demonstrate proper self-administration of the medication (e.g., dose, timing, and when to notify the provider).

Implementation

Interventions and (Rationales)	Patient-Centered Care
Ensuring therapeutic effects:	• Teach the patient to supplement drug therapy with nonpharmacologic measures such as increased fluid intake to liquefy and mobilize mucus, and to reduce exposure to allergens where possible.
• Continue assessments as above for therapeutic effects. (Increased ease of breathing, lessened adventitious breath sounds, improved signs of tissue oxygenation, and normal appetite and eating and sleeping patterns should occur.)	• Advise the patient to carry a wallet identification card or wear medical identification jewelry indicating the presence of asthma or a respiratory condition, any significant allergies or anaphylaxis, and use of inhaler therapy.
• Monitor pulmonary function periodically with pulse oximeter, peak expiratory flow meter, and/or arterial blood gases. (Periodic monitoring is necessary to assess drug effectiveness.)	• Teach the patient how to use the peak expiratory flow meter or other equipment ordered to monitor pulmonary function.
	• Instruct the patient to immediately report symptoms of deteriorating respiratory status such as increased dyspnea, breathlessness with speech, increased anxiety, or orthopnea.

(continued)

- For treatment of acute asthmatic attacks, inhaler therapy should be started at first sign of respiratory difficulty to abort the attack. For preventive therapy, long-term bronchodilation by inhaler or orally will be used to maintain bronchodilation. *LABAs and long-acting bronchodilators are not to be used to abort an acute attack.* (Acute asthmatic attacks are managed with quick-acting bronchodilation such as beta$_2$ agonists. For maintaining bronchodilation and preventing attacks, LABAs, anticholinergics, mast cell stabilizers, and glucocorticoid or methylxanthine therapy may be used. It is crucial to know and recognize the difference between quick-acting and long-acting inhalers.)

- Provide explicit instructions on the use of quick-acting versus long-acting inhalers. Teach the patient to use quick-acting inhalers at the earliest possible appearance of symptoms. Long-acting inhalers or oral therapy may be used to maintain bronchodilation but *do not discard quick-acting inhalers if on long-term maintenance therapy.* They may still be needed for periodic acute attacks.

Minimizing adverse effects:

- Continue to monitor respirations, rate, depth, breath sounds, mucus production, and for increasing dyspnea, adventitious breath sounds, and signs of tissue hypoxia (e.g., cyanosis), anxiety, confusion, or decreasing pulmonary function (e.g., pulse oximeter, peak expiratory flow). Immediately notify the provider if symptoms continue to increase, especially if respiratory involvement worsens or fever is present. (Increasing dyspnea, adventitious breath sounds, diminished oxygenation, or increasing anxiety or confusion may indicate inadequate drug therapy, worsening disease process, or respiratory infection and should be reported immediately.)

- Instruct the patient to report immediately symptoms of deteriorating respiratory status such as increased dyspnea, breathlessness with speech, increased anxiety, or orthopnea.

- Provide explicit instruction on the use of quick-acting and long-acting inhalers. Ensure that the patient is able to identify the appropriate inhaler for the treatment of acute asthmatic attacks or for preventive therapy. (Acute asthmatic attacks are managed with quick-acting bronchodilation such as beta$_2$ agonists and the patient must be able to identify the appropriate inhaler to use. Provide written instructions, including drug name and when to use if both quick-acting and long-acting inhalers are ordered.)

- Teach the patient to use the quick-acting inhaler at the earliest possible appearance of symptoms. Long-acting inhalers or oral therapy may be used to maintain bronchodilation but *do not discard quick-acting inhalers if on long-term maintenance therapy.* They may still be needed for periodic acute attacks.
- Teach the patient not to rely on the color of the inhaler to indicate quick-acting versus long-acting inhalers. Depending on the manufacturer and trade versus generic drugs, the color may change. If the patient desires to color-code, suggest individual color stickers or tape be used per patient preference. Instruct the patient not to obscure the drug name with the sticker.

- Monitor eating and sleep patterns and ability to maintain functional ADLs. Provide for calorie-rich, nutrient-dense foods, frequent rest periods between eating or activity, and a cool room for sleeping. (Respiratory difficulty and fatigue associated with hypoxia and the work of breathing may affect appetite, ability to eat during dyspnea, and maintenance of required ADLs. Adequate nutrition, fluids, rest, and sleep are essential to support optimal health.)

- Teach the patient to supplement drug therapy with nonpharmacologic measures including:
  - Increased fluid intake to liquefy and assist in mobilizing mucus
  - Small, frequent meals of calorie-rich, nutrient-dense foods to prevent fatigue and maintain normal nutrition
  - Adequate rest periods between eating and activities
  - Decreased room temperature for ease of breathing during sleep
  - Reduced exposure to allergens where possible.
- Instruct the patient to immediately report any significant change in appetite, inability to maintain normal intake, inadequate sleep periods, or inability to carry out required ADLs.

- Eliminate smoking, limit exposure to secondhand smoke, and limit caffeine intake, especially if methylxanthines are prescribed. (Cigarette smoke irritates respiratory mucous membranes, increasing the risk of adverse effects and increasing bronchoconstriction. Caffeine may increase the risk of tachycardia in addition to the drugs' adverse effects, and both smoking and caffeine affect the metabolism of methylxanthines.)

- Teach the patient about smoking cessation programs, to avoid environments with secondhand smoke, and to limit or abstain from caffeine intake while taking bronchodilator therapy.

- Maintain consistent dosing of long-acting bronchodilators. LABAs, anticholinergics, mast cell stabilizers, and corticosteroids are used to prevent or limit acute bronchoconstrictive attacks. Regular, consistent dosing must be maintained for best results.)

- Teach the patient the importance of continuing regular and consistent administration of all bronchodilation therapy to prevent acute attacks. Irregular use may increase the risk or severity of bronchoconstrictive events.

- Utilize the appropriate spacer between the inhaler and mouth and rinse mouth after using the inhaler, especially after corticosteroids. (Spacers between metered-dose inhalers may be ordered to assist in coordination and timing of inhalation and to prevent medication being delivered to the back of the pharynx. Rinsing the mouth after the use of inhalers prevents systemic absorption or localized reactions to the drug such as ulceration.)

- Instruct the patient in the proper use of spacers if ordered, followed by return demonstration.
- Teach the patient to rinse the mouth after each use of the inhaler and not to swallow after rinsing.

Patient understanding of drug therapy:	• The patient should be able to state the reason for drug, appropriate dose and scheduling, what adverse effects to observe for, and when to report them.
• Use opportunities during administration of medications and during assessments to discuss the rationale for drug therapy, desired therapeutic outcomes, commonly observed adverse effects, parameters for when to call the health care provider, and any necessary monitoring or precautions. (Using time during nursing care helps to optimize and reinforce key teaching areas.)	
Patient self-administration of drug therapy:	• The patient, family, or caregiver is able to discuss appropriate dosing and administration needs.
• When administering the medication, instruct the patient, family, or caregiver in proper self-administration of the drug, e.g., take the drug at the first appearance of symptoms before they are severe. (Utilizing time during nurse-administration of these drugs helps to reinforce teaching.)	• The patient recognizes the difference between quick-acting and long-acting inhalers, and knows when each is to be used.
	• Instruct the patient in proper administration techniques for inhalers, followed by return demonstration, including:
	• Use a spacer if instructed between the metered-dose inhaler and the mouth.
	• Shake the inhaler or load it with a tablet or powder as instructed.
	• If using a bronchodilator and corticosteroid inhalers, use the bronchodilator first, wait 5 min, then use the corticosteroid to ensure the drug reaches deeply into the bronchial area.
	• Rinse mouth after using any inhaler.
	• Clean the inhaler at least weekly by running warm water through the plastic mouthpiece after removing the drug canister, shaking out excess water, and allowing to air dry.

Evaluation of Outcome Criteria

Evaluate the effectiveness of drug therapy by confirming that patient goals and expected outcomes have been met (see "Planning").

Chronic Obstructive Pulmonary Disease

12 Chronic obstructive pulmonary disease may be treated with bronchodilators, anti-inflammatory agents, and mucolytics.

Chronic obstructive pulmonary disease (COPD) is a progressive pulmonary disorder characterized by chronic and recurrent obstruction of airflow. The two most common examples of conditions that cause chronic pulmonary obstruction are chronic bronchitis, a condition in which excess mucus is produced in the lower respiratory tract, and emphysema, a condition in which there is loss of bronchiolar elasticity and destruction of alveolar walls.

The clinical distinction between chronic bronchitis and emphysema is sometimes unclear because patients may exhibit symptoms of both conditions concurrently. Both conditions are strongly associated with smoking tobacco products (cigarette smoking accounts for 85% to 90% of all cases of non-asthmatic COPD) and, secondarily, breathing air pollutants. In chronic bronchitis, excess mucus is produced in the lower respiratory tract due to the inflammation and irritation from cigarette smoke or pollutants. The airway becomes partially obstructed with mucus, resulting in the classic signs of dyspnea and coughing. An early sign of bronchitis is often a productive cough that occurs on awakening. Gas exchange may be impaired; thus wheezing and decreased exercise tolerance are additional clinical signs. Microbes thrive in the mucus-rich environment, and pulmonary infections are common.

Because most patients with COPD are lifelong tobacco users, they often have serious comorbid cardiovascular conditions such as heart failure and HTN. Emphysema is most often the result of years of chronic inflammation and is characterized by loss of elasticity of the bronchioles and damage and loss of alveolar wall structures. The loss of elasticity results in partial collapse of the airways on exhalation, leading to air trapping, and the destruction of alveolar walls leads to decreased perfusion and gas exchange at the alveolus. The patient with emphysema may experience extreme dyspnea from even the slightest physical activity.

Drugs may be used to bring symptomatic relief to patients with COPD, but they do not alter the progression of COPD or cure the disorder. The goals of pharmacotherapy of COPD are to relieve symptoms and avoid complications of the condition. Various classes of drugs are used to treat infections, control cough, and relieve bronchospasm. Most patients receive the same classes of bronchodilators and anti-inflammatory agents that are prescribed for asthma. One of the newest treatments for severe COPD is roflumilast (Daliresp), a drug approved in 2011 that exhibits anti-inflammatory effects on the airways by inhibiting the enzyme phosphodiesterase-4. Roflumilast is only indicated to reduce the incidence of COPD exacerbations and the drug should not be used to treat acute bronchospasms.

Mucolytics, which are agents given to loosen thick viscous bronchial secretions, and expectorants, which are agents given to aid in the removal of mucus, are sometimes prescribed. Long-term oxygen therapy is prescribed in later stages and it has been shown to decrease mortality in patients with advanced COPD. Antibiotics may be prescribed for patients who experience multiple bouts of pulmonary infections.

Patients with COPD should not receive drugs that have beta-adrenergic antagonist activity because these agents cause bronchoconstriction. Respiratory depressants such as opioids and barbiturates should also be avoided when possible. An important teaching point for the nurse is to strongly encourage smoking cessation in these patients. Smoking cessation has been shown to slow the progression of COPD and to result in fewer respiratory symptoms; however, it cannot undo damage that has already occurred.

UNDERSTANDING THE CHAPTER

Key Concepts Summary

1 The physiology of the respiratory system involves two main processes: perfusion and ventilation.

2 Asthma is a chronic disease that has both inflammatory and bronchospasm components.

3 Inhalation is a common route of administration for pulmonary drugs because it delivers drugs directly to their sites of action.

4 The goals of asthma pharmacotherapy are to terminate acute bronchospasms and to reduce the frequency of asthma attacks.

5 Beta$_2$-adrenergic agonists are the most effective drugs for relieving acute bronchospasm.

6 The inhaled anticholinergics are used for preventing bronchospasm.

7 Inhaled corticosteroids are the most effective drugs for the long-term control of asthma.

8 Mast cell stabilizers are used for the prophylaxis of asthma and act by preventing the release of histamine.

9 The leukotriene modifiers, which are primarily used for asthma prophylaxis, act by reducing the inflammatory component of asthma.

10 Methylxanthines were once the mainstay of asthma pharmacotherapy but are now rarely prescribed for that disorder.

11 Monoclonal antibodies are a newer form of therapy for the prevention of asthma symptoms.

12 Chronic obstructive pulmonary disease may be treated with bronchodilators, anti-inflammatory agents, and mucolytics.

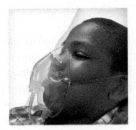

Making the PATIENT Connection

Remember the patient "Nathan Geisel" at the beginning of the chapter? Now read the remainder of the case study. Based on the information presented within this chapter, respond to the critical thinking questions that follow.

Nathan is a 12-year-old with a history of asthma, diagnosed 2 years ago. He is an outgoing, active boy and participates in a swim club and a basketball team, but he has had a difficult time adjusting to the limitations of his asthma. He has learned to control acute attacks by using an albuterol (Proventil) metered-dose inhaler, and because his asthma is often triggered by exercise, he has also been using a budesonide (Pulmicort) inhaler and taking montelukast (Singulair).

After competing in his swim meet at the local indoor pool, Nathan began experiencing respiratory distress. He alerted his coach, who retrieved the albuterol inhaler from Nathan's backpack. After two inhalations, Nathan was still in distress and the rescue squad was called.

On admission to the emergency department, Nathan is in obvious distress with pulse oximeter readings of 90% to 91%. He has nasal flaring and bilateral wheezing is heard in his lung fields, pulse rate is 122 beats/min, and he is orthopneic. While treatment is started, the nurse asks him questions that he can nod or shake his head to answer. He shakes his head "no" when asked if he used his budesonide inhaler today and shrugs when asked about his last dose of montelukast.

Critical Thinking Questions

1. Considering his history, medications, and the location where Nathan's asthma attack occurred, what might explain his acute attack?

2. What medications would you anticipate will be prescribed to treat Nathan's acute asthmatic attack and why?

3. What changes might be made to Nathan's medications? What teaching will Nathan and his family need prior to discharge?

See Answers to Critical Thinking Questions on student resource website.

NCLEX-RN® Review

1 A client with asthma asks which of the prescribed medications should be used in the event of an acute episode of bronchospasm. The nurse will instruct the client to use:

1. Albuterol, a beta agonist bronchodilator, by inhalation.
2. Beclomethasone, a glucocorticoid anti-inflammatory drug, by inhalation.
3. Ipratropium, an anticholinergic bronchodilator, by inhalation.
4. Zafirlukast, a leukotriene modifier, by mouth.

2 A client is prescribed beclomethasone (Qvar), a glucocorticoid inhaler. Education by the nurse will include:

1. "Check your heart rate because this may cause tachycardia."
2. "Limit your coffee intake while on this drug."
3. "Rinse your mouth out well after each use."
4. "You may feel shaky and nervous after using this drug."

3 The nurse should inform the client who is prescribed a nebulizer treatment with albuterol (Proventil, VoSpire) that a common adverse effect is:

1. An increased heart rate with palpitations.
2. A predisposition to infection.
3. Sedation.
4. Temporary dyspnea.

4 The nurse should monitor the client who is taking beclomethasone (Qvar) for evidence of: Select all that apply.

1. Infection.
2. Hyperglycemia.
3. Urinary retention.
4. Tachycardia.
5. Photophobia.

5 A 4-year-old child with respiratory distress secondary to asthma has an order for a nebulizer treatment. The type of medication most likely to be given for asthma management is a:

1. Beta agonist.
2. Beta antagonist.
3. Corticosteroid.
4. Leukotriene modifier.

6 Despite repeated demonstrations of proper inhaler use by the nurse, the client is unable to return a proper demonstration on the training inhaler. The client is becoming frustrated. What is the best action for the nurse to take?

1. Encourage the client to keep practicing just a little longer.
2. Notify the health care provider that the client is incompetent.
3. Provide a spacer for use with the inhaler.
4. Switch to an oral form of a beta agonist.

Additional Case Study

As the home health nurse, you visit with Mr. Jonas Maxwell weekly to assess his pulmonary status and his adherence to his medication regimen. Jonas has end-stage COPD. He was diagnosed with the disease many years ago and his pulmonary status has deteriorated slowly during the past few years. Despite his health care provider's recommendation to change to another medication, Jonas insists that theophylline (Theo-Dur) is the only medication that helps him to breathe. He also uses several MDIs with spacers several times per day.

1. What symptoms would you expect to observe in Jonas if he is experiencing early signs of toxicity?
2. Create a list of things to avoid for an individual who is receiving theophylline therapy.
3. In your own words, how would you describe the function of the spacer used with Jonas's MDI?

See Answers to Additional Case Study on student resource website.

References

Asthma and Allergy Foundation of America. (n.d.). *Asthma facts and figures.* Retrieved from http://www.aafa.org/display .cfm?id=9&sub=42#disp

Bloom, B., Cohen, R. A., & Freeman, G. (2010). Summary health statistics for U.S. children: National health interview survey, 2009. National Center for Health Statistics. *Vital Health Statistics, 10*(247). Retrieved from http://www.cdc.gov/nchs/data/ series/sr_10/sr10_247.pdf

Bruzzese, J. M., Unikel, L. H., Evans, D., Bornstein, L., Surrence, K., & Mellins, R. B. (2010). Asthma knowledge and asthma management behavior in urban elementary school teachers. *Journal of Asthma, 47*(2), 185–191. doi:10.3109/02770900903519908

Colbert, B. J., Gonzales, L. S., & Kennedy, B. J. (2012). *Integrated cardiopulmonary pharmacology* (3rd ed.). Upper Saddle River, NJ: Pearson Education.

Lemanske, R. F., & Busse, W. W. (2010). The U.S. Food and Drug Administration and long-acting ß₂ agonists: The importance of striking the right balance between risks and benefits of therapy? *Journal of Allergy and Clinical Immunology, 126*(3), 449–452.

National Asthma Education and Prevention Program Coordinating Committee. (2007). *Expert panel report 3 (EPR3): Guidelines for the diagnosis and management of asthma.* Coordinated by the National Heart, Lung, and Blood Institute of the National Institutes of Health. Retrieved from http://www.nhlbi.nih.gov/guidelines/ asthma/asthgdln.htm

O'Connor, R. D., Patrick, D. L., Parasuraman, B., Martin, P., & Goldman, M. (2010). Comparison of patient-reported outcomes during treatment with adjustable- and fixed-dose budesonide/formoterol pressurized metered-dose inhaler versus fixed-dose fluticasone propionate/ salmeterol dry powder inhaler in patients with asthma. *Journal of Asthma, 47*(2), 217–223.doi:10.3109/02770900903497154

Shah, S. (2011). Exogenous surfactant: Intubated present, nebulized future? *World Journal of Pediatrics, 7*(1), 11–15. doi:10.1007/ s12519-010-0201-4

Selected Bibliography

Akinbami, L. (2010). *Asthma prevalence, health care use and mortality: United States 2003–2005.* Retrieved from http://www .cdc.gov/nchs/data/hestat/asthma03-05/ asthma03-05.htm

American Lung Association. (2010). *Trends in asthma: Morbidity and mortality.* Retrieved from http://www.lungusa.org/ finding-cures/our-research/trend-reports/ asthma-trend-report.pdf

American Lung Association. (2010). *Trends in COPD (chronic bronchitis and emphysema): Morbidity and mortality.* Retrieved from http://www.lungusa.org/finding-cures/ our-research/trend-reports/copd-trend- report.pdf

Banasiak, N. (2007). Childhood asthma part one: Initial assessment, diagnosis, and education. *Journal of Pediatric Health Care, 21*(1), 44–48.

Centers for Disease Control and Prevention. (2010). *Asthma.* Retrieved from http:// www.cdc.gov/nchs/fastats/asthma.htm

D'Amatol, G., Perticone, M., Bucchioni, E., Salzillo1, A., D'Amato, M., & Liccardi, G. (2010). Treating moderate-to-severe allergic asthma with anti-IgE monoclonal antibody (omalizumab). An update. *European Annals of Allergy and Clinical Immunology, 42*(4), 135–140.

George, M., Birck, K., Hufford, D. J., Jemmott, L. S., & Weaver, T. E. (2006). Beliefs about asthma and complementary and alternative medicine in low-income inner-city African-American adults. *Journal of General Internal Medicine, 21*, 1317–1325.

Hurst, J. R., & Wedzicha, J. A. (2009). Management and prevention of chronic obstructive pulmonary disease exacerbations: A state of the art review. *Biomed Central Medicine, 7*, 40. doi:10.1186/1741-7015-7-40

Kelly-Shanovich, K., Pulvermacher, A., Sorkness, C., Bhattacharya, A., & Gustafson, B. (2007). The integration of web-based asthma education with nurse case management. *Journal of Allergy and Clinical Immunology, 119*(1), S80.

McIvor, A. R. (2011). Inhaler blues? *CMAJ, 183*(4), 464. doi:10.1503/cmaj.111-2025

Answers to NCLEX-RN® Review

1 Answer: 1 Rationale: A quick-acting inhaled beta agonist such as albuterol is used to abort bronchospasm. Options 2, 3, and 4 are incorrect. Beclomethasone, ipratropium, and zafirlukast are drugs used to prevent and control bronchospastic attacks and will not cause bronchodilation quickly enough to abort an attack. Cognitive Level: Applying; Client Need: Physiological Integrity; Nursing Process: Implementation

2 Answer: 3 Rationale: Corticosteroids can decrease the beneficial oral flora that will allow for an overgrowth of fungal infections such as *Candida*. Rinsing the mouth removes any corticosteroid drug deposited there and prevents it from being swallowed, decreasing the likelihood of systemic absorption. Options 1, 2, and 4 are incorrect. Inhaled corticosteroids such as beclomethasone do not cause tachycardia, nervousness, or tremors, and caffeine does not need to be avoided while the drug is used. Cognitive Level: Applying; Client Need: Health Promotion and Maintenance; Nursing Process: Implementation

3 Answer: 1 Rationale: Bronchodilators such as albuterol may have an adverse effect on heart rate elevation and palpitations related to dosage. Options 2, 3, and 4 are incorrect. Bronchodilators do not decrease the immune response or increase alertness. While some bronchodilators have been known to cause unexpected problems and paradoxical bronchospasm, this is uncommon. Cognitive Level: Applying; Client Need: Physiological Integrity; Nursing Process: Implementation

4 Answer: 1, 2 Rationale: Because corticosteroids such as beclomethasone decrease the immune response, the likelihood of infections is increased. Corticosteroids also increase blood glucose thus increasing the likelihood of hyperglycemia. Options 3, 4, and 5 are incorrect. Corticosteroids do not cause urinary retention, do not increase the likelihood of tachycardia, and do not cause photophobia. Cognitive Level: Applying; Client Need: Physiological Integrity; Nursing Process: Assessment

5 Answer: 1 Rationale: Beta agonists are agents that may be given to children younger than age 5 to manage asthma. They are available in formulations suitable for nebulizer treatments. Options 2, 3, and 4 are incorrect. Beta-antagonists, corticosteroids, and leukotriene modifiers will not cause the rapid bronchodilation required in an acute asthma attack. Cognitive Level: Applying; Client Need: Physiological Integrity; Nursing Process: Planning

6 Answer: 3 Rationale: Some clients have difficulty mastering the coordination between inhalation and activation of the medication. In these instances, a spacer will hold the medication cloud so that this is not a concern. The spacer has additional advantages because it results in more effective delivery of the drug to the site of action and less drug deposition in the mouth and oropharynx. Options 1, 2, and 4 are incorrect. Additional practice may help in the long term, but it is not the priority for an immediate solution to the problem and may only serve to frustrate the client further. The health care provider would not need to be contacted because the client has difficulty learning, provided that a solution is readily available. Substitution of an oral form of the drug is not within the nursing scope of practice. Cognitive Level: Analyzing; Client Need: Health Promotion and Maintenance; Nursing Process: Planning

Basic Principles of Anti-Infective Pharmacotherapy

From Chapter 49 of *Pharmacology: Connections to Nursing Practice*, Second Edition. Michael Patrick Adams, Carol Quam Urban. Copyright ©
2013 by Pearson Education, Inc. All rights reserved.

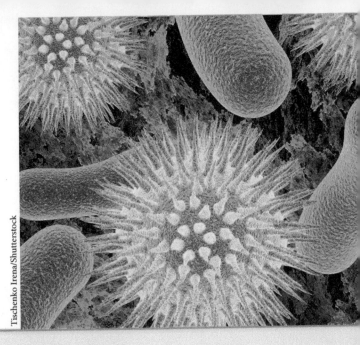

Tischenko Irena/Shutterstock

Basic Principles of Anti-Infective Pharmacotherapy

Learning Outcomes

After reading this chapter, the student should be able to:

1. Explain the mechanisms by which pathogens infect the body.
2. Describe methods for classifying bacteria.
3. Explain the mechanisms by which anti-infective drugs act to kill pathogens or restrict their growth.
4. Describe the clinical significance of bacterial resistance.
5. Identify steps that the nurse can take to limit the development of resistance.
6. Describe the clinical rationale for selecting specific antibiotics.
7. Identify the role of the nurse in preventing, identifying, and treating adverse effects due to antibiotic therapy.
8. Explain how the patient's immune status, history of allergic reactions, age, pregnancy status, genetics, or local tissue conditions influence anti-infective pharmacotherapy.
9. Explain the clinical importance of selecting the correct antibiotic for the individual patient.
10. Describe the development of superinfections.

Chapter Outline

The human body has adapted quite well to living in a world teeming with microorganisms (microbes). In the air, water, food, and soil, microbes have been essential components of life on the planet for billions of years. In some cases, these microorganisms coexist in intimate contact with human beings. It is estimated that 10^{14} bacterial cells reside inside or on the surface of the body, which is more than the total number of human cells in an average person. Fortunately, of the millions of species of microbes, only a relative few are harmful to human health. The purpose of this chapter is to present the fundamental principles that apply to the pharmacotherapy of infectious diseases.

PharmFACT

In 1900, 5 of the 10 most frequent causes of death in the United States were infectious diseases. In 2010, only influenza or pneumonia and septicemia were in the top 10 causes of death (Madigan, Martinko, Stahl, & Clark, 2012).

Pathogenicity and Virulence

1 Pathogens cause disease due to their ability to invade tissues or secrete toxins.

The first challenge in studying the pharmacotherapy of infectious disease is to understand the terminology that is used to describe the organisms and drugs. Microbes that are capable of causing human disease, or **pathogens**, include viruses, bacteria, fungi, unicellular organisms (protozoans), and multicellular animals (e.g., fleas, mites, and worms).

Some pathogens are extremely infectious and life threatening to humans, whereas others simply cause annoying symptoms or none at all. **Pathogenicity**, the ability of an organism to cause disease, depends on an organism's speed of reproduction and its skill in bypassing or overcoming body defenses. Organisms that usually infect only when the body's immune system is suppressed are called *opportunistic pathogens*.

Virulence is a quantitative measure of an organism's pathogenicity. A highly virulent microbe is one that can produce disease when present in very small numbers. Virulent pathogens produce their devastating effects through two primary characteristics: invasiveness and toxicity.

Invasiveness is the ability of a pathogen to grow extremely rapidly and cause direct damage to surrounding tissues by their sheer numbers. Because a week or more may be needed to mount an immune response against the organism, this exponential growth can rapidly overwhelm body defenses and disrupt normal cellular function. Some streptococci, staphylococci, and clostridia secrete hyaluronidase, an enzyme that digests the matrix between human cells, allowing the bacteria to penetrate anatomic barriers more easily. *Staphylococcus aureus* secretes the enzyme coagulase, causing fibrin to be deposited on its cells, thereby protecting it from phagocytes.

The second characteristic of virulence is the production of toxins, or toxicity. **Exotoxins** are proteins released by bacteria into surrounding tissues that have the ability to inactivate or kill host cells. *Clostridium botulinum*, the organism responsible for botulism, produces one of the most potent toxins known that binds to presynaptic motor neurons to prevent the release of acetylcholine. Cholera toxin from *Vibrio cholerae* causes large amounts of fluid to be secreted into the intestinal lumen. Symptoms of exotoxin-producing bacteria are usually caused by the toxin itself, not the bacteria. For example, patients experience food poisoning by ingesting food containing the toxins produced by the organisms; growth of the bacteria in the body is not required. Most exotoxins are water soluble and can readily enter the blood to cause systemic toxemia.

Endotoxins are harmful nonprotein chemicals that are part of the outer layer of the normal cell wall of gram-negative bacteria. After the bacterial cell dies, endotoxins are liberated into the surrounding tissue and induce macrophages to release large amounts of cytokines, causing generalized inflammation, fever, and chills. Rapid decreases in the number of lymphocytes, leukocytes, and platelets may occur. The initial doses of antibiotic therapy may actually worsen symptoms by lysing bacteria and releasing larger amounts of endotoxins. Even very small amounts of some bacterial endotoxins may disrupt normal cellular activity and, in extreme cases, result in death. Examples of organisms producing endotoxins include *Proteus*, a common cause of urinary tract infections (UTIs), and *Neisseria meningitidis*, the agent that causes meningitis.

CONNECTION Checkpoint 49.1

If your patient has a particularly virulent infection, which route of administration would likely be used during antibiotic therapy to most rapidly kill the organisms? *See Answer to Connection Checkpoint 49.1 on student resource website.*

Describing and Classifying Bacteria

2 Bacteria are described by their staining characteristics, shape, and ability to utilize oxygen.

Because of the enormous number of bacterial species, several descriptive systems have been developed to simplify their study. It is important for nurses to learn these classification

Key Terms

acquired resistance

aerobic

anaerobic

antibiotic

anti-infective

bacteriocidal

bacteriostatic

broad-spectrum antibiotic

conjugation

culture and sensitivity (C&S) testing

endotoxins

exotoxins

gram negative

gram positive

host flora

invasiveness

microbial antagonism

mutations

narrow-spectrum antibiotic

nosocomial infections

pathogenicity

pathogens

peptidoglycan

superinfections

virulence

schemes, because drugs that are effective against one organism in a class are likely to be effective against other pathogens in the same class. Common bacterial pathogens and their associated diseases are listed in Table 1.

One of the simplest methods of classifying microbes is to examine them microscopically after a crystal violet Gram stain has been applied to the microbes. Some bacteria contain a thick cell wall composed of peptidoglycan and retain the violet color after staining. These bacteria are called **gram positive** and include *Staphylococcus*, *Streptococcus*, and *Enterococcus*. Bacteria that have thinner cell walls will lose the violet stain and are called **gram negative**. Examples of gram-negative bacteria

TABLE 1 Common Bacterial Pathogens		
Name of Organism	**Disease(s)**	**Description**
Gram-Positive Bacilli		
Bacillus anthracis	Anthrax	Aerobe; appears in cutaneous and respiratory forms
Clostridium	Food poisoning, gas gangrene, tetanus	Anaerobe
Corynebacterium	Diphtheria	Aerobe or anaerobe
Gram-Positive Cocci		
Enterococci	Wounds, UTI, endocarditis, bacteremia	Aerobe; part of host flora of the genitourinary and intestinal tracts; common opportunistic pathogen
Staphylococcus aureus	Pneumonia, food poisoning, impetigo, wounds, bacteremia, endocarditis, toxic shock syndrome, osteomyelitis, UTI	Aerobe; some species are part of host flora on the skin and mucous membranes
Streptococci	Pharyngitis, pneumonia, skin infection, septicemia, endocarditis, otitis media, meningitis in children	Aerobe; some species are part of host flora of the respiratory, genital, and intestinal tracts
Gram-Negative Bacilli		
Bacteroides	Peritonitis, abdominal abscess	Anaerobe; part of host flora of the intestinal, respiratory, and genitourinary tracts
Campylobacter	Gastroenteritis, diarrhea	One of the most common causes of diarrheal illness in the United States
Enterobacter	UTI, blood or lung infections	Aerobe or anaerobe
Escherichia coli	Traveler's diarrhea, UTI, meningitis in children, bacteremia	Part of host flora of the intestinal tract
Haemophilus influenzae	Pneumonia, meningitis in children, bacteremia, otitis media, sinusitis	Some species are part of host flora of the upper respiratory tract
Klebsiella pneumoniae	Pneumonia, UTI	Common opportunistic pathogen; often fatal if not treated aggressively
Proteus mirabilis	UTI, skin infection	Part of host flora of the intestinal tract
Pseudomonas aeruginosa	UTI, skin infection, septicemia	Common opportunistic pathogen
Salmonella enteritides	Food poisoning	Acquired from infected animal products: raw eggs, undercooked meat or chicken
Salmonella typhi	Enteric (typhoid) fever	Acquired from contaminated food or water supplies
Serratia	Nosocomial infections of wounds and UTI	Aerobic or anaerobic
Shigella	Dysentery	Aerobic or anaerobic; part of host flora of the gastrointestinal (GI) tract
Vibrio cholerae	Cholera	Gram-negative aerobe; acquired from contaminated food or water
Gram-Negative Cocci		
Neisseria gonorrhoeae	Gonorrhea, urethritis, anorectal infection, pelvic inflammatory disease, neonatal eye infection	Gram-negative aerobe; some species are part of host flora of the upper respiratory tract
Neisseria meningitides	Meningitis, particularly in children	Gram-negative aerobe; may result in death within hours of onset of symptoms
Spirilla/Spirochetes		
Borrelia burgdorferi	Lyme disease	Acquired from tick bites
Treponema	Syphilis	Sexually transmitted infection (STI)
Other Organisms		
Chlamydia trachomatis	Venereal disease, eye infection	Gram-negative; most common cause of STIs in the United States
Mycobacterium leprae	Leprosy	Most cases in the United States occur in immigrants from Africa or Asia
Mycobacterium tuberculosis	Tuberculosis	Very high incidence in patients with human immunodeficiency virus (HIV) or acquired immunodeficiency syndrome (AIDS)
Mycoplasma pneumoniae	Pneumonia	Most common cause of pneumonia in patients ages 5–35
Rickettsia rickettsii	Rocky mountain spotted fever	Gram-negative; acquired from tick bites

include *Bacteroides*, *Escherichia*, *Klebsiella*, *Pseudomonas*, and *Salmonella*. The distinction between gram-positive and gram-negative bacteria is a profound one that reflects important biochemical and physiological differences between the two groups. Many antibiotics are effective against only one of the two groups. For example, gram-negative bacteria are generally susceptible to the tetracycline class but are resistant to the sulfonamides. This generalization, however, quickly breaks down when resistant strains develop.

Bacteria are often described by their basic shape, which can be readily determined microscopically. Those with rod shapes are called bacilli, those that are spherical are called cocci, and those that are spiral are called spirilla. The shape, along with the Gram stain, helps pathologists to identify organisms that are isolated from infectious specimens.

A third factor used to categorize bacteria is their ability to use oxygen. Those that thrive in an oxygen-rich environment are called **aerobic**; those that grow optimally without oxygen are called **anaerobic**. Some organisms have the ability to change their metabolism and survive in either aerobic or anaerobic conditions, depending on their external environment. Antibiotics are often selective for either aerobes or anaerobes.

Classification of Anti-Infectives

3 Anti-infective drugs are classified by their susceptible organisms, chemical structures, and mechanisms of action.

Anti-infective is a general term that applies to any medication that is effective against pathogens. In its broadest sense, an anti-infective drug may be used to treat bacterial, fungal, viral, or parasitic infections. To distinguish among the various anti-infectives, these medications are classified as antibacterial, antifungal, antiviral, antiprotozoan, and antihelminthic based on the susceptible organism they treat.

The most frequent term used to describe an antibacterial drug is antibiotic. Technically, **antibiotic** refers to a natural substance produced by a microorganism that can kill other microorganisms. However, many of the newer drugs that are available to treat bacterial infections are now produced synthetically. In clinical practice, the terms *antibacterial* and *antibiotic* are used interchangeably to refer to any drug that is effective against bacteria. In this text, antibiotic and antibacterial are used interchangeably.

Classifying drugs only by their susceptible organism, such as an antibacterial, tells us nothing about the properties, actions, or adverse effects of a drug. With over 300 antibacterials available, it is helpful to group these drugs into subclasses that share similar therapeutic properties. Two means of grouping are widely used: chemical classes and pharmacologic classes.

Class names such as aminoglycosides, fluoroquinolone, and sulfonamides refer to the fundamental chemical structure shared by a group of anti-infectives. Anti-infectives that belong to the same chemical class have close structural similarities and usually share similar antibacterial properties and adverse effects. Although chemical names are sometimes long and difficult to pronounce, placing drugs into chemical classes

TABLE 2 Classification of Anti-Infective Drugs

Mechanism of Action	Chemical Class	Examples
Inhibition of cell wall synthesis	Penicillins Cephalosporins Carbapenems	penicillin G cefotaxime (Claforan) imipenem (Primaxin) isoniazid (INH) vancomycin (Vancocin)
Inhibition of protein synthesis	Aminoglycosides Tetracyclines Macrolides Oxazolidinones	gentamicin (Garamycin) tetracycline (Achromycin) erythromycin (E-mycin) linezolid (Zyvox)
Disruption of plasma membrane	Azoles Polyenes	amphotericin B (Fungizone) fluconazole (Diflucan) nystatin (Fungizone)
Inhibition of nucleic acid synthesis	Fluoroquinolones	ciprofloxacin (Cipro)
Inhibition of metabolic pathways	Sulfonamides	dapsone (DDS) trimethoprim-sulfamethoxazole (Bactrim, Septra)

will assist the student in mentally organizing these drugs into distinct therapeutic groups.

Pharmacologic classes are used to group anti-infectives by their mechanism of action. Like chemical classes, placing an antibiotic into a pharmacologic class allows the nurse to develop a mental framework on which to organize these medications and to predict similar actions and adverse effects. Examples of pharmacologic classes along with their prototype drugs are listed in Table 2. It is important that the nurse learn both the chemical class and the pharmacologic class for each antibiotic because this will provide a deeper understanding of the drug's therapeutic action and potential adverse effects.

Mechanisms of Action of Anti-Infectives

4 Anti-infective drugs act by selectively targeting a pathogen's metabolism or life cycle.

Although the immune system provides elaborate defenses against microbial invaders, there are times when the body defenses become overwhelmed by an infection. Furthermore, there are times when acquiring an infection could be a serious health challenge for a patient, and it is best to prevent it. Whether it is used for treating or preventing disease, the primary goal of anti-infective therapy is to assist the body in eliminating a pathogen. Drugs that accomplish this goal by killing bacteria are called **bacteriocidal**. Some drugs do not kill pathogens but instead slow their growth, allowing natural body defenses to eliminate the microorganisms. These growth-slowing drugs are called **bacteriostatic**.

Bacterial cells have distinct anatomic and physiological differences compared to human cells. Bacteria incorporate different chemicals into their membranes and use unique biochemical pathways and enzymes to manage their rapid growth. Even the more complex pathogens such as fungi and protozoans have different cell structures and use certain metabolic pathways not found in human cells. Antibiotics exert selective toxicity by targeting these unique differences between human and bacterial, fungal, and protozoan cells. Through this selective action, these pathogens can be killed, or their growth severely hampered, without any major effects on human cells. Of course, there are limits to this selective toxicity, depending on the specific antibiotic and the dose employed. Adverse effects can be expected from all the anti-infectives. There are five major methods by which antibacterials exert their selective toxicity: inhibition of cell wall synthesis, inhibition of protein synthesis, disruption of the plasma cell membrane, inhibition of nucleic acid synthesis, and inhibition of metabolic pathways (antimetabolites).

Inhibition of Cell Wall Synthesis

Unlike human cells, bacteria have rigid cell walls that create a high osmotic pressure within the cells. The cell wall primarily consists of **peptidoglycan**, a strong, repeating network of carbohydrate and protein chains found only in bacteria and that contains sugars bound to peptides. Disruption of this wall causes the cell to absorb water and eventually lyse. The presence of a unique cell wall gives several means by which antibiotics may act. Fungi also have a unique cell wall that contains lipids that are not used in human cells.

The penicillins and cephalosporins bind to specific proteins that are essential to building the bacterial cell wall. Vancomycin acts by preventing the formation of peptide chains that are used in the construction of the cell wall. Several drugs that are effective against *Mycobacterium tuberculosis*, including isoniazid, act by inhibiting the incorporation of mycolic acid, an important component of the cell wall of this mycobacterium.

Inhibition of Protein Synthesis

Both bacterial and human cells conduct protein synthesis, so this may seem an unlikely target for antibiotics. However, proteins are constructed on the surface of ribosomes, and these organelles have different structures in humans and bacteria. This difference in ribosomal structure accounts for the selective toxicity of certain antibiotics for bacterial cells.

The fact that protein synthesis occurs in several steps affords different mechanisms by which antibiotics may act. For example, the tetracyclines interfere with the transfer of ribonucleic acid (RNA), which carries the amino acids to the ribosome. The aminoglycosides change the shape of the ribosome so that protein synthesis is impeded.

Disruption of the Plasma Cell Membrane

A few antibacterial and antifungal agents act by interfering with the pathogen's plasma membrane. For example, when polymyxin B attaches to the phospholipids in bacterial plasma membranes, the permeability of the membrane changes and substances escape from the cell. The antifungal drug amphotericin B shuts down the synthesis of ergosterol, a lipid essential to the integrity of fungal plasma membranes.

Inhibition of Nucleic Acid Synthesis

Although deoxyribonucleic acid (DNA) and RNA synthesis are complex processes that occur in both human and bacterial cells, the molecular structures of the various enzymes required for these processes differ considerably. The largest group of antibiotics that inhibits DNA synthesis is the fluoroquinolones. These drugs affect bacterial DNA gyrase, an enzyme that uncoils DNA during the replication process.

Inhibition of Metabolic Pathways (Antimetabolites)

Because they divide rapidly, bacterial cells need a steady supply of nutrients and metabolites. A few drugs structurally resemble these building blocks and "fool" the bacterial cell into using them for growth. The sulfonamide antibiotics resemble para-amino benzoic acid (PABA), a precursor to folic acid. Folic acid, a B vitamin that is essential to human metabolism, is also essential to bacteria. When the bacteria attempt to use the sulfonamides, bacterial protein synthesis is blocked.

Other Mechanisms of Action

Anti-infectives act by a number of other miscellaneous mechanisms. The antifungal drug griseofulvin inhibits the formation of mitotic microtubules. Antiretrovirals such as zidovudine block the synthesis of viral DNA by inhibiting the enzyme reverse transcriptase. Mebendazole kills parasitic worms by preventing their absorption of nutrients.

Many other possible mechanisms exist. As the understanding of bacterial physiology increases, it is likely that pharmacologists will develop anti-infectives with entirely new mechanisms of action. The primary mechanisms of action of antibacterial drugs are shown in Pharmacotherapy Illustrated 1.

Acquired Resistance

5 Acquired resistance is a major clinical problem that is worsened by improper use of anti-infectives.

In the 1950s, health care providers called antibiotics "miracle drugs" and predicted that all infectious disease would one day be eliminated. It did not take long, however, to discover that these miracle drugs were rapidly becoming ineffective. How could a drug that once killed nearly 100% of a species of bacteria soon prove to be ineffective? The answer is acquired resistance.

Acquired resistance is the ability of an organism to become unresponsive over time to the effects of an anti-infective. Resistance occurs in antibacterials, antifungals, antivirals, and antiprotozoal drugs. It is a major clinical problem that is growing in importance.

PHARMACOTHERAPY ILLUSTRATED   1

Mechanisms of Action of Antimicrobial Drugs

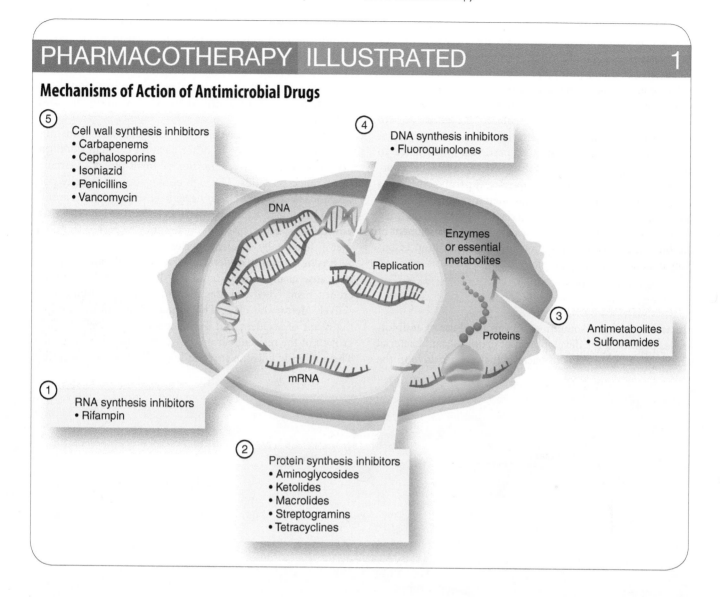

⑤ Cell wall synthesis inhibitors
- Carbapenems
- Cephalosporins
- Isoniazid
- Penicillins
- Vancomycin

④ DNA synthesis inhibitors
- Fluoroquinolones

③ Antimetabolites
- Sulfonamides

① RNA synthesis inhibitors
- Rifampin

② Protein synthesis inhibitors
- Aminoglycosides
- Ketolides
- Macrolides
- Streptogramins
- Tetracyclines

DNA

Replication

Enzymes or essential metabolites

Proteins

mRNA

Mechanisms of Resistance

How can an organism become insensitive to a drug that kills other members of its species? Medicine has discovered a number of mechanisms by which pathogens acquire resistance:

- **Destruction of the drug.** Organisms can produce an enzyme that destroys or deactivates the drug. For example, some bacteria are able to produce beta lactamase, an enzyme that splits the active portion of the drug molecule. Organisms that produce beta lactamase are resistant to many of the penicillin and cephalosporin antibiotics.

- **Prevention of drug entry into the pathogen.** Some antibiotics must enter the pathogen to cause their action. Some bacteria have developed enzymes that inactivate the drug as it crosses the cell wall. Others have changed the structure of the channels or pores that the antibiotic normally uses to enter the cell. Resistance to penicillins and tetracyclines can occur by these methods.

- **Removal by resistance pumps.** Some bacteria have developed a system that rapidly pumps the antibiotic out of the bacterial cell before it can reach intracellular targets such as

ribosomes. Resistant bacteria have developed several types of pumps, each of which is used to remove different antibiotics.

- **Alteration of the drug's target site.** Most antibiotics bind to a specific receptor that is located on the cell surface or inside the bacteria. Certain bacteria have changed the shape of these receptors, so they no longer bind the drug. This mechanism of resistance is common for the sulfonamides. For the macrolide antibiotics, mutations have resulted in changes to the structure of the bacterial ribosome, which is the receptor for macrolide binding.

- **Development of alternative metabolic pathways.** Some antibiotics act by depleting the pathogen of an essential substance necessary for growth. Some resistant organisms have survived antibiotic application by synthesizing larger amounts of the essential substance or by finding an alternative means of obtaining it from the environment.

How do bacteria change their physiology to become resistant to antibiotics? The answer lies in the nature of bacterial cell division. Microorganisms have the ability to replicate extremely rapidly. Under ideal conditions *Escherichia coli* can produce a million cells every 20 minutes, or 1×10^{21} cells in only 24 hours. During exponential division, bacteria make frequent errors, or **mutations**, while duplicating their genetic code. These mutations, which occur spontaneously and randomly, occasionally result in a change in physiology that gives a bacterial cell a reproductive advantage over its neighbors. For example, the mutated bacterium may be able to survive in harsher conditions, change the shape of its organelles, or perhaps grow faster than other bacterial cells.

One such mutation that is of particular importance to medicine is that which confers drug resistance on a microorganism. Once a resistant strain appears, it permanently loses sensitivity to that specific drug and often to other drugs in the same pharmacologic and chemical class. Over several decades, these drug-resistant mutants may colonize a large segment of the human population, thus making the medication essentially useless as a first-line antibiotic.

Promotion of Resistance

The widespread and sometimes unwarranted use of antibiotics has promoted the development of drug-resistant bacterial strains. By killing strains of bacteria that are sensitive to the drug, the only bacteria remaining to replicate are those that acquire the mutations that make them insensitive to the effects of the antibiotic. These drug-resistant bacteria are then free to grow, unrestrained by their neighbors that are killed by the antibiotic. Soon the patient develops an infection that is resistant to conventional drug therapy. This concept is shown in Figure 1.

After acquiring resistance, the mutated bacterium may pass its resistance gene to other bacteria through **conjugation**, which is the direct transfer of small pieces of circular DNA called plasmids. Through conjugation, it is quite possible for a bacterium that has never been exposed to the antibiotic to become resistant. Furthermore, because conjugation is not species specific, resistance genes may be passed from one species to a totally different species.

It is important to understand that the antibiotic itself does not cause changes in bacterial physiology, nor does the microorganism have a master plan to become resistant or to actively defeat the drug. The mutation occurs randomly—the result of accident and pure chance. The promotion and growth of the resistant strain, however, is not due to chance. The antibiotic kills the surrounding cells that are susceptible

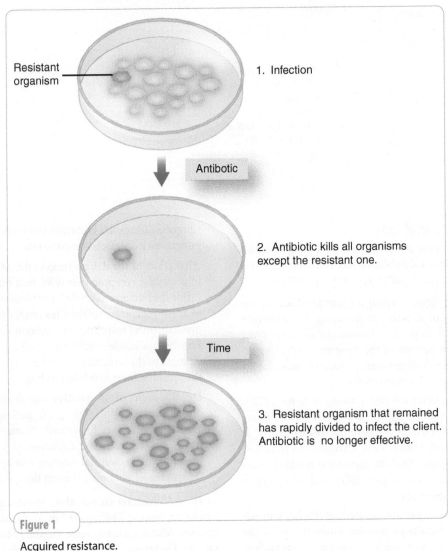

Resistant organism

1. Infection

Antibotic

2. Antibiotic kills all organisms except the resistant one.

Time

3. Resistant organism that remained has rapidly divided to infect the client. Antibiotic is no longer effective.

Figure 1

Acquired resistance.

to the drug, leaving the mutated bacterium plenty of room to divide and infect. It should also be understood that it is the bacteria that become resistant, not the patient.

Prevention of Resistant Strains

Patients and their health care providers play important roles in delaying the emergence of resistance to antibiotics. The Centers for Disease Control and Prevention (CDC) has developed a set of guidelines for preventing antimicrobial resistance in the health care setting:

- **Prevent infections when possible.** Nurses must always teach their patients that it is always easier to prevent an infection than to treat one. One important aspect of prevention is getting immunizations to protect against diseases such as influenza, tetanus, polio, measles, and hepatitis B. Prevention also includes proper care and hygiene of catheters, which are significant sources of microorganisms and provide portals of entry into the body.

- **Diagnose and treat the infection properly.** Infections should be cultured so that the offending organism can be identified and the correct drug chosen, as discussed in Section 7.

- **Use antimicrobials wisely.** Antibiotics should only be prescribed when there is a clear rationale for their use. The drugs should be taken for the full length of therapy, and the prescription should not be renewed if the infection has been eliminated or prevented. The more often an antibiotic is prescribed in the population, the larger will be the percentage of resistant strains.

- **Prevent transmission.** Nurses can contain infections and stop the spread of the disease in their work settings by using proper infection control procedures. Additionally, nurses should teach their patients the methods of proper hygiene to prevent the transmission of infectious disease in the home and community settings.

CONNECTION Checkpoint 49.2

Explain the difference between resistance and tolerance. *See Answer to Connection Checkpoint 49.2 on student resource website.*

6 Several resistant strains are major clinical challenges due to the lack of therapeutic options.

Infections that are acquired in a health care setting, known as **nosocomial infections**, are often resistant to common antibiotics. Recently, the term *health care–associated infection* (HAI) has begun to replace the term *nosocomial*. The most common site of HAIs is the urinary tract, followed by surgical wounds, respiratory tract, and bacteremia. Table 3 lists the organisms that are frequently responsible for HAI infections.

There are four general sources of HAIs:

- **Patient flora.** Bacteria normally residing on the skin and in the lung or genitourinary tract
- **Invasive devices.** Urinary catheters, vascular catheters, endotracheal tubes, and endoscopes

TABLE 3 Common Pathogens Associated with Health Care-Associated Infections

Pathogen	Infection
Acinetobacter species (spp)	Bacteremia
Enterobacter spp	Pneumonia
Enterococcus spp	Urinary tract
Escherichia coli	Urinary tract, primary bacteremia, pneumonia
Klebsiella pneumoniae	Pneumonia, urinary tract
Pseudomonas aeruginosa	Pneumonia, urinary tract
Staphylococcus aureus	Surgical wounds, pneumonia, bacteremia
Staphylococci (coagulase negative)	Bacteremia

- **Medical personnel.** Infected health care workers or non-infectious carriers
- **Medical environment.** Contaminated instruments, air, food, or fluids

Many times, patients are at risk for HAIs caused by resistant organisms. Two types of resistant strains are especially important to pharmacotherapy: methicillin-resistant *Staphylococcus aureus* and vancomycin-resistant enterococci.

Methicillin-resistant *Staphylococcus aureus* (MRSA): MRSA is a type of bacterium that is resistant to certain antibiotics such as methicillin, amoxicillin, and penicillin. At least 60% of *S. aureus* infections are now resistant to penicillin. The term "methicillin resistant" is still used for these infections despite the fact that methicillin was removed from the market many years ago.

MRSA infections are most frequently acquired in hospitals and long-term care facilities. These hospital-acquired infections (HA-MRSA) occur primarily in patients with weakened immune systems. MRSA infections that occur in nonhospitalized settings are called community-acquired infections. Community-acquired MRSA (CA-MRSA) infections occur in otherwise healthy people and are usually manifested as skin and soft tissue infections, such as pimples and boils. The strains that are responsible for HA-MRSA infections appear to be distinctly different from those that cause CA-MRSA infections; thus the pharmacotherapy of the two infections differs somewhat.

Therapeutic options for patients with serious MRSA infections are limited. In recent years, MRSA strains have developed resistance to most classes of antimicrobials, including fluoroquinolones, macrolides, aminoglycosides, tetracyclines, and clindamycin. In general, the HA-MRSA strains are resistant to more classes than the CA-MRSA infections. Until recently, vancomycin was the only antibiotic effective for treating serious MRSA infections. Unfortunately, MRSA strains that are also resistant to vancomycin have appeared. Several newer antibiotics, including linezolid (Zyvox), quinupristin-dalfopristin, and daptomycin, are now available to treat multidrug-resistant strains of MRSA.

Vancomycin-resistant enterococci (VRE): Enterococci are normal inhabitants of the human GI tract and the female genital tract. Enterococci are also frequently found in wounds and pressure ulcers in hospitalized patients or nursing home residents. Patients with compromised immune systems are at greatest risk. Because enterococci are hardy organisms, they can survive for prolonged periods on environmental surfaces, and health care workers using poor infection control techniques can easily spread them. More than 95% of VRE strains in the United States are *Enterococcus faecium*.

Like MRSA, VRE infections represent a major therapeutic challenge, and treatment options are limited. Strains that are resistant to the most commonly used classes of antibiotics have been isolated. Virtually all are resistant to high levels of ampicillin, which is the conventional treatment for enterococci infections. In the 1990s, vancomycin became the only antibiotic effective against multidrug-resistant VRE strains. Unfortunately, each year finds more VRE strains becoming resistant to vancomycin, and newer antibiotics must be used for these infections.

PharmFACT

Up to 90% of all *S. aureus* organisms isolated from individuals are now resistant to penicillin G. Over half of these are also methicillin resistant (Gumbo, 2011).

7 Careful selection of the correct antibiotic is essential for effective pharmacotherapy and to limit adverse effects.

It is essential for the health care provider to select an antibiotic that will be effective against the specific pathogen that is causing the patient's infection. Selecting an incorrect drug will delay proper treatment, giving the microorganisms more time to invade or secrete toxins. For some infections, treatment delays of just a few hours or days can lead to poorer patient prognosis and even death. Prescribing ineffective antibiotics also promotes the development of resistance and may cause unnecessary adverse effects in the patient.

For the correct antibiotic to be chosen, identification of the causative agent is necessary. Although gathering data on symptoms is important, many infections produce the same signs early in their course; thus more exact laboratory means of diagnosis are necessary.

Specimens such as urine, sputum, blood, or pus are examined in the laboratory for the purpose of isolating and identifying specific pathogens. After isolation, the microbe is exposed in the laboratory to different antibiotics to determine the most effective ones. This process of isolating the infectious organism and identifying the most effective antibiotic is called **culture and sensitivity (C&S) testing**. Other laboratory techniques include examination of the blood for specific antibodies, direct antigen detection, and DNA probe hybridization.

Ideally, the pathogen should be identified before anti-infective therapy is begun. However, laboratory testing and identification may take several days and, in the case of viruses, several weeks. Indeed, some pathogens cannot be cultured at all. If the infection is severe, therapy is often begun with a **broad-spectrum antibiotic**, which is one that is effective against a wide variety of different microbial species. After C&S testing is completed, the drug may be changed to a **narrow-spectrum antibiotic**, which is one that is effective against a smaller group of microbes or only the isolated species. In general, narrow-spectrum antibiotics have less effect on **host flora**, thus causing fewer adverse effects. Host flora are microorganisms that normally inhabit the human body.

Anti-infectives should not be prescribed for infections such as the common cold or for disorders for which antibiotics serve no therapeutic advantage. Antibiotics do not affect viral diseases such as the common cold, although many patients with this self-limiting disorder believe that these drugs will speed their recovery. Another example of anti-infective misuse is prescribing antibiotics to patients who have a cough due to chronic bronchitis. It should be understood, however, that health care providers may prescribe anti-infectives to prevent a secondary infection from developing. For example, an elderly patient with a severe cold may develop a weakened immune response. Thus the health care provider may order an antibiotic not for the viral infection, but to prevent a secondary bacterial infection from developing.

Indications and Selection of Specific Anti-Infectives

8 Depending on the pathogen, anti-infective therapy may be conducted with a single drug or a combination of drugs.

If C&S testing confirms that an infection is caused by a single species of microbe, antibiotic therapy is usually begun with one drug. In some cases, combining two antibiotics may actually decrease each drug's effectiveness, a phenomenon known as *antagonism*. For example, giving a drug that slows bacterial growth may interfere with an antibiotic that depends on a high bacterial growth rate to produce its bacteriocidal effect. Use of multiple antibiotics can also promote the emergence of multidrug-resistant strains and produce unnecessary adverse effects.

In well-defined circumstances combination therapy with multiple antibiotics is warranted. For example, multiple anti-infective drugs are indicated if several different species of pathogens are causing the infection. Patients may present with a life-threatening infection of unknown etiology and the health care provider may need to prescribe several antibiotics until the specific pathogens can be identified. In some cases, two antibiotics have been shown through clinical research to work synergistically, producing a greater kill rate than would be achieved by either antibiotic given alone. Examples of situations where multidrug therapy is clearly warranted are for the pharmacotherapy of tuberculosis and HIV-AIDS.

CONNECTION Checkpoint 49.3

Why would there probably be fewer adverse effects in a patient if two antibiotics are given at lower doses, rather than a single antibiotic given at a higher dose? *See Answer to Connection Checkpoint 49.3 on student resource website.*

9 Anti-infectives may be administered to prevent infections.

In most cases, anti-infectives are given when there is clear evidence of infection. This is because health care providers have developed clear rationales for prescribing these drugs to discourage the emergence of resistant strains.

However, anti-infectives are administered to prevent infections in certain high-risk patients. In these cases, research has demonstrated that the benefits of infection prophylaxis outweigh the increased risk of adverse effects or the potential for producing resistant strains. Prophylactic anti-infectives are indicated for the following clinical situations:

- Antibiotics for patients with suppressed immune systems, including those with HIV-AIDS or profound neutropenia
- Antibiotics for patients with deep puncture wounds such as from dog bites
- Antibiotics for patients with prosthetic heart valves, prior to receiving medical or dental surgery, to prevent bacterial endocarditis
- Antibiotics for patients who are undergoing specific types of surgery, such as cardiovascular surgery, orthopedic surgery, and surgery of the alimentary canal, where it has been shown that antibiotic use decreases the risk of postoperative infections
- Antimalarial drugs for patients who are entering areas of the world where malaria is endemic
- Antitubercular drugs for close personal contacts of patients who have confirmed or suspected active tuberculosis
- Antiretrovirals to prevent the transmission of HIV to newborns when the mother is HIV positive
- Antiretrovirals for health care workers who have a confirmed exposure to HIV-contaminated body fluids

Prophylactic therapy with anti-infectives is usually conducted using specific protocols that designate the duration of therapy. For example, chloroquine (Aralen) is given 1 week before expected exposure to malaria and continues for 4 weeks following exposure. Zidovudine (AZT) is given to the HIV-positive mother beginning by week 14 of pregnancy until birth, after which the drug is given to the neonate for 6 weeks. Only in rare cases are anti-infectives given prophylactically for indefinite time periods. Examples include the prevention of infections in patients with suppressed immune systems such as those with HIV infection, or those receiving immunosuppressants following an organ transplant.

Host Factors Affecting Anti-Infective Selection

10 Patient factors such as host defenses, local tissue conditions, history of allergic reactions, age, pregnancy status, and genetics influence the choice of anti-infective.

The most important factor in selecting an appropriate antibiotic is to be certain that the microbe is sensitive to the bacteriocidal or bacteriostatic effects of the drug. Once the appropriate drug has been chosen, the nurse must consider a number of host factors that have the potential to significantly influence the success of anti-infective therapy.

Host Defenses

Remember that the primary goal of antibiotic therapy is to kill enough of the pathogen or slow its growth such that natural body defenses can overcome the invading agents. An anti-infective is rarely able to eliminate a pathogen without help from a functioning immune system. Patients with weakened immune defenses often require the administration of prophylactic antibiotics. Should an infection occur in these patients, anti-infective therapy is more aggressive and prolonged. Examples of patients who may require this type of antibiotic therapy include those with AIDS and those with neutropenia caused by immunosuppressive or antineoplastic medications.

Local Tissue Conditions

Anti-infectives must be able to reach the area of infection in sufficient concentrations to be effective; thus local conditions at the infection site are important to the success of pharmacotherapy. Infections of the central nervous system (CNS) are particularly difficult to treat because many medications are unable to cross the blood–brain barrier to reach the brain and associated tissues. Injury or inflammation at an infection site can cause tissues to become acidic or anaerobic and have poor circulation. Excessive pus formation or large hematomas can impede drugs from reaching their targets. Pathogens such as mycobacteria, salmonella, toxoplasma, and listeria can reside intracellularly and thus be resistant to antibacterial action.

Factors that hinder the drug from reaching microbes will limit therapeutic success, and adjustments in treatment may be necessary. Increasing the dosage or switching to a different route of drug administration may be indicated. Occasionally, it is necessary to switch to a different antibiotic that is more effective for conditions specific to the infection site.

Allergy History

Although not common, serious hypersensitivity reactions to antibiotics may be fatal. The penicillins are the class of antibacterials that have the highest incidence of allergic reactions: Between 0.7% and 10% of all patients who receive these drugs exhibit some degree of hypersensitivity.

Patient assessment must always include a thorough medication history. A previous acute allergic incident with a drug is highly predictive of future hypersensitivity to the same medication. Because the patient may have been exposed to an antibiotic unknowingly, such as through food products or molds, allergic reactions can occur without any apparent previous exposure. If severe allergy to a drug is established, it is best to avoid all drugs in the same chemical class.

Other Host Factors

Age, pregnancy status, and genetics are additional factors that influence anti-infective pharmacotherapy. Infants and older adults are less able to metabolize and excrete antibiotics; thus doses are generally decreased. Because of polypharmacy in older patients, this group is more likely to be taking multiple drugs that could interact with antibiotics.

Some antibiotics are readily secreted in breast milk or cross the placenta. For example, tetracyclines taken by the mother can cause teeth discoloration in the newborn, and aminoglycosides can affect hearing. Some anti-infectives are pregnancy category D, such as minocycline, doxycycline, neomycin, and streptomycin. The benefits of antibiotic use in pregnant or lactating women must be carefully weighed against the potential risks to the fetus and neonate.

A genetic absence of certain enzymes can lead to an inability of a patient to metabolize antibiotics to their inactive forms. For example, patients with a deficiency of the enzyme glucose-6-phosphate dehydrogenase should not receive sulfonamides, chloramphenicol, or nalidixic acid due to the possibility of erythrocyte rupture.

CONNECTION Checkpoint 49.4

What classes of drugs are administered to boost immune function so that the patient is less likely to experience an opportunistic infection? *See Answer to Connection Checkpoint 49.4 on student resource website.*

Superinfections

11 Superinfections can occur when an anti-infective antibiotic kills host flora.

Microorganisms that normally inhabit the human body, or host flora, are present on the surface of the skin and in the upper respiratory, genitourinary, and intestinal tracts. Some of these microbes serve useful purposes by producing natural antibacterial substances or by breaking down toxic agents. The various host flora are in competition with each other for physical space and nutrients. This **microbial antagonism** helps protect the host from being overrun by pathogenic organisms.

Antibiotics are unable to distinguish between host flora and pathogenic organisms. When an antibiotic kills the host's normal flora, additional nutrients and space are available for pathogenic microorganisms to grow unchecked. These new, secondary infections caused by antibiotic use are called **superinfections**, or suprainfections. The appearance of a new infection while receiving anti-infective therapy is highly suspicious of a superinfection. Signs and symptoms of superinfection commonly include diarrhea, bladder pain, painful urination, or abnormal vaginal discharges.

Broad-spectrum antibiotics are more likely to cause superinfections because they kill many microbial species, which sometimes includes host flora. Organisms that commonly cause superinfections are *Clostridium albicans* in the vagina, streptococci in the oral cavity, and *Clostridium difficile* in the colon.

UNDERSTANDING THE CHAPTER

Key Concepts Summary

1 Pathogens cause disease due to their ability to invade tissues or secrete toxins.

2 Bacteria are described by their staining characteristics, shape, and ability to utilize oxygen.

3 Anti-infective drugs are classified by their susceptible organisms, chemical structures, and mechanisms of action.

4 Anti-infective drugs act by selectively targeting a pathogen's metabolism or life cycle.

5 Acquired resistance is a major clinical problem that is worsened by improper use of anti-infectives.

6 Several resistant strains are major clinical challenges due to the lack of therapeutic options.

7 Careful selection of the correct antibiotic is essential for effective pharmacotherapy and to limit adverse effects.

8 Depending on the pathogen, anti-infective therapy may be conducted with a single drug or a combination of drugs.

9 Anti-infectives may be administered to prevent infections.

10 Patient factors such as host defenses, local tissue conditions, history of allergic reactions, age, pregnancy status, and genetics influence the choice of anti-infective.

11 Superinfections can occur when an anti-infective antibiotic kills host flora.

Pearson Nursing Student Resources

Find additional review materials at
nursing.pearsonhighered.com
Prepare for success with additional NCLEX®-style practice
questions, interactive assignments and activities, web links,
animations, videos, and more!

References

Gumbo, T. (2011). General principles of antimicrobial therapy. In L. L. Brunton, B. A. Chabner, & B. C. Knollman (Eds.), *The pharmacological basis of therapeutics* (12th ed., pp. 1365–1382). New York, NY: McGraw-Hill.

Madigan, M. T., Martinko, J. M., Stahl, A. A., & Clark, D. P. (2012). *Brock biology of microorganisms* (13th ed.). San Francisco, CA: Benjamin Cummings.

Selected Bibliography

Barnes, B. E., & Sampson, D., A. (2011). A literature review on community-acquired methicillin-resistant *Staphylococcus aureus* in the United States: Clinical information for primary care nurse practitioners. *Journal of the American Academy of Nurse Practitioners, 23*(1), 23–32. doi:10.1111/j.1745-7599.2010.00571.x

Bauman, R. W. (2012). *Microbiology with diseases by body system* (3rd ed.). San Francisco, CA: Benjamin Cummings.

Cole, L. M. (2010). Prophylactic antibiotics: What's your game plan? *Nursing Management, 41*(4), 46–47. doi:10.1097/01.NUMA.0000370879.55842.ae

Estes, K. (2010). Methicillin-resistant *Staphylococcus aureus* skin and soft tissue infections. *Critical Care Nursing Quarterly, 34*(2), 101–109. doi:10.1097/CNQ.0b013e31820f6f9e

Furtado, G. H., & Nicolau, D. P. (2010). Overview perspective of bacterial resistance. *Expert Opinion on Therapeutic Patents, 20*(10), 1273–1276. doi:10.1517/13543776.2010.507193

Gilbert, D. N., Moellering, R. C., & Sande, M. A. (2011). *The Sanford guide to antimicrobial therapy 2011* (41st ed.). Sperryville, VA: Antimicrobial Therapy.

Kunz, A. M., & Brook, I. (2010). Emerging resistant gram-negative aerobic bacilli in hospital-acquired infections. *Chemotherapy, 56*(6), 492–500. doi:10.1159/000321018

Parsons, L., & Krau, S. (2007). Bacterial infections: Management by acute and critical care nurses. *Critical Care Nursing Clinics of North America, 19*(1), 17–26. doi:10.1016/j.ccell.2006.10.011

Tortora, G. J., Funke, B. R., & Case, C. L. (2010). *Microbiology: An introduction* (10th ed.). San Francisco, CA: Benjamin Cummings.

Antibiotics Affecting the Bacterial Cell Wall

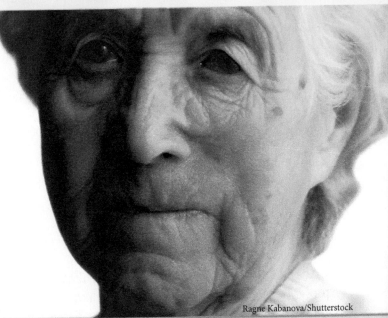

"Last month I underwent surgery for the removal of a skin lesion from my left arm. Unfortunately, I think the wound has become infected. The area is red, swollen, and painful and has a yellowish drainage."

Patient "Katie Dennison"

Antibiotics Affecting the Bacterial Cell Wall

Learning Outcomes

After reading this chapter, the student should be able to:

1. Explain the structure of a bacterial cell wall and its importance to pharmacotherapy.
2. Identify the classes of antibiotics that act by affecting the synthesis of the bacterial cell wall.
3. Explain the mechanisms by which antibiotics affect the bacterial cell wall.
4. Compare and contrast the four classes of penicillins.
5. Compare and contrast the five generations of cephalosporins.
6. Identify similarities and differences among drugs in the carbapenem class.
7. For each of the classes shown in the chapter outline, identify the prototype and representative drugs and explain the mechanism(s) of drug action, primary indications, contraindications, significant drug interactions, pregnancy category, and important adverse effects.
8. Apply the nursing process to care for patients who are receiving pharmacotherapy with bacterial cell wall inhibitors.

Chapter Outline

Structure of Bacterial Cell Walls

Penicillins

Natural Penicillins
PROTOTYPE **Penicillin G**

Broad-Spectrum Penicillins (Aminopenicillins)
PROTOTYPE **Ampicillin (Principen)**

Extended-Spectrum (Antipseudomonal) Penicillins

Penicillinase-Resistant (Antistaphylococcal) Penicillins

Cephalosporins
PROTOTYPE **Cefazolin (Ancef, Kefzol)**

Carbapenems
PROTOTYPE **Imipenem-Cilastatin (Primaxin)**

Miscellaneous Cell Wall Inhibitors
PROTOTYPE **Vancomycin (Vancocin)**

The discovery and development of the first anti-infective drugs in the mid-1900s was a milestone in the field of medicine. Humans no longer die in massive numbers from infectious organisms such as *Yersinia pestis*, which killed 25% of the known human population in the 14th century due to the bubonic plague. This chapter examines the penicillins, cephalosporins, and other antibiotic agents that kill bacteria by disrupting their cell walls.

Structure of Bacterial Cell Walls

1 Bacterial cell walls consist of layers of carbohydrate and protein chains, which are constructed by enzymes called penicillin-binding proteins.

The cell wall is a structure that sets people apart from the bacterial world. Humans do not have them, but all bacteria do. The osmotic pressure is so high within a bacterial cell that the cell would rupture without the containment of this rigid structure. The cell wall also serves as a barrier to substances that try to enter the cell, including antibiotics. Simply, it protects the bacterial cell from a hostile environment. The cell walls of gram-positive bacteria are very thick, whereas the walls of gram-negative bacteria are thinner. The structure of a bacterial cell wall is illustrated in Figure 1.

The primary material in a bacterial cell wall is peptidoglycan, a strong, repeating network of carbohydrate and protein chains that contains sugars bound to peptides. In gram-positive bacteria, peptidoglycan is laid down in repeated layers that are cross-linked to each other to provide greater stability to the wall. The layers may be compared to a fort that is built to provide protection from invaders. A single wall could be easily destroyed, but five or six repeated walls would provide almost impenetrable protection to those inside.

Because of the critical importance of their cell walls, bacteria spend a lot of time and energy building them. At least 30 different bacterial enzymes participate in their construction. Some of these enzymes are targets for penicillins and related antibiotics and are called **penicillin-binding proteins (PBPs)**. Most penicillins affect transpeptidase, which is the final PBP enzyme in the construction of the cell wall that adds the cross-links to the peptidoglycan layers. Without the cross-linking, the cell wall becomes weakened and bulges due to the high osmotic pressure inside the cell. The bacterial cell eventually lyses (disintegrates). This process is illustrated in Figure 2. Because humans do not construct cell walls, they do not have PBPs. Therefore, antibiotics that affect the cell wall have selective toxicity to bacteria.

The PBPs are located on the outside of the plasma membrane of the bacterial cell. This location allows antibiotics to

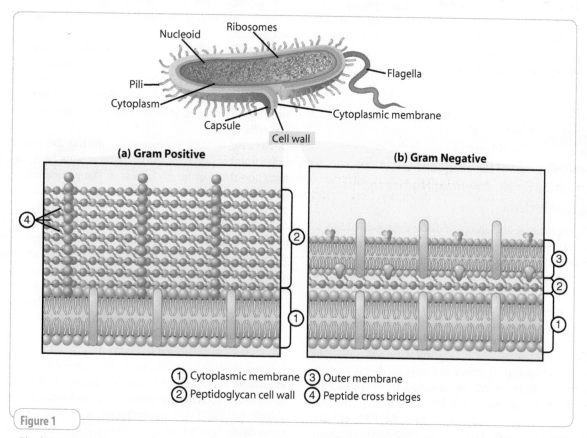

Nucleoid
Ribosomes
Pili
Cytoplasm
Capsule
Cell wall
Flagella
Cytoplasmic membrane

(a) Gram Positive

(b) Gram Negative

4

2

3
2
1

1

① Cytoplasmic membrane   ③ Outer membrane
② Peptidoglycan cell wall   ④ Peptide cross bridges

Figure 1

The bacterial cell wall: (a) gram-positive bacterium; (b) gram-negative bacterium.

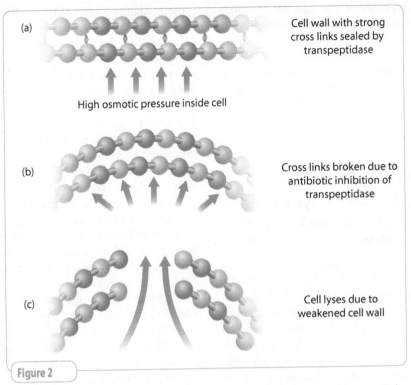

Figure 2

Mechanism of penicillin: (a) Bacterial cell wall strengthened by peptide cross-links. (b) Penicillin breaks cross-links. (c) Cell death due to weakened cell walls.

exert their bacteriocidal effect without actually entering the cell. Although all bacteria have a cell wall, the materials and PBPs used in their construction differ among species. Even slight structural changes to a PBP can cause lack of antibiotic binding to the enzyme. This explains why penicillins are not effective against all species of microorganisms. This also provides an explanation as to how an organism develops resistance to the penicillins.

Penicillins

2 The penicillins, one of the oldest and safest groups of antibacterials, are primarily active against gram-positive bacteria.

Although not the first anti-infective discovered, penicillin was the first mass-produced antibiotic. Discovered in cultures of the common fungus *Penicillium* in 1929, penicillin was first administered therapeutically in 1941. The medication quickly gathered a reputation as a miracle drug by preventing thousands of deaths from what are now considered minor infections. Penicillins are the most extensively studied of all the antibiotic classes. Doses of the penicillins are listed in Table 1.

Penicillins kill bacteria by disrupting their cell walls. The portion of the chemical structure of penicillin that is responsible for its antibacterial activity is called the **beta-lactam ring**. The beta-lactam ring resembles one of the chemical building blocks of peptidoglycan. When the PBP enzyme attempts to add the next "link" in the peptidoglycan chain, it binds to the beta-lactam ring, and construction of the cell

wall is terminated. Other antibiotic classes that contain a beta-lactam ring include the cephalosporins, monobactams, and carbapenems, as shown in Figure 3. These classes are sometimes grouped together and referred to as beta-lactam antibiotics.

Penicillin lyses the growing bacterial cells that are building cell walls; therefore, it is considered bacteriocidal. It has much less toxicity, however, on bacterial cells that have already constructed their cell walls. Like all infections, the body's immune defenses are needed to eliminate stable, slow-growing bacterial cells.

Because of their extensive use during the past 70 years, large numbers of resistant bacterial strains have emerged to limit the therapeutic usefulness of the penicillins. There are several mechanisms by which bacteria may become resistant to penicillins. Through mutations, the structures of PBPs have changed such that they no longer bind penicillin. Indeed, many species of bacteria are inherently insensitive to penicillins because they lack the target binding protein for these antibiotics.

Another mechanism of resistance is that some bacteria secrete enzymes that split the beta-lactam ring, rendering the antibiotic ineffective. **Beta lactamase** is the general term used for any of several enzymes produced by bacteria that can split the four-atom beta-lactam ring structure. The action of this enzyme is illustrated in Figure 4.

Scientists who first discovered this enzyme named it **penicillinase**, a name that is still frequently used in medicine. Although the terms are sometimes used interchangeably, it should be noted that penicillinase is only one type of beta lactamase—that which splits the ring in penicillin antibiotics. Other forms of beta lactamase exist that can inactivate

TABLE 1 Penicillins

Drug	Route and Adult Dose (maximum dose where indicated)	Adverse Effects
Natural Penicillins		
penicillin G benzathine (Bicillin)	IM: 1.2 million units as a single dose (max: 2.4 million units/day)	*Rash, pruritus, diarrhea, nausea, fever*
penicillin G potassium	IM/IV: 2–24 million units divided every 4–6 h (max: 80 million units/day)	
penicillin G procaine (Wycillin)	IM: 600,000–1.2 million units daily (max: 4.8 million units/day)	Anaphylaxis symptoms, including angioedema, circulatory collapse, and cardiac arrest; nephrotoxicity
penicillin V	PO: 125–250 mg qid (max: 7.2 g/day)	
Broad-Spectrum Penicillins (Aminopenicillins)		
amoxicillin (Amoxil, Trimox)	PO: 250–500 mg tid (max: 1,750 mg/day)	
amoxicillin-clavulanate (Augmentin)	PO: 250- or 500-mg tablet (each with 125 mg clavulanic acid) every 8–12 h	
ampicillin (Principen)	PO/IV/IM: 250–500 mg every 6 h (max: 4 g/day PO or 14 g/day IV/IM)	
ampicillin and sulbactam (Unasyn)	IV/IM: 1.5–3 g every 6 h	
Extended-Spectrum (Antipseudomonal) Penicillins		
piperacillin	IM/IV: 2–4 g tid–qid (max: 24 g/day)	
piperacillin-tazobactam (Zosyn)	IV: 3.375 g qid over 30 min	
ticarcillin-clavulanate (Timentin)	IV: 3.1 g every 4–6 h	
Penicillinase-Resistant (Antistaphylococcal) Penicillins		
dicloxacillin	PO: 125–500 mg qid (max: 4 g/day)	
nafcillin	PO: 250 mg–1 g qid (max: 12 g/day)	
oxacillin	PO: 250 mg–1 g qid (max: 12 g/day)	

Note: Italics indicate common adverse effects. Underline indicates serious adverse effects.

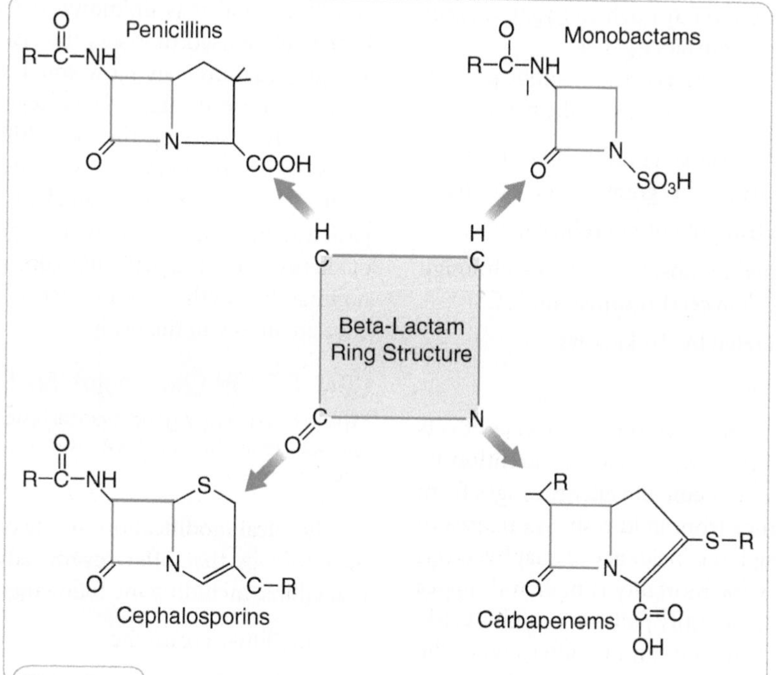

Figure 3

Beta-lactam antibiotics: The beta-lactam ring is common to many different classes of antibiotics.

cephalosporins, carbapenems, and other antibiotics with this ring structure. In this text, the term *penicillinase* is used when referring to this enzyme's action on penicillins; the term *beta lactamase* is used when referring to other antibiotics. It should be understood, however, that these are two forms of the same enzyme.

To overcome the killing effects of penicillin, some bacteria secrete larger amounts of penicillinase when exposed to

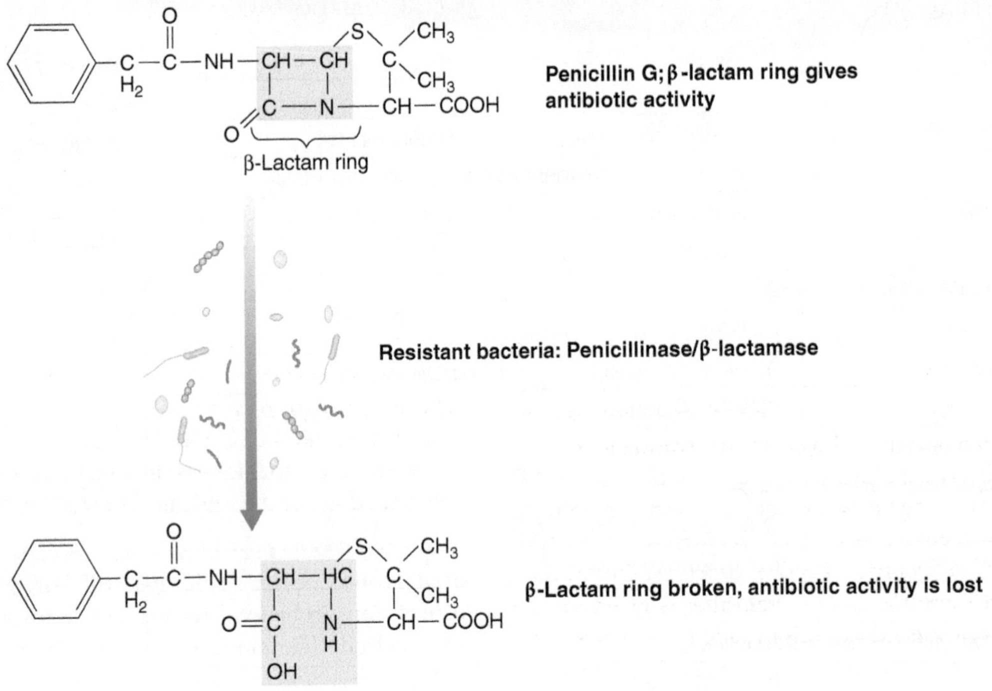

Figure 4

Action of penicillinase.

antibiotics. In addition, the genes encoding for penicillinase can be transferred to other bacteria through conjugation, thus spreading the development of resistance genes.

Although each drug in this class has certain unique properties, some generalizations may be made about the penicillins:

- Most are more effective against gram-positive bacteria, although a few have activity against gram-negative bacteria.
- Most have a narrow spectrum of antimicrobial activity.
- They are widely distributed to most body tissues, although only small amounts reach the cerebrospinal fluid (CSF).
- Nearly all are rapidly excreted by the kidneys.
- Most have short half-lives.

Allergic reactions are the most common adverse effects of the penicillins and ones that require careful attention by nurses. The overall incidence of penicillin allergy ranges from 0.7% to 10%. Symptoms range from mild rash and nausea to fever or anaphylaxis. Although the incidence of anaphylaxis is low, ranging from 0.04% to 2%, mortality is high and nurses must take every precaution to identify patients at highest risk. Allergic reactions may occur within minutes after taking the drug, or they may be delayed for several days or weeks.

Prior exposure to penicillin is necessary for an allergic reaction, although this exposure may have occurred inadvertently through exposure to mold or by eating animal products that contain small amounts of penicillin. Allergy to one penicillin increases the risk of allergy to other drugs in this class. There is also a degree of cross-hypersensitivity between penicillins and cephalosporins. The nurse should not give penicillin to a patient who has a medical history of serious penicillin allergy. If penicillin must be given due to a patient's condition, and it is unknown if the patient is allergic, skin tests may be used to assess the risk of experiencing a severe allergic reaction. Giving a small amount of penicillin and waiting to see if anaphylaxis develops is not an acceptable method for assessing the probability of allergy. The size of a dose is not related to the severity of the response, because even very small amounts can elicit anaphylaxis in susceptible patients. Nurses must always be vigilant in observing for signs of allergy following penicillin administration, because there is no infallible method for predicting which patient will experience an allergy to the drug.

CONNECTION Checkpoint 50.1

Explain how taking a good medical history can eliminate some allergic reactions to antibiotics. *See Answer to Connection Checkpoint 50.1 on student resource website.*

Chemical modifications to the original molecule have produced drugs that offer several advantages over the natural penicillins, including the following:

- Penicillinase resistance
- Broader antimicrobial spectrum
- Extended spectrum

PharmFACT

The U.S. Food and Drug Administration's Nonprescription Drugs Advisory Committee has determined that there is a lack of evidence to support the benefit of using consumer products, including hand washes, body washes, and others, that contain antibacterial additives (Centers for Disease Control and Prevention [CDC], 2010).

Natural Penicillins

The natural penicillins were the first to be isolated from the fungus *Penicillium*. They are inexpensive and the drugs of choice for susceptible infections.

PROTOTYPE DRUG | Penicillin G

Classification: **Therapeutic:** Antibacterial
Pharmacologic: Cell wall inhibitor, natural penicillin

Therapeutic Effects and Uses: Approved in 1943, penicillin G has a narrow spectrum of activity that includes most gram-positive bacteria. Many gram-negative organisms are resistant to penicillin G. It is a drug of choice for the treatment of infections shown to be susceptible by culture and sensitivity (C&S) testing because it is inexpensive and exhibits few adverse effects. These include susceptible strains of *Staphylococcus*, *Streptococcus*, *Neisseria*, *Actinomyces*, *Bacillus anthracis*, *Clostridium*, *Treponema*, and *Corynebacterium*. Penicillin is given for the prophylaxis of bacterial endocarditis in patients with prosthetic heart valves or congenital heart disease and for those at risk for recurrent bouts of rheumatic fever.

Penicillin G is available as a benzathine, potassium, or a procaine salt; each has slightly different pharmacokinetics. For example, while the intramuscular (IM) administration of penicillin G potassium is rapid, the benzathine and procaine salts are absorbed from an IM site very slowly, over a 24-hour period. However, there is no difference in effectiveness among the three salts because they all dissociate to penicillin G. Penicillin G benzathine and penicillin G procaine are administered IM; penicillin G potassium may be administered by either the IV or IM routes. Penicillin G potassium was once available by the oral (PO) route, but the drug had low bioavailability due to destruction by gastric acid. Penicillin V and amoxicillin are more stable in acid and are used when oral penicillin therapy is desired.

Mechanism of Action: This drug inhibits bacterial wall synthesis by binding PBPs. Penicillin G is bacteriocidal and destroyed by penicillinase.

Pharmacokinetics:

Route(s)	IM, IV
Absorption	Rapid absorption (IM)
Distribution	Widely distributed; only small amounts cross the blood–brain barrier; secreted in breast milk; approximately 60% bound to plasma proteins
Primary metabolism	15–30% metabolized, primarily hepatic
Primary excretion	Renal
Onset of action	IM: 15–30 min; IV: immediate
Duration of action	4–6 h; half-life: 20–60 min

Adverse Effects: Penicillin G is well tolerated by most patients and adverse effects are uncommon. Urticaria and delayed skin reactions occasionally occur. The most serious adverse effect is severe hypersensitivity reaction. The anaphylactic response may include cardiovascular collapse; edema of the mouth, tongue, pharynx, and larynx; confusion; seizures; and hallucinations. While most allergic reactions to penicillin occur with minutes after administration, late hypersensitivity reactions may occur several weeks into the regimen.

Contraindications/Precautions: Penicillin G is contraindicated in patients who are allergic to any drug in the penicillin class and is used cautiously in those with hypersensitivity to cephalosporins. In cases where penicillin G is the only effective antibiotic in a patient with a known allergy to the drug, penicillin may be given via a desensitization procedure whereby the dose begins very small and gradually increases. Because 90% of a dose of penicillin G is excreted unchanged by the kidneys through tubular secretion, patients with significant renal impairment must be carefully monitored. Patients with heart failure should not receive the penicillin sodium salt. Hyperkalemia may result with high doses of the penicillin G potassium salt.

Drug Interactions: Penicillin G may decrease the effectiveness of oral contraceptives. Colestipol will decrease the absorption of penicillin. Probenecid decreases the excretion of penicillin G and can lead to antibiotic toxicity. Potassium-sparing diuretics such as spironolactone may cause hyperkalemia when administered with penicillin G potassium. Because penicillins can antagonize the actions of aminoglycoside antibiotics, drugs from these two classes are not administered concurrently. The bacteriostatic action of tetracyclines may inhibit the bacteriocidal action of penicillin G. **Herbal/Food:** Unknown.

Pregnancy: Category B.

Treatment of Overdose: No specific therapy is available. Patients are treated symptomatically.

Nursing Responsibilities: Key nursing implications for patients receiving penicillin G are included in the Nursing Practice Application for Patients Receiving Penicillin, Cephalosporin, or Vancomycin Therapy.

Lifespan and Diversity Considerations:

- Monitor hepatic and renal function laboratory values more frequently in the older adult because normal physiological changes related to aging may affect the drug's metabolism and excretion.

- Monitor cardiac status in the older adult receiving penicillin G. Undetected cardiac disease may increase the likelihood of adverse effects related to the sodium or potassium salt base.

- Carefully monitor for diarrhea in the infant and young child as well as the older adult. Cases of *Clostridium difficile*–associated diarrhea (CDAD) and pseudomembranous colitis (PMC) have been reported with antibiotic use, greatly increasing the risk of fluid and electrolyte imbalances and a risk for severe bowel effects in all patients, but especially in these populations.

Patient and Family Education:

- Immediately report severe or persistent diarrhea accompanied by fever to the health care provider. Do not attempt to treat antibiotic-related diarrhea with over-the-counter (OTC) products.

Drugs Similar to Penicillin G

Other natural penicillins include penicillin G benzathine, penicillin G procaine, and penicillin V.

Penicillin G benzathine (Bicillin): Approved in 1943, penicillin G benzathine dissociates to form penicillin G; thus they share the same actions, indications, and adverse effects. Penicillin G benzathine is given only by the IM route and is absorbed very slowly, resulting in low peak serum levels with a prolonged duration of action that can last up to 26 days. Neurologic adverse effects have been reported with penicillin G benzathine, including severe agitation, confusion, hallucinations, and seizures. Injections of this drug are painful and injection-site reactions may occur. Permanent neurologic damage occurs if this drug is injected near a nerve. This drug is pregnancy category B.

Penicillin G procaine (Wycillin): Approved in 1943, penicillin G procaine is a repository form of penicillin given only by the IM route. Like the benzathine salt, it is absorbed slowly from its injection site and has a prolonged duration of action (15–20 hours). It shares the same actions, indications, and adverse effects as penicillin G. The procaine salt is less painful on administration than penicillin G administered by the IM route. Penicillin G procaine can cause neurotoxicity if the drug is accidentally injected near a nerve. Like the benzathine salt, neurologic adverse effects can occur with penicillin G procaine, including severe agitation, confusion, hallucinations, and seizures. Patients with allergies to the local anesthetic procaine (Novocain) should not receive this drug. This drug is pregnancy category B.

Penicillin V: Penicillin V is nearly identical to penicillin G, except that it is more acid stable, which allows it to be administered by the PO route. However, it should be taken on an empty stomach to maximize absorption. Approved in 1956, it shares the same actions, indications, and adverse effects as penicillin G. Some patients experience nausea, vomiting, and diarrhea. This drug is pregnancy category B.

Broad-Spectrum Penicillins (Aminopenicillins)

A major limitation of the natural penicillins is their lack of activity against gram-negative organisms. The aminopenicillins, amoxicillin and ampicillin, are effective against gram-positive and certain gram-negative bacilli such as *Haemophilus influenzae*, *Escherichia coli*, *Salmonella*, and *Shigella*. This distinction is responsible for them being placed into a separate class called broad-spectrum penicillins.

Aminopenicillins are rapidly inactivated by penicillinase, which limits their therapeutic usefulness, particularly against *Staphylococcus aureus* infections. Despite this limitation, the aminopenicillins are some of the most widely prescribed antibiotics for sinus and upper respiratory and genitourinary tract infections. Their widespread use over many decades has resulted in the emergence of a large number of resistant strains.

Combination drugs have been developed that offer certain advantages over single-drug therapy with aminopenicillins. The fixed-dose combination of Augmentin combines amoxicillin with clavulanate, a beta-lactamase (penicillinase) inhibitor.

Another fixed-dose product, Unasyn, contains ampicillin and the beta-lactamase inhibitor sulbactam. By inhibiting penicillinase, these combined agents allow a greater percentage of the aminopenicillin molecules to reach pathogens and affect cell wall synthesis. The beta-lactamase inhibitors are ineffective when used alone and therefore are always used in fixed combination formulations with other drugs.

PROTOTYPE DRUG	Ampicillin (Principen)

Classification: **Therapeutic:** Antibacterial
Pharmacologic: Cell wall inhibitor, aminopenicillin

Therapeutic Effects and Uses: Approved in 1963, the actions of ampicillin are similar to those of penicillin G except that ampicillin has a broader spectrum that includes enhanced activity over enterococci, *E. coli*, *Proteus mirabilis*, *Neisseria gonorrhoeae*, *H. influenzae*, *Salmonella*, *Shigella*, and *Bordetella pertussis*. Because a large percentage of resistant strains have developed, ampicillin is no longer a drug of choice for the treatment of gonococcal infections, childhood meningitis, or *Salmonella* or *Shigella* enteritis.

Mechanism of Action: Ampicillin inhibits bacterial wall synthesis by binding PBPs. This drug is bacteriocidal and inactivated by penicillinase.

Pharmacokinetics:

Route(s)	PO, IM, and IV
Absorption	50% absorbed PO
Distribution	Widely distributed; only small amounts cross the blood–brain barrier; secreted in breast milk; plasma protein binding is about 15–20%
Primary metabolism	Largely unmetabolized, 10% hepatic
Primary excretion	Renal
Onset of action	PO: 30–60 min; IM: 15–30 min
Duration of action	Half-life: 1–2 h

Adverse Effects: Ampicillin is a safe drug that rarely produces serious adverse effects. Rash and diarrhea are the most common adverse effects, and diarrhea occurs more frequently with ampicillin than with the other aminopenicillins. Pain at the injection site is common. Like all penicillins, anaphylaxis is rare, though potentially fatal. Anaphylactic response may include cardiovascular collapse; edema of the mouth, tongue, pharynx, and larynx; confusion; seizure; and hallucinations. Pseudomembranous colitis is an additional rare, though serious, severe adverse effect. Very high doses may produce confusion and seizures.

Contraindications/Precautions: Ampicillin is contraindicated in patients who are allergic to any drug in the penicillin class and used cautiously in those with hypersensitivity to cephalosporins. Ampicillin is excreted primarily by the kidneys; therefore, drug therapy must be monitored carefully in patients with renal disease.

Drug Interactions: Ampicillin may decrease the effectiveness of oral contraceptives. Probenecid (Benemid) decreases the excretion of ampicillin and can lead to antibiotic toxicity. Penicillins can antagonize the actions of aminoglycoside antibiotics and must be administered at least 2 hours apart. The antibacterial actions of ampicillin are diminished when it is taken concurrently with chloramphenicol, erythromycin, or tetracyclines. **Herbal/Food:** Because food decreases its absorption, ampicillin should be taken on an empty stomach.

Pregnancy: Category B.

Treatment of Overdose: No specific therapy is available. Patients are treated symptomatically.

Nursing Responsibilities: Key nursing implications for patients receiving ampicillin are included in the Nursing Practice Application for Patients Receiving Penicillin, Cephalosporin, or Vancomycin Therapy.

Lifespan and Diversity Considerations:

- Monitor renal function laboratory values more frequently in the older adult because normal physiological changes related to aging may affect the drug's excretion.

- Monitor renal function laboratory values and urine output more frequently in the neonate or young infant because normal renal immaturity in these stages may increase the risk of adverse renal effects.

- Carefully monitor for diarrhea in the infant and young child as well as the older adult. Cases of CDAD and PMC have been reported with antibiotic use, greatly increasing the risk of fluid and electrolyte imbalances and the risk for severe bowel effects in all patients, but especially in these populations.

Patient and Family Education:

- Immediately report severe or persistent diarrhea accompanied by fever to the health care provider. Do not attempt to treat antibiotic-related diarrhea with OTC products.

- Immediately report any disorientation or confusion to the provider. These may be symptoms of an excessive dose or other adverse effects.

Drugs Similar to Ampicillin (Principen)

The only other aminopenicillin is amoxicillin.

Amoxicillin (Amoxil, Trimox): Approved in 1974, amoxicillin is closely related structurally to ampicillin and has many of the same characteristics. The drug is destroyed by penicillinase-producing organisms. It is more acid stable than ampicillin and offers greater gastrointestinal (GI) absorption with peak serum levels twice as high. It exhibits a lower incidence of diarrhea than ampicillin. Amoxicillin has largely replaced ampicillin, and it is one of the most frequently prescribed antibiotics. Amoxicillin should not be administered to patients with hypersensitivity to any penicillin. An extended release form of the drug (Moxatag) was approved in 2008 for treating *Streptococcus pyogenes* infections. This drug is pregnancy category B.

Extended-Spectrum (Antipseudomonal) Penicillins

Piperacillin and ticarcillin have broad spectrums of antimicrobial activity similar to those of the aminopenicillins. Their primary advantage is their additional activity against *Pseudomonas aeruginosa*; thus they are called extended-spectrum or antipseudomonal penicillins. A third drug in this class, carbenicillin, is no longer marketed in the United States.

P. aeruginosa is an opportunistic pathogen found in air, soil, and water. It can persist on environmental surfaces such as soap residues and hot tubs and can even survive in some antiseptic solutions. *P. aeruginosa* infections may occur anywhere in the body, primarily causing disease in patients whose health is already compromised in some manner. It is responsible for about 10% of all health care–associated infections (HAIs), including serious pneumonia in debilitated patients and a large number of infections in wounds and in patients with extensive burns.

P. aeruginosa has natural resistance to most antibiotics due in part to its ability to rapidly pump out antibiotic molecules that enter its cells. Because *Pseudomonas* infections are often persistent, aggressive combination anti-infective therapy is often indicated. A typical combination includes an aminoglycoside antibiotic with an antipseudomonal penicillin. Because penicillins inactivate aminoglycosides, they must be administered at least 2 hours apart. Other antibiotics such as ceftazidime (Ceptaz, Fortaz, Tazicef), ciprofloxacin (Cipro), or imipenem (Primaxin) may be needed.

As with the other penicillins, drugs in this class inhibit bacterial wall synthesis by binding PBPs. The antipseudomonal penicillins achieve their extended spectrum because they have greater penetration through the outer membrane of gram-negative bacteria and a higher affinity for penicillin-binding proteins. The two drugs in this class are similar, and there are few differences on which to distinguish them. Like most penicillins, the antipseudomonal penicillins are widely distributed to tissues and rapidly excreted mostly unchanged in the urine.

Because penicillinase-producing bacteria can inactivate the antipseudomonal penicillins, they are usually combined with a beta-lactamase inhibitor. Fixed-dose combinations with beta-lactamase inhibitors include piperacillin with tazobactam (Zosyn) and ticarcillin with clavulanate (Timentin).

Rash and diarrhea are the most common adverse effects of the antipseudomonal penicillins. These drugs prevent the aggregation of platelets, which can prolong bleeding time. Caution must therefore be used when using these drugs concurrently with agents that modify coagulation. Sodium salts of the antipseudomonal penicillins cause sodium overload in patients with heart failure. Like all penicillins, anaphylaxis is rare, though potentially fatal. PMC is an additional severe adverse effect. Very high doses may produce confusion and seizures. The antipseudomonal penicillins are pregnancy category B.

Piperacillin: Approved in 1981, piperacillin has one of the broadest spectrums of any of the penicillins and is effective against most gram-negative and many gram-positive anaerobic and aerobic microbes. It has been used to treat a variety of serious infections, including those of the skin, blood, sinuses, central nervous system (CNS), respiratory tract, and genitourinary tract. Available by the IM and IV routes, piperacillin is often used in combination with an aminoglycoside antibiotic because together they exert synergistic action on gram-negative microbes. High doses can lead to platelet dysfunction, although piperacillin seems to have less effect than other anti-pseudomonal penicillins. Electrolytes should be regularly monitored to prevent hypokalemia and hypernatremia. Piperacillin should not be administered to patients with hypersensitivity to any penicillin. Localized injection-site reactions include pain, inflammation, phlebitis, and hematomas. Zosyn is a fixed-dose combination of piperacillin and tazobactam.

Ticarcillin-clavulanate (Timentin): As with piperacillin, ticarcillin has one of the broadest spectrums of any penicillin. Approved in 1976, it has been used to treat moderate to severe gram-negative infections of the skin, blood, bone and joints, CNS, respiratory tract, and genitourinary tract. Available by the IV route, high doses can lead to hypernatremia, platelet dysfunction, and hypokalemia. Electrolytes should be regularly monitored to prevent hypokalemia and hypernatremia. Ticarcillin has a high sodium content that could affect patients with preexisting heart disease. Ticarcillin should not be administered to patients with hypersensitivity to any penicillin. Pain and phlebitis with thrombosis may occur at the injection site. To increase its effectiveness, it is combined with clavulanate.

Penicillinase-Resistant (Antistaphylococcal) Penicillins

The final subclass of penicillins includes dicloxacillin, nafcillin, and oxacillin, which are drugs that are effective against penicillinase-producing bacteria. These agents are less effective than penicillin G against non-penicillinase-producing strains and are ineffective against gram-negative bacteria. This narrow spectrum of activity has largely restricted their use to penicillinase-producing strains of *Staphylococcus*. Because they are often the preferred drugs for infections by this organism, they are referred to as antistaphylococcal penicillins. An older drug in this class, cloxacillin (Cloxapen), is no longer marketed in the United States.

The emergence of many methicillin-resistant *S. aureus* (MRSA) strains has limited the use of this class of drugs. As discussed in Chapter 49, the appearance of MRSA strains that are resistant to all penicillins is an emerging clinical problem. The first drug developed in the penicillinase-resistant class, called methicillin, was removed from the U.S. market for producing an unacceptable incidence of interstitial nephritis.

Drugs in the penicillinase-resistant class share similar actions and properties with penicillin G. They are only administered by the PO route, where they are readily absorbed, especially on an empty stomach. They are rapidly excreted by the kidneys, having a half-life of 30 to 60 minutes. As with all penicillins, hypersensitivity reactions may occur. Some of

these agents are sodium salts, which may cause sodium overload in susceptible patients. PMC has been reported in a small number of patients taking these drugs. All are pregnancy category B drugs.

Dicloxacillin: Approved in 1968, dicloxacillin is a penicillinase-resistant penicillin available by the PO route. As with other drugs in this class, its use is primarily limited to the treatment of susceptible staphylococcal infections. It is not effective against MRSA. It exhibits more reliable GI absorption than nafcillin, but nausea and vomiting are commonly reported adverse effects. It should be taken on an empty stomach to enhance absorption. Other adverse effects and contraindications are the same as those of other penicillins. This drug should not be given to a patient with hypersensitivity to any penicillin.

Nafcillin: Approved in 1964, nafcillin is used to treat susceptible infections of the blood, skin, upper and lower respiratory tract, bone and joints, and urinary tract. It is ineffective against MRSA infections. Unlike most penicillins, nafcillin undergoes enterohepatic circulation and is excreted primarily in the bile; thus dosage adjustments for patients with hepatic disease are necessary. It is available in both oral and parenteral formulations. Because only 10% to 20% of the drug is absorbed when given PO, it should be taken on an empty stomach. The complete blood count (CBC) must be regularly monitored because nafcillin can cause neutropenia and other blood abnormalities in 10% to 20% of the patients taking it. This drug should not be given to a patient with hypersensitivity to any penicillin.

Oxacillin: Approved in 1962, oxacillin is used to treat a variety of staphylococcal infections of the blood, skin, upper and lower respiratory tract, bone and joints, and urinary tract. It is ineffective against MRSA infections. Because oxacillin causes fewer injection-site reactions than nafcillin, it is sometimes the parenteral agent of choice in its class. It is also available

Lifespan Considerations
Antibiotic Use in the Older Adult

Older adults may forego filling an expensive antibiotic prescription due to lack of adequate drug coverage on their insurance. Studies have noted that as the cost of the drug and the amount of cost sharing (copay) required increases, the number of prescriptions filled decreases. As with other drugs, newer antibiotics may be costly, and an older generic version may not be available to treat the infection. Because the older adult may not exhibit the same symptoms of an infection as a younger patient will, an untreated infection may quickly become more serious. Recent changes to Medicare and the implementation of the drug benefit (Part D) portion may increase the number of prescriptions filled. In a recent study, Zhang, Lee, and Donohue (2010) noted that as Medicare drug coverage improved, older adults increased their use of broad-spectrum, newer, and more expensive antibiotics. While this may be a double-edged sword with inappropriate use also occurring, it lessens the chance that an infection will remain untreated due to cost concerns.

by the PO route, but absorption is poor and it should be taken on an empty stomach. Indications and adverse effects are similar to those of other penicillinase-resistant penicillins. This drug should not be given to a patient with hypersensitivity to any penicillin.

Cephalosporins

3 The cephalosporins are similar in structure and function to the penicillins and are widely prescribed for gram-negative infections.

Isolated shortly after penicillin, the cephalosporins comprise the largest antibiotic class. Like the penicillins, many cephalosporins contain a beta-lactam ring that is responsible for their antimicrobial activity. In some cephalosporins, the structure of the beta-lactam ring is quite stable and resistant to enzyme destruction. The cephalosporins are bacteriocidal and inhibit cell wall synthesis by binding to PBPs. Growing bacterial cells are unable to build their cell walls properly, and lysis occurs in the same manner as penicillins. The cephalosporins are listed in Table 2.

The primary therapeutic use of the cephalosporins is for gram-negative infections and for patients who are allergic to penicillin or who have penicillin-resistant infections. Over 20 cephalosporins are available, all having similar sounding names that can challenge even the best memory. Selection of a specific cephalosporin is first based on the sensitivity of the pathogen, and secondly on possible adverse effects.

The cephalosporins are classified chronologically by their generations, which are loosely based on differences in their spectrums of microbial activity. It is important to note that the placement of a drug in a particular generation is somewhat arbitrary and has little therapeutic usefulness. Drugs within each generation have different chemical structures, routes of administration, and spectrums of activity. Scientists do not always agree on placement. The following generalizations may be made regarding the generations:

- First-generation cephalosporins contain a beta-lactam ring; bacteria that produce beta lactamase are usually resistant to these drugs. They are the most effective cephalosporins against gram-positive bacteria, including staphylococci and streptococci and are sometimes the drugs of choice for these organisms. First-generation cephalosporins have

TABLE 2 Cephalosporins		
Drug	**Route and Adult Dose (maximum dose where indicated)**	**Adverse Effects**
First Generation		
cefadroxil (Duricef)	PO: 500 mg–1 g once or twice a day (max: 2 g/day)	*Diarrhea, abdominal cramping, nausea, fatigue, rash, pruritus, pain at injection sites, oral or vaginal candidiasis*
cefazolin (Ancef, Kefzol)	IM: 250 mg–2 g tid (max: 12 g/day)	
cephalexin (Keflex)	PO: 250–500 mg qid (max: 4 g/day)	
Second Generation		Pseudomembranous colitis, nephrotoxicity, anaphylaxis
cefaclor (Ceclor)	PO: 250–500 mg tid (max: 2 g/day)	
cefotetan (Cefotan)	IV/IM: 1–2 g every 12 h (max: 6 g/day)	
cefoxitin (Mefoxin)	IV/IM: 1–2 g every 6–8 h (max: 12 g/day)	
cefprozil (Cefzil)	PO: 250–500 mg 1–2 times/day (max: 1 g/day)	
cefuroxime (Ceftin, Zinacef)	PO (Ceftin): 250–500 mg bid (max: 1 g/day) IM/IV (Zinacef): 750 mg–1.5 g every 8 h (max: 9 g/day)	
Third Generation		
cefdinir (Omnicef)	PO: 300 mg bid (max: 600 mg/day)	
cefditoren (Spectracef)	PO: 400 mg bid for 10 days (max: 800 mg/day)	
cefixime (Suprax)	PO: 400 mg/day or 200 mg bid (max: 800 mg/day)	
cefotaxime (Claforan)	IM: 1–2 g bid–tid (max: 12 g/day)	
cefpodoxime (Vantin)	PO: 200 mg every 12 h for 10 days (max: 800 mg/day)	
ceftazidime (Fortaz, Tazicef)	IV/IM: 1–2 mg every 8–12 h (max: 6 g/day)	
ceftibuten (Cedax)	PO: 400 mg/day for 10 days (max: 400 mg/day)	
ceftizoxime (Cefizox)	IV/IM: 1–2 g every 8–12 h, up to 2 g every 4 h (max: 12 g/day)	
ceftriaxone (Rocephin)	IV/IM: 1–2 g every 12–24 h (max: 4 g/day)	
Fourth Generation		
cefepime (Maxipime)	IV/IM: 0.5–1 g every 12 h for 7–10 days (max: 6 g/day)	
Fifth Generation		
ceftaroline (Teflaro)	IV: 600 mg every 12 h for 5–14 days	

Note: Italics indicate common adverse effects. <u>Underline</u> indicates serious adverse effects.

only moderate activity against gram-negative bacteria. First-generation drugs do not cross the blood–brain barrier to any appreciable extent.

- Second-generation cephalosporins exhibit a broader spectrum against gram-negative organisms than do the first-generation agents. They are more potent and less sensitive to beta lactamase than the first-generation drugs. Like the first-generation agents, however, they are unable to enter the CSF in sufficient concentration to treat infections of the CNS. In general, the second-generation agents have largely been replaced by third-generation cephalosporins.

- Third-generation cephalosporins exhibit an even broader spectrum against gram-negative bacteria than the second-generation agents. They generally have a longer duration of action and are resistant to beta lactamase. These cephalosporins are sometimes the drugs of choice against infections by *Pseudomonas, Klebsiella, Neisseria, Salmonella, Proteus,* and *H. influenzae.* Third-generation drugs are able to enter the CSF to treat CNS infections.

- Fourth-generation cephalosporins have a similar antimicrobial spectrum to third-generation agents but are more effective against organisms that have developed resistance to earlier cephalosporins. Fourth-generation drugs are capable of entering the CSF in sufficiently high concentrations to treat CNS infections.

- Fifth-generation cephalosporins are broad-spectrum drugs with extended gram-positive effectiveness. They are designed to be effective against MRSA infections. This generation is still in development and the first drug, ceftaroline, was approved in 2010.

CONNECTION Checkpoint 50.2

What is the primary difference in physiology that distinguishes a gram-positive organism from a gram-negative organism? *See Answer to Connection Checkpoint 50.2 on student resource website.*

Over decades of use, many bacterial strains have developed resistance to the cephalosporins. Like the penicillins, the primary mechanism of resistance is the secretion of beta-lactamase enzymes (sometimes called cephalosporinases). Although third-generation agents were initially unaffected by beta lactamase, resistant strains that can inactivate drugs in this generation have been identified. None of the cephalosporins has significant activity against MRSA or penicillin-resistant *Streptococcus pneumoniae.*

In general, the cephalosporins are safe drugs with adverse effects similar to those of the penicillins. Allergic reactions are the most common adverse effect. Although sometimes prescribed for patients who are allergic to penicillin, nurses must be aware that 5% to 10% of the patients who are allergic to penicillin will also exhibit hypersensitivity to cephalosporins. Despite this small incidence of cross-allergy, the cephalosporins offer a reasonable alternative for patients who are unable to take penicillin. Cephalosporins are contraindicated, however, for patients who have experienced anaphylaxis following penicillin exposure.

In addition to allergy, rash and GI complaints are common adverse effects of cephalosporins. Nurses should continually assess for the presence of superinfections. Because cephalosporins are secreted in small amounts in breast milk, they should be used with caution in nursing mothers.

Nearly all cephalosporins are eliminated by the kidneys. Earlier-generation cephalosporins exhibited kidney toxicity but this is diminished with the later-generation drugs in this class. Patients with preexisting renal impairment or those who are concurrently receiving nephrotoxic drugs should be monitored carefully during therapy with any cephalosporin. Kidney function tests should be evaluated on a regular basis.

Other adverse effects are specific to particular cephalosporins. For example, cefotetan interferes with vitamin K metabolism and increases the risk of bleeding due to hypoprothrombinemia. Nurses must carefully monitor prothrombin time (PT) in patients taking these drugs, particularly those who are concurrently taking anticoagulants. Cefotetan produces a disulfiram-like reaction when taken concurrently with alcohol. Cephalosporins cause pain at IM injection sites, and thrombophlebitis can occur when given IV. Over half of the cephalosporins are only administered parenterally.

PROTOTYPE DRUG | Cefazolin (Ancef, Kefzol)

Classification: **Therapeutic:** Antibacterial
Pharmacologic: Cell wall inhibitor, first-generation cephalosporin

Therapeutic Effects and Uses: Approved in 1973, cefazolin is a beta-lactam antibiotic used for the treatment and prophylaxis of bacterial infections, particularly those that are caused by susceptible gram-positive organisms. Its effectiveness extends to nonpencillinase- and penicillinase-producing *S. aureus* and streptococci (except enterococci). Cefazolin is not effective against MRSA. Cefazolin has been used to treat infections of the respiratory tract, urinary tract, skin structures, biliary tract, bones, and joints. It has also been useful in the pharmacotherapy of genital infections, septicemia, and endocarditis. This drug is sometimes used for infection prophylaxis in patients who are undergoing surgical procedures. Cefazolin has a longer half-life than other first-generation cephalosporins, which allows for less frequent dosing. It is one of the most frequently prescribed parenteral antibiotics.

Mechanism of Action: Cefazolin inhibits bacterial wall synthesis by binding to specific PBPs. The drug is bacteriocidal, exhibits a broad spectrum, and is sensitive to beta lactamase.

Pharmacokinetics:

Route(s)	IM and IV
Absorption	Well absorbed when given IM
Distribution	Widely distributed; only small amounts cross the blood–brain barrier; crosses the placenta; secreted in breast milk; about 85% bound to plasma protein
Primary metabolism	Not metabolized
Primary excretion	Renal
Onset of action	Immediate
Duration of action	Half-life: 90–135 min

Adverse Effects: Like the penicillins, the cephalosporins are well tolerated by most patients. Rash and diarrhea are the most common adverse effects, and superinfections are likely when the antibiotic is used for prolonged periods. Approximately 1% to 4% of patients will experience some kind of an allergic reaction. Severe hypersensitivity reactions are rare, though potentially fatal. Anaphylactic response may include cardiovascular collapse; edema of the mouth, tongue, pharynx, and larynx; confusion; seizures; and hallucinations. Pain and phlebitis can occur at IM injection sites. However, cefazolin causes less pain than do other cephalosporins. Seizures are a rare, though potentially serious, adverse effect of cephalosporin therapy.

Contraindications/Precautions: Cefazolin is contraindicated in patients who are allergic to any drug in the cephalosporin class and is used cautiously in those with hypersensitivity to penicillins. Because most cefazolin is excreted unchanged by the kidneys, patients with significant renal impairment must be carefully monitored.

Drug Interactions: Probenecid decreases the excretion of cefazolin and can lead to antibiotic toxicity. Concurrent use of cefazolin with nephrotoxic drugs, such as aminoglycosides or vancomycin, increases the risk of nephrotoxicity. Cefazolin may have additive or synergistic antimicrobial action with other antibiotics such as aztreonam, carbapenems, and the penicillins. The anticoagulant effect of warfarin may be increased if given concurrently with cefazolin. **Herbal/Food**: None known.

Pregnancy: Category B.

Treatment of Overdose: No specific therapy is available. Patients are treated symptomatically.

Nursing Responsibilities (includes all generations of cephalosporins): Key nursing implications for patients receiving cefazolin are included in the Nursing Practice Application for Patients Receiving Penicillin, Cephalosporin, or Vancomycin Therapy.

Lifespan and Diversity Considerations:
* Monitor renal function laboratory values more frequently in the older adult because normal physiological changes related to aging may affect the drug's excretion.
* Monitor renal function laboratory values and urine output more frequently in the neonate or young infant because normal renal immaturity in these stages may increase the risk of adverse renal effects.
* Carefully monitor for diarrhea in the infant and young child as well as the older adult. Cases of CDAD and PMC have been reported with antibiotic use, greatly increasing the risk of fluid and electrolyte imbalances and the risk for severe bowel effects in all patients, but especially in these populations.

Patient and Family Education:
* Consult the health care provider or pharmacist before drinking alcoholic beverages. For some cephalosporins, this can cause a disulfiram-like reaction with symptoms that include flushing, throbbing in the head and neck, respiratory difficulty, nausea, vomiting, sweating, thirst, chest pain, blurred vision, and confusion.
* Immediately report severe or persistent diarrhea accompanied by fever to the health care provider. Do not attempt to treat antibiotic-related diarrhea with OTC products.

Drugs Similar to Cefazolin (Ancef, Kefzol)

First generation: Other first-generation cephalosporins include cefadroxil (Duricef) and cephalexin (Keflex). These drugs are administered parenterally and have the same spectrum of microbial activity. They have the same basic indications (primarily gram-positive bacteria) and are eliminated by the kidneys. Cephradine (Velosef) is no longer available in the United States.

Second generation: Second-generation cephalosporins include cefaclor (Ceclor), cefotetan (Cefotan), cefoxitin (Mefoxin), cefprozil (Cefzil), and cefuroxime (Ceftin, Zinacef). All have the same spectrum of microbial activity and there is little difference among the drugs other than the route of administration (see Table 2). The kidneys eliminate all second-generation cephalosporins. Cefoxitin and cefotetan are the most active against *Bacteroides fragilis*.

Third generation: Third-generation cephalosporins are the largest group and include cefdinir (Omnicef), cefditoren (Spectracef), cefixime (Suprax), cefotaxime (Claforan), cefpodoxime (Vantin), ceftazidime (Fortaz, Tazicef), ceftibuten (Cedax), ceftizoxime (Cefizox), and ceftriaxone (Rocephin). The differences among third-generation cephalosporins are minor. Some are available by the PO route, whereas others are given only parenterally (see Table 2). Cefixime and ceftriaxone have longer durations that allow for once-daily dosing. Ceftazidime is one of the few third-generation drugs with significant activity against *P. aeruginosa*. Cefotaxime is a preferred drug for certain types of meningitis and for infection prophylaxis in patients who are undergoing surgical procedures. Cefoperazone (Cefobid) is no longer available in the United States.

Fourth generation: Cefepime (Maxipime) is the only drug in this generation. It is very similar to the third-generation drugs but appears to have a slightly broader spectrum of activity and is more stable against beta lactamase–producing organisms. It has been used for the treatment of serious infections in hospitalized patients with gram-positive microorganisms such as *Enterobacteriaceae*, and *Pseudomonas*. It is not effective against MRSA.

Fifth Generation: Ceftaroline (Teflaro), the first drug in this generation, was approved by the FDA in 2010 for acute bacterial skin and skin structure infections and community-acquired bacterial pneumonia. It is effective against a broad spectrum of both gram-positive and gram-negative organisms, including MRSA. Available by the IV route, it is relatively safe, with the most common adverse effects being diarrhea, nausea, and rash.

CONNECTIONS: NURSING PRACTICE APPLICATION

Patients Receiving Penicillin, Cephalosporin, or Vancomycin Therapy

Assessment	Potential Nursing Diagnoses
Baseline assessment prior to administration: • Understand the reason the drug has been prescribed in order to assess for therapeutic effects. • Obtain a complete health history including neurologic, cardiovascular, respiratory, hepatic, or renal disease, and the possibility of pregnancy. Obtain a drug history including allergies, specific reactions to drugs, current prescription and OTC drugs, herbal preparations, and alcohol use. Be alert to possible drug interactions. • Assess signs and symptoms of the current infection noting location, characteristics (what it looks like), presence or absence of drainage and the character of drainage, duration, and the presence or absence of fever or pain. • Evaluate appropriate laboratory findings (e.g., CBC, C&S, hepatic and renal function studies). • Assess the patient's ability to receive and understand instructions. Include family and caregivers as needed. **Assessment throughout administration:** • Assess for desired therapeutic effects (e.g., diminished signs and symptoms of infection and fever). • Continue periodic monitoring of CBC, hepatic and renal function, urinalysis, and C&S as ordered. • Assess for adverse effects: nausea, vomiting, abdominal cramping, diarrhea, drowsiness, or dizziness. Severe diarrhea, especially containing mucus, blood, or pus, yellowing of the sclera or skin, decreased urine output, or darkened urine should be reported immediately.	• *Acute Pain* • *Hyperthermia* • *Deficient Knowledge* (Drug Therapy) • *Risk for Injury*, related to adverse drug effects • *Risk for Deficient Fluid Volume*, related to fever and/or diarrhea caused by adverse drug effects

Planning: Patient Goals and Expected Outcomes

The patient will:

• Experience therapeutic effects dependent on the reason the drug is being given (e.g., diminished signs and symptoms of infection, decreased fever).
• Be free from or experience minimal adverse effects.
• Verbalize an understanding of the drug's use, adverse effects, and required precautions.
• Demonstrate proper self-administration of the medication (e.g., dose, timing, and when to notify the provider).

Implementation

Interventions and (Rationales)	Patient-Centered Care
Ensuring therapeutic effects: • Continue assessments as above for therapeutic effects. (Diminished fever, pain, or signs and symptoms of infection should begin after taking the first dose and continue to improve. The provider should be notified if fever and signs and symptoms of infection remain or increase after 3 days or if the entire course of antibacterial has been taken and signs of infection are still present.)	• Teach the patient to report fever that does not diminish below 37.8°C (100°F) or per parameters set by the health care provider within 3 days, increasing signs and symptoms of infection, or symptoms that remain after taking the entire course of antibacterial therapy. • Teach the patient *not* to stop taking the antibacterial when feeling better but to take the entire course of antibacterial therapy; to not share doses with other family members with similar symptoms; and to return to the provider if symptoms have not resolved after an entire course of therapy.
Minimizing adverse effects: • Continue to monitor vital signs, especially temperature if fever is present. Immediately report undiminished fever, changes in level of consciousness (LOC), or febrile seizures to the health care provider. (Fever should begin to diminish within 1–3 days after starting the drug. Continued fever may be a sign of worsening infection, adverse drug effects, or antibiotic resistance.)	• Teach the patient to report a fever that does not diminish below 37.8°C (100°F) or per the parameters set by the health care provider. Immediately report febrile seizures, changes in behavior, or changes in LOC to the health care provider.
• Continue to monitor periodic laboratory work: renal function tests, CBC, urinalysis, and C&S as ordered. (Penicillins and cephalosporins may be renal toxic and laboratory values should be monitored to prevent adverse effects. Periodic C&S tests may be ordered if infections are severe or are slow to resolve to confirm appropriate therapy.)	• Instruct the patient on the need for periodic laboratory work.
• Monitor for hypersensitivity and allergic reactions, especially with the first dose of the drug. Continue to monitor the patient for up to 2 weeks after completing antibacterial therapy. (Anaphylactic reactions are possible, particularly with the first dose of an antibacterial. As sensitivity occurs, reactions may continue to develop. Post-use, residual drug levels, dependent on length of half-life, may cause delayed reactions.)	• Teach the patient to immediately report any itching, rashes, swelling (particularly of tongue or face), urticaria, flushing, dizziness, syncope, wheezing, throat tightness, or difficulty breathing. • Instruct the patient with known antibacterial allergies to carry a wallet identification card or wear medical identification jewelry indicating allergy.

• Continue to monitor for renal toxicity; e.g., darkened urine, diminished urine output, or weight gain greater than 1 kg (2.2 lbs) in 24 hours. (Penicillins and cephalosporins may require frequent monitoring to prevent adverse effects. Increasing fluid intake will prevent drug accumulation in the kidneys.)	• Teach the patient to immediately report any diminished urine output, weight gain of more than 1 kg (2.2 lbs) in a 24 h period, darkening of urine, ringing, humming, or buzzing in the ears, dizziness, or vertigo. • Advise the patient to increase fluid intake to 2–3 L/day if permitted.
• Monitor for severe diarrhea, especially if mucus, blood, or pus is present. (Severe diarrhea may indicate the presence of CDAD or PMC, superinfections caused by *C. difficile*.)	• Instruct the patient to report any diarrhea that increases in frequency, amount, or contains mucus, blood, or pus. • Instruct the patient to consult the health care provider before taking any antidiarrheal drugs, which cause the retention of harmful bacteria. • Teach the patient to increase intake of dairy products containing live active cultures such as yogurt, kefir, or buttermilk, to help restore normal intestinal flora.
• Monitor for development of superinfections, e.g., PMC, fungal or yeast infections. (Superinfections with opportunistic organisms may occur when normal host flora are diminished or killed by the antibacterial drug and no longer hold pathogens in check. Appropriate treatment may be needed.)	• Teach the patient to observe for changes in stool, white patches in the mouth, whitish thick vaginal discharge, itching in the urogenital area, or blistering itchy rash, and to immediately report severe diarrhea. • Teach the patient infection control measures such as frequent hand washing, allowing for adequate drying after showering or bathing, and to increase intake of live-culture dairy foods.
• Monitor for significant GI effects, including nausea, vomiting, abdominal pain, or cramping. Give the drug with food or milk to decrease adverse GI effects. (Cephalosporins are associated with significant adverse GI effects.)	• Teach the patient to take the drug with food or milk but to avoid acidic foods and beverages or carbonated drinks, which may cause GI distress.
• Monitor for signs and symptoms of neurotoxicity, e.g., dizziness, drowsiness, severe headache, changes in LOC, or seizures. (Penicillins and cephalosporins have an increased risk of neurotoxicity. Previous seizure disorders or head injuries may increase this risk. Frequent monitoring is needed to prevent adverse effects.)	• Instruct the patient to immediately report increasing headache, dizziness, drowsiness, changes in behavior or LOC, or seizures. • Caution the patient that drowsiness may occur and to be cautious with driving or other activities requiring mental alertness until the effects of the drug are known.
• Monitor for development of red man syndrome in patients receiving vancomycin. Report any significantly large area of reddening such as trunk, head, neck, limbs, or gluteal area, especially if associated with decreased blood pressure or tachycardia. (Vancomycin hypersensitivity may cause the release of large amounts of histamine. If a significant area is involved, vasodilation from histamine may cause hypotension and reflex tachycardia. Prevancomycin antihistamines, e.g., diphenhydramine, may be required. Running the IV drip more slowly may prevent or decrease the effects of the syndrome.)	• Instruct the patient to immediately report unusual flushing, especially involving a large body area, dizziness, dyspnea, or palpitations.
• Monitor for signs and symptoms of blood dyscrasias, e.g., low-grade fevers, bleeding, bruising, or significant fatigue. (Penicillins may cause blood dyscrasias with resulting decreases in RBCs, WBCs, and/or platelets. Periodic monitoring of CBC may be required.)	• Teach the patient to report any low-grade fevers, sore throat, rashes, bruising, nosebleeds, increased bleeding, unusual fatigue, or shortness of breath, especially after taking the antibiotic for a prolonged period.
• Monitor electrolytes, pulse, and ECG if indicated in patients on penicillin. (Some preparations of penicillin may be based in sodium or potassium salts and may cause hypernatremia and hyperkalemia.)	• Teach the patient to promptly report any palpitations, lightheadedness, dizziness, or swelling of feet or ankles.
• Women of childbearing age taking oral contraceptives and penicillin antibiotics should use an alternative form of birth control to prevent pregnancy. (Some penicillins may significantly reduce the effectiveness of oral contraceptives.)	• Teach women of childbearing age on oral contraceptives to consult their health care provider about birth control alternatives if penicillin antibiotics are ordered.
Patient understanding of drug therapy: • Use opportunities during administration of medications and during assessments to discuss the rationale for drug therapy, desired therapeutic outcomes, commonly observed adverse effects, parameters for when to call the health care provider, and any necessary monitoring or precautions. (Using time during nursing care helps to optimize and reinforce key teaching areas.)	• The patient, family, or caregiver should be able to state the reason for the drug, appropriate dose and scheduling, what adverse effects to observe for and when to report them, and the anticipated length of medication therapy.

Patient self-administration of drug therapy:
• When administering medications, instruct the patient, family, or caregiver in proper self-administration techniques followed by return demonstration. (Utilizing time during nurse-administration of these drugs helps to reinforce teaching.)
	• Teach the patient to take the medication:
	  • Complete the entire course of therapy unless otherwise instructed. Do not share with other family members, and do not stop the medicine when starting to feel better.
	  • Avoid or eliminate alcohol. Cephalosporins may cause significant reactions when taken with alcohol, and alcohol increases adverse GI effects of the drug.
	  • Take the drug with food or milk, but avoid acidic or carbonated beverages to decrease adverse GI effects.
	  • Take the medication as evenly spaced throughout each day as feasible.
	  • Increase overall fluid intake while taking the antibacterial drug.
	  • Discard outdated medications or those no longer in use. Review medicine cabinet twice a year for old medications (e.g., at beginning and end of daylight saving time).

Evaluation of Outcome Criteria

Evaluate the effectiveness of drug therapy by confirming that patient goals and expected outcomes have been met (see "Planning").

To the Community — Risk Factors for Pseudomembranous Colitis

Clostridium difficile–associated diarrhea (CDAD) and pseudomembranous colitis (PMC), progressing from CDAD, are significant infections related to antibiotic use. They account for the majority of HAI diarrheal infections with an increase in mortality rate associated with these infections. PMC may be recurrent and the older adult is particularly at risk for CDAD and PMC. Symptoms include watery diarrhea with up to 5 to 10 or more occurrences per day, abdominal cramping, fever, blood and mucus in the stool, and dehydration. While it has long been recognized that the overuse of antibiotics, either prophylactically, at high doses, or beyond the time required to adequately treat the infection, contributes to CDAD and PMC, there are other risk factors. Proton pump inhibitors (PPIs), which lower gastric acidity, contribute to a favorable environment for *C. difficile*. Patients receiving tube feedings with elemental diets (i.e., without fiber, fructose, starches, or probiotics) are also at risk. O'Keefe (2010) recommends that the critically ill ICU patient be assessed for the need for prophylactic antibiotics, PPIs, or elemental tube feedings and that there be judicious use of broad-spectrum antibiotics as methods to reduce CDAD and PMC. When necessary, elemental tube feeding diets should be changed to those containing more healthful ingredients such as fiber, and PPIs should be limited to confirmed cases of hyperacidity. All patients on high-dose, broad-spectrum, or long-term antibiotics should be carefully monitored for the development of CDAD and PMC.

TABLE 3 Carbapenems and Miscellaneous Cell Wall Inhibitors

Drug	Route and Adult Dose (maximum dose where indicated)	Adverse Effects
Carbapenems		
doripenem (Doribax)	IV: 500 mg every 8 h for 5–14 days (max: 500 mg every 8 h)	*Nausea, diarrhea, headache*
ertapenem (Invanz)	IV/IM: 1 g/day	Anaphylaxis, superinfections, PMC, confusion, seizures
imipenem-cilastatin (Primaxin)	IV: 250–500 mg tid–qid (max: 4 g/day)	
meropenem (Merrem)	IV: 1–2 g tid (max: 2 g tid)	
Miscellaneous Cell Wall Inhibitors		
aztreonam (Azactam, Cayston)	IM (Azactam): 0.5–2 g bid–qid (max: 8 g/day) Inhalation (Cayston): one vial in nebulizer tid for 28 days	*Nausea, vomiting, rash, thrombophlebitis (Azactam); cough, nasal congestion, wheezing (Cayston)* Anaphylaxis, superinfections, bronchospasm (Cayston)
fosfomycin (Monurol)	PO: 3 g sachet dissolved in 3–4 oz of water as a single dose	*Nausea, diarrhea, back pain, headache* Anaphylaxis, superinfections
telavancin (Vibativ)	IV: 10 mg administered over 60 min, once daily for 7–10 days	*Nausea, vomiting and foamy urine* Nephrotoxicity, QT interval prolongation, infusion-related reactions, birth defects
vancomycin (Vancocin)	IV: 500 mg qid; 1 g bid PO: 500 mg–2.0 g in three to four divided doses for 7–10 days	*Nausea, vomiting* Anaphylaxis, superinfections, nephrotoxicity, ototoxicity, red man syndrome

Note: Italics indicate common adverse effects. Underline indicates serious adverse effects.

Carbapenems

4 The carbapenems are resistant to beta lactamase and are broad-spectrum alternatives to penicillin.

Although the penicillins and cephalosporins comprise the largest groups of drugs affecting the bacterial cell wall, several other antibacterials also act by this mechanism. Doses of these agents are listed in Table 3.

Imipenem (Primaxin), ertapenem (Invanz), doripenem (Doribax), and meropenem (Merrem IV) belong to a class of antibiotics called carbapenems. These drugs are bacteriocidal and have some of the broadest antimicrobial spectrums of any class of antibiotics. They contain a beta-lactam ring and kill bacteria by inhibiting construction of the cell wall. Though similar, the ring in carbapenems has a slightly different structure than other beta-lactam antibiotics that makes it very resistant to destruction by beta lactamase. These factors allow the carbapenems to provide better activity against serious gram-negative and multidrug-resistant infections than most cephalosporins or penicillins. A disadvantage is that they can only be given parenterally.

All the carbapenems exhibit a low incidence of adverse effects. Diarrhea, nausea, rashes, and thrombophlebitis at injection sites are the most common adverse effects.

PROTOTYPE DRUG | Imipenem-Cilastatin (Primaxin)

Classification: **Therapeutic:** Antibacterial
Pharmacologic: Cell wall inhibitor, carbapenem

Therapeutic Effects and Uses: Approved in 1985, imipenem is used for the treatment and prophylaxis of susceptible bacterial infections. Imipenem has a very broad antimicrobial spectrum and is the most widely used carbapenem. Because of its broad spectrum and beta-lactamase resistance, it is effective against most gram-positive and gram-negative microbes, including anaerobic bacteria. It is particularly useful for mixed infections containing both aerobic and anaerobic organisms, including those with *S. aureus. P. aeruginosa* and strains of MRSA are also susceptible to imipenem.

Although imipenem contains a beta-lactam ring, it is resistant to the actions of beta lactamase. This drug, however, is rapidly destroyed by dipeptidase, an enzyme found in the kidney tubules. Concurrent administration of the drug cilastatin, a renal dipeptidase inhibitor, with imipenem prevents the destruction of imipenem and allows for higher serum levels of the antibiotic. Cilastatin possesses no antimicrobial activity of its own. Imipenem is only marketed with cilastatin in a fixed-dose combination (Primaxin).

Primaxin is sometimes combined with antibiotics from other classes, such as the aminoglycosides or cephalosporins, when treating *P. aeruginosa* infections. Primaxin has a short half-life that requires administration every 6 hours.

Mechanism of Action: Imipenem inhibits bacterial wall synthesis by binding to specific PBPs. Cilastatin blocks renal dipeptidase, which is the enzyme primarily responsible for the excretion of imipenem. The combination of imipenem-cilastatin is bacteriocidal.

Pharmacokinetics:

Route(s)	IM and IV
Absorption	Not absorbed PO
Distribution	Widely distributed, including in the CSF; secreted in breast milk; both imipenem and cilastatin cross the placenta
Primary metabolism	Hepatic
Primary excretion	Renal
Onset of action	IM: rapid; IV: immediate
Duration of action	Half-life: 1 h

Adverse Effects: The most frequent adverse effects of imipenem-cilastatin include nausea, vomiting, diarrhea, rash, and pain and phlebitis at the injection site. Rare, though serious, reactions include confusion, seizures, hallucinations, PMC, and anaphylaxis. Anaphylactic response may include cardiovascular collapse and edema of the mouth, tongue, pharynx, and larynx.

Contraindications/Precautions: Imipenem-cilastatin is contraindicated in patients who have experienced a severe allergic reaction to this drug, other carbapenems, cephalosporins, or penicillins. Because the kidneys excrete imipenem-cilastatin, patients with significant renal impairment must be carefully monitored and dosages lowered. This drug should be used cautiously in patients with brain lesions, head trauma, or a history of seizures due to an increased risk of seizures.

Drug Interactions: Certain other antibiotics, including penicillins, cephalosporins, and aztreonam antagonize the antimicrobial effects of imipenem-cilastatin; therefore, they should not be given concurrently. Concurrent use with cyclosporine, tramadol, theophylline, or ganciclovir may increase the risk of seizures and other CNS effects. **Herbal/Food:** None known.

Pregnancy: Category C.

Treatment of Overdose: Overdose may result in ataxia and seizures. Patients are treated symptomatically.

Nursing Responsibilities: Key nursing implications for patients receiving imipenem-cilastin are included in the Nursing Practice Application for Patients Receiving Penicillin, Cephalosporin, or Vancomycin Therapy.

Lifespan and Diversity Considerations:

- Monitor renal function laboratory values more frequently in the older adult because normal physiological changes related to aging may affect the drug's excretion.
- Monitor renal function laboratory values and urine output more frequently in the neonate or young infant because normal renal immaturity in these stages may increase the risk of adverse renal effects.
- Carefully monitor for diarrhea in the infant and young child as well as the older adult. Cases of CDAD and PMC have been reported with antibiotic use, greatly increasing the risks of fluid and electrolyte imbalances and severe bowel effects in all patients, but especially in these populations.

Patient and Family Education:

- Immediately report severe or persistent diarrhea accompanied by fever to the health care provider. Do not attempt to treat penicillin-related diarrhea with OTC products.
- Immediately report disorientation, confusion, or seizures to the health care provider.
- Immediately notify the health care provider of any known or suspected pregnancy.
- Do not breast-feed while taking this drug without approval of the health care provider.

Drugs Similar to Imipenem-Cilastatin (Primaxin)

Other carbapenems include doripenem, ertapenem, and meropenem.

Doripenem (Doribax): Doripenem (Doribax) is a newer drug in this class that was approved in 2007. It is similar to meropenem and has activity against both gram-positive and gram-negative organisms. It is approved to treat complicated intra-abdominal infections and urinary tract infections (UTIs). It is administered by IV infusion over 60 minutes. Common adverse effects include headache, rash, nausea, vomiting, diarrhea, and phlebitis. Doripenem is contraindicated in patients who have experienced a severe allergic reaction to other carbapenems, cephalosporins, or penicillins. This drug is pregnancy category B.

Ertapenem (Invanz): A newer drug in this class, ertapenem, has a narrower spectrum than the other carbapenems, being active primarily against gram-negative aerobes. Its major advantage is its longer half-life, which allows for once-daily dosing. It is approved for the treatment of serious abdominopelvic and skin infections, community-acquired pneumonia, complicated

UTIs, and diabetic foot infections without concomitant osteomyelitis. It is administered by the IV and IM routes. Adverse effects are similar to those of other carbapenems. Ertapenem is contraindicated in patients who have experienced a severe allergic reaction to other carbapenems, cephalosporins, or penicillins. This drug is pregnancy category B.

Meropenem (Merrem): Approved in 1996, meropenem has a similar spectrum of activity to imipenem, although it is only approved for peritonitis and skin and skin structure infections in adults and bacterial meningitis in children. The drug is used off-label for other indications. The antimicrobial spectrum of activity of meropenem is similar to that of imipenem. Meropenem may be more active against *Enterobacteriaceae*, gonococcus, *H. influenzae*, and *P. aeruginosa*. This drug is not destroyed by renal dipeptidase, so it is not administered with cilastatin. Adverse effects are similar to those of imipenem. Meropenem is contraindicated in patients who have experienced a severe allergic reaction to other carbapenems, cephalosporins, or penicillins. It is only available by the IV route. Bolus injections are given IV over 3 to 5 minutes, and infusions over 15 to 30 minutes. This drug is pregnancy category B.

PharmFACT

Central-line associated bloodstream infections are a deadly form of HAI with a mortality rate of 12% to 24%. The number of these infections declined from 43,000 in 2001 to 18,000 in 2009 (CDC, 2011).

Miscellaneous Cell Wall Inhibitors

5 Several miscellaneous cell wall inhibitors have activity against resistant microbes.

Several other cell wall inhibitors have important roles in the pharmacotherapy of infections. These agents are either new drugs or the only agent in a class.

PROTOTYPE DRUG | Vancomycin (Vancocin)

Classification: **Therapeutic:** Antibacterial
Pharmacologic: Cell wall inhibitor

Therapeutic Effects and Uses: Approved in 1964, vancomycin (Vancocin) is used for the treatment and prophylaxis of susceptible bacterial infections. It is effective against most gram-positive organisms, including *Streptococcus*, *Corynebacterium*, *Clostridium*, *Listeria*, and *Bacillus* species. Vancomycin is usually administered by slow IV infusion for systemic infections because it is not well absorbed from the GI tract. It has been administered off-label by the intrathecal or intraventricular route to treat meningitis. Oral vancomycin is approved for the treatment of antibiotic-induced PMC, which is caused by a toxin produced by *C. difficile*. When given orally, the drug acts locally in the intestine and very little is absorbed into the systemic circulation.

Current protocols restrict the use of vancomycin to severe infections that have become resistant to safer antibiotics. It is anticipated that this restriction will discourage or delay the appearance of resistant strains. Because vancomycin was used infrequently during the first 30 years following its discovery, the incidence of vancomycin-resistant organisms has been less than that of other antibiotics. Vancomycin is the most effective drug for treating MRSA infections. Vancomycin-resistant strains of *S. aureus*, however, have begun to appear in recent years. Vancomycin is often considered the "last chance" antibiotic. Therapeutic options for vancomycin-resistant infections are limited.

Mechanism of Action: Although vancomycin kills bacteria mainly by inhibiting bacterial cell wall synthesis, it also affects the plasma membrane and interferes with ribonucleic acid (RNA) synthesis. The fact that it has multiple mechanisms is probably responsible for the low rate of resistance from the drug. It is bacteriocidal and only effective against gram-positive organisms such as *S. aureus* and *S. pneumoniae*.

Pharmacokinetics:

Route(s)	IV, PO
Absorption	Poorly absorbed PO
Distribution	Oral form does not usually enter systemic circulation; IV form is widely distributed with small amounts in the CSF; secreted in breast milk; 55% bound to plasma proteins
Primary metabolism	Probably not metabolized
Primary excretion	Renal
Onset of action	IV: immediate
Duration of action	Half-life: 4–8 h

Adverse Effects: Vancomycin may cause a syndrome of flushing, hypotension, tachycardia, and rash on the upper body, a condition called the red man syndrome. This syndrome can be minimized by infusing the drug over at least 60 minutes. Other common adverse effects include nausea, rash, fever, and chills. Serious adverse effects include confusion, seizures, and hallucinations. If extravasation occurs, it may lead to tissue necrosis. Ototoxicity is associated with serum concentrations of vancomycin above 60 to 80 mcg/mL. Tinnitus and high-tone hearing loss precede deafness and may progress even after this drug is discontinued. The most susceptible are older adults and those on high doses. Nephrotoxicity can occur in patients with therapeutic concentrations but is more common if trough serum concentrations are kept above 10 mcg/mL. Anaphylactic response may include cardiovascular collapse or edema of the mouth, tongue, pharynx, and larynx.

Contraindications/Precautions: Vancomycin is contraindicated in patients who have experienced previous hypersensitivity to this drug. The nurse must monitor drug therapy carefully in patients with impaired renal function and those with a history of hearing loss.

Drug Interactions: Vancomycin adds to toxicity of aminoglycosides, amphotericin B, cisplatin, cyclosporine, polymyxin B, and other ototoxic and nephrotoxic medications. Vancomycin may increase the risk of lactic acidosis when administered with metformin, especially in patients with renal impairment.
Herbal/Food: Unknown.

Pregnancy: Category C.

Treatment of Overdose: Because overdose may result in renal impairment, patients are treated supportively to maintain kidney function.

Nursing Responsibilities: Key nursing implications for patients receiving vancomycin are included in the Nursing Practice Application for Patients Receiving Penicillin, Cephalosporin, or Vancomycin Therapy.

Lifespan and Diversity Considerations:

* Monitor renal function laboratory values more frequently in the older adult because normal physiological changes related to aging may affect the drug's excretion.

* Monitor renal function laboratory values and urine output more frequently in the neonate or young infant because normal renal immaturity in these stages may increase the risk of adverse renal effects.

* Monitor hearing and balance, especially in the older adult, to detect early symptoms of ototoxicity.

* Carefully monitor for diarrhea in the infant and young child as well as the older adult. Cases of CDAD and PMC have been reported with antibiotic use, greatly increasing the risk of fluid and electrolyte imbalances and severe bowel effects in all patients, but especially in these populations.

Patient and Family Education:

* Notify the health care provider immediately of any known or suspected pregnancy.

* Do not breast-feed while taking this drug without prior approval of the health care provider.

* Maintain adequate fluid intake (2–3 L/day).

Drugs Similar to Vancomycin (Vancocin)

Other miscellaneous cell wall inhibitors include aztreonam, fosfomycin, and telavancin.

Aztreonam (Azactam, Cayston): Approved in 1986, aztreonam has a beta-lactam ring and belongs to a newer class of antibiotics known as monobactams. Like other cell wall inhibitors, aztreonam binds to specific penicillin-binding proteins to cause a bacteriocidal effect. Although considered narrow-spectrum antibiotics, monobactams are particularly useful against certain gram-negative aerobes, such as *P. aeruginosa*. Other organisms considered susceptible to aztreonam include *Citrobacter, Enterobacter, E. coli, H. influenzae, Neisseria, Proteus, Providencia rettgeri,* and *Shigella.* Monobactams have little or no activity against gram-positive bacteria or anaerobes. Although they have beta-lactam rings, they do not exhibit cross-hypersensitivity with penicillins or cephalosporins. Azactam is administered by the parenteral route and exhibits similar adverse effects as those of other cell wall inhibitors including nausea, vomiting, diarrhea, superinfections such as vaginal candidiasis, and local pain or phlebitis at the injection site. Anaphylaxis and PMC are rare. An inhalation form of the drug, Cayston, was approved in 2010 to improve respiratory symptoms in patients with cystic fibrosis who have *P. aeruginosa* infection. This drug is pregnancy category B.

Fosfomycin (Monurol): Approved in 1996, fosfomycin is a cell wall inhibitor that is currently approved for the treatment of uncomplicated UTI and bladder infections in women caused by *E. coli* and *Enterococcus faecalis*. It is given as an oral powder, which is mixed with water and taken PO as a single dose. Adverse effects are minor and include asthenia, nausea, vomiting, diarrhea, headache, and vaginitis. This drug is pregnancy category B.

Telavancin (Vibativ): Approved in 2009, telavancin is a synthetic derivative of vancomycin that acts by inhibiting the polymerization and cross-linking of peptidoglycan in bacterial cell walls. It is approved as a once-daily IV infusion for the treatment of complicated skin and skin structure infections caused by gram-negative bacteria, including MRSA. Common adverse effects include taste disturbances, nausea, vomiting, and foamy urine. Telavancin is nephrotoxic and kidney function should be monitored during therapy. Telavancin prolongs the QT interval and it should be used with caution with other medications that cause this effect. This drug is pregnancy category B.

UNDERSTANDING THE CHAPTER

Key Concepts Summary

1 Bacterial cell walls consist of layers of carbohydrate and protein chains, which are constructed by enzymes called penicillin-binding proteins.

2 The penicillins, one of the oldest and safest groups of antibacterials, are primarily active against gram-positive bacteria.

3 The cephalosporins are similar in structure and function to the penicillins and are widely prescribed for gram-negative infections.

4 The carbapenems are resistant to beta lactamase and are broad-spectrum alternatives to penicillin.

5 Several miscellaneous cell wall inhibitors have activity against resistant microbes.

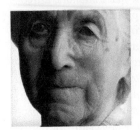

Making the PATIENT Connection

Remember the patient "Katie Dennison" at the beginning of the chapter? Now read the remainder of the case study. Based on the information presented within this chapter, respond to the critical thinking questions that follow.

Katie Dennison is an 83-year-old retired school teacher. She was recently seen by her health care provider for removal of a noncancerous skin lesion. Now she suspects that the wound on her arm has become infected. She has attempted to report this condition to her health care provider. However, due to the holidays she has been unable to reach him. Ms. Dennison presents to a local urgent care center for treatment.

The physical examination and diagnostic tests reveal the following findings. Vital signs are temperature, 38°C (100.9°F); pulse, 110 beats/min; respiratory rate, 20 breaths/min; and blood pressure, 108/68 mmHg. The large dressing on her left arm is saturated with dried yellow-green exudates. She states that it is painful to move her left arm and that the pain has limited her range of motion in the affected extremity. She is pale and has "paper thin" fragile skin.

Katie reports that she accidentally got the dressing wet while taking a shower. She did not change the dressing because she was not told to do so by her health care provider when the skin lesion was removed. A series of laboratory tests were completed. A sterile dressing was applied to the wound. Ms. Dennison was given an injection of cefazolin (Ancef) and a prescription for antibiotics. She was also instructed to follow up with her health care provider within the next 2 to 3 days.

Critical Thinking Questions

1. What factors possibly contributed to the wound infection in this patient?
2. What laboratory tests were probably obtained during this visit to the urgent care center?
3. What information should the nurse provide to the patient concerning the antibiotic?
4. Discuss the mechanism of action for cefazolin.

See Answers to Critical Thinking Questions on student resource website.

NCLEX-RN® Review

1. Which instruction should the nurse give a 21-year-old female client being treated with ampicillin (Principen)?
   1. Stop taking oral contraceptives because serious adverse effects could occur.
   2. Use oral contraceptives as prescribed because antibiotics do not react with birth control pills.
   3. The antibiotic may decrease the effectiveness of oral contraceptives.
   4. The antibiotic when taken with oral contraceptives causes toxicity.

2. The nurse is caring for a client who is receiving intravenous vancomycin (Vancocin). Which symptom, if present, may indicate that the client is experiencing drug-induced ototoxicity?
   1. Erythema of the earlobes and ear canal
   2. Inner ear pruritus after infusion is completed
   3. Tinnitus and dizziness when remaining still
   4. Ocular pain with purulent drainage

3. The client reports abnormal vaginal discharge after completing a prescription of cefotaxime (Claforan). For which condition is the client most likely exhibiting symptoms?
   1. Hypersensitivity reaction
   2. Superinfection
   3. Pseudomembranous colitis
   4. Antibiotic toxicity

4. The client who has been taking cefixime (Suprax) for the past week and a half returns to the provider with reports of "explosive diarrhea," up to eight times in the last 2 days. The diarrhea is described as "very watery, sometimes with a lot of mucus" and the client reports significant weakness. For which condition is the client describing symptoms?
   1. Antibiotic-induced peptic ulcer disease
   2. Antibiotic-associated malabsorption
   3. GI-associated hypersensitivity
   4. *Clostridium difficile*–associated diarrhea

5. The client who is taking imipenem-cilastatin (Primaxin) reports shortness of breath, mouth and tongue swelling, and generalized itching. For which of the following does the nurse initially assess the client?
   1. Hypersensitivity reaction
   2. Blood dyscrasias
   3. Beta-lactamase induction
   4. Drug toxicity

6. The nurse is teaching a client who recently was diagnosed with an upper respiratory infection and is prescribed ampicillin (Principen). The nurse would evaluate the session as being successful if the client states which of the following?
   1. "I should take this medication on an empty stomach with a full glass of water."
   2. "I can expect my tongue to become black and furry."
   3. "Once I stop coughing, I should stop taking this medication."
   4. "If I miss a dose, I should take two doses together to catch up."

Additional Case Study

Mrs. Murphy is 80 years old and lives in a retirement community for lower income older adults. You are the community health nurse visiting with her. As part of your assessment, you ask Mrs. Murphy how she obtains her prescribed medications. The patient explains that most of the time, her neighbor will pick up prescriptions for her. She further explains that in some cases, however, she has "stockpiled" medicines she has been prescribed. When you investigate, you find that the patient has multiple bottles of various types of unused antibiotics. Some of the drugs were prescribed 5 or 6 years ago.

1. Describe how you should respond to this situation.

2. Identify the health teaching needs of this patient regarding "stockpiling" (saving) antibiotics.

See Answers to Additional Case Study on student resource website.

Pearson Nursing Student Resources

Find additional review materials at nursing.pearsonhighered.com

Prepare for success with additional NCLEX®-style practice questions, interactive assignments and activities, web links, animations, videos, and more!

References

Centers for Disease Control and Prevention. (2010). *Get smart: Know when antibiotics work. Antibiotic resistance questions and answers.* Retrieved from http://www.cdc.gov/getsmart/antibiotic-use/anitbiotic-resistance-faqs.html

Centers for Disease Control and Prevention. (2011). Vital signs: Central line-associated blood stream infections—United States, 2001, 2008, and 2009. *Morbidity and Mortality Weekly Report, 60*(8), 243–248.

O'Keefe, S. J. D. (2010). Tube feeding, microbiota, and *Clostridium difficile* infection. *World Journal of Gastroenterology, 16*(2), 139–142. doi:10.3748/wjg.v16.i2.139

Zhang, Y., Lee, B. Y., & Donohue, J. M. (2010). Ambulatory antibiotic use and prescription drug coverage in older adults. *Archives of Internal Medicine, 170*(5), 1308–1314. doi:10.1001/archinternmed.2010.235

Selected Bibliography

Baughman, R. P. (2009). The use of carbapenems in the treatment of serious infections.

Journal of Intensive Care Medicine, 24(4), 230–241. doi:10.1177/0885066609335660

Bosquet, P. J., Demoly, P., & Romano, A. (2009). Drug allergy and hypersensitivity: Still a hot topic. *Allergy, 64*(2), 179–182. doi:10.1111/j.1398-9995.2008.01960.x

Chen, L. F., Chopra, T., & Kaye, K. S. (2010). Pathogens resistant to antibacterial agents. *Medical Clinics of North America, 95*(4), 647–676. doi:10.1016/j.mcna.2011.03.005

El-Shaboury, S. R., Saleh, G. A., Mohamed, F. A., & Rageh, A. H. (2007). Analysis of cephalosporin antibiotics. *Journal of Pharmaceutical and Biomedical Analysis, 45*(1), 1–19. doi:10.1016/j.jpba.2007.06.002

Goedken, A. M., Urmie, J. M., Farris, K. B., & Doucette, W. R. (2009). Effect of cost sharing on prescription drug use by Medicare beneficiaries prior to the Medicare drug benefit and potential adverse selection in the benefit. *Journal of American Pharmacists Association, 49*(1), 18–25. doi:10.1331/JAPhA.2009.08001

Matteo, B., Ginocchio, F., Giacobbe, D. R., & Malgorzata, M. (2011). Development of

antibiotics for gram-negatives: Where now? *Clinical Investigation, 1*(2), 221–227. doi:10.4155/cli.10.31

Nicolau, D. P. (2008). Carbapenems: A potent class of antibiotics. *Expert Opinion on Pharmacotherapy, 9*(1), 23–27. doi:10.1517/14656566.9.1.23

Smith, S. M. (2010). Update on *Clostridium difficile* infection and its management. *Nursing for Women's Health, 14*(5), 391–397. doi:10.1111/j.1751-486X.2010.01578.x

Tacconelli, E., De Angelis, G., Cataldo, M. A., Pozzi, E., & Cauda, R. (2008). Does antibiotic exposure increase the risk of methicillin-resistant *Staphylococcus aureus* (MRSA) isolation? A systematic review and meta-analysis. *Journal of Antimicrobial Chemotherapy, 61*(1), 26–38.

Answers to NCLEX-RN® Review

1 Answer: 3   Rationale: Ampicillin may decrease the effectiveness of oral contraceptives, and the client should be instructed to use a barrier method to avoid unwanted pregnancies while on the antibiotic and until the next cycle of oral contraceptives is started. Options 1, 2, and 4 are incorrect. The combination of ampicillin and oral contraceptives will not increase the risk of adverse effects related to the antibiotic. Oral contraceptive effectiveness may be reduced during ampicillin therapy, and ampicillin will not create serious toxicity related to the use of oral contraceptives. Cognitive Level: Applying; Client Need: Health Promotion and Maintenance; Nursing Process: Implementation

2 Answer: 3   Rationale: Ototoxicity is associated with serum concentrations of vancomycin above 60 to 80 mcg/mL and manifests with tinnitus and dizziness or balance and coordination effects. Options 1, 2, and 4 are incorrect. Redness of the ears, itching of the ears, and ocular pain are not symptoms related to ototoxicity caused by vancomycin. Cognitive Level: Analyzing; Client Need: Physiological Integrity; Nursing Process: Evaluation

3 Answer: 2   Rationale: A vaginal yeast infection with discharge may be a symptom of a superinfection. Superinfection is a possible adverse effect associated with all antibiotics and particularly with fungal and viral infections. Options 1, 3, and 4 are incorrect. A hypersensitivity reaction is not usually manifested by vaginal discharge. The symptoms associated with pseudomembranous colitis (PMC) are significant GI effects. Vaginal discharge is not a symptom of antibiotic toxicity. Cognitive Level: Applying; Client Need: Physiological Integrity; Nursing Process: Evaluation

4 Answer: 4   Rationale: Watery diarrhea containing mucus, blood, or pus is symptomatic of *Clostridium difficile*–associated diarrhea (CDAD) and must be monitored closely for progressing to PMC; both are adverse effects related to antibiotic use. Options 1, 2, and 3 are incorrect. These symptoms are not related to peptic ulcers, malabsorption, and hypersensitivity reactions. Cognitive Level: Analyzing; Client Need: Physiological Integrity; Nursing Process: Evaluation

5 Answer: 1   Rationale: Shortness of breath, mouth and tongue swelling, and generalized itching are signs of hypersensitivity reaction. Options 2, 3, and 4 are incorrect. Blood dyscrasias include such problems as thrombocytopenia and neutropenia, and the drug does not cause these symptoms. Beta lactamase is a substance secreted by some bacteria that renders the antibiotic ineffective. Drug toxicity may result from an excessive level of the medication, or adverse effects on body organ systems related to age or other changes. Hypersensitivity is associated with antigen and antibody reactions. Cognitive Level: Analyzing; Client Need: Physiological Integrity; Nursing Process: Assessment

6 Answer: 1   Rationale: Ampicillin should be taken on an empty stomach to ensure adequate absorption. Options 2, 3, and 4 are incorrect. A black and furry tongue is the symptom of an oral superinfection and should be reported. The client should be taught to take the full prescription even if the symptoms subside. Clients should never take two doses because this will place them at risk for toxicity. Cognitive Level: Analyzing; Client Need: Health Promotion and Maintenance; Nursing Process: Evaluation

Antibiotics Affecting Bacterial Protein Synthesis

From Chapter 51 of *Pharmacology: Connections to Nursing Practice*, Second Edition. Michael Patrick Adams, Carol Quam Urban. Copyright © 2013 by Pearson Education, Inc. All rights reserved.

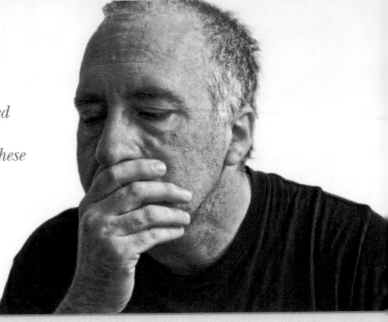

"*Today is the fifth day since I started taking the medication and I'm still having chills and fever. I thought these antibiotics were supposed to get rid of this!*"

Patient "John Talley"

Stephen Orsillo/Shutterstock

Antibiotics Affecting Bacterial Protein Synthesis

Learning Outcomes

After reading this chapter, the student should be able to:

1. Explain the steps in the synthesis of bacterial proteins.
2. Identify the classes of antibiotics that act by inhibiting bacterial protein synthesis.
3. Explain mechanisms by which antibiotics inhibit bacterial protein synthesis.
4. Explain how protein synthesis inhibitors exert selective toxicity toward bacterial, rather than human, cells.
5. Describe means by which bacteria become resistant to protein synthesis inhibitors.
6. For each of the classes shown in the chapter outline, identify the prototype and representative drugs and explain the mechanism(s) of drug action, primary indications, contraindications, significant drug interactions, pregnancy category, and important adverse effects.
7. Apply the nursing process to care for patients who are receiving pharmacotherapy with bacterial protein synthesis inhibitors.

Chapter Outline

Mechanisms of Antibiotic Inhibition of Bacterial Protein Synthesis

Tetracyclines

PROTOTYPE **Tetracycline (Sumycin, Others)**

Macrolides

PROTOTYPE **Erythromycin (EryC, Erythrocin, Others)**

Aminoglycosides

PROTOTYPE **Gentamicin (Garamycin, Others)**

Miscellaneous Inhibitors of Bacterial Protein Synthesis

To maintain the extreme metabolic rate required for exponential reproduction, bacteria must synthesize huge amounts of protein. Antibacterial drugs that inhibit this high rate of protein metabolism can either kill the bacterial cell or slow its replication rate. Tetracyclines, macrolides, and a few miscellaneous drugs are bacteriostatic inhibitors of protein synthesis. The aminoglycosides are bacteriocidal inhibitors.

Mechanisms of Antibiotic Inhibition of Bacterial Protein Synthesis

1 Antibiotics inhibit microbial protein synthesis by binding to the bacterial ribosome.

The importance of protein to a microbe is illustrated by the fact that up to 50% of the dry weight of a bacterial cell consists of protein. Bacterial proteins serve many of the same functions as human proteins. For example, the bacterial enzymes required for all biochemical reactions are proteins. Proteins are studded in the plasma membrane and serve as channels, pores, or transporters, assisting substances as they move into and out of cells. Like human proteins, bacterial proteins are composed of long chains of amino acids.

Several types of proteins, however, are unique to bacteria. Bacterial cells produce protein toxins, which kill other bacteria and can cause serious injury to human cells. The sticky gel-like substance that allows bacterial cells to cling to human epithelial cells on the skin surface, in bronchi, in the gastrointestinal (GI) tract, or in the genitourinary tract consists of proteins combined with carbohydrates. The structure of the bacterial cell wall consists of peptidoglycan layers of protein and carbohydrates that protect the bacterium from

its environment. From these examples, it is easy to understand why proteins are critical to bacterial cells.

Knowledge of how proteins are synthesized by bacterial cells is important to understanding how antibiotics act. The basic steps in protein synthesis, or **translation**, are the same in bacteria as they are in humans. Knowledge of translation, which is illustrated in Figure 1, is necessary to understand the mechanisms of action of antibiotics that inhibit protein synthesis.

Protein synthesis occurs in the cytoplasm and requires the following three components:

- Messenger ribonucleic acid (mRNA)
- Transfer ribonucleic acid (tRNA)
- Ribosomes, which consist of one large and one small subunit

The mRNA carries the encoded message for making a protein from the deoxyribonucleic acid (DNA) to the ribosome, which serves as the site for protein construction. The strand of mRNA squeezes between the two ribosomal subunits and begins to move through the subunits. As it does, a tRNA molecule arrives, carrying the specific amino acid that was encoded in the mRNA strand. As the mRNA proceeds through the ribosome, subsequent amino acids are added one at a time to the growing protein chain. This growing chain is known as a polypeptide. Eventually, a "stop signal" is reached on the mRNA strand,

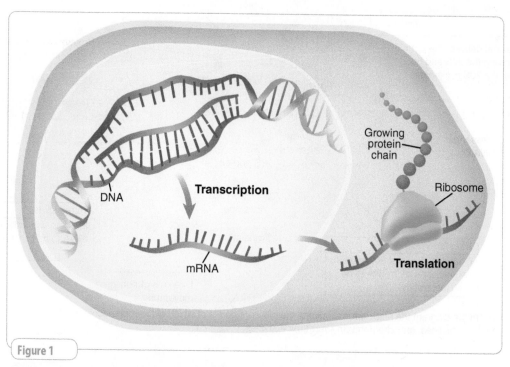

Figure 1

Steps in protein synthesis: The DNA is used as a template to make mRNA (transcription). The mRNA is sent to the ribosome to make the protein chain (translation).

which tells the ribosome that the last amino acid has been added and the protein is ready to be released. The protein may be active immediately, or it may be processed to its active form in the Golgi body. The finished protein may be used within the bacterial cell (enzymes) or be exported outside (toxins).

All cells, including bacteria, are able to quickly increase protein synthesis to meet their growth demands or to respond to environmental challenges. For example, a bacterium may receive a message that other competitive bacteria are in the vicinity. The gene coding for a toxin or antibiotic may become active, producing large amounts of mRNA and eventually protein toxin, which serves as a defense against the invader.

If both humans and bacteria conduct continuous protein synthesis, why are antibiotics that inhibit protein synthesis not also toxic to human cells? The answer lies in differences in the structures of the bacterial and human ribosomes. Ribosomes are composed of two subunits, one of which is larger and less dense than the other. In bacteria, these ribosomal components are referred to as 30S and 50S subunits. The letter "S" is a unit of measurement, the **Svedberg unit**, which reflects the ribosome's size or sedimentation rate in a high-speed centrifuge. The

entire bacterial ribosome is called a 70S ribosome (Svedberg units are not additive). Antibiotics that inhibit protein synthesis do so by affecting subunits of the bacterial ribosome. Humans have ribosomes that are larger and denser than the 70S bacterial ribosome. The 80S human ribosome is mostly unaffected by antibiotics that bind to the bacterial 70S ribosome, thus providing a degree of selective toxicity. Interestingly, human mitochondria do contain a 70S ribosome that is affected by several of these antibiotics, thus explaining some of the adverse effects of these drugs.

About 20 drugs that affect the synthesis of bacterial proteins have been discovered. The different steps at which antibiotics inhibit the production of bacterial proteins are shown in Figure 2.

Tetracyclines

2 Tetracyclines have broad antimicrobial activity against many gram-positive and gram-negative bacteria.

The first tetracyclines were extracted from *Streptomyces* in soil samples in 1948. Unfortunately, their widespread use in the 1950s and 1960s resulted in a large number of resistant

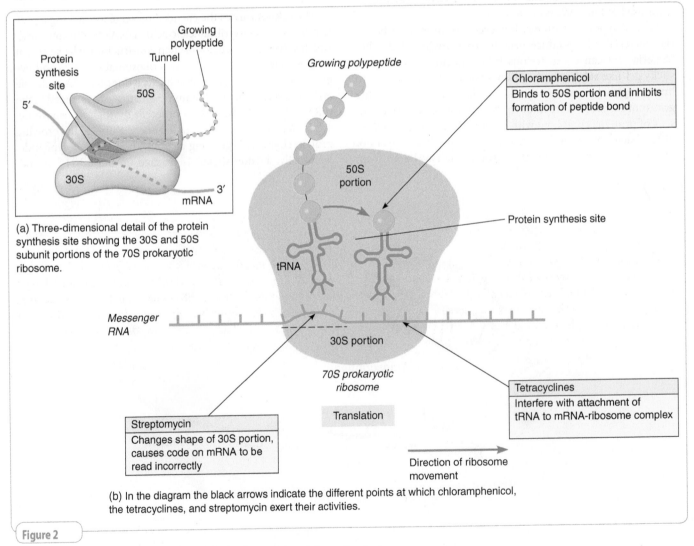

(a) Three-dimensional detail of the protein synthesis site showing the 30S and 50S subunit portions of the 70S prokaryotic ribosome.

(b) In the diagram the black arrows indicate the different points at which chloramphenicol, the tetracyclines, and streptomycin exert their activities.

Figure 2

Mechanisms of action of antibiotics inhibiting bacterial protein synthesis.
Source: From *Microbiology: An Introduction* (10th ed., p. 558), by G. Tortora, B. Funke, & C. Case, 2010. Reprinted by permission of Pearson Education, Inc., Upper Saddle River, NJ.

Evidence-Based Practice   Traveler's Diarrhea

Clinical Question

What are the current recommendations for prevention or treatment of traveler's diarrhea?

Evidence

Traveler's diarrhea (TD) is an unpleasant but rarely fatal infection that affects travelers going to developing regions of the world, especially tropical or semitropical areas. *E. coli, Shigella, Campylobacter, Salmonella,* and the noroviruses are common causes of traveler's diarrhea. As many as 4 out of every 10 travelers going to a high-risk region will develop TD (Greenwood et al., 2008) and while mortality is low, the diarrhea may ruin a trip and result in long-term complications. Risk factors include age (toddler or adolescent), infrequent travel to developing regions, lack of infection control practices such as hand washing or care in eating or drinking, and daily use of a proton pump inhibitor (de la Cabada Bauche & DuPont, 2011). Chronic, postinfection inflammatory bowel syndrome (IBS) persisting for up to 5 years has been noted following TD infections.

Three antibiotics have shown the most promise in treating TD infections, dependent on the endemic pathogens in the area of travel: fluoroquinolones (ciprofloxacin [Cipro] or levofloxacin [Levaquin]), rifaximin (Xifaxan, Salix), and azithromycin (Zithromax, Zmax). While the time for initiation of treatment, after the first loose stool or after the classic TD definition of three loose stools, has not been determined, it is recommended that travelers visiting high-risk countries bring an antibiotic for self-treatment of TD.

Implications

More people are traveling to foreign countries than ever before. Nurses can be instrumental in teaching methods to avoid traveler's diarrhea. Travelers can decrease their risk by practicing frequent hand cleansing with hand sanitizers or antiseptic cloths; avoiding beverages with ice, not drinking water that has not been boiled, and not using tap water for teeth brushing; and not consuming raw fruits or vegetables that cannot be peeled because they may be contaminated. Over-the-counter (OTC) medications such as bismuth subsalicylate (Pepto-Bismol) or probiotics such as *Lactobacillus* and *Saccharomyces boulardii* may confer some protection against TD.

Depending on the area of the world that the traveler will be visiting and endemic pathogens most likely to be encountered there, an antibiotic may be prescribed to have on hand in case of TD. The nurse should assess for allergies and provide patient education on when the antibiotic should be used (e.g., after one or more loose stools). The nurse should teach that local health authorities should be contacted if the diarrhea worsens, is accompanied by severe abdominal pain or fever, or if blood is present in the stool. Upon returning home, the traveler should consult a health care provider, and any continued diarrhea or GI symptoms should be monitored for the development of postinfection IBS.

Critical Thinking Question

In what specific patient populations would TD be most serious? Why?

See Answers to Critical Thinking Questions on student resource website.

---

strains, limiting the therapeutic usefulness of the drugs in this class.

The five tetracyclines are effective against a large number of aerobic and anaerobic gram-negative and gram-positive organisms: They have one of the broadest antimicrobial spectrums of any class of antibiotics. They are effective against some species that are resistant to penicillins and other cell wall inhibitors. Because of widespread bacterial resistance, however, they are the drugs of choice for only a few diseases: Rocky Mountain spotted fever, typhus, cholera, Lyme disease, peptic ulcers caused by *Helicobacter pylori*, and chlamydial infections. In addition, *Treponema pallidum* (syphilis) responds well to tetracycline therapy for patients who are allergic to penicillin. Although traditionally used for gonorrhea, most strains of *Neisseria gonorrhoeae* are now resistant to tetracyclines. Drugs in this class are occasionally used for the treatment of acne vulgaris, for which they are given topically or

orally (PO) at low doses. Almost all strains of *Pseudomonas aeruginosa* are resistant to tetracyclines. Once resistance develops to one tetracycline, it usually extends to all drugs in this class. Doses for the tetracyclines are listed in Table 1.

Tetracyclines exert a bacteriostatic effect by selectively inhibiting bacterial protein synthesis. As illustrated in Figure 2, the tetracyclines bind to the 30S bacterial ribosome, thereby preventing the addition of amino acids to the growing polypeptide chain. Resistance to tetracyclines develops when bacteria prevent tetracyclines from concentrating inside their cells, or when their ribosome shape is altered so the antibiotic can no longer bind. In addition to having ribosomes with different structures, human cells lack the active transport system required for tetracyclines to enter their cells. At high doses, however, tetracyclines begin to exert toxicity on human cells.

All tetracyclines have the same spectrum of antimicrobial activity and similar adverse effects. All except tigecycline may

TABLE 1 Tetracyclines

Drug	Route and Adult Dose (maximum dose where indicated)	Adverse Effects
demeclocycline (Declomycin)	PO: 150 mg every 6 h or 300 mg every 12 h (max: 2.4 g/day)	*Nausea, vomiting, abdominal cramping, flatulence, diarrhea, mild phototoxicity, rash, dizziness, stinging or burning with topical applications*
doxycycline (Vibramycin, Others)	PO: 100 mg bid on day 1, then 100 mg daily (max: 200 mg/day)	
minocycline (Minocin, Others)	PO: 200 mg as one dose followed by 100 mg bid	
tetracycline (Sumycin, Others)	PO: 250–500 mg bid–qid (max: 2 g/day)	Anaphylaxis, superinfections, hepatotoxicity, exfoliative dermatitis, permanent teeth discoloration in children
tigecycline (Tygacil)	IV: 100 mg, followed by 50 mg every 12 h	

Note: Italics indicate common adverse effects. Underline indicates serious adverse effects.

To the Community — Photosensitivity and Antibiotics

C O N N E C T I O N S

Having fun in the sun may be hazardous to some patients. Photosensitivity is a relatively common adverse reaction to some medications, especially antibiotics. Many pharmacologic therapies have photosensitivity as a possible adverse effect. Nurses should counsel patients on the risk of medication-induced photosensitivity and ways to avoid this problem.

Any skin reaction to light is generally defined as photosensitivity. However, this medication-induced adverse effect can present in two categories: phototoxicity and photoallergic reactions. The more common of the two conditions is phototoxicity, which encompasses both sunburn and reactions caused by chemical photosensitizers such as medications. Both reactions are typically manifested by delayed redness and edema

followed by hyperpigmentation. Phototoxicity may occur after first exposure to a drug.

Photoallergic reactions are less common. These reactions present as variations of contact dermatitis and are the result of hypersensitivity. In photoallergic reactions, the drug forms an immunogenic complex with cutaneous proteins due to the presence of light energy. Photoallergic reactions tend to become more pronounced with repeat exposures.

Nurses should educate patients about various methods to protect the skin from damage and severe reactions to the sun. The proper use of protective clothing and sunscreens and restrictions on the amount of time spent in direct sunlight are needed to avoid these problems.

---

be given PO. Several have topical and parenteral formulations. They are sometimes classified by their duration of action as short acting, intermediate acting, or long acting.

Most PO tetracyclines should be taken on an empty stomach to maximize their absorption. Because gastric distress is relatively common with drugs in this class, patients will often take tetracyclines with food. However, these drugs bind metal ions such as calcium and iron, and tetracyclines should not be taken with milk or iron supplements. Food, milk, or other dairy products can reduce drug absorption by 50% or more. Food does not interfere with absorption of the longer acting drugs doxycycline and minocycline.

Because most tetracyclines are incompletely absorbed, they remain in the GI tract in high concentrations, often killing normal flora in the colon. Tetracycline-induced diarrhea is common and could indicate toxic effects on normal flora or a bowel superinfection. The presence of diarrhea must be monitored carefully due to the possibility of **pseudomembranous colitis (PMC)**. Caused by *Clostridium difficile*, this is a rare though potentially severe disorder resulting from therapy with tetracyclines and other classes of antibiotics.

When administered parenterally or in high doses, certain tetracyclines can cause hepatotoxicity, especially in patients with preexisting liver disease. Some patients experience photosensitivity during therapy, making their skin especially susceptible to sunburn. Photosensitivity may appear as exaggerated sunburn within minutes to hours of exposure and is often accompanied by a tingling, burning sensation. Because of their broad spectrum, superinfections due to *Candida albicans* are relatively common. Women who are on oral contraceptives may be more susceptible to vaginal candidiasis. Tetracyclines are usually contraindicated in pregnant or lactating women and in children under the age of 8 because these drugs cause yellow-brown teeth discoloration and may slow the overall growth rate in fetuses or children.

PROTOTYPE DRUG	Tetracycline (Sumycin, Others)

Classification: **Therapeutic:** Antibacterial
Pharmacologic: Bacterial protein synthesis inhibitor, tetracycline

Therapeutic Effects and Uses: Approved in 1953, tetracycline is used for the treatment and prophylaxis of susceptible gram-positive and gram-negative bacteria as well as chlamydiae, rickettsiae, mycoplasmas, and certain protozoa. Tetracycline has one of the broadest spectrums of any antibiotic. Its use has increased during the past decade due to its effectiveness against *H. pylori* in the treatment of peptic ulcer disease. Oral and topical preparations are available for treating inflammatory acne vulgaris.

Mechanism of Action: Tetracycline inhibits bacterial protein synthesis by binding to the 30S ribosomal subunit, interfering with the attachment of the tRNA to the mRNA-ribosome complex. The growing amino acid chain is prematurely terminated and protein synthesis is inhibited. Tetracycline is usually considered bacteriostatic, although it can be bacteriocidal at high concentrations.

Pharmacokinetics:

Route(s)	PO, topical
Absorption	80% is absorbed PO
Distribution	Widely distributed; only small amounts cross the blood–brain barrier; crosses the placenta; secreted in breast milk
Primary metabolism	15–30% metabolized, primarily in the liver
Primary excretion	60% renal, small amounts excreted into bile
Onset of action	1–2 h
Duration of action	Half-life: 6–12 h

Adverse Effects: Being a broad-spectrum antibiotic, tetracycline has a tendency to affect vaginal, oral, and intestinal flora and cause superinfections. Other frequent adverse effects include nausea, vomiting, epigastric burning, diarrhea, discoloration of the teeth, and photosensitivity. Serious adverse reactions include anaphylaxis; fatty degeneration of the liver, producing jaundice; and exfoliative dermatitis. Although not nephrotoxic, tetracycline can worsen kidney impairment in patients with preexisting disease.

Contraindications/Precautions: Tetracycline is contraindicated in patients who are allergic to any drug in the tetracycline class. As a pregnancy category D agent, tetracycline should not be used during pregnancy. Drug therapy must be monitored carefully in patients with impaired hepatic or renal function, because this drug is excreted by these routes.

Drug Interactions: Calcium or iron supplements, magnesium-containing laxatives, and antacids reduce the absorption and serum levels of oral tetracycline. Tetracycline binds with colestipol and cholestyramine, thereby decreasing the antibiotic's absorption. Tetracyclines decrease the effectiveness of oral contraceptives. **Herbal/Food:** Dairy products interfere with tetracycline absorption. Tetracycline eliminates vitamin K–producing bacteria in the intestines; patients taking warfarin may experience an increased anticoagulant effect.

Pregnancy: Category D.

Treatment of Overdose: No specific therapy is available. Patients are treated symptomatically.

Nursing Responsibilities: Key nursing implications for patients receiving tetracycline are included in the Nursing Practice Application for Patients Receiving Tetracycline, Macrolide, or Aminoglycoside Therapy.

Lifespan and Diversity Considerations:

* Monitor hepatic and renal function laboratory values more frequently in the older adult because normal physiological changes related to aging may affect the drug's metabolism and excretion.

* Do not administer tetracycline to children under the age of 8 without confirming the order with the prescriber.

* Carefully monitor for diarrhea in the infant and young child as well as the older adult. Cases of *C. difficile*–associated diarrhea (CDAD) and PMC have been reported with antibiotic use, greatly increasing the risk of fluid and electrolyte imbalances and the risk for severe bowel effects which is a concern for all patients, but especially these populations.

Patient and Family Education:

* Before application of the topical drug, clean the affected skin area with soap and water, rinse, and dry well. Protect the eyes, nose, and mouth from topical medication. Topical tetracycline may stain clothing.

* Be aware that maximal results for treating acne may take up to 12 weeks.

* Note that skin color may appear bright fluorescent yellow to green under ultraviolet light and black light when treated with the topical drug.

* Immediately notify the health care provider of any known or suspected pregnancy.

* Do not breast-feed while taking this drug without approval of the health care provider.

Drugs Similar to Tetracycline (Sumycin, Others)

Other tetracyclines include demeclocycline, doxycycline, minocycline, and tigecycline. Oxytetracycline (Terramycin) was discontinued in the United States in 2003.

Demeclocycline (Declomycin): Approved in 1960, demeclocycline has the same spectrum of action and indications as other drugs in this class. Unrelated to its anti-infective properties, demeclocycline is the only drug in this class that has the ability to stimulate urine flow by blocking the reabsorption of water in the distal renal tubule. Because of this blocking action on antidiuretic hormone (ADH), demeclocycline is used to produce a diuresis in patients with excess ADH secretion. Photosensitivity is more severe with demeclocycline than with any other drug in this class. Demeclocycline undergoes extensive enterohepatic recirculation and is excreted in the bile; thus doses should be reduced for patients with hepatic impairment. This drug is pregnancy category D.

Doxycycline (Vibramycin, Others): Approved in 1967, doxycycline is the safest tetracycline for patients with impaired renal function because it is excreted primarily by nonrenal routes. Normally administered PO, an IV form is available for treating severe infections. It is absorbed well, with or without food, and offers the advantage of once- or twice-daily dosing. Doxycycline is included in the *CDC* "Sexually Transmitted Diseases: Treatment Guidelines" (2010) for treating syphilis, chlamydial infections, and pelvic inflammatory disease. Doxycycline is recommended as an alternative to ciprofloxacin for the prophylactic treatment of *Bacillus anthracis* (anthrax). Adverse effects and contraindications are the same as those of other tetracyclines.

Two doxycycline products are available for the treatment of chronic periodontitis in adults. Atridox is administered as a topical, subgingival controlled release product, and Periostat is given as an oral tablet. Several newer formulations of doxycycline have been approved. In 2005, Doryx, an extended release enteric-coated oral formulation was approved. Approved in 2006, Oracea is a dual-release capsule, containing immediate and delayed release beads for the treatment of inflammatory lesions of the skin associated with rosacea. Oracea is not intended for the treatment or prevention of infections. Doxycycline is pregnancy category D.

Minocycline (Minocin, Others): Approved in 1971, minocycline offers the advantage of once or twice a day dosing and may be administered without regard to meals or dairy products. It is the only tetracycline that can cause reversible vestibular toxicity, resulting in dizziness, vertigo, and weakness that can limit therapy. Minocycline is active against some strains of bacteria that are resistant to other drugs in the tetracycline class. Hepatic function laboratory values should be monitored during therapy to assess for hepatotoxicity. Other adverse effects and contraindications are the same as those of other tetracyclines. A microsphere powder formulation, called Arestin, is introduced subgingivally to treat periodontitis. In 2006, Solodyn, an extended release tablet, was approved for the treatment of inflammatory lesions associated with moderate to severe acne vulgaris in patients over 12 years of age. This drug is pregnancy category D.

Tigecycline (Tygacil): Tigecycline is a tetracycline that was approved in 2005. Available only by the intravenous (IV) route, it has more limited indications than other drugs in this class: complicated skin and skin structure infections and complicated intra-abdominal infections in patients over age 18. Tigecycline is effective against certain bacterial strains resistant to other antibiotics, including methicillin-resistant *Staphylococcus aureus* (MRSA) and vancomycin-resistant enterococci (VRE). It has not yet shown any cross-resistance with other antibiotics. Nausea and vomiting are the most frequent adverse effects, and these may be severe enough to cause discontinuation of therapy. Life-threatening anaphylaxis and pancreatitis have been reported. A slight increase in mortality has been reported with the use of tigecycline, although its cause remains unknown. Other adverse effects and contraindications are the same as those of other tetracyclines. Hepatic function laboratory values should be monitored during therapy to assess for hepatotoxicity. This drug is pregnancy category D.

PharmFACT

The bubonic plague caused by the bacterium *Yersinia pestis* was responsible for killing approximately 50% of the population during the 5th and 6th centuries AD, and 40% of the population between the 8th and 14th centuries. If antibiotics had been available back then, most of the estimated 200 million people who died would likely have survived after a 10-day treatment with tetracyclines or aminoglycosides (Dufel, 2011).

Macrolides

3 The macrolides are alternatives to penicillin for many gram-positive infections.

Erythromycin (EryC, Erythrocin, Others), the first macrolide antibiotic, was isolated from *Streptomyces* organisms in a soil sample in 1952. The name *macrolide* was chosen for this drug class because they all possess an unusually large 14- to 15-atom ring as part of their chemical structure. Doses for the macrolides are listed in Table 2.

Macrolides are considered alternative drugs for patients who are allergic to penicillin. They are widely prescribed although they are the drugs of first choice for relatively few diseases. Most effective against gram-positive bacteria, common indications for macrolides include the treatment of whooping cough, diphtheria, Legionnaire's disease, and infections by streptococci, *Haemophilus influenzae*, *Mycoplasma pneumoniae*, and chlamydia. Clarithromycin is one of several antibiotics used to treat peptic ulcer disease due

to its activity against *H. pylori*. The macrolides are preferred drugs for the prophylaxis of recurring rheumatic fever in patients who are allergic to penicillins. Fidaxomicin (Dificid) was approved in 2011 for treatment of *C. difficile*–associated diarrhea.

The macrolides inhibit bacterial protein synthesis by binding to the 50S ribosomal subunit, thus preventing movement of the ribosome along the mRNA. Macrolides do not bind to human ribosomes, thus offering a degree of selective toxicity. These agents are usually bacteriostatic, though they may be bacteriocidal depending on the dose and the target organism.

The newer macrolides have longer half-lives and generally cause less GI irritation than erythromycin, which is the original drug from which macrolides were synthesized. Azithromycin (Zithromax) has an extended half-life such that it can be administered for only 5 days rather than the 10-day therapy required for most antibiotics. A single dose of azithromycin is effective against *N. gonorrhoeae*. The brief duration of therapy is thought to increase patient adherence and to offset the added cost of azithromycin.

Like most of the older antibiotics, macrolide-resistant strains are becoming more common. Many organisms develop resistance to macrolides by pumping it out of the cell before the antibiotic has a chance to reach an effective concentration. In some cases, bacteria have modified the shape of their 50S ribosomal subunit so that it no longer binds the drug.

The macrolides are well tolerated and considered to be one of the safest antibiotic classes. The most common adverse effects are GI related and include nausea, vomiting, abdominal cramping, and diarrhea. These GI symptoms occur whether the drug is administered PO or IV. Taking the drug with food can significantly inhibit the absorption of troleandomycin and azithromycin suspension. Thus these drugs should be taken on an empty stomach.

Many macrolides have an enteric coating, which serves two purposes. First, the coating allows the drug to dissolve in the small intestine rather than the stomach, causing less gastric irritation. Second, the macrolides are inactivated in gastric acid, and the enteric coating allows it to avoid destruction and reach the small intestine where they are readily absorbed in the alkaline environment.

Macrolides are metabolized and concentrated in the liver and excreted into bile. Because macrolides decrease the hepatic metabolism of other drugs, a number of drug–drug

TABLE 2 Macrolides		
Drug	**Route and Adult Dose** (maximum dose where indicated)	**Adverse Effects**
azithromycin (Zithromax, Zmax)	PO: 500 mg for one dose, then 250 mg/day for 4 days	*Nausea, vomiting, diarrhea, abdominal cramping, dry skin or burning (topical route)*
clarithromycin (Biaxin)	PO: 250–500 mg bid	
erythromycin (EryC, Erythrocin, Others)	PO: 250–500 mg bid or 333 mg tid	Anaphylaxis, ototoxicity, PMC, hepatotoxicity, superinfections, dysrhythmias
fidaxomicin (Dificid)	PO: 200 mg bid for 10 days	*Nausea, vomiting, abdominal pain* GI bleeding, anemia, neutropenia

Note: Italics indicate common adverse effects. Underline indicates serious adverse effects.

interactions are possible. When macrolides prevent the conversion of drugs to their less active form, the serum levels of these other drugs will increase and cause potential toxicity. For example, warfarin (Coumadin) is extensively metabolized to its inactive form in the liver. If given concurrently with erythromycin, the destruction of warfarin is diminished and greater amounts of "active" warfarin remain in the blood for longer periods. Because warfarin increases bleeding time, this could result in prolonged bleeding in a patient. In general, doses of drugs that are metabolized in the liver should be reduced, or at least carefully monitored, if they are given concurrently with macrolides.

CONNECTION Checkpoint 51.1

What type of laboratory monitoring should be done for a patient who is taking warfarin concurrently with a macrolide? *See Answer to Connection Checkpoint 51.1 on student resource website.*

| PROTOTYPE DRUG | Erythromycin (EryC, Erythrocin, Others) |

Classification: **Therapeutic:** Antibacterial
Pharmacologic: Bacterial protein synthesis inhibitor, macrolide

Therapeutic Effects and Uses: Erythromycin (also called erythromycin base) is indicated for the treatment and prophylaxis of susceptible bacterial infections. The main application for erythromycin is for patients who are allergic to penicillins or who may have a penicillin-resistant infection. It has a spectrum similar to that of the penicillins and is effective against most gram-positive bacteria, including susceptible strains of *Staphylococcus* and *Streptococcus*. Susceptible gram-negative strains include *N. gonorrhea* and *H. influenzae*. It is a drug of choice for infections from *Bordetella pertussis* (whooping cough), *Legionella pneumophila* (Legionnaire's disease), *M. pneumoniae,* and *Corynebacterium diphtheriae.*

All oral forms of erythromycin are considered to have equal effectiveness. Topical and ophthalmic formulations are also available. Erythromycin is available in a number of salts:

- Erythromycin stearate (Erythrocin) and erythromycin ethylsuccinate (EryPed, Pediamycin) are acid stable and more readily absorbed in the stomach than erythromycin base. These forms are converted to the base form in the liver before they become bacteriostatic. The stearate salt should be taken on an empty stomach, whereas the ethylsuccinate salt may be taken without regard to food.

- Erythromycin lactobionate is given IV when the patient is unable to take oral medications, or when the infection is severe enough to warrant a faster onset of action.

Mechanism of Action: Erythromycin inhibits bacterial protein synthesis by binding to the 50S ribosomal subunit. Erythromycin is considered bacteriostatic but may be bacteriocidal in high doses.

Pharmacokinetics:

Route(s)	PO, topical, IV (gluceptate and lactobionate salts)
Absorption	Readily absorbed PO; enteric coated
Distribution	Widely distributed; only small amounts cross the blood–brain barrier; secreted in breast milk
Primary metabolism	Hepatic metabolism (CYP3A); concentrates in the liver and bile
Primary excretion	Bile
Onset of action	1 h
Duration of action	Half-life: 1.5–2 h

Adverse Effects: The most common adverse effects from erythromycin are nausea, vomiting, and abdominal cramping, although these are rarely serious enough to cause discontinuation of therapy. Concurrent administration with food reduces these adverse effects. When given by the IV route, phlebitis and intense pain at the injection site are common. Anaphylaxis is possible. Hearing loss, vertigo, and dizziness may be experienced when using high doses, particularly in older adults and in those with impaired hepatic or renal excretion. High doses of IV erythromycin may be cardiotoxic and pose a risk for torsades de pointes, which is a type of dysrhythmia that is potentially fatal. Like nearly all other antibiotics, PMC is possible with the use of erythromycin.

Contraindications/Precautions: Erythromycin is contraindicated in patients with hypersensitivity to drugs in the macrolide class and for those who are taking terfenadine, astemizole, or cisapride. Drug therapy must be monitored carefully in patients with impaired hepatic or biliary function, due to the possibility of **cholestatic hepatitis**, a type of liver inflammation caused by obstruction of the bile ducts.

Drug Interactions: Erythromycin inhibits hepatic CYP450 metabolic enzymes and can interact with many drugs. When used concurrently with erythromycin, the serum levels and toxicities of alfentanil, carbamazepine, cyclosporine, fentanyl, theophylline, and methadone may increase. Because erythromycin may increase the effects of digoxin or warfarin, leading to abnormal bleeding, the doses of these anticoagulants may need to be lowered. Erythromycin competes with clindamycin and chloramphenicol for binding sites on the 50S bacterial ribosomal subunit, causing an antagonistic effect. Thus these antibiotics should not be taken concurrently. The concurrent use of erythromycin with lovastatin or simvastatin is not recommended because it may increase the risk of myopathy and rhabdomyolysis. Because fluconazole also inhibits CYP3A4, especially at high dosages, its concurrent use with erythromycin should be avoided. **Herbal/Food:** Grapefruit juice may increase the bioavailability of erythromycin.

Pregnancy: Category B.

Treatment of Overdose: No specific therapy is available. Patients are treated symptomatically.

Nursing Responsibilities: Key nursing implications for patients receiving erythromycin are included in the Nursing Practice

Application for Patients Receiving Tetracycline, Macrolide, or Aminoglycoside Therapy.

Lifespan and Diversity Considerations:

- Monitor hepatic function laboratory values more frequently in the older adult because normal physiological changes related to aging may affect the drug's metabolism.

- Because erythromycin is metabolized through one of the P450 system pathways, monitor ethnically diverse populations frequently to ensure optimal therapeutic effects and minimize the risk of adverse effects.

- Carefully monitor for diarrhea in the infant and young child as well as the older adult. Cases of CDAD and PMC have been reported with antibiotic use, greatly increasing the risk of fluid and electrolyte imbalances and the risk for severe bowel effects, which is a concern for all patients, but especially these populations.

Patient and Family Education:

- Shake liquid and pediatric drops well before each use to mix the medication evenly. Use the bottle dropper to measure the dose of pediatric drops.

- Do not breast-feed while taking this drug without approval of the health care provider.

Drugs Similar to Erythromycin (EryC, Erythrocin, Others)

Other macrolides include azithromycin and clarithromycin. The macrolide dirithromycin (Dynabac) is no longer available in the United States.

Azithromycin (Zithromax, Zmax): Approved in 1991, azithromycin has a long duration of action that allows for less frequent dosing. A "Tri-pak" consists of three 500 mg tablets (taken over 3 days) and a "Z-pak" contains six 250 mg tablets (taken over 5 days). For acute otitis media in children, a single dose has been found to be as effective as 3- or 5-day regimens. An IV form for infusions is available for the treatment of pelvic inflammatory disease and community-acquired pneumonia. An ophthalmic solution (AzaSite) was approved in 2007 for treating bacterial conjunctivitis. Azithromycin demonstrates greater activity over gram-negative organisms than erythromycin.

Azithromycin causes less nausea than erythromycin and may be taken with or without food. The extended release oral suspension should be administered on an empty stomach. Because azithromycin does not inhibit liver metabolism, it is safer for patients with hepatic impairment and causes fewer drug–drug interactions than erythromycin base. The most common adverse effects are diarrhea, nausea, and abdominal pain. Patients with a known hypersensitivity to any macrolide should not receive azithromycin. This drug is pregnancy category B.

Clarithromycin (Biaxin): Approved in 1991, clarithromycin is similar to erythromycin but causes significantly less nausea, and the regular release tablets may be taken with or without food. The drug is commonly prescribed for infections of the respiratory tract, sexually transmitted infections, H. pylori–associated peptic ulcer disease, and otitis media. An extended release (XL) formulation is used to treat sinusitis, chronic bronchitis, and community-acquired pneumonia. The XL form should be administered with food because its absorption is increased. The most frequent adverse effects with clarithromycin are diarrhea, nausea, abnormal taste, dyspepsia, abdominal discomfort, and headache. Like erythromycin, clarithromycin is metabolized by CYP 450 enzymes and a significant number of drug–drug interactions may occur. Patients with a known hypersensitivity to any macrolide should not receive clarithromycin. This drug is pregnancy category C.

Fidaxomicin (Dificid): The newest of the macrolides, fidaxomicin was approved in 2011 specifically for infections proven or strongly suspected to be caused by C. difficile. The drug should only be prescribed for this indication because other uses could encourage the development of resistant strains. Taken as an oral tablet, the drug is not significantly absorbed and remains in the digestive tract where it produces its effects on C. difficle. Fidaxomicin appears to have equal efficacy to vancomycin, the primary antibiotic used to treat C. difficile diarrhea. Relapses are less frequent than with vancomycin. The drug is well tolerated with the most frequent adverse effects being nausea, vomiting, abdominal pain and GI bleeding. This drug is pregnancy category B.

Aminoglycosides

4 The aminoglycosides are effective against aerobic gram-negative organisms but have the potential to cause ototoxicity and nephrotoxicity.

The first aminoglycoside, streptomycin, was named after *Streptomyces griseus*, the soil organism from which it was isolated in 1943. Once widely used, streptomycin is now usually reserved for the treatment of tuberculosis (TB) due to the development of safer alternatives and the appearance of a large number of resistant strains. Other aminoglycosides have since been isolated, and several have been produced semisynthetically. All have a common chemical structure of two or more amino sugars with a glycosidic, or sugar, link. The differences in spelling of some of these drugs, *-mycin* and *-micin*, reflects the different organisms from which the drugs were originally isolated. Doses for the aminoglycosides are listed in Table 3.

Aminoglycosides bind irreversibly to the 30S ribosomal subunit of bacteria, changing its shape and preventing the initiation stage of protein synthesis. Some drugs in this class also affect the 50S subunit. In addition, these antibiotics cause mRNA to be read incorrectly, resulting in abnormal proteins that are subsequently inserted into the bacterial plasma membrane, causing it to leak. Whereas most antibiotics that affect protein synthesis are bacteriostatic, aminoglycosides are bacteriocidal.

Although they have the ability to kill many different bacterial species, the aminoglycosides are considered narrow-spectrum drugs because they are normally reserved for serious systemic infections caused by aerobic gram-negative organisms, such as *Pseudomonas* and members of the Enterobacteriaceae family, which includes *E. coli*, *Serratia*, *Proteus*, and *Klebsiella*.

TABLE 3 Aminoglycosides

Drug	Route and Adult Dose (maximum dose where indicated)	Adverse Effects
amikacin	IV/IM: 5–7.5 mg/kg as a loading dose, then 7.5 mg/kg bid	*Pain or inflammation at the injection site, rash, fever, nausea, diarrhea, dizziness, tinnitus*
gentamicin (Garamycin, Others)	IV/IM: 1.5–2 mg/kg as a loading dose, then 1–2 mg/kg bid–tid	
kanamycin	IV/IM: 5–7.5 mg/kg bid–tid	Anaphylaxis, nephrotoxicity, irreversible ototoxicity, superinfections
neomycin	PO: 4–12 g/day in divided doses	
paromomycin (Humatin)	PO: 7.5–12.5 mg/kg tid	
streptomycin	IM: 15 mg/kg up to 1 g as a single dose	
tobramycin	IV/IM: 1 mg/kg tid (max: 5 mg/kg/day)	

Note: Italics indicate common adverse effects. <u>Underline</u> indicates serious adverse effects.

Aminoglycosides are ineffective against most gram-positive bacteria. Because oxygen is required for aminoglycoside antibiotics to be transported inside bacterial cells, this class of drugs does not affect anaerobes.

Most aminoglycosides are polar compounds that are poorly absorbed from the GI tract. Less than 1% of an oral dose is absorbed; therefore they must be administered parenterally to treat systemic infections. Because aminoglycosides travel through the alimentary canal unchanged, they are occasionally given PO to sterilize the bowel prior to intestinal surgery. Neomycin is available for topical infections of the skin, eyes, and ears. Paromomycin (Humatin) is given orally for the treatment of parasitic infections.

Due to their polar nature, aminoglycosides cannot enter most human cells. Although distributed to most body fluids, not enough of the drugs enter the cerebrospinal fluid (CSF) for them to treat central nervous system infections. Aminoglycosides can, however, cross the placenta. If taken late in pregnancy, streptomycin can cause hearing loss in the child. In addition, aminoglycosides concentrate in renal tissue, which leads to potential nephrotoxicity.

Resistance develops quickly when aminoglycosides are administered as monotherapy. Resistance occurs when a species acquires an ability to degrade the antibiotic. Once degraded by the bacterial enzymes, these drugs are unable to bind with the bacterial ribosome. Some resistance also occurs when mutations change the shape of the bacterial ribosome so that it no longer binds the aminoglycoside. The emergence of aminoglycoside-resistant strains of *Enterococcus faecalis* and *Enterococcus faecium* has become a serious clinical problem because there are few therapeutic alternatives to treat these infections. Once resistance develops to an aminoglycoside, the mutant strain is usually resistant to the other drugs in this class. An exception is amikacin, which appears to have some activity against gentamicin-resistant strains.

Several techniques have been used to increase the effectiveness of the aminoglycosides. Administering these drugs in one large dose per day rather than smaller divided doses results in a greater bacteriocidal effect and fewer resistant microbes. A second technique is to administer aminoglycosides and penicillins concurrently (though not mixed in the same IV solution). The penicillin weakens the cell wall, allowing a greater amount of aminoglycoside to enter and reach its ribosomal targets.

Aminoglycosides are excreted almost exclusively by the kidneys. Because certain tissues bind the drugs very tightly, renal excretion may be prolonged up to 20 days after discontinuation of the drug. Although serum drug levels may fall below what is considered a minimally effective concentration, some antimicrobial activity continues during this time. This is known as a **postantibiotic effect**.

The clinical applications of the aminoglycosides are limited by their potential to cause serious adverse effects. The degree and types of toxicity are similar for all drugs in this class. For example, all aminoglycosides can impair both hearing and balance. Damage to sensory cells in the cochlea causes hearing loss. Balance is affected by damage to sensory cells in the vestibular apparatus of the inner ear. As many as 25% of patients who are taking aminoglycoside antibiotics may experience some ototoxicity. This effect is more prominent when the medications are used for longer than 10 days, or when the patient has preexisting kidney impairment, causing high serum drug levels. The damage to sensory cells is cumulative; repeated doses of the drug can damage increasing numbers of cells. Because many older adults have some degree of preexisting hearing impairment, permanent deafness may occur in this group. Signs of impending inner ear damage include high-pitched tinnitus, headache, nausea, vomiting, and vertigo. Signs of ototoxicity may continue for several weeks after the drugs are discontinued. If hearing and balance functions are not carefully monitored during therapy and proper interventions are not implemented, the ototoxicity may become irreversible.

One of the most serious adverse effects of aminoglycosides is their potential to cause nephrotoxicity. Aminoglycosides directly injure renal tubule cells, and this nephrotoxicity may be severe, affecting up to 26% of patients receiving these antibiotics. As expected, patients who are receiving higher doses for longer periods are most affected. Those with preexisting renal impairment or who are receiving concurrent therapy with other nephrotoxic agents must be monitored carefully: Regular evaluation of urinalysis, blood urea nitrogen (BUN), and serum creatinine results is essential. Serum drug concentrations should be obtained regularly and doses adjusted accordingly to prevent permanent damage. If recognized early, renal damage caused by aminoglycosides is reversible. Impaired kidney function may cause drug serum levels to rise, thus increasing the risk or worsening of ototoxicity.

A less common, though serious adverse effect of aminoglycosides is neuromuscular blockade. Aminoglycosides inhibit the release of acetylcholine at synapses. Giving other drugs that affect acetylcholine release, such as anesthetics or neuromuscular blockers, can result in profound apnea and prolonged muscle paralysis. Because they have fewer acetylcholine receptors, patients with myasthenia gravis are especially at risk. To avoid the problem, aminoglycosides may be discontinued prior to surgery. IV calcium salts have been found to reverse aminoglycoside-induced neuromuscular blockade.

CONNECTION Checkpoint 51.2

Name the prototype drugs classified as neuromuscular blockers. Is muscle paralysis occurring at a nicotinic or muscarinic synapse? *See Answer to Connection Checkpoint 51.2 on student resource website.*

PROTOTYPE DRUG | Gentamicin (Garamycin, Others)

Classification: **Therapeutic:** Antibacterial
Pharmacologic: Bacterial protein synthesis inhibitor, aminoglycoside

Therapeutic Effects and Uses: Approved in 1966, gentamicin is used for the treatment and prophylaxis of susceptible bacterial infections. It is prescribed primarily for serious infections caused by aerobic, gram-negative bacilli. Activity includes *Enterobacter, E. coli, Klebsiella, Citrobacter, Pseudomonas,* and *Serratia.* Gentamicin is effective against a few gram-positive bacteria, including some strains of MRSA. It has no activity against anaerobes. This drug is not absorbed by the PO route. A topical formulation (Genoptic) is available for infections of the external eye.

Therapy with gentamicin is generally limited to those cases in which a less toxic alternative is not available. Resistance to gentamicin is increasing, and some patients show cross-resistance to other aminoglycosides such as tobramycin. Gentamicin is sometimes given concurrently with a beta-lactam antibiotic such as a penicillin or cephalosporin to improve bacterial kill and to delay resistance.

Mechanism of Action: Gentamicin inhibits bacterial protein synthesis by binding to the 30S ribosomal subunit. Gentamicin is bacteriocidal in that it causes premature termination of the growing polypeptide chain.

Pharmacokinetics:

Route(s)	Intramuscular (IM), IV, topical (ophthalmic)
Absorption	Not absorbed PO; readily absorbed IM
Distribution	Distributed to most body tissues and fluids, except the CSF; concentrates in the kidney and inner ear; crosses the placenta; small amounts secreted in breast milk;
Primary metabolism	Not metabolized
Primary excretion	Renal
Onset of action	Rapid
Duration of action	Half-life: 3–4 h

Adverse Effects: Resistance to gentamicin is increasing and some cross-resistance among aminoglycosides has been reported. Rash, nausea, vomiting, and fatigue are the most common adverse effects. **Black Box Warnings:** Adverse effects from parenteral gentamicin may be severe and include the following:

- Neurotoxicity may manifest as ototoxicity and produce a loss of hearing or balance, which may become permanent with continued use. Tinnitus, vertigo, and persistent headaches are early signs of ototoxicity. The risk of neurologic effects is higher in patients with impaired renal function. Other signs of neurotoxicity include paresthesias, muscle twitching, and seizures. Concurrent use with other neurotoxic drugs should be avoided.

- Neuromuscular blockade and respiratory paralysis are possible and the drug may cause severe neuromuscular weakness that lasts for several days.

- Nephrotoxicity is possible. Signs of reduced kidney function include oliguria, proteinuria, and elevated BUN and creatinine levels. Nephrotoxicity is of particular concern to patients with preexisting kidney disease and may limit pharmacotherapy. Concurrent use with other nephrotoxic drugs should be avoided.

Contraindications/Precautions: Gentamicin is contraindicated in patients who are hypersensitive to aminoglycosides. Drug therapy must be monitored carefully in patients with impaired renal function or in those with preexisting hearing loss. Gentamicin should not be used in pregnant or breast-feeding patients.

Drug Interactions: Concurrent use with other nephrotoxic drugs such as acyclovir, amphotericin B, capreomycin, cisplatin, cyclosporine, salicylates, polymyxin B, or vancomycin increases the risk of nephrotoxicity. Other drugs affecting the eighth cranial nerve such as ethacrynic acid and furosemide will increase the risk of ototoxicity if given concurrently with gentamicin. Penicillins can inactivate aminoglycosides if they are mixed together in the same solution. Antiemetics such as dimenhydrinate, meclizine, promethazine, and scopolamine may block the nausea characteristic of vestibular toxicity or motion sickness, thus masking the signs of aminoglycoside-induced ototoxicityV. **Herbal/Food:** No significant interactions are known.

Pregnancy: Category D (parenteral).

Treatment of Overdose: Overdose can result in serious kidney damage and ototoxicity. No specific therapy is available. Patients are treated symptomatically.

Nursing Responsibilities: Key nursing implications for patients receiving gentamicin are included in the Nursing Practice Application for Patients Receiving Tetracycline, Macrolide, or Aminoglycoside Therapy.

Lifespan and Diversity Considerations:

- Monitor renal function laboratory values more frequently in the older adult because normal physiological changes related to aging may affect the drug's excretion.

- Monitor for changes in hearing or balance frequently in the older adult because normal changes in hearing, balance, or gait related to aging may mask ototoxic drug effects.

- Carefully monitor for diarrhea in the infant and young child as well as the older adult. Cases of CDAD and PMC have been reported with antibiotic use, greatly increasing the risk of fluid and electrolyte imbalances and the risk for severe bowel effects, which is a concern for all patients, but especially these populations.

Patient and Family Education:

- Immediately notify your health care provider of any known or suspected pregnancy.

- Do not breast-feed while taking this drug without prior approval of the health care provider.

Drugs Similar to Gentamicin (Garamycin, Others)

Other aminoglycosides include amikacin, kanamycin, neomycin, paromomycin, streptomycin, and tobramycin. All aminoglycosides have similar spectrums of activity and adverse effects. They all carry the same black box warning as gentamicin.

Amikacin: Approved in 1976, amikacin has the broadest spectrum in this class, and is sometimes effective against organisms that have developed resistance to other aminoglycosides. Amikacin has been used to treat multidrug-resistant TB. It is administered by the IV and IM routes. Indications, contraindications, and adverse effects (including the black box warning) are nearly the same as those for gentamicin. This is a pregnancy category D drug.

Kanamycin: Approved in 1958, kanamycin is the most toxic aminoglycoside, and resistant strains are common. Its use is limited to the adjunctive treatment of hepatic coma and for the short-term treatment of serious infections. Like amikacin, kanamycin may be used to treat multidrug-resistant TB after first-line agents have failed. Kanamycin can be delivered IV, IM, by inhalation, or by intraperitoneal instillation. Contraindications and adverse effects (including the black box warning) are the same as for gentamicin. This is a pregnancy category D drug. Concurrent therapy with other nephrotoxic and neurotoxic drugs should be avoided due to the potential for additive adverse effects.

Neomycin: Approved in 1952, neomycin is widely used for topical infections as an OTC ointment combined with polymyxin B and bacitracin (Neosporin). It is also combined in OTC creams with hydrocortisone for minor skin irritations and insect bites. Not available in parenteral form due to toxicity, neomycin may be used orally to sterilize the bowel. Oral neomycin can cause headache, lethargy, nausea, and vomiting. Oral neomycin carries a black box warning regarding neurotoxicity, nephrotoxicity, and ototoxicity. This is a pregnancy category C drug.

Paromomycin (Humatin): Approved in 1959, paromomycin is most active against gram-negative aerobic bacteria (with the exception of *Pseudomonas*). When administered orally, the drug is not absorbed and 100% is recovered in the feces. The primary use of this drug is for sterilizing the bowel and treating intestinal parasitic infections caused by protozoans and tapeworms. Because this drug is not absorbed systemically, it does not carry the same black box warnings as other aminoglycosides. This is a pregnancy category C drug.

Streptomycin: The use of streptomycin, the first aminoglycoside approved by the U.S. Food and Drug Administration (FDA) in 1945, was generally discontinued in 1993, but it is still available on a case-by-case basis. It is rarely used due to a large number of resistant strains and its high risk for ototoxicity. It is most often used in combination with other drugs in the pharmacotherapy of multidrug-resistant TB. Streptomycin carries a black box warning regarding neurotoxicity and nephrotoxicity. This is a pregnancy category D drug.

Tobramycin: Approved in 1975, tobramycin has a spectrum of activity similar to that of gentamicin, but it is more effective against *P. aeruginosa* than gentamicin. Most often administered parenterally, tobramycin is also available as an ophthalmic solution (Tobrex) and in nebulizer form for patients with cystic fibrosis who have *Pseudomonas* infections. Adverse effects (including the black box warning) and contraindications are similar to those of gentamicin. This is a pregnancy category D drug.

PharmFACT

This chapter discussed antibiotics selective for bacterial protein synthesis. However, bacteria can fight back. *Corynebacterium diphtheriae* produces a toxin that targets human protein synthesis (Madigan, Martinko, Stahl, & Clark, 2012).

CONNECTIONS: NURSING PRACTICE APPLICATION

Patients Receiving Tetracycline, Macrolide, or Aminoglycoside Therapy

Assessment	Potential Nursing Diagnoses
Baseline assessment prior to administration: • Understand the reason the drug has been prescribed in order to assess for therapeutic effects. • Obtain a complete health history including neurologic, cardiovascular, respiratory, hepatic, or renal disease, and the possibility of pregnancy. Obtain a drug history including allergies, specific reactions to drugs, current prescription and OTC drugs, herbal preparations, and alcohol use. Be alert to possible drug interactions. • Assess signs and symptoms of the current infection noting location, characteristics, presence or absence of drainage and the characteristics of drainage, duration, and presence or absence of fever or pain. • Evaluate appropriate laboratory findings (e.g., CBC, culture and sensitivity [C&S], hepatic and renal function studies). • Assess the patient's ability to receive and understand instructions. Include family and caregivers as needed.	• *Infection* (bacterial) • *Acute Pain* • *Hyperthermia* • *Deficient Knowledge* (Drug Therapy) • *Risk for Injury*, related to adverse drug effects • *Risk for Deficient Fluid Volume*, related to diarrhea caused by adverse drug effects

Assessment throughout administration:

- Assess for desired therapeutic effects (e.g., diminished signs and symptoms of infection and fever).
- Continue periodic monitoring of CBC, hepatic and renal function, urinalysis, and C&S as ordered.
- Assess for adverse effects: nausea, vomiting, abdominal cramping, diarrhea, drowsiness, tinnitus, or dizziness. Severe diarrhea, especially that containing mucus, blood, or pus, yellowing of the sclera or skin, decreased urine output or darkened urine should be reported immediately.

Planning: Patient Goals and Expected Outcomes

The patient will:

- Experience therapeutic effects dependent on the reason the drug is being given (e.g., diminished signs and symptoms of infection, decreased fever).
- Be free from or experience minimal adverse effects.
- Verbalize an understanding of the drug's use, adverse effects, and required precautions.
- Demonstrate proper self-administration of the medication (e.g., dose, timing, and when to notify the provider).

Implementation

Interventions and (Rationales)	Patient-Centered Education
Ensuring therapeutic effects: • Continue assessments as above for therapeutic effects. (Diminished fever, pain, or signs and symptoms of infection should begin after taking the first dose and continue to improve. The provider should be notified if fever and signs and symptoms of infection remain or increase after 3 days, or if the entire course of antibacterial has been taken and signs of infection are still present.)	• Teach the patient to report fever that does not diminish below 37.8°C (100°F) or per parameters set by the health care provider within 3 days, increasing signs and symptoms of infection, or symptoms that remain present after taking the entire course of the antibacterial drug. • Teach the patient *not* to stop taking the antibacterial when feeling better but to take the entire course of the antibacterial drug; do not share doses with other family members with similar symptoms; and return to the provider if symptoms have not resolved after an entire course of therapy.
Minimizing adverse effects: • Continue to monitor vital signs, especially temperature if fever is present. Immediately report undiminished fever, changes in level of consciousness, or febrile seizures to the health care provider. (Fever should begin to diminish within 1–3 days after starting the drug. Continued fever may be a sign of worsening infection, adverse drug effects, or antibiotic resistance.)	• Teach the patient to report fever that does not diminish below 37.8°C (100°F) or per parameters set by the health care provider. Immediately report febrile seizures, changes in behavior, or changes in level of consciousness to the health care provider.
• Continue to monitor periodic laboratory work: hepatic and renal function tests, CBC, urinalysis, C&S, and peak and trough drug levels as ordered. (Tetracyclines and aminoglycosides may be renal toxic; macrolides may be hepatotoxic. Laboratory values should be monitored to prevent adverse effects. Periodic C&S tests may be ordered if infections are severe or are slow to resolve to confirm appropriate therapy. Peak and trough drug levels will be monitored for aminoglycosides to prevent severe adverse effects.)	• Instruct the patient on the need for periodic laboratory work.
• Monitor for hypersensitivity and allergic reactions, especially with the first dose of the drug. Continue to monitor the patient for up to 2 weeks after completing antibacterial therapy. (Anaphylactic reactions are possible, particularly with the first dose of an antibacterial. As sensitivity occurs, reactions may continue to develop. Post-use, residual drug levels, dependent on the length of half-life, may cause delayed reactions.)	• Teach the patient to immediately report any itching, rashes, or swelling, particularly of the face or tongue, urticaria, flushing, dizziness, syncope, wheezing, throat tightness, or difficulty breathing. • Instruct the patient with known antibacterial allergies to carry a wallet identification card or wear medical identification jewelry indicating the allergy.
• Continue to monitor for renal toxicity; e.g., diminished urine output, or weight gain greater than 1 kg (2.2 lb) in 24 h. (Tetracyclines and aminoglycosides may require frequent monitoring to prevent adverse effects. Increasing fluid intake will help prevent drug accumulation in the kidneys.)	• Teach the patient to immediately report any diminished urine output, visible swelling of feet or ankles, or weight gain greater than 1 kg (2.2 lbs) in 24 h. • Advise the patient to increase fluid intake to 2–3 L/day.
• Monitor for severe diarrhea, especially if mucus, blood, or pus is present. (Severe diarrhea may indicate the presence of CDAD or PMC.)	• Instruct the patient to report any diarrhea that increases in frequency, amount, or contains mucus, blood, or pus. • Instruct the patient to consult the health care provider before taking any antidiarrheal drugs, because they cause the retention of harmful bacteria. • Teach the patient to increase the intake of dairy products containing live active cultures such as yogurt, kefir, or buttermilk, to help restore normal intestinal flora. Do not take dairy products at the same time as a tetracycline antibiotic. Take the tetracycline 1 h before or 2 h after a meal containing dairy.
• Monitor for the development of superinfections, e.g., PMC, fungal or yeast infections. (Superinfections with opportunistic organisms may occur when normal host flora are diminished or killed by the antibacterial drug and no longer hold pathogens in check. Appropriate treatment may be needed.)	• Teach the patient to observe for changes in the color, consistency, or frequency of stool, white patches in the mouth, whitish thick vaginal discharge, itching in the genital area, or blistering itchy rash, and to immediately report severe diarrhea. • Teach the patient infection control measures such as frequent hand washing, adequate drying after showering or bathing, and to increase the intake of live-culture dairy foods.

CONNECTIONS: NURSING PRACTICE APPLICATION *(continued)*

• Monitor for significant GI effects, including nausea, vomiting, abdominal pain or cramping, difficulty swallowing, or throat pain. Give tetracycline or erythromycin with 240 mL (8 oz) of water on an empty stomach or with a small amount of food if the patient cannot tolerate the drug on an empty stomach. (Some forms of erythromycin may be given with food. Carbonated or acidic beverages should be avoided to prevent further GI upset or irritation. Do not give tetracyclines with milk products or concurrently with iron preparations or antacids. Immediately report any difficulty swallowing or throat or epigastric pain, which may indicate esophagitis or esophageal ulceration secondary to tetracycline use.)	• Teach the patient to take the drug with a full glass of water on an empty stomach, and to avoid acidic beverages or carbonated drinks that may increase the chance of GI distress. • Teach the patient taking tetracycline to immediately report any difficulty in swallowing or throat or epigastric pain.
• Monitor for signs and symptoms of neurotoxicity, e.g., dizziness, drowsiness, severe headache, tinnitus, increasing muscle weakness, paresthesias, twitching, or seizures. (Aminoglycosides have an increased risk of neurotoxicity. Previous seizure disorders or head injuries may increase this risk. Frequent monitoring is needed to prevent adverse effects. Tinnitus, vertigo, and persistent headaches are early symptoms and should be immediately reported.)	• Instruct the patient to immediately report increasing headache, dizziness, vertigo, tinnitus (ringing, humming, or buzzing in the ears), twitching, or seizures.
• Monitor for signs and symptoms of ototoxicity, e.g., dizziness, vertigo, tinnitus, or diminished hearing. (Erythromycin and aminoglycosides have an increased risk of ototoxicity. Frequent monitoring is needed to prevent adverse effects.)	• Instruct the patient to immediately report dizziness, vertigo, tinnitus, or diminished hearing.
• Monitor for the effects of other drugs if the patient is on erythromycin. (Erythromycin inhibits CYP 450 enzymes and is known to increase the effects of some drugs such as anticoagulants and digoxin and decrease others. Grapefruit juice taken concurrently with erythromycin may increase drug levels.)	• Teach the patient to report any unusual effects related to other drugs taken concurrently. If the patient is taking anticoagulants, an increase in bleeding should be immediately reported. • Teach the patient not to consume grapefruit or grapefruit juice while taking erythromycin.
• Continue to monitor for dermatologic effects including red or purplish skin rash, blisters, or sunburn. Immediately report severe rashes, especially when accompanied by blistering. (Tetracyclines may cause significant dermatologic effects including Stevens–Johnson syndrome. Sunscreens and protective clothing should be used to prevent photosensitivity and photoallergic reactions.)	• Teach the patient to wear sunscreen and protective clothing for sun exposure and to avoid tanning beds. Immediately report any severe sunburn or rashes.
• Assess for the possibility of pregnancy or breast-feeding in patients prescribed tetracycline antibiotics. Women of childbearing age who are taking erythromycin antibiotics should use an alternative form of birth control to prevent pregnancy. (Tetracyclines affect fetal bone growth and teeth development, causing permanent yellowish-brown staining of teeth. Tetracycline use in children under age 8 or 9 should also be avoided. Erythromycin antibiotics may significantly reduce the effectiveness of oral contraceptives, and a secondary method to prevent conception should be used.)	• Advise women who are pregnant, breast-feeding, or attempting to become pregnant to inform their health care provider before receiving any tetracycline antibiotic. • Teach women of childbearing age on oral contraceptives to consult their health care provider about birth control alternatives if erythromycin antibiotics are ordered.
Patient understanding of drug therapy: • Use opportunities during administration of medications and during assessments to discuss the rationale for drug therapy, desired therapeutic outcomes, commonly observed adverse effects, parameters for when to call the health care provider, and any necessary monitoring or precautions. (Using time during nursing care helps to optimize and reinforce key teaching areas.)	• The patient, family, or caregiver should be able to state the reason for the drug, appropriate dose and scheduling, what adverse effects to observe for and when to report them, and the anticipated length of medication therapy.

Patient self-administration of drug therapy:
• When administering the medications, instruct the patient, family, or caregiver in proper self-administration techniques followed by return demonstration. (Utilizing time during nurse-administration of these drugs helps to reinforce teaching.)
	• Teach the patient to take the medication:
	  • Complete the entire course of therapy unless otherwise instructed. Do not share with other family members and do not stop taking the medicine when starting to feel better.
	  • Take the drug with food or milk and avoid acidic or carbonated beverages to decrease GI effects.
	  • Do not take tetracycline with milk products, iron-containing preparations such as multivitamins, or with antacids. Take the tetracycline 1 h before or 2 h after consuming these products.
	  • Take the medication as evenly spaced throughout each day as feasible.
	  • Increase overall fluid intake while taking the antibacterial drug.
	  • Discard outdated medications or those no longer in use. Review the medicine cabinet twice a year for old medications (e.g., at the beginning and end of daylight saving time).

Evaluation of Outcome Criteria

Evaluate the effectiveness of drug therapy by confirming that patient goals and expected outcomes have been met (see "Planning").

Miscellaneous Inhibitors of Bacterial Protein Synthesis

5 Several inhibitors of protein synthesis are effective against resistant infections but may have significant adverse effects that limit their use.

Several bacterial protein synthesis inhibitors do not belong to the tetracycline, macrolide, or aminoglycoside classes. These miscellaneous agents, listed in Table 4, have varying spectrums of activity and adverse effect profiles and thus must be considered individually. One of the drugs in the miscellaneous class, spectinomycin (Trobicin), has been discontinued in the United States.

Chloramphenicol: Chloramphenicol is an older, broad-spectrum antibiotic that was approved in 1960 and has been available for nearly 60 years. It binds to the 50S subunit of the bacterial ribosome and may be bacteriostatic or bacteriocidal, depending on species and dose. Chloramphenicol is administered PO or IV as chloramphenicol succinate for serious infections. A topical form is available for ophthalmic and otic infections.

Effective in treating salmonellae, rickettsiae, streptococci, typhoid fever, and meningitis caused by *H. influenzae*, this agent was widely used before it was found to be associated with bone marrow suppression and a very small, though fatal, incidence of aplastic anemia. This drug carries a black box warning that serious and fatal blood dyscrasias have been reported with chloramphenicol. Peak and trough serum levels should be monitored regularly during therapy to avoid serious adverse effects. Chloramphenicol is now reserved for meningitis and other infections in which the benefits of the drug clearly outweigh the risks of serious drug toxicity.

Another serious toxicity from chloramphenicol is **gray baby syndrome**. Most often seen in premature or newborn infants, this syndrome occurs when the baby's liver is unable to metabolize or excrete this drug. Symptoms include failure to feed, abdominal distention, cyanosis, and cardiovascular collapse. The syndrome is rapidly fatal and can cause death in a just few hours. If done early, discontinuing chloramphenicol therapy can reverse the syndrome. This is a pregnancy category C drug.

Clindamycin (Cleocin, Others): Approved in 1970, clindamycin acts on the 50S bacterial ribosomal subunit in a manner similar to that of the macrolides. It is usually bacteriostatic. A drug of choice for abdominal infections caused by *Bacteroides fragilis*, it is also effective against *Fusobacterium, Actinomyces,* and *Clostridium.*

Three salts of clindamycin are available: clindamycin hydrochloride (PO), clindamycin palmitate (PO), and clindamycin phosphate (parenteral or topical). In 2004, an aerosol topical foam of 1% clindamycin (Evoclin) was approved for the treatment of acne vulgaris, and a single-dose suppository vaginal cream (Clindesse) was marketed for bacterial vaginosis.

Once widely prescribed as a penicillin alternative, the use of clindamycin has become limited due to the development of resistant strains, a high incidence of diarrhea, and a potential risk of drug-induced PMC caused by *C. difficile,* which can be fatal (black box warning). It is generally only used when safer alternatives are not effective. The nurse must advise patients to report incidences of diarrhea during clindamycin therapy. If PMC is suspected, clindamycin is discontinued and the patient is placed on a drug that is effective against *C. difficile* such as vancomycin. This is a pregnancy category B drug.

Lincomycin (Lincocin): Approved in 1964, lincomycin is chemically similar to clindamycin. Lincomycin may be used for patients who cannot take penicillins or cephalosporins but it offers no therapeutic advantages over clindamycin. The drug is rarely prescribed due to a relatively high incidence of serious adverse effects, especially PMC (black box warning). It is available by both PO and parenteral routes. This is a pregnancy category B drug.

TABLE 4 Miscellaneous Inhibitors of Bacterial Protein Synthesis

Drug	Route and Adult Dose (maximum dose where indicated)	Adverse Effects
chloramphenicol	PO: 12.5 mg/kg qid	*Nausea, vomiting, diarrhea* Anaphylaxis, superinfections, pancytopenia, bone marrow depression, aplastic anemia
clindamycin (Cleocin, Others)	PO: 150–450 mg qid IV: 600–1,200 mg/day in divided doses	*Nausea, vomiting, diarrhea, rash, burning, or pruritus (topical forms)* Anaphylaxis, superinfections, cardiac arrest, PMC, blood dyscrasias
lincomycin (Lincocin)	PO: 500 mg tid–qid (max: 8 g/day) IM: 600 mg every 12–24 h (max: 8 g/day)	*Nausea, vomiting, diarrhea* Anaphylaxis, superinfections, cardiac arrest, PMC, blood dyscrasias
linezolid (Zyvox)	PO/IV: 600 mg every 12 h (max: 1,200 mg/day)	*Nausea, diarrhea, headache* Anaphylaxis, superinfections, PMC, blood dyscrasias
quinupristin-dalfopristin (Synercid)	IV: 7.5 mg/kg infused over 60 min every 8 h	*Pain and inflammation at the injection site, myalgia, arthralgia, diarrhea* Superinfections, PMC
telithromycin (Ketek)	PO: 800 mg once a day	*Nausea, vomiting, diarrhea* Visual disturbances, hepatotoxicity, dysrhythmias

Note: Italics indicate common adverse effects. <u>Underline</u> indicates serious adverse effects.

Linezolid (Zyvox): Approved in 2000, linezolid is in a class of antibiotics, the **oxazolidinones**, that act by binding to a part of the bacterial 50S ribosome known as the 23S portion. It is unique among antibiotics in that it prevents the first event in protein synthesis, which is the formation of an initiation complex. It is believed to be bacteriocidal. Linezolid is important because it is effective against infections that have become resistant to most other antibiotics, including MRSA and VRE. It is less effective against gram-negative organisms. Oral and IV formulations are available.

Adverse effects are usually minor and related to GI distress. Because this drug can cause transient dose-related myelosuppression, laboratory blood counts should be frequently monitored during therapy. Linezolid is a nonselective inhibitor of monoamine oxidase (MAO) and may cause hypertension in some patients. Risk for hypertension and palpitations is increased if the patient is taking sympathomimetics concurrently with linezolid; thus these medications should be avoided. This is a pregnancy category C drug.

Quinupristin-dalfopristin (Synercid): Approved in 1999, quinupristin-dalfopristin is a fixed-dose bacteriocidal combination used for therapy of life-threatening *E. faecium* infections that are vancomycin resistant and for complicated infections caused by MRSA or *Streptococcus pyogenes*. It belongs to a class of antibiotics called **streptogramins** that act by binding the 50S bacterial ribosome in a manner similar to that of the macrolides. The combination of the two antibiotics is truly synergistic: The combination has 16 times more antimicrobial activity compared to either drug used alone. Synercid is bacteriocidal and only available by the IV route.

Joint and muscle pain, diarrhea, rash, and pain at the infusion site are common adverse effects. Venous irritation may be severe enough to cause the drug to be discontinued. Synercid inhibits hepatic drug metabolism enzymes, resulting in numerous drug–drug interactions. The nurse should use caution when administering drugs concurrently with Synercid, because those that rely on hepatic metabolism for detoxification may build to toxic levels in the blood. In addition, some cases of PMC have been reported. Despite its potential for adverse effects, quinupristin-dalfopristin serves an important role in treating multidrug-resistant gram-positive pathogens, which have become a major clinical challenge. Cross-resistance has not yet developed between Synercid and other antibiotic classes. This is a pregnancy category B drug.

Telithromycin (Ketek): Approved in 2004, telithromycin is a newer, broad-spectrum antibiotic. Structurally similar to the macrolides, telithromycin is the sole member of a class called *ketolides*. Ketolides inhibit bacterial protein synthesis by the same mechanism as the macrolides: by binding to the 50S ribosomal subunit. However, telithromycin binds more tightly to the ribosome than other protein synthesis inhibitors and is capable of causing greater bacterial kill. It also exhibits a significant postantibiotic effect in some organisms. Indications for telithromycin are similar to those of the macrolides except it has greater activity against *S. pneumoniae*. Because of this, its primary use is to treat bronchitis, sinusitis, and community-acquired pneumonia. It is effective against many other bacterial strains, including those that show macrolide resistance. This drug is available as oral tablets.

Although most adverse effects are minor and GI related, telithromycin has the potential to cause several serious adverse effects. Hepatotoxicity has occurred in a small number of patients. Telithromycin can cause blurred vision, double vision, and difficulty focusing, which can be severe enough to cause discontinuation of therapy. Telithromycin carries a black box warning that patients with myasthenia gravis should not take this drug because life-threatening respiratory failure may occur. As with some of the macrolides, telithromycin may increase the risk for ventricular dysrhythmias such as torsade de pointes and is contraindicated in patients with prolonged QT intervals. This is a pregnancy category C drug.

UNDERSTANDING THE CHAPTER

Key Concepts Summary

1 Antibiotics inhibit microbial protein synthesis by binding to the bacterial ribosome.

2 Tetracyclines have broad antimicrobial activity against many gram-positive and gram-negative bacteria.

3 The macrolides are alternatives to penicillin for many gram-positive infections.

4 The aminoglycosides are effective against aerobic gram-negative organisms but have the potential to cause ototoxicity and nephrotoxicity.

5 Several inhibitors of protein synthesis are effective against resistant infections but may have significant adverse effects that limit their use.

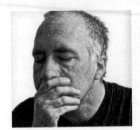

Making the PATIENT Connection

Remember the patient "John Talley" at the beginning of the chapter? Now read the remainder of the case study. Based on the information presented within this chapter, respond to the critical thinking questions that follow.

John Talley, a 51-year-old truck driver, has had an upper respiratory infection for the past 2 weeks. Although he has seen his health care provider, he does not seem to be improving. He is convinced that if he takes the antibiotic just 1 more day, he will surely improve. However, after 5 days of drug therapy, John continues to experience chills, fever, and a productive cough. His wife insisted that he return to the clinic for further evaluation and treatment.

At the clinic the patient's physical examination and diagnostic tests reveal the following findings: Temperature is 39.2°C (102.6°F), pulse rate is 112 beats/min, respiratory rate is 30 breaths/min, and blood pressure is 134/88 mmHg. He is visibly short of breath and is experiencing intermittent coughing episodes. On auscultation of his lung fields, bilateral crackles and wheezes are discovered. His WBC count is 14,400 mm^3. A chest x-ray is taken to confirm a diagnosis of pneumonia and reveals right lower lobe infiltrates (white areas in the lung that indicate infection).

The patient is diagnosed with bacterial pneumonia. He is hospitalized and prescribed IV antibiotic therapy. On the second hospital day you are assigned to care for John. He and his wife have multiple questions about the drug therapy prescribed.

Critical Thinking Questions

1. Why did the first antibiotic prescribed not cure the infection?
2. The patient has been told that a sputum specimen is needed for a "C and S" and asks what that is. What will the nurse teach him about this test and why it is needed?
3. John has been told that laboratory personnel will be collecting blood for a peak and trough level this afternoon and in the morning. How would the nurse explain this laboratory test to the patient?
4. What symptoms would indicate that the patient's condition is worsening?

See Answers to Critical Thinking Questions on student resource website.

NCLEX-RN® Review

1. While teaching the client about taking oral tetracycline, which of the following does the nurse advise the client to do?
   1. Consume calcium-rich products to decrease the duration of the antibacterial effect.
   2. Use a soft toothbrush and floss teeth gently to remove staining on teeth.
   3. Report any ringing in the ears or dizziness
   4. Avoid direct exposure to sunlight and apply sun block when outdoors.

2. The nurse determines that the client understands the use of azithromycin (Zithromax) when the client makes which statement?
   1. "It only needs to be taken once-daily because it lasts longer."
   2. "It causes more nausea than most other antibiotics in this classification."
   3. "It must be taken on an empty stomach."
   4. "It is ineffective if taken with calcium-rich foods."

3. The client is receiving amikacin (Amikin) for a bacterial infection. Which adverse effects does the nurse include in the plan of care to monitor the client's status?
   1. Weight gain
   2. Visual disturbances
   3. Mental depression
   4. Urinary frequency

4. The health care provider orders gentamicin (Garamycin) for a client with a postoperative wound infection. Which laboratory result should prompt the nurse to consult with the prescriber about possible nephrotoxicity of this drug?
   1. Elevated serum creatinine level
   2. Decreased blood urea nitrogen (BUN) level
   3. Increased white blood cell (WBC) count
   4. Elevated serum iron level

5. The client has received a prescription for tetracycline (Sumycin) for treatment of acne. The nurse will teach the client to avoid taking the tetracycline concurrently with

   _____.

6. The client is receiving gentamicin (Garamycin) IV for a significant infection. While the client is receiving this drug, what assessment data will the nurse gather to monitor for adverse effects? Select all that apply.
   1. Serum creatinine
   2. Signs of muscle weakness
   3. Liver function studies
   4. Urine output
   5. Hearing and balance assessments

Additional Case Study

Mr. Klein is an 85-year-old man seen in the outpatient clinic for an acute infection. He has informed the health care provider that he is allergic to a variety of antibiotics and is subsequently prescribed erythromycin estolate. The patient is a recovering alcoholic who has been abstinent for 10 years.

1. What is the significance of Mr. Klein's history of alcoholism?
2. What possible adverse effect should the nurse instruct the patient to watch for?
3. What laboratory diagnostic studies may be indicated in this patient?

See Answers to Additional Case Study on student resource website.

Pearson Nursing Student Resources

Find additional review materials at
nursing.pearsonhighered.com

Prepare for success with additional NCLEX®-style practice
questions, interactive assignments and activities, web links,
animations, videos, and more!

References

Centers for Disease Control and Prevention. (2010). Sexually transmitted diseases: Treatment guidelines 2010. *Morbidity and Mortality Weekly Report, 59.* Retrieved from http://www.uphs.upenn.edu/bugdrug/antibiotic_manual/cdcstdrx2010.pdf

de la Cabada Bauche, J., & DuPont, H. L. (2011). New developments in traveler's diarrhea. *Gastroenterology and Hepatology, 7*(2), 88–95.

Dufel, S. E. (2011). CBRNE—Plague. *Medscape Reference.* Retrieved from http://emedicine.medscape.com/article/829233-overview

Greenwood, Z., Black, J., Weld, L., O'Brien, D., Leder, K., VonSonnenburg, F., et al. (2008). Gastrointestinal infection among international travelers globally. *Journal of Travel Medicine, 15*(4), 221–228. doi:10.111/j.1708-8305.2008.00203.x

Madigan, M. T., Martinko, J. M., Stahl, D. A., & Clark, D. P. (2012). *Brock biology of microorganisms* (13th ed.). San Francisco, CA: Benjamin Cummings.

Tortora, G. J., Funke, B. R., & Case, C. L. (2010). *Microbiology: An introduction* (10th ed.). San Francisco, CA: Benjamin Cummings.

Selected Bibliography

Barnes, B. E., & Sampson, D. A. (2011). A literature review on community-acquired methicillin-resistant *Staphylococcus aureus* in the United States: Clinical information for primary care nurse practitioners. *Journal of the American Academy of Nurse Practitioners, 23,* 23–32. doi:10.1111/j.1745-7599.2010.00571.x

Davey, P., Sneddon, K., & Nathwani, D. (2010). Overview of strategies for overcoming the challenge of antimicrobial resistance. *Expert Review of Clinical Pharmacology, 3*(5), 667–686. doi:10.1586/ecp.10.46

Guilbeau, J. R., & Fordham, P. N. (2010). Evidence-based management and treatment of outpatient community-associated MRSA. *Journal for Nurse Practitioners, 6*(2), 140–145. doi:10.1016/j.nurpra.2009.07.011

McFarland, L., Beneda, H., Clarridge, J., & Raugi, G. (2007). Implications of the changing face of *Clostridium difficile* disease for health care practitioners. *American Journal of Infection Control, 35*(4), 237–253.

Rodriguez, A., Mendia, A., Sirvent, J., Barcenilla, F., de la Torre-Prados, M. V., Sole-Violan, & Rello, J. (2007). Combination antibiotic therapy improves survival in patients with community-acquired pneumonia and shock. *Critical Care Medicine, 35*(6), 1493–1498.

Rossolini, G. M., Mantengoli, E., Mantagnani, F., & Pollini, S. (2010). Epidemiology and clinical relevance of microbial resistance determinants versus anti-gram-positive agents. *Current Opinion in Microbiology, 13*(5), 582–588. doi:10.1016/j.mib.2010.08.006

Silva, J. G., & Carvalho, I. (2007). New insights into aminoglycoside antibiotics and derivatives. *Current Medicinal Chemistry, 14*(10), 1101–1119.

Answers to NCLEX-RN® Review

1 Answer: 4 Rationale: This drug potentially causes photosensitivity. Options 1, 2, and 3 are incorrect. Calcium products should be avoided with tetracycline therapy. Brushing will not remove teeth staining caused by the drug. The staining of the teeth due to medication can only be removed by a dental specialist. Ototoxicity is not associated with tetracycline use, and any tinnitus or dizziness may be related to other causes. Cognitive Level: Applying; Client Need: Health Promotion and Maintenance; Nursing Process: Implementation

2 Answer: 1 Rationale: Longer duration of action is one of the benefits of azithromycin therapy. Options 2, 3, and 4 are incorrect. There is no evidence that azithromycin causes any more nausea than other antibiotics. Azithromycin is not affected by the gastric content and can be taken any time. Azithromycin is not affected by calcium-based foods. Cognitive Level: Analyzing; Client Need: Physiological Integrity; Nursing Process: Evaluation

3 Answer: 1 Rationale: Weight gain will be one of the first signs associated with renal damage secondary to amikacin toxicity. Options 2, 3, and 4 are incorrect. Adverse effects of amikacin are not manifested by visual disturbances, mental depression, or urinary frequency. Cognitive Level: Applying; Client Need: Physiological Integrity; Nursing Process: Planning

4 Answer: 1 Rationale: Drug-induced renal toxicity would cause an elevated serum creatinine level and should be reported to the health care provider. Options 2, 3, and 4 are incorrect. BUN level is more commonly associated with hepatic toxicity but would be elevated and not decreased if renal toxicity is present. Nephrotoxicity is not typically indicated via the WBC levels or changes in serum iron levels. Cognitive Level: Analyzing; Client Need: Physiological Integrity; Nursing Process: Assessment

5 Answer: Tetracycline antibiotics should not be taken concurrently with dairy products, iron-containing preparations such as multivitamins, or with antacids. If these products are to be consumed, they should be taken 1 h before or 2 h after the tetracycline. Cognitive Level: Applying; Client Need: Health Promotion and Maintenance; Nursing Process: Implementation

6 Answer: 1, 2, 4, 5 Aminoglycosides are renal, oto-, and neurotoxic. They may also cause neuromuscular blockade. Increases in serum creatinine may indicate renal toxicity. Urine output should also be monitored. Dizziness, vertigo, or tinnitus may be signs of ototoxicity. Muscle weakness may indicate neuromuscular blockade and may last for several days. Option 3 is incorrect. Gentamicin is not metabolized, and changes in liver function tests would not be drug related. Cognitive Level: Analyzing; Client Need: Physiological Integrity; Nursing Process: Assessment

Fluoroquinolones
and Miscellaneous Antibacterials

From Chapter 52 of *Pharmacology: Connections to Nursing Practice*, Second Edition. Michael Patrick Adams, Carol Quam Urban. Copyright © 2013 by Pearson Education, Inc. All rights reserved.

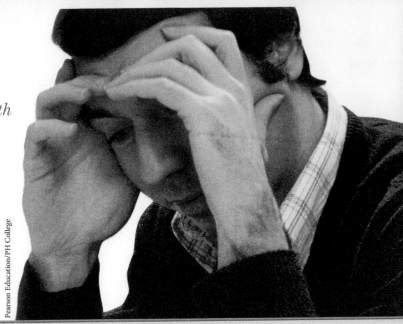

"Every morning for the last month I have had terrible headaches with pain directly on my forehead. Then my upper jaw and cheeks became tender to touch and my teeth ached."

Patient "Mike Springs"

Fluoroquinolones and Miscellaneous Antibacterials

Learning Outcomes

After reading this chapter, the student should be able to:

1. Explain the steps in bacterial DNA replication.
2. Identify the classes of drugs that act by affecting bacterial DNA replication.
3. Explain mechanisms by which fluoroquinolones inhibit bacterial DNA replication.
4. Describe means by which bacteria become resistant to fluoroquinolones.
5. For each of the classes shown in the chapter outline, identify the prototype and representative drugs and explain the mechanism(s) of drug action, primary indications, contraindications, significant drug interactions, pregnancy category, and important adverse effects.
6. Explain the nurse's role in the safe administration of fluoroquinolones.
7. Apply the nursing process to care for patients who are receiving pharmacotherapy with fluoroquinolones and miscellaneous antibacterials.

Chapter Outline

Bacterial DNA Replication

Inhibition of DNA Replication

Fluoroquinolones

PROTOTYPE **Ciprofloxacin (Cipro)**

Miscellaneous Antibacterials

Bacitracin
Daptomycin (Cubicin)
Metronidazole (Flagyl)
Polymyxin B
Rifampin (Rifadin, Rimactane)
Telithromycin (Ketek)

With resistance to other antibacterials developing rapidly, drugs in the fluoroquinolone class have become increasingly important in the pharmacotherapy of infectious diseases. Fluoroquinolones are bacteriocidal and are effective against many gram-positive and gram-negative microbes. They affect bacterial deoxyribonucleic acid (DNA) synthesis, and are particularly useful in the management of respiratory, genitourinary, and gastrointestinal (GI) infections.

Bacterial DNA Replication

1 Bacterial DNA replication requires several different enzymes to uncoil, unwind, and duplicate the DNA.

Under optimal conditions, many pathogenic bacteria can divide every 1 to 3 hours. Under highly favorable conditions, *Escherichia coli* divides every 20 minutes, producing a billion cells in only 10 hours. The most critical step in bacterial reproduction is duplicating the DNA so that each daughter cell contains the same genetic material. Thus, bacteria are in the process of continuously replicating their DNA, as well as constructing cell walls and synthesizing proteins.

Like human DNA, bacterial DNA uses the four bases, adenine, guanine, cytosine, and thymidine, and is arranged in a double-helical formation. Most bacteria, however, contain a single circular chromosome as illustrated in Figure 1. The helix is then twisted and coiled. This highly twisted arrangement is called a **supercoil**. This supercoiled arrangement is necessary for all the DNA to fit into the small bacterial cell. However, this supercoil must be relaxed and the two helices unwound immediately prior to replicating its DNA, so that duplication enzymes can reach the bases.

A large number of enzymes are needed for DNA replication, and some of these enzymes are targets for antibiotics. This is a complex process but may be simplified in four steps. The enzymes involved in this four-step process afford different sites at which drugs may act.

1. Relax: Supercoil is relaxed by the enzyme **DNA gyrase** (also called **topoisomerase II**).

2. Unwind: After the supercoil is relaxed, the enzyme **DNA helicase** unwinds the two strands.

3. Replicate: The enzyme **DNA polymerase** adds the precursor bases to replicate the original DNA and form new DNA strands.

4. Migrate: The two newly formed strands are interlocked until the enzyme **topoisomerase IV** frees them to migrate to opposite sides of the cell, where they are segregated into the two daughter cells.

Inhibition of DNA Replication

2 Drugs have been discovered that inhibit different steps in bacterial DNA replication.

Blocking the DNA replication of a pathogen is a common mechanism used by drugs across several different therapeutic classes. Drugs can block bacterial DNA replication in three basic ways:

- Drugs can inhibit the synthesis or availability of precursor bases or nucleotides.
- Drugs can bind to bacterial DNA, preventing the relaxation and uncoiling processes required for replication.
- Drugs can bind to enzymes of DNA replication, halting the formation of new DNA strands.

A number of drugs employed in cancer chemotherapy act by mimicking precursor molecules or by interacting with DNA. Cytarabine (Cytosar-U) and fluorouracil (5-FU) resemble nucleotides and are mistakenly incorporated into newly formed DNA strands. Daunorubicin (Cerubidine) and bleomycin (Blenoxane) are highly toxic antibiotics that interact with DNA to physically block replication. Although classified as antibiotics, these agents

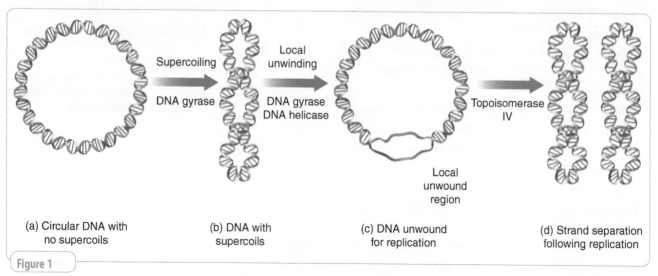

(a) Circular DNA with no supercoils

Supercoiling
DNA gyrase

(b) DNA with supercoils

Local unwinding
DNA gyrase
DNA helicase

(c) DNA unwound for replication

Local unwound region

Topoisomerase IV

(d) Strand separation following replication

Figure 1

Bacterial DNA.

are too toxic to be used for infections, but have therapeutic indications in the chemotherapy of specific types of cancer.

Several drugs act by inhibiting enzymes involved in DNA replication. Acyclovir (Zovirax) inhibits the DNA polymerase of herpesvirus, and is a leading drug for treating this infection. Teniposide (Vumon) and etoposide (VePesid) are antineoplastic agents that act by inhibiting topoisomerase I, an enzyme that helps repair DNA damage. By binding in a complex with topoisomerase and DNA, these antineoplastics cause strand breaks that accumulate and permanently damage the DNA.

The fluoroquinolone antibiotics act on two enzymes in the DNA replication process. First, they bind to DNA gyrase, inhibiting its ability to relax the supercoiling of the bacterial DNA. When the replication enzymes reach an area still in a supercoiled state, replication terminates. A second mechanism is binding to topoisomerase IV. When this occurs, the two daughter DNA strands cannot migrate to opposite sides of the cell, and division cannot be completed. It is thought that fluoroquinolones inhibit DNA gyrase in gram-negative organisms, and inhibit topoisomerase IV in gram-positive organisms. However, this is likely an oversimplification of their exact mechanism. These drugs have no effect on human enzymes involved in DNA replication because of significant differences in the chemical structures of the human and bacterial enzymes. These differences account for their selective toxicity on bacteria, and their favorable safety profile.

Fluoroquinolones

3 Fluoroquinolones are antibiotics whose therapeutic applications have expanded in recent years to treat many gram-positive and gram-negative infections.

The first drug in this class, nalidixic acid (NegGram), was approved in 1962. Classified as a quinolone, the use of nalidixic acid was restricted to treating urinary tract infections (UTIs) due to its narrow spectrum of activity and a high incidence of bacterial resistance. Nalidixic acid is still used for the pharmacotherapy of UTIs, although it is not a drug of first choice. Nalidixic acid is important because it served as a building block for the synthesis of other drugs in this class.

In the late 1980s, the development of quinolones with a fluorine side chain resulted in drugs with wider spectrums of activity and longer durations of action. The fluoroquinolones, listed in Table 1, have become an increasingly important class of antibiotics in the past two decades. Fluoroquinolones are bacteriocidal, and affect bacterial DNA synthesis by inhibiting both DNA gyrase and topoisomerase IV.

Four generations of fluoroquinolones are available, based on their antibacterial spectrums. All fluoroquinolones have activity against gram-negative pathogens, with the newer drugs being significantly more effective against gram-positive bacteria. The distinctions among the generations are listed in Table 2. The newer fluoroquinolones were developed and approved primarily for the treatment of respiratory infections.

Clinical applications of fluoroquinolones include infections of the respiratory, GI, and genitourinary tracts, and some skin and soft tissue infections. Their effectiveness against gram-negative organisms makes them drugs of choice in the treatment of uncomplicated UTIs. A newer agent, moxifloxacin (Avelox), is effective against anaerobes, a group of bacteria that are often difficult to treat. Ciprofloxacin (Cipro) is the fluoroquinolone usually selected for infections by *Pseudomonas aeruginosa*. Recent studies have suggested that some fluoroquinolones may be effective against *Mycobacterium tuberculosis*, although the U.S. Food and Drug Administration (FDA) has not approved these drugs for this indication.

Along with doxycycline, streptomycin, and penicillin, several fluoroquinolones are indicated for pathogens that could potentially be used in a bioterrorism incident. Ciprofloxacin (Cipro) is a drug of choice for postexposure prophylaxis to *Bacillus anthracis*, the causative agent of anthrax. Ciprofloxacin is also indicated for postexposure prophylaxis to other

TABLE 1 Fluoroquinolones and Quinolones		
Drug	Route and Adult Dose (maximum dose where indicated)	Adverse Effects
First Generation		*Nausea, headache, diarrhea, rash, insomnia, pain and inflammation at injection site, local burning, stinging, corneal irritation (ophthalmic)*
nalidixic acid (NegGram)	PO: Acute therapy: 1 g qid PO: Chronic therapy: 500 mg qid	
Second Generation		Anaphylaxis, tendon rupture, superinfections, photosensitivity, pseudomembranous colitis (PMC), seizure, peripheral neuropathy, hepatotoxicity
ciprofloxacin (Cipro)	PO: 250–750 mg bid (max: 1,500 mg/day)	
norfloxacin (Noroxin)	PO: 400 mg bid or 800 mg once daily	
ofloxacin (Floxin)	PO/IV: 200–400 mg bid (max: 800 mg/day)	
Third Generation		
gatifloxacin (Zymar, Zymaxid)	Drops (ophthalmic solution): 1 drop in each affected eye every 2–4 h	
levofloxacin (Levaquin)	PO/IV: 250–750 mg/day (max: 750 mg/day)	
Fourth Generation		
besifloxacin (Besivance)	Drops (ophthalmic solution): 1 drop in each affected eye every 8 h	
gemifloxacin (Factive)	PO: 320 mg/day (max: 320 mg/day)	
moxifloxacin (Avelox)	PO/IV: 400 mg/day once daily (max: 400 mg/day)	

Note: *Italics* indicate common adverse effects. <u>Underline</u> indicates serious adverse effects.

TABLE 2 Generations of Fluoroquinolones

Generation	Example	Route of Administration	Spectrum of Activity	Indications
First generation	nalidixic acid	Oral	Enterobacteriaceae	Uncomplicated UTI
Second generation	ciprofloxacin	Oral and IV	Enterobacteriaceae, atypical pathogens, *P. aeruginosa*	Complicated UTI, gastroenteritis with severe diarrhea, sexually transmitted infections (STIs)
Third generation	levofloxacin	Oral and IV	Enterobacteriaceae, atypical pathogens, some streptococci	Complicated UTI, gastroenteritis with severe diarrhea, STIs, community-acquired pneumonia
Fourth generation	moxifloxacin	Oral	Enterobacteriaceae, atypical pathogens, some streptococci, MRSA, anaerobes	Bacterial conjunctivitis (ophthalmic drops), acute bacterial sinusitis, exacerbations of chronic bronchitis, community-acquired pneumonia, skin and skin structure infections

potential biologic warfare pathogens such as *Yersinia pestis* (plague), *Francisella tularensis* (tularemia), and *Brucella melitensis* (brucellosis).

Fluoroquinolones are well absorbed orally and may be administered either once or twice a day, making them ideal for outpatient therapy. The serum levels of these drugs after oral (PO) administration are nearly equivalent to the levels achieved during IV administration. This allows for a rapid, smooth transition from IV therapy to oral therapy, potentially decreasing the length of the hospital stay. Like aminoglycosides, fluoroquinolones exhibit a postantibiotic effect. Their bacteriocidal actions continue after serum levels fall to below minimum inhibitory concentrations.

Adverse Effects

In the 1990s, fluoroquinolones came into widespread use because they were well tolerated and few serious adverse effects were reported. Over time, several uncommon, although very serious, adverse effects were discovered. Since that time, almost half the fluoroquinolones approved by the FDA have been discontinued in the United States due to safety concerns.

Cartilage toxicity: Animal studies have suggested that fluoroquinolones can affect the extracellular matrix of cartilage during development, and tendon toxicity has been reported in children using these drugs. Although these abnormalities ceased upon termination of antibiotic therapy, fluoroquinolones are not approved for patients under age 18, and their use in children is restricted to instances where the benefits of pharmacotherapy clearly outweigh the potential risks.

Although rare, tendon abnormalities have also been reported in adults. Tendinitis and rupture of the shoulder, hand, and Achilles tendons have occurred several months after discontinuation of therapy. In 2007, the FDA approved safety labeling revisions that state patients older than 65 years are at increased risk for severe tendon disorders and that this risk is further increased by concurrent use of corticosteroids. Musculoskeletal complaints should be carefully monitored during therapy with fluoroquinolones, and patients should be advised to report unexplained joint or tendon pain.

GI toxicity: GI symptoms such as nausea, vomiting, and diarrhea occur in as many as 20% of patients taking fluoroquinolones. Although food does not affect their absorption, certain multivitamins or mineral supplements containing calcium, zinc, iron, aluminum, and magnesium can delay absorption

of the antibiotic by as much as 90%. Substances containing these minerals should not be administered at the same time as fluoroquinolones.

In 2007, the FDA approved safety labeling revisions for certain antimicrobials to warn of the risk for *Clostridium difficile*–associated diarrhea (CDAD). This safety labeling applied to most fluoroquinolones, as well as drugs from most other antibiotic classes.

Hypersensitivity reactions: Certainly not unique to fluoroquinolones, hypersensitivity may occur to any antibiotic. Although the FDA has always required label warnings on quinolones for the risk of hypersensitivity reactions that occur after the first dose, new labels warn of the rare risk for serious, and sometimes fatal, events after multiple doses.

Cardiotoxicity: Some of the most serious adverse effects of drugs in this class are dysrhythmias (moxifloxacin). Several of the drugs in this class were removed from the market due to the potential for fatal dysrhythmias. Nearly all fluoroquinolones prolong the QT interval.

Central nervous system toxicity: Central nervous system (CNS) effects such as dizziness, headache, and sleep disturbances affect 1% to 8% of patients. Seizures, hallucinations, high intracranial pressure, confusion, and toxic psychoses have been reported in patients taking fluoroquinolones. These drugs should be used with caution in patients with preexisting seizure disorders.

Phototoxicity: Moderate to severe phototoxicity may occur in patients exposed to direct or indirect sunlight, or to sunlamps during or following treatment with fluoroquinolones. Recovery may take several weeks.

Hepatotoxicity: Some of the fluoroquinolones elevate hepatic enzymes, which usually return to normal 1 to 2 months following completion of therapy. Trovafloxacin mesylate (Trovan) was discontinued due to an unacceptable incidence of liver damage, including fatal hepatic failure.

Resistance: Like other antibiotics, resistance of bacterial species to fluoroquinolones has been increasing and can occur by multiple mechanisms. Mutations to DNA gyrase can alter its ability to bind fluoroquinolones, thus rendering the drug less effective. Some bacteria have developed resistance pumps that remove fluoroquinolones from inside their cells, while others have developed a cell wall structure that is less permeable to the drugs. Fluoroquinolones were drugs of choice for treating *Neisseria gonorrhoeae* from 1993 to 2005. Because of the large number of resistant strains, however, the Centers for Disease Control and Prevention no longer recommends fluoroquinolones for the treatment of gonorrhea. Because resistance to one fluoroquinolone sometimes confers resistance to all drugs in this class, resistance is becoming a limiting factor in the clinical utility of these drugs.

PharmFact

Someone who is taking a fluoroquinolone antibiotic has a three times greater risk of tendon rupture than someone in the general population. If the person is over age 60 and also taking a corticosteroid, the risk is six times greater (Doyle, 2010).

| PROTOTYPE DRUG | Ciprofloxacin (Cipro) |

Classification: **Therapeutic:** Antibacterial
Pharmacologic: Bacterial DNA replication inhibitor, fluoroquinolone

Therapeutic Effects and Uses: Ciprofloxacin is a second-generation fluoroquinolone approved in 1987 that is the most widely used drug in this class. It is prescribed for UTI, sinusitis, pneumonia, skin, bone and joint infections, infectious diarrhea, and certain eye infections. It is a broad-spectrum antibiotic that is more effective against gram-negative organisms. It is active against *Enterobacter, Citrobacter, E. coli, Haemophilus, Klebsiella, Proteus, Staphylococcus, Shigella, Salmonella, Neisseria,* and *Serratia.* It is poorly effective against *Streptococcus pneumoniae* and is inactive against most anaerobic bacteria. Ciprofloxacin is a preferred drug for postexposure prophylaxis of inhalational *B. anthracis* spores.

Ciprofloxacin is available by multiple routes, including oral, IV, ophthalmic, and otic. As an ophthalmic solution (Ciloxan), it is used to treat corneal ulcers and conjunctivitis due to *Staphylococcus, Haemophilus* and *Pseudomonas.* An otic suspension (Ciprodex otic) is a combination of ciprofloxacin and dexamethasone to treat acute otitis media and acute otitis externa in children ages 6 months and older. Cipro HC otic combines ciprofloxacin with hydrocortisone to treat adults and children with acute otitis media.

Several extended release (XR) formulations are available that permit once-daily dosing, usually for treating UTI. Cipro XR contains two different ciprofloxacin salts: ciprofloxacin hydrochloride and ciprofloxacin betaine. Approved in 2005, Proquin XR contains only the hydrochloride salt and has been formulated to cause less nausea, vomiting, and diarrhea than other formulations. Proquin XR is administered for only 3 days and is only approved for uncomplicated UTI (acute cystitis).

Mechanism of Action: By inhibiting bacterial DNA gyrase and topoisomerase, ciprofloxacin affects bacterial replication and DNA repair. Ciprofloxacin is usually considered bacteriocidal and exhibits a prolonged postantibiotic effect.

Pharmacokinetics:

Route(s)	PO, IV, ophthalmic and otic drops
Absorption	60–80% absorbed
Distribution	Widely distributed to all body fluids; crosses the placenta; secreted in breast milk; small amounts in cerebrospinal fluid; 20–40% bound to plasma proteins
Primary metabolism	Mostly unchanged; small amounts of hepatic metabolism
Primary excretion	Primarily renal; 15% by biliary route
Onset of action	Rapid
Duration of action	12 h

Adverse Effects: Ciprofloxacin is well tolerated by most patients, and serious adverse effects are uncommon. GI adverse effects, such as nausea, vomiting, and diarrhea, may occur in as many as 20% of patients taking high doses. Ciprofloxacin may be administered with food to diminish adverse GI effects. The patient should not, however, take this drug with antacids or mineral supplements, because drug absorption will be diminished. Some patients report phototoxicity, headache, and dizziness. Like most antibiotics, ciprofloxacin can cause serious pseudomembranous colitis (PMC). Although rare, seizures and toxic psychosis have been reported in patients receiving fluoroquinolones. **Black Box Warning:** Tendinitis and tendon rupture may occur in patients of all ages. Risk is especially high in patients over age 60, in kidney, heart, and lung transplant recipients, and in those receiving concurrent corticosteroid therapy. Fluoroquinolones may cause extreme muscle weakness in patients with myasthenia gravis.

Contraindications/Precautions: Ciprofloxacin is contraindicated in patients who are hypersensitive to fluoroquinolones, and in pregnant patients. Drug therapy must be monitored carefully in patients with suspected CNS disorders, because this drug can be neurotoxic at high doses, and can cause seizures when given by rapid IV infusion. Although prescribed for patients with UTIs, the drug should be used with caution in patients with serious renal impairment, because this drug is excreted by this route and may accumulate to toxic levels.

Drug Interactions: Concurrent administration with warfarin may increase anticoagulant effects and result in bleeding due to the decreased metabolism of warfarin. Antacids and vitamin supplements containing calcium or aluminum, iron or zinc sulfate, and sucralfate decrease the absorption of ciprofloxacin, thus causing decreased effectiveness of the antibiotic. Ciprofloxacin slows the hepatic metabolism of xanthines, including caffeine, theophylline, and theobromine. Theophylline levels may increase 15% to 30%. **Herbal/Food:** Patients ingesting large quantities of caffeinated products may experience excessive nervousness, anxiety, or tachycardia. Calcium-fortified juices may interfere with absorption of the antibiotic.

Pregnancy: Category C.

Treatment of Overdose: No specific therapy is available; patients are treated symptomatically.

Nursing Responsibilities: Key nursing implications for patients receiving ciprofloxacin are included in the Nursing Practice Application for Patients Receiving Fluoroquinolone Therapy.

- Monitor older adults frequently for joint pain, tendon pain, or difficulty with gait. An increased risk of tendinitis and tendon rupture has been noted in this population.
- Carefully monitor for diarrhea in the older adult. Cases of CDAD and PMC have been reported with antibiotic use, greatly increasing the risk of fluid and electrolyte imbalances and the risk for severe bowel adverse effects, which is of concern for all patients, but especially for this population.

Patient and Family Education:

- Do not take any products containing magnesium or calcium (such as antacids), iron, or aluminum with this drug, or within 2 hours of this drug.
- Report sudden, unexplained joint or tendon pain, tendinitis, or difficulty with walking or movement.
- Do not breast-feed while taking this drug without approval of the health care provider.

Drugs Similar to Ciprofloxacin (Cipro)

Other fluoroquinolones include besifloxacin, gatifloxacin, gemifloxacin, levofloxacin, moxifloxacin, norfloxacin, and ofloxacin. With few exceptions, these drugs have very similar actions and adverse effects to ciprofloxacin. A black box warning regarding possible tendon rupture is included for all oral and parenteral drugs in this class. Cinoxacin (Cinobac), Enoxacin (Penetrex), lomefloxacin (Maxaquin), sparfloxacin (Zagam), and trovafloxacin (Trovan)/alatrofloxacin (Trovan IV) are drugs in this class that have been discontinued in the United States.

Besifloxacin (Besivance): Besifloxacin is one of the newer fluoroquinolones, approved in 2009 for the treatment of bacterial conjunctivitis. It is available as a 0.6% ophthalmic suspension. The most frequently reported adverse reaction is conjunctival redness. If used for a prolonged time period, the patient should be examined for the possibility of overgrowth of resistant microbes. Patients should be advised to discontinue use of contact lenses during therapy. This drug is pregnancy category C.

Gatifloxacin (Zymar, Zymaxid): In 2006, the drug manufacturer discontinued the distribution of the oral and parenteral forms of gatifloxacin. However, it is still available as an ophthalmic solution for the treatment of bacterial conjunctivitis. The most frequently reported adverse reactions after ophthalmic administration include increased worsening of conjunctivitis, eye irritation, dysgeusia, and eye pain. Patients should be advised to discontinue use of contact lenses during therapy. This drug is pregnancy category C.

Gemifloxacin (Factive): Gemifloxacin was approved in 2003 for acute bacterial exacerbations of chronic bronchitis and community-acquired pneumonia. It is primarily effective against gram-positive bacteria, most importantly *S. pneumoniae* and *Staphylococcus aureus*, than many other drugs in this class. It is only available orally. The drug undergoes only minimal metabolism by the liver and is excreted almost equally by the kidneys and in the feces. Diarrhea, rash, and nausea are the most common adverse effects. It is contraindicated in patients

with certain dysrhythmias, due to its effects on cardiac conduction. Other contraindications and adverse effects (including the black box warning) are similar to those of ciprofloxacin. This drug is pregnancy category C.

Levofloxacin (Levaquin): Approved in 1996, levofloxacin is prescribed for UTI, acute pyelonephritis, chronic bacterial prostatitis, pneumonia (nosocomial and community-acquired), acute bacterial sinusitis, acute bacterial exacerbations of chronic bronchitis, skin infections, and bacterial conjunctivitis. It is available for PO, IV, and ophthalmic (Iquix, Quixin) administration. Levofloxacin has a long half-life that allows for once-daily dosing. The most common adverse effects are nausea, headache, diarrhea, insomnia, constipation, and dizziness. Adverse effects of ophthalmic levofloxacin include transient blurred vision, foreign body sensation, headache, burning, pharyngitis, and photophobia. Caution should be used for patients with certain dysrhythmias, due to its effects on cardiac conduction. Although rare, hematologic toxicity, including agranulocytosis and thrombocytopenia, and renal toxicity may occur after multiple doses. Other contraindications and adverse effects for the oral and IV forms (including the black box warning) are similar to those of ciprofloxacin. This drug is pregnancy category C.

Moxifloxacin (Avelox): Approved in 1999, moxifloxacin is prescribed for skin infections, community-acquired pneumonia, acute sinusitis, and acute bacterial exacerbations of chronic bronchitis. It is available by oral and IV routes, and as an ophthalmic preparation (Moxeza, Vigamox) for bacterial conjunctivitis. The most common adverse effects are dizziness, diarrhea, nausea, and vomiting. For the ophthalmic drops, eye irritation, pyrexia, and conjunctivitis are the common adverse effects. Like gemifloxacin, it is contraindicated in patients with certain dysrhythmias, due to its effects on cardiac conduction. Other contraindications and adverse effects for the oral and IV forms (including the black box warning) are similar to those of ciprofloxacin. This drug is pregnancy category C.

Norfloxacin (Noroxin): Norfloxacin was approved in 1986 and is indicated for UTI and prostatitis. It has the shortest half-life of all fluoroquinolones and is available only by the PO route. The most common adverse effects are nausea, headache, asthenia, rash, and abdominal cramping. Other contraindications and adverse effects (including the black box warning) are similar to those of ciprofloxacin. An ophthalmic solution once used for bacterial conjunctivitis is no longer available in the United States. This drug is pregnancy category C.

Ofloxacin (Ocuflox, Floxin Otic): Approved in 1990, ofloxacin is indicated for acute bacterial exacerbations of chronic bronchitis, community-acquired pneumonia, chlamydial infections of the reproductive tract, cystitis, complicated UTI, prostatitis, superficial ocular infections (Ocuflox), and otitis media (Floxin Otic). The most common adverse effects are nausea, headache, insomnia, dizziness, and rash. The otic preparation can cause otic pruritus. Other contraindications and adverse effects for the oral and IV forms (including the black box warning) are similar to those of ciprofloxacin. It is available for the PO, IV, ophthalmic, and otic routes. This drug is pregnancy category C.

Patients Receiving Fluoroquinolone Therapy

Assessment	Potential Nursing Diagnoses
Baseline assessment prior to administration: • Understand the reason the drug has been prescribed in order to assess for therapeutic effects. • Obtain a complete health history including neurologic, cardiovascular, respiratory, hepatic, or renal disease, myasthenia gravis, and the possibility of pregnancy. Assess for previous organ transplantation surgery. Obtain a drug history including allergies, noting specific reactions to drugs, current prescriptions, particularly corticosteroids, and OTC drugs, herbal preparations, and alcohol use. Be alert to possible drug interactions. • Assess signs and symptoms of current infection noting location, characteristics, presence or absence of drainage and character of drainage, duration, and presence or absence of fever or pain. • Evaluate appropriate laboratory findings (e.g., CBC, culture and sensitivity [C&S], hepatic function studies). • Assess the patient's ability to receive and understand instructions. Include family and caregivers as needed.	• *Infection* (bacterial) • *Acute Pain* • *Hyperthermia* • *Impaired Physical Mobility*, related to adverse drug effects • *Deficient Knowledge* (Drug Therapy) • *Risk for Injury*, related to adverse drug effects • *Risk for Deficient Fluid Volume*, related to diarrhea caused by adverse drug effects
Assessment throughout administration: • Assess for desired therapeutic effects (e.g., diminished signs and symptoms of infection and fever). • Continue periodic monitoring of CBC, renal function, urinalysis, and C&S as ordered. • Assess for adverse effects: nausea, vomiting, abdominal cramping, diarrhea, headache, or dizziness. Severe diarrhea, especially containing mucus, blood, or pus, or decreased urine output should be reported immediately.	

Planning: Patient Goals and Expected Outcomes

The patient will:

• Experience therapeutic effects dependent on the reason the drug is being given (e.g., diminished signs and symptoms of infection, decreased fever).
• Be free from or experience minimal adverse effects.
• Verbalize an understanding of the drug's use, adverse effects, and required precautions.
• Demonstrate proper self-administration of the medication (e.g., dose, timing, and when to notify the provider).

Implementation

Interventions and (Rationales)	Patient-Centered Care
Ensuring therapeutic effects: • Continue assessments as above for therapeutic effects. (Diminished fever, pain, or signs and symptoms of infection should begin after taking the first dose and continue to improve. The provider should be notified if fever and signs and symptoms of infection remain or increase after 3 days or if the entire course of antibacterial has been taken and signs of infection are still present.)	• Teach the patient to report a fever that does not diminish below 37.8°C (100°F) or per the parameters set by the health care provider within 3 days, increasing signs and symptoms of infection, or symptoms that remain after taking the entire course of the antibacterial drug. • Teach the patient *not* to stop the antibacterial drug when feeling better but to take entire course of the antibacterial therapy; do not share doses with other family members with similar symptoms; and return to the provider if symptoms have not resolved after an entire course of therapy.
Minimizing adverse effects: • Continue to monitor vital signs, especially temperature if fever is present. Immediately report undiminished fever, changes in level of consciousness, or febrile seizures to the health care provider. (Fever should begin to diminish within 1–3 days after starting drug. Continued fever may be a sign of worsening infection, adverse drug effects, or antibiotic resistance.)	• Teach the patient to report fever that does not diminish below 37.8°C (100°F) or per the health care provider parameters. Immediately report febrile seizures, changes in behavior, or changes in level of consciousness to the provider.
• Continue to monitor periodic laboratory work: renal function tests, CBC, urinalysis, and C&S as ordered. (Fluoroquinolones may be renal toxic and laboratory values should be monitored to prevent adverse effects. Periodic C&S tests may be ordered if infections are severe or are slow to resolve to confirm appropriate therapy.)	• Instruct the patient on the need for periodic laboratory work.
• Monitor for hypersensitivity and allergic reactions, especially with the first dose of the drug. Continue to monitor the patient for up to 2 weeks after completing antibacterial therapy. (Anaphylactic reactions are possible, particularly with the first dose of an antibacterial. As sensitivity occurs, reactions may continue to develop. Post-use, residual drug levels may cause delayed reactions, dependent on the length of half-life.)	• Teach the patient to immediately report any itching, rashes, or swelling, particularly of the tongue or face, urticaria, flushing, dizziness, syncope, wheezing, throat tightness, or difficulty breathing. • Instruct the patient with known antibacterial allergies to carry a wallet identification card or wear medical identification jewelry indicating allergy.
• Continue to monitor for renal toxicity, e.g., diminished urine output, or weight gain greater than 1 kg (2.2 lb) in 24 h. (Fluoroquinolones may require frequent monitoring to prevent adverse effects. Increasing fluid intake will help prevent drug accumulation in the kidneys.)	• Teach the patient to immediately report any diminished urine output, visible swelling of feet or ankles, or weight gain greater than 1 kg (2.2 lb) in 24 h. • Advise the patient to increase fluid intake to 2–3 L/day.

• Monitor for severe diarrhea, especially if mucus, blood, or pus is present. (Severe diarrhea may indicate the presence of CDAD or PMC.)	• Instruct the patient to report any diarrhea that increases in frequency or amount, or that contains mucus, blood, or pus. • Instruct the patient to consult the health care provider before taking any antidiarrheal drugs, because they cause the retention of harmful bacteria. • Teach the patient to increase the intake of dairy products containing live active cultures such as yogurt, kefir, or buttermilk, to help restore normal intestinal flora. Do not consume dairy products at the same time as a fluoroquinolone antibiotic. Take the antibiotic 1 h before or 2 h after a meal containing dairy.
• Monitor for development of superinfections, e.g., PMC, fungal, or yeast infections. (Superinfections with opportunistic organisms may occur when normal host flora are diminished or killed by the antibacterial drug and no longer hold pathogens in check. Appropriate treatment may be needed.)	• Teach the patient to observe for changes in stool, white patches in the mouth, whitish thick vaginal discharge, itching in the genital area, blistering itchy rash, and to immediately report severe diarrhea. • Teach the patient infection control measures such as frequent hand washing, adequate drying after showering or bathing, and to increase the intake of live-culture dairy foods.
• Monitor for significant GI effects, including nausea, vomiting, and abdominal pain or cramping. Fluoroquinolones may be taken with food, but consumption of dairy products at the same time as the drug will inhibit absorption. (Excessive use of beverages containing caffeine should be avoided because they may cause adverse effects such as nervousness or anxiety. Taking the drug along with calcium-fortified juices should also be avoided because it may inhibit the drug's absorption.)	• Teach the patient that the drug may be taken with food, but to avoid concurrent consumption of dairy or calcium-fortified juices, which may inhibit absorption. Do not take antacids or preparations such as vitamins containing iron or zinc at the same time as the fluoroquinolones dose. • Teach the patient to avoid consuming beverages with caffeine to decrease the chance of adverse effects such as nervousness or anxiety.
• Monitor for signs and symptoms of neurotoxicity, e.g., dizziness, severe headache, or seizures. (Fluoroquinolones have an increased risk of neurotoxicity. Previous seizure disorders or head injuries may increase this risk. Frequent monitoring is needed to prevent adverse effects. Persistent or increasing headaches should be immediately reported.)	• Instruct the patient to immediately report persistent or increasing headache, dizziness, or seizures.
• Monitor for joint, tendon, leg, or heel pain, or difficulty with movement or walking in patients on fluoroquinolones. (Fluoroquinolones have been associated with tendinitis and tendon rupture, especially of the Achilles tendon.)	• Instruct the patient to immediately report any significant or increasing joint, tendon, heel, lower leg or calf pain, or difficulty moving or walking to the health care provider.
• Monitor for the anticoagulation effects if the patient is on warfarin. (Fluoroquinolones decrease the metabolism of warfarin and may increase the anticoagulation effect and risk of bleeding.)	• Teach the patient to report any increase in bruising or bleeding while on warfarin. More frequent laboratory work may be needed.
• Continue to monitor for dermatologic effects including red or purplish skin rash, blisters, or sunburning. Immediately report severe rashes, especially associated with blistering. (Fluoroquinolones may cause significant dermatologic effects including Stevens–Johnson syndrome. Sunscreens and protective clothing should be used to prevent photosensitivity and photoallergic reactions.)	• Teach the patient to wear sunscreens and protective clothing for sun exposure and to avoid tanning beds. Immediately report any severe sunburn or rashes.
Patient understanding of drug therapy: • Use opportunities during administration of the medications and during assessments to discuss the rationale for drug therapy, desired therapeutic outcomes, commonly observed adverse effects, parameters for when to call the health care provider, and any necessary monitoring or precautions. (Using time during nursing care helps to optimize and reinforce key teaching areas.)	• The patient, family, or caregiver should be able to state the reason for the drug, appropriate dose and scheduling, what adverse effects to observe for and when to report them, and the anticipated length of medication therapy.

Patient self-administration of drug therapy:
• When administering medications, instruct the patient, family, or caregiver in proper self-administration techniques followed by return demonstration. (Utilizing time during nurse-administration of these drugs helps to reinforce teaching.)
	• Teach the patient to take the medication:
	  • Complete the entire course of therapy unless otherwise instructed. Do not share with other family members and do not stop the medicine when starting to feel better.
	  • Take the drug with food but avoid taking the drug concurrently with dairy products or calcium-fortified juices, which may decrease absorption. Take the fluoroquinolone 1 h before or 2 h after consuming these products.
	  • Do not take antacids or preparations such as vitamins containing iron or zinc at the same time as the fluoroquinolones dose.
	  • Avoid excess consumption of beverages or foods containing caffeine, which may increase the chance of nervousness or anxiety.
	  • Take the medication as evenly spaced throughout each day as feasible.
	  • Increase overall fluid intake while taking the antibacterial drug.
	  • Discard outdated medications or those no longer in use. Review the medicine cabinet twice a year for old medications (e.g., at beginning and end of daylight saving time).

Evaluation of Outcome Criteria

Evaluate the effectiveness of drug therapy by confirming that patient goals and expected outcomes have been met (see "Planning").

Patient Saftey

Levofloxacin (Levaquin)

Yesterday, Mrs. Rackey received the first dose of IV levofloxacin (Levaquin). While receiving the medication, she reported itching and a slight swelling of the tongue and lips (angioedema). However, later that day she had no discomfort or presence of the previous symptoms. She will receive the second dose of the medication again this morning. What should the nurse do?

See Answers to Patient Safety Questions on student resource website.

Miscellaneous Antibacterials

4 A number of miscellaneous antibacterials have specific clinical indications.

Several drugs act by miscellaneous mechanisms or are the only drugs in their class. Doses for the miscellaneous agents are listed in Table 3.

Bacitracin: Bacitracin is an older antibiotic, approved in 1948, that acts by inhibiting cell wall synthesis. It is combined with polymyxin B in over-the-counter (OTC) first aid products (Neosporin, Polysporin), and is also available as monotherapy in OTC products such as Bacitracin First Aid. It is effective against a variety of gram-positive and a few gram-negative microbes. Although an intramuscular (IM) form is available, bacitracin is almost always used topically due to potential nephrotoxicity (black box warning). In addition to creams and ointments, bacitracin solutions may be used to soak compresses that can be applied to large areas of the skin. This drug is pregnancy category C.

Daptomycin (Cubicin): Approved in 2003, daptomycin belongs to a class of antibiotics known as the **cyclic lipopeptides**. The spectrum of activity of daptomycin includes a wide variety of gram-positive pathogens. It is indicated for the treatment of complicated skin infections caused by organisms such as *S. aureus*, including methicillin-resistant *S. aureus* (MRSA), *Streptococcus pyogenes*, and *Enterococcus faecalis* (vancomycin-susceptible strains only). Daptomycin is bacteriocidal and its mechanism of action is clearly distinct from that of any other antibiotic. When binding to bacterial membranes, daptomycin causes a rapid depolarization of membrane potential, leading to inhibition of protein, DNA, and ribonucleic acid (RNA) synthesis. It is given only by IV infusion. The most clinically significant adverse effects are abnormal liver function tests, elevated creatine phosphokinase (CPK), dyspnea, and pneumonia. Myopathy has been recorded in a small percentage of patients taking daptomycin; therefore, the nurse should carefully monitor for muscle pain or weakness. The drug should be withheld if the CPK becomes elevated above 1,000 units/L. This drug is pregnancy category B.

Metronidazole (Flagyl): Metronidazole is another older anti-infective, approved in 1963, that is effective against a large number of anaerobes. It acts by interfering with the DNA

TABLE 3 Miscellaneous Antibacterials

Drug	Route and Adult Dose (maximum dose where indicated)	Adverse Effects
bacitracin	Topical: Apply thin layer of ointment bid or tid or as solution of 250–1,000 units/mL in wet dressing	*Anorexia, nausea, vomiting* Nephrotoxicity, anaphylaxis
daptomycin (Cubicin)	IV: 4–6 mg/kg once every 24 h for 7–14 days	*Nausea, diarrhea, constipation, headache* Anaphylaxis, superinfections, renal failure, myopathy, jaundice, PMC
metronidazole (Flagyl)	Anaerobic infections: PO: 7.5 mg/kg every 6 h (max: 4 g/day) IV loading dose: 15 mg/kg IV maintenance dose: 7.5 mg/kg every 6 h (max: 4 g/day)	*Dizziness, headache, anorexia, abdominal pain, metallic taste and nausea, Candida infections* Seizures, peripheral neuropathy, leukopenia
polymyxin B	IV: 15,000–25,000 units/kg/day divided every 12 h IM: 25,000–30,000 units/kg/day divided every 4–6 h	*Urticaria* Nephrotoxicity, neurotoxicity (confusion, blurred vision, paresthesias, paralysis), superinfections
rifampin (Rifadin, Rimactane)	PO/IV: 600 mg/day	*Nausea, vomiting, heartburn, anorexia, diarrhea, orange discoloration of the urine, sweat, and tears* PMC, acute renal failure, hepatotoxicity, blood dyscrasias
telithromycin (Ketek)	PO: 800 mg once daily	*Nausea, diarrhea, dizziness, headache, blurred vision* Superinfections, PMC, hepatotoxicity, dysrhythmias, respiratory failure, loss of consciousness

Note: Italics indicate common adverse effects. Underline indicates serious adverse effects.

and RNA synthesis of pathogens. Metronidazole is one of only a few drugs that have dual activity against both bacteria and multicellular parasites. It is a preferred drug for trichomoniasis, giardiasis, and amebiasis. Unlike most antibiotics, resistance to metronidazole is uncommon. When given orally, adverse effects are generally minor, and include nausea, dry mouth, and headache. High doses can produce neurotoxicity.

As an antibacterial, metronidazole has two indications: serious infections due to anaerobic bacteria, and peptic ulcer disease. Few antibacterials are effective against anaerobes because the organisms reside in sites that have tissue destruction and a poor blood supply. Anaerobic bacteria are common causes of abscesses, gangrene, diabetic skin ulcers, and deep wound infections. Serious intra-abdominal infections or septicemia due to *Bacteroides* and streptococci often respond well to IV infusions of the drug. It is a preferred drug for managing CDAD. Metronidazole has found a relatively new use in the treatment of *Helicobacter pylori* infections of the stomach associated with peptic ulcer disease. This drug is pregnancy category B.

Polymyxin B: Approved in 1951, polymyxin B is an older, bacteriocidal drug that acts by disrupting the bacterial cell membrane. The drug is able to penetrate the phospholipid layer, make the membrane leaky, and cause the death of the bacterium. Although parenteral formulations are available, polymyxin B is rarely prescribed by these routes due to potential nephrotoxicity and neurotoxicity (black box warnings). Its primary application is in the treatment of topical infections of the skin, mucous membranes, or eye, caused by gram-negative organisms. It is not effective against gram-positive microbes. It is combined with bacitracin and neomycin in common OTC first aid products such as Neosporin Ointment, Bactine Antibiotic, and Polysporin. Topical application, including to denuded skin, results in negligible systemic absorption. Polymyxin B is combined with neomycin and hydrocortisone in prescription otic preparations. Topical polymyxin B is pregnancy category B.

Rifampin (Rifadin, Rimactane): Approved in 1958, rifampin is administered PO or IV, and is usually associated with the pharmacotherapy of tuberculosis. The drug, however, is effective against a wide range of both gram-positive and gram-negative organisms. As an antibacterial, it is used for prophylaxis in contacts of patients with *Haemophilus influenzae* type B and for the prophylaxis of asymptomatic carriers of meningococcal disease. Occasionally, it is used for Legionnaire's disease, or when therapy with other antibiotics is unsuccessful. The reason its applications are limited is because of the rapid development of resistance, which can appear after only a few days of therapy. A flulike syndrome develops in about half the patients receiving the drug. Rifampin acts by inhibiting bacterial RNA polymerase, the enzyme that makes bacterial RNA. This drug is pregnancy category C.

Telithromycin (Ketek): In 2004, the FDA approved telithromycin for respiratory infections, the first in a class of antibiotics known as the **ketolides**. Telithromycin blocks bacterial protein synthesis by binding to two different sites on the 50S ribosomal subunit. Telithromycin is an oral drug, with the most common adverse effects being diarrhea, nausea, and headache. The primary indication for this drug is community-acquired pneumonia due to *S. pneumoniae*, *H. influenzae*, *Moraxella catarrhalis*, or *Mycoplasma pneumoniae*. When post–market surveillance discovered several cases of hepatic failure in patients receiving this drug, the FDA withdrew its approval for the treatment of acute bacterial sinusitis and acute bacterial exacerbations of chronic bronchitis. Hepatic function tests must be monitored during therapy. Telithromycin has the potential to prolong the QT interval, which represents an increased risk for ventricular dysrhythmias. The drug may cause mild to moderate visual disturbances, including blurred vision, diplopia, and difficulty focusing. Telithromycin carries a black box warning that it should not be used in patients with myasthenia gravis because fatal respiratory depression may occur. This drug is pregnancy category C.

UNDERSTANDING the CHAPTER

Key Concepts Summary

1 Bacterial DNA replication requires several different enzymes to uncoil, unwind, and duplicate the DNA.

2 Drugs have been discovered that inhibit different steps in bacterial DNA replication.

3 Fluoroquinolones are antibiotics whose therapeutic applications have expanded in recent years to treat many gram-positive and gram-negative infections.

4 A number of miscellaneous antibacterials have specific clinical indications.

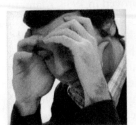

Making the PATIENT *Connection*

Remember the patient "Mike Springs" at the beginning of the chapter? Now read the remainder of the case study. Based on the information presented within this chapter, respond to the critical thinking questions that follow.

Mike Springs presents to the local health clinic. He is a 38-year-old male who has no history of chronic illness. His vital signs are normal with the exception of a slight increase in body temperature, 37.3°C (99.2°F). He denies shortness of breath. However, his nasal passages are congested, causing him to "mouth breathe." Mike is busy with work and family responsibilities. Until this most recent illness, he had started efforts toward a healthier lifestyle and weight reduction. Mike is now jogging for exercise and taking vitamin tablets. He is diagnosed with acute sinusitis, and the health care provider orders ciprofloxacin PO 500 mg twice daily for 10 days. Additional medications prescribed include a nasal decongestant and a mild analgesic.

As Mike is leaving the health clinic, he comments that he is responsible for multiple corporate offices and will soon be traveling. He is worried about remembering to take the medication, and admits to a history of nonadherence with medication regimens because he sometimes forgets to take medications.

Critical Thinking Questions

1. Prepare a patient teaching handout for Mike that provides him with information about the antibiotics he is being prescribed.

2. Mike asks you, the nurse, if he should continue jogging and taking vitamins. What would you advise?

3. What tips can you provide someone who forgets to take scheduled medication?

See Answers to Critical Thinking Questions on student resource website.

NCLEX-RN® Review

1 The client is prescribed ciprofloxacin (Cipro) and is instructed to take each dose of medication as evenly spaced apart during the day as possible. The nurse recognizes that this instruction is essential because:

1. The medication can cause sleep pattern disturbances.
2. Pathogenic bacteria have extremely rapid growth and reproduction rates.
3. Superinfections may develop if a dose of the medication is missed.
4. Allergic reactions are more likely to occur if a dose is missed.

2 The client is prescribed ofloxacin (Floxin) for treatment of acute bronchitis. The client tells the nurse that he experienced an allergic reaction when he took ciprofloxacin (Cipro) previously. As reported by the client, which of the following would be most indicative of an allergic reaction to this drug group? Select all that apply.

1. Headache
2. Nausea and vomiting
3. Itching without visible rash
4. Swelling of lips or tongue
5. Nervousness or anxiety

3 The nurse is instructing a client on a new prescription for ciprofloxacin (Cipro), and will include which instructions? Select all that apply.

1. Increase fluid intake to 2–3 liters per day.
2. Avoid consuming dairy products or antacids when you take the antibiotic.
3. Limit vitamin C intake in both dietary and oral vitamin forms.
4. Take the pill with an antihistamine to avoid adverse effects.
5. Coffee or tea without milk, cream, or coffee-lightener are the preferred beverages for taking the antibiotic dose.

4 A client has been receiving levofloxacin (Levaquin) IV for septicemia for 2 weeks and will be given the drug orally at home. Which discharge instruction would be most appropriate for the nurse to give this client?

1. Report any unusual joint or tendon pain or difficulty with movement or walking.
2. Take a daily multivitamin supplement with the levofloxacin.
3. Exposure to direct sunlight will help increase absorption of vitamin D, which is impaired by this medication.
4. Limit fluid intake to less than 1,500 mL per day.

5 A client has been given a prescription for ciprofloxacin (Cipro). The nurse checks the client's history because this drug should be used cautiously, or is contraindicated, in clients with what condition?

1. A history of anxiety disorder and nervousness
2. Clients over the age of 65
3. A history of penicillin allergy
4. Clients with myasthenia gravis

6 Which is the most important goal of nursing care for a client receiving polymyxin B ointment on a laceration?

1. Promote wound healing.
2. Sterilize the skin and mucous membranes.
3. Prevent allergic reaction.
4. Maximize pain relief.

Additional Case Study

Carolyn Ijams is doing her spring cleaning. As she is arranging the content in her medicine cabinet, she notices that there a tube of bacitracin antibiotic ointment, about half-used. She wonders whether she should keep it or not and asks you, the nurse who lives next door, what she should do with the tube.

1. Should Carolyn keep the antibiotic ointment? What would you want to know before making a recommendation?

2. What would you teach Carolyn about the use of topical antibiotic ointments such as the bacitracin?

See Answers to Additional Case Study on student resource website.

Pearson Nursing Student Resources

Find additional review materials at nursing.pearsonhighered.com

Prepare for success with additional NCLEX®-style practice questions, interactive assignments and activities, web links, animations, videos, and more!

References

Doyle, H. E. (2010). *Tendinopathy resulting from the use of fluoroquinolones: Managing risks.* Retrieved from http://media.jaapa.com/documents/19/cme_tendinopathy_1210_4543.pdf

Selected Bibliography

Albertson, T. E., Dean, N. C., El Solh, A. A., Gotfried, M. H., Kaplan, C., & Niederman, M. S. (2010). Fluoroquinolones in the management of community-acquired pneumonia. *International Journal of Clinical Practice, 64,* 378–388. doi:10.1111/j.1742-1241.2009.02239.x

Bouziana, D. G. (2010). Current and future medical approaches to combat the anthrax threat. *Journal of Medicinal Chemistry, 53*(11), 4505–4531. doi:10.1021/jm901024b

Bradbury, B. J., & Pucci, M. J. (2008). Recent advances in bacterial topoisomerase inhibitors.

Current Opinion in Pharmacology, 8(3), 132–145.

Deshpande, A., Pant, C., Jain, A., Fraser, T. G., & Rolston, D. (2008). Do fluoroquinolones predispose patients to *Clostridium difficile* associated disease? A review of the evidence. *Current Medical Research and Opinion, 24*(2), 329–333.

Frei, C. R., Labreche, M. J., & Attridge, R. T. (2011). Fluoroquinolones in community-acquired pneumonia: Guide to selection and appropriate use. *Drugs, 71*(6), 757–770. doi:10.2165/11585430-000000000-00000

Gerboc, J., Metro, M., Ginsberg, P., & Harkaway, R. (2008). *Rapidly developing fluoroquinolone resistance of common uropathogens.* Paper presented at the annual meeting of the American Urological Association, Orlando, FL.

Henderson, D. A., Inglesby, T. V., & O'Toole, T. (2002). *Bioterrorism: Guidelines for medical*

and public health management. Chicago, IL: American Medical Association.

Madigan, M. T., Martinko, J. M., Stahl, D. A., & Clark, D. P. (2012). *Brock biology of microorganisms* (13th ed.). San Francisco, CA: Benjamin Cummings.

Parry, C. M. (2010). Fluoroquinolone resistance: Challenges for disease control. In T. J. Weber (Ed.), *Antimicrobial resistance: Beyond the breakpoint.* Basil, Switzerland: Karger.

Smith, S. M. (2010). An update on *Clostridium difficile* infection and its management. *Nursing for Women's Health, 14*(5), 391–397. doi:10.1111/j.1751-486X.2010.01578.x

Stahlman, R., & Hartmut, L. (2010). Safety considerations of fluoroquinolones in the elderly: An update. *Drugs and Aging, 27*(3), 193–209. doi:10.2165/11531490-000000000-00000

Answers to NCLEX-RN® Review

1 Answer: 2 Rationale: Because pathogens grow rapidly and are constantly proliferating, all antibiotic therapies should be taken around the clock. Taking the drug as evenly spaced apart during the day as possible will help ensure a steady serum drug level to fight the bacteria. Options 1, 3, and 4 are incorrect. Ciprofloxacin is not known to cause problems with clients' sleep patterns. Superinfections occur when an antibiotic eradicates normal flora and an opportunistic organism invades. This is a problem associated with antibiotic therapy in general and is not caused by not adhering to the prescribed schedule. Allergic reactions are very common with antibiotic therapy, but they do not result from failing to adhere to the medication schedule. Cognitive Level: Applying; Client Need: Physiological Integrity; Nursing Process: Implementation

2 Answers: 3, 4, 5 Rationale: Itching, even without the presence of a rash, may indicate histamine release from a drug allergy. Swelling of the face, lips or tongue, known as angioedema, is also a symptom of allergy. Nervousness or anxiety may indicate an adrenergic response secondary to an allergic reaction and while they may have other causes, should be investigated further to rule out a developing allergic reaction. Options 1 and 2 are incorrect. Common adverse effects of ofloxacin are headache, nausea, and vomiting. Cognitive Level: Analyzing; Client Need: Physiological Integrity; Nursing Process: Assessment

3 Answers: 1, 2 Rationale: Ciprofloxacin is excreted renally and increasing fluid intake will help to prevent drug accumulation in the kidneys. Dairy products and antacids taken concurrently may inhibit absorption of the ciprofloxacin. Options 3, 4, and 5 are incorrect. Vitamin C does not need to be avoided while on ciprofloxacin. An antihistamine does not need to be taken concurrently and may mask the symptoms of adverse effects such as allergy. Excessive caffeine intake may increase the chance of nervousness or anxiety and should be avoided. Cognitive Level: Applying; Client Need: Physiological Integrity; Nursing Process: Implementation

4 Answer: 1 Rationale: Fluoroquinolones such as levofloxacin have been associated with tendonitis and tendon rupture, especially in patients over age 65. Any unusual joint or tendon pain or difficulty moving or walking should be reported to the provider. Options 2, 3, and 4 are incorrect. Many multivitamins contain iron and zinc, and concurrent administration with levofloxacin will impair the antibiotic's absorption. Fluoroquinolones do not impair vitamin D absorption and may cause dermatologic toxicities such as photosensitivity and photoallergy. Sunscreens and protective clothing should be used if sun exposure is anticipated. Fluoroquinolones may be renal toxic and *increased* fluid intake is advised. Cognitive Level: Applying; Client Need: Physiological Integrity; Nursing Process: Implementation

5 Answer: 4 Rationale: Fluoroquinolones such as ciprofloxacin may cause profound muscle weakness in clients with myasthenia gravis. Options 1, 2, and 3 are incorrect. Anxiety and nervousness do not require cautious use and are not contraindications to ciprofloxacin. While the incidence of tendonitis and tendon rupture is higher in the adult over age 65, the drug is not contraindicated in this population. However, more frequent monitoring may be needed. Cross-allergy to penicillins is not known for the fluoroquinolones and a history of penicillin is not a contraindication to ciprofloxacin. Cognitive Level: Analyzing; Client Need: Physiological Integrity; Nursing Process: Assessment

6 Answer: 1 Rationale: Polymyxin B is a topical antibiotic used to promote wound healing. Options 2, 3, and 4 are incorrect. Skin and mucous membranes cannot be made sterile. Polymyxin B will cause cell death of the invading pathogenic bacteria but will not completely sterilize the skin. Polymyxin B does not prevent allergic reaction, nor does it provide pain relief to wounds. Cognitive Level: Applying; Client Need: Physiological Integrity; Nursing Process: Planning

Review of the Endocrine System

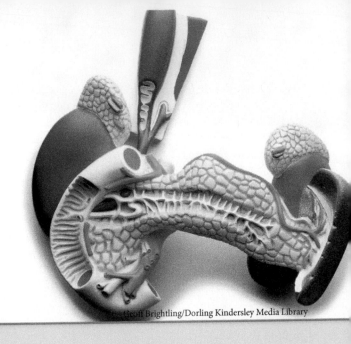

Review of the Endocrine System

Learning Outcomes

After reading this chapter, the student should be able to:

1. Describe the general structure and functions of the endocrine system.
2. Compare and contrast the nervous and endocrine systems in the control of homeostasis.
3. Explain circumstances in which hormone receptors may be up-regulated or down-regulated.
4. Through the use of a specific example, explain the concept of negative feedback in the endocrine system.
5. Explain the three primary types of stimuli that regulate hormone secretion.
6. Identify indications for hormone pharmacotherapy.

Chapter Outline

Like the nervous system, the endocrine system is a major controller of homeostasis. Whereas a nerve exerts instantaneous control over a single muscle fiber or gland, a hormone from the endocrine system may affect all body cells and take as long as several days to produce an optimum response. Hormonal balance is kept within a narrow range: Too little or too much of a hormone may produce profound physiological changes. This chapter reviews endocrine anatomy and physiology and its relevance to pharmacotherapy. For a more detailed review of the endocrine system, the student should refer to an anatomy and physiology textbook.

Overview of the Endocrine System

1 The endocrine system controls homeostasis through the secretion of hormones.

The **endocrine system** consists of various glands that secrete **hormones**, chemical messengers that the body releases in response to a change in the body's internal environment. The role of hormones is to maintain homeostasis in the body. For example, when the level of glucose in the blood rises above normal, the pancreas secretes insulin to return glucose levels to normal. The various endocrine glands and their hormones are illustrated in Figure 1.

After secretion from an endocrine gland, hormones enter the blood and are transported throughout the body. Compared to the nervous system, which reacts to body changes within milliseconds, the endocrine system responds relatively slowly. A few hormones, such as epinephrine, act within seconds, whereas others, such as testosterone, may take several days or even months to produce noticeable changes. Although slower in onset, the effects of hormones have a longer duration than those of the nervous system.

Hormone Receptors

2 Hormones must bind to specific receptors to cause physiological changes.

The cells affected by a hormone are called its target cells. **Target cells** have specific protein receptors on their plasma membrane that bind to the hormone. For some hormones, the receptors are in the cytoplasm or nucleus of the target cell. Once binding occurs, a change is produced in the cell, resulting in an action that is characteristic for the hormone. For example, when epinephrine binds to receptors on smooth muscle cells, they contract. When prolactin binds to secretory cells in the breast, milk production occurs.

Although a hormone travels throughout the body via the circulation, it only affects cells that have receptors for that specific hormone. Epinephrine does not affect breast secretory cells, because these cells have no epinephrine receptors. Prolactin does not cause muscular contraction because smooth muscle cells do not have prolactin receptors. This concept is illustrated in Figure 2.

In some cases, the target cells for a hormone are limited and specific. For example, the only receptors for thyroid-stimulating hormone are in the thyroid gland. However, some hormones, such as insulin and cortisol, have receptors on nearly every cell in the body; thus, these hormones have widespread effects.

The number of protein receptors for a hormone is dynamic, and changes with the needs of the body. Cells can create more receptors on their plasma membrane to capture hormone molecules as they pass by, a process called **up-regulation**. This may occur if the cell is receiving signals that a hormone action is needed, such as the need for production of more breast milk or additional secretion of thyroid hormone. Once the hormone is up-regulated (secreted in large quantities), the cell no longer needs to capture every hormone molecule so it makes fewer receptors on its surface, a process called **down-regulation**. Receptors are very efficient at capturing hormone molecules; although most hormones are secreted only in small amounts, they produce profound changes.

Down-regulation has important implications for pharmacotherapy. When a hormone is administered as pharmacotherapy for long periods, the body recognizes an abundance of the hormone, and cells will down-regulate the number of receptors for that hormone. This causes a desensitization of the target cells; that is, they are less responsive to the effects of the hormone. When therapy is discontinued, the cells will need time, usually several days, to synthesize more protein receptors and adjust to the new hormone level.

It is important to understand that the amount of hormone secreted by an endocrine gland is only partially responsible for the therapeutic response. Other critical components include the number of receptors and their sensitivity. During pharmacotherapy, increasing the dose of a hormone will produce little additional pharmacologic effect if all the receptors are already occupied, or if they are no longer sensitive to the hormone.

Negative Feedback Mechanisms

3 Most hormone action is regulated through negative feedback.

Because hormones can produce profound effects on the body, their secretion and release is carefully regulated by several levels of control. The most important mechanism is **negative feedback**, which is illustrated in Figure 3. A hormone causes an output or action in its target cell or tissue. As the levels of hormone rise, so does its action. The increased output or action is monitored by sensors. Once homeostasis is restored, the sensor signals the endocrine tissue to stop secreting the hormone; that is, the target tissue provides negative feedback.

Depending on the specific hormone, the negative feedback mechanism may be based on three primary types of stimuli: neuronal, humoral, and hormonal. In some cases, regulation involves multiple stimuli. The various hormones and their regulation are summarized in Table 1.

Key Terms

down-regulation

endocrine system

hormones

negative feedback

replacement therapy

target cells

up-regulation

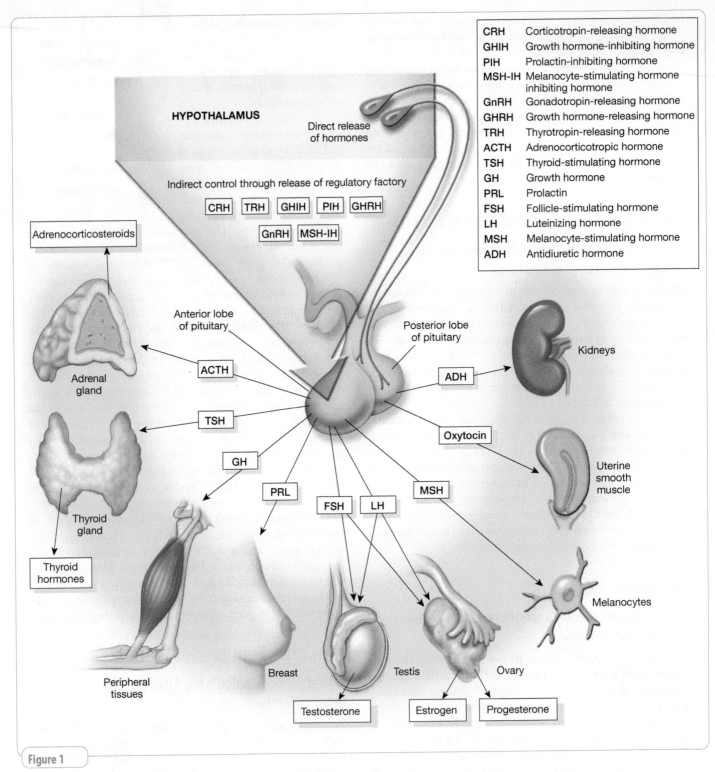

CRH Corticotropin-releasing hormone
GHIH Growth hormone-inhibiting hormone
PIH Prolactin-inhibiting hormone
MSH-IH Melanocyte-stimulating hormone inhibiting hormone
GnRH Gonadotropin-releasing hormone
GHRH Growth hormone-releasing hormone
TRH Thyrotropin-releasing hormone
ACTH Adrenocorticotropic hormone
TSH Thyroid-stimulating hormone
GH Growth hormone
PRL Prolactin
FSH Follicle-stimulating hormone
LH Luteinizing hormone
MSH Melanocyte-stimulating hormone
ADH Antidiuretic hormone

HYPOTHALAMUS

Direct release of hormones

Indirect control through release of regulatory factory

CRH TRH GHIH PIH GHRH

GnRH MSH-IH

Adrenocorticosteroids

Anterior lobe of pituitary

Posterior lobe of pituitary

Kidneys

Adrenal gland

ACTH

ADH

TSH

Oxytocin

Uterine smooth muscle

GH

PRL

MSH

Thyroid gland

FSH LH

Thyroid hormones

Melanocytes

Peripheral tissues

Breast

Testis

Ovary

Testosterone

Estrogen

Progesterone

Figure 1

Hormones and the endocrine system.

Neuronal stimuli: A few hormones are regulated by nerve impulses. The best example is epinephrine, which is released when a neuronal impulse from the sympathetic nervous system reaches the adrenal medulla. Another example is the release of oxytocin from the pituitary gland.

Humoral stimuli: Some endocrine glands sense the levels of specific substances in the blood and release the hormone when

the substance rises above or falls below the normal range. For example, pancreatic islet cells can sense the level of glucose in the blood. If glucose levels become too high, insulin is secreted. Another example is the release of parathyroid hormone when blood calcium levels fall.

Hormonal stimuli: In the endocrine system, it is common for one hormone to control the secretion of another hormone. In some

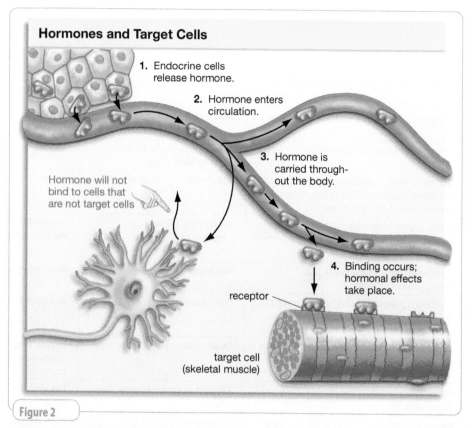

Figure 2

Hormones and their target cells.
Source: From *KROGH, DAVID, BIOLOGY: A GUIDE TO THE NATURAL WORLD,* 5th Ed., (c) 2011. Reprinted and Electronically reproduced by permission of Pearson Education, Inc., Upper Saddle River, New Jersey.

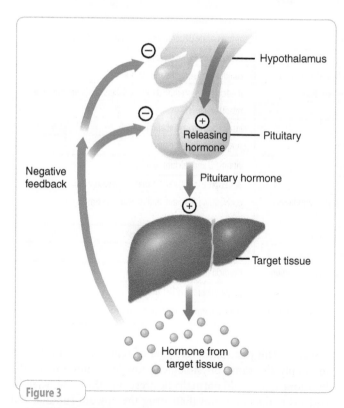

Figure 3

Negative feedback mechanism.

cases, the sequence involves three hormones. For example, thyrotropin-releasing hormone (TRH, from the hypothalamus) stimulates thyroid-stimulating hormone (TSH, from the pituitary), which causes the release of thyroid hormone (TH, from the thyroid gland). In a loop typical of the endocrine system, the last hormone in the pathway (TH) provides negative feedback to shut off secretion of the initial hormone (TRH).

CONNECTION Checkpoint 67.1

Identify indications for epinephrine pharmacotherapy. *See Answer to Connection Checkpoint 67.1 on student resource website.*

PharmFACT

Light at night on a regular basis interferes with melatonin, the "darkness hormone" secreted by the pineal gland. Studies suggested that working the late shift may increase your risk of cancer, probably caused by immune suppression (Blask, 2009).

Hormone Pharmacotherapy

4 Hormone pharmacotherapy is indicated for a diverse variety of conditions.

The goals of hormone pharmacotherapy vary widely. In many cases, a hormone is administered as **replacement therapy** for patients who are unable to secrete sufficient quantities of

TABLE 1 Selected Hormones and Their Regulation

Hormone	Target Organ(s) and Action	REGULATION	
		Stimulation	Inhibition
Adrenocorticotropic hormone (ACTH)	Adrenal cortex: stimulates release of glucocorticoids	Corticotropin-releasing hormone	Negative feedback from corticosteroids
Aldosterone	Kidneys: promotes reabsorption of sodium and water	Renin-angiotensin-aldosterone pathway, decreased blood volume, hypotension	Increased blood volume or hypertension
Antidiuretic hormone (ADH)	Kidneys: increases water reabsorption	Increased osmolarity of blood or decreased blood volume	Adequate hydration
Corticosteroids (glucocorticoids)	Most tissues: increases protein breakdown and glucose metabolism, provides resistance to stress, suppresses inflammation and immune response	Adrenocorticotropic hormone (ACTH)	Negative feedback from corticosteroids
Follicle-stimulating hormone (FSH)	Ovaries: promotes maturation of ovarian follicles and estrogen production Testes: increases sperm production	Gonadotropin-releasing hormone (GnRH)	Negative feedback from estrogen (females) or testosterone (males)
Growth hormone (GH)	Most tissues: including bone, muscle, liver: stimulates growth and mobilizes lipids	Gonadotropin-releasing hormone (GnRH)	Negative feedback from growth hormone
Insulin	Most tissues: promotes movement of glucose into cells, lowers blood glucose, decreases glycogen synthesis, and increases lipogenesis and protein synthesis	Hyperglycemia	Hypoglycemia
Luteinizing hormone (LH)	Ovaries: stimulates ovulation and production of estrogen Testes: produces testosterone	Gonadotropin-releasing hormone (GnRH)	Negative feedback from estrogen and progesterone (females) or testosterone (males)
Oxytocin	Uterus: stimulates contractions Breasts: ejects milk	Stretching of uterus or infant suckling	Lack of stretching of the uterus or discontinuation of breast-feeding
Parathyroid hormone	Kidneys, gastrointestinal tract, bone: increases calcium levels in blood	Hypocalcemia	Hypercalcemia
Prolactin	Breast: promotes lactation	Prolactin-releasing hormone	Prolactin-inhibiting hormone
Thyroid hormone	Most tissues: increases basal metabolic rate and growth	Thyroid-stimulating hormone	Negative feedback from thyroid hormone

TABLE 2 Selected Endocrine Disorders and Their Pharmacotherapy

Gland	Hormone(s)	Disorder	Drug Therapy Examples
Adrenal cortex	Corticosteroids	Hypersecretion: Cushing's syndrome	ketoconazole (Nizoral) and mitotane (Lysodren)
		Hyposecretion: Addison's disease	hydrocortisone, prednisone
Gonads	Ovaries: estrogen	Hyposecretion: menstrual and metabolic dysfunction	conjugated estrogens and estradiol
	Ovaries: progesterone	Hyposecretion: dysfunctional uterine bleeding	medroxyprogesterone (Provera, Others) and norethindrone
	Testes: testosterone	Hyposecretion: hypogonadism	testosterone
Pancreatic islets	Insulin	Hyposecretion: diabetes mellitus	insulin and oral antidiabetic agents
Parathyroid	Parathyroid hormone	Hypersecretion: hyperparathyroidism	surgery (no drug therapy)
		Hyposecretion: hypoparathyroidism	vitamin D and calcium supplements
Pituitary	Antidiuretic hormone	Hyposecretion: diabetes insipidus	desmopressin (DDAVP, Stimate) and vasopressin
		Hypersecretion: syndrome of inappropriate antidiuretic hormone (SIADH)	conivaptan (Viprostol) and tolvaptan (Samsca)
	Growth hormone	Hyposecretion: small stature	somatropin (Genotropin, others)
		Hypersecretion: acromegaly (adults)	octreotide (Sandostatin)
	Oxytocin	Hyposecretion: delayed delivery or lack of milk ejection	oxytocin (Pitocin)
Thyroid	Thyroid hormone (T$_3$ and T$_4$)	Hypersecretion: Grave's disease	propylthiouracil (PTU) and I-131
		Hyposecretion: myxedema (adults), cretinism (children)	thyroid hormone and levothyroxine (T4)

their own endogenous hormones. Examples of replacement therapy include the administration of thyroid hormone after the thyroid gland has been surgically removed, supplying insulin to patients whose pancreas is not functioning, or administering growth hormone to children with short-stature disorder. The pharmacologic goal of replacement therapy is to supply the same physiological, low-level amounts of the hormone that would normally be present in the body. Selected endocrine disorders and their drug therapy are summarized in Table 2.

Some hormones are used in cancer chemotherapy to shrink the size of hormone-sensitive tumors. For example, certain breast cancers are strongly dependent on estrogen for their growth. Giving the "opposite" hormone, testosterone, will shrink the tumor. In a similar manner, estrogen is used to shrink the size of testicular cancer, which is dependent on testosterone for its growth. Exactly how these hormones produce their antineoplastic action is largely unknown. When hormones are used as antineoplastics, their doses far exceed physiological levels normally present in the body. Hormones are nearly always used in combination with other antineoplastic medications.

Another goal of hormonal pharmacotherapy may be to produce an exaggerated response that is part of the normal action of the hormone. Administering hydrocortisone to suppress inflammation takes advantage of the normal action of the corticosteroids, but at higher amounts than would normally be present in the body. Hydrocortisone is indicated for acute inflammatory disorders such as lupus or rheumatoid arthritis. As another example, supplying estrogen or progesterone at specific times during the uterine cycle can prevent ovulation and pregnancy. In this example, the patient is given natural hormones; however, they are taken at a time when levels in the body are normally low.

Endocrine pharmacotherapy also involves the use of "antihormones." These hormone antagonists block the actions of endogenous hormones. For example, propylthiouracil (PTU) is given to block the effects of an overactive thyroid gland. Tamoxifen is given to block the actions of estrogen in estrogen-receptor dependent breast cancers (see Chapter 60).

CONNECTION Checkpoint 67.2

Glucocorticoids, or corticosteroids, are important drugs in treating inflammation. Explain their role in treating autoimmune disease. *See Answer to Connection Checkpoint 67.2 on student resource website.*

UNDERSTANDING THE CHAPTER

Key Concepts Summary

1. The endocrine system controls homeostasis through the secretion of hormones.

2. Hormones must bind to specific receptors to cause physiological changes.

3. Most hormone action is regulated through negative feedback.

4. Hormone pharmacotherapy is indicated for a diverse variety of conditions.

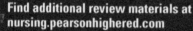

Pearson Nursing Student Resources

Find additional review materials at nursing.pearsonhighered.com

Prepare for success with additional NCLEX®-style practice questions, interactive assignments and activities, web links, animations, videos, and more!

References

Blask, D. E. (2009). Melatonin, sleep disturbance and cancer risk. *Sleep Medicine Reviews, 13*(4), 257–264. doi:10.1016/j.smrv.2008.07.007

Colbert, J. B., Ankney, J., & Lee, K. T. (2011). *Anatomy and physiology for health professionals: An interactive journey* (2nd ed.). Upper Saddle River, NJ: Pearson Education.

Krogh, D. (2011). *Biology: A guide to the natural world* (5th ed.). San Francisco, CA: Benjamin Cummings.

Selected Bibliography

Greenstein, B., & Wood, D. (2011). *The endocrine system at a glance* (3rd ed.). Malden, MA: Wiley-Blackwell.

Marieb, E. N., & Hoehn, K. (2010). *Human anatomy and physiology* (8th ed.). San Francisco, CA: Benjamin Cummings.

Martini, F. H., Nath, J. L., & Bartholomew, E. F. (2012). *Fundamentals of human anatomy and physiology* (9th ed.). San Francisco, CA: Benjamin Cummings.

Silverthorn, D. U. (2010). *Human physiology: An integrated approach* (5th ed.). San Francisco, CA: Benjamin Cummings.

Pharmacotherapy of Diabetes Mellitus

From Chapter 69 of *Pharmacology: Connections to Nursing Practice*, Second Edition. Michael Patrick Adams, Carol Quam Urban. Copyright © 2013 by Pearson Education, Inc. All rights reserved.

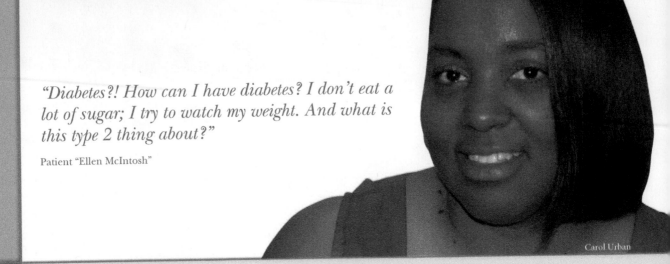

"Diabetes?! How can I have diabetes? I don't eat a lot of sugar; I try to watch my weight. And what is this type 2 thing about?"

Patient "Ellen McIntosh"

Carol Urban

Pharmacotherapy of Diabetes Mellitus

Learning Outcomes

After reading this chapter, the student should be able to:

1. Explain how blood glucose levels are maintained within narrow limits by insulin and glucagon.

2. Compare and contrast the etiology and pathogenesis of type 1, type 2, and gestational diabetes.

3. Describe the signs and diagnosis of diabetes.

4. Describe the acute complications of diabetes.

5. Identify the chronic complications of diabetes.

6. Compare and contrast the pharmacotherapy of the different types of diabetes.

7. For each type of insulin, identify the onset of action, peak action and duration of action, administration routes, when it is given related to meals, compatibility with other insulins, and adverse effects.

8. For each of the classes shown in the chapter outline, identify the prototype and representative drugs and explain the mechanism(s) of drug action, primary indications, contraindications, significant drug interactions, pregnancy category, and important adverse effects.

9. Apply the nursing process to the care of patients receiving pharmacotherapy for diabetes.

Chapter Outline

Physiology of Serum Glucose Control

Pathophysiology of Diabetes Mellitus: Types of Diabetes

Symptoms and Diagnosis of Diabetes

Complications of Diabetes Mellitus

PROTOTYPE **Glucagon (GlucaGen)**

Insulin Therapy

PROTOTYPE **Human Regular Insulin (Humulin R, Novolin R)**

Antidiabetic Agents for Type 2 Diabetes

Sulfonylureas

PROTOTYPE **Glyburide (DiaBeta, Glynase, Micronase)**

Biguanides

PROTOTYPE **Metformin (Glucophage, Glumetza, Others)**

Meglitinides

PROTOTYPE **Repaglinide (Prandin)**

Thiazolidinediones

PROTOTYPE **Rosiglitazone (Avandia)**

Alpha-Glucosidase Inhibitors

PROTOTYPE **Acarbose (Precose)**

Incretin Enhancers

PROTOTYPE **Sitagliptin (Januvia)**

Miscellaneous Antidiabetic Drugs

It is estimated that nearly 21 million people in the United States have diabetes mellitus, with more than 6 million of those being undiagnosed. Diabetes is one of the leading causes of death in the United States. Mortality has risen in recent years, causing some public health officials to refer to it as an epidemic. Diabetes can lead to serious acute and chronic complications, including heart disease, stroke, blindness, kidney failure, and amputations. Because nurses frequently care for patients with diabetes, it is imperative that they thoroughly understand the disorder, its treatment, and possible complications. There is an unrelated disorder, diabetes insipidus, which results from a deficiency of antidiuretic hormone. When the term *diabetes* is used in this chapter, it is referring to diabetes mellitus.

Physiology of Serum Glucose Control

1 Serum glucose is maintained within a narrow range by the hormones insulin and glucagon.

Because diabetes is essentially a disorder of carbohydrate metabolism, it is important to understand the way the body obtains, metabolizes, and stores glucose. Of all the different molecules available, the body prefers to use glucose as its primary energy source. The brain relies almost exclusively on glucose for its energy needs because it is unable to synthesize glucose and it will exhaust its supply after just a few minutes of activity. Most other tissues can use fatty acids and proteins for energy production, if necessary, but they too prefer to use glucose. The primary role of the liver and pancreas is to regulate the body's fuel supply.

Although the normal range for serum glucose is considered to be 60 to 100 mg/dL, it is usually tightly regulated by the body to remain between 80 and 90 mg/dL. Two pancreatic hormones contribute to maintaining a stable serum glucose level: **insulin**, which acts to decrease blood glucose levels, and glucagon, which acts to increase blood glucose levels.

Following a meal, glucose is rapidly absorbed from the gastrointestinal (GI) tract, and serum levels rise. Some of the glucose is taken up by cells and used for immediate energy needs, but about two thirds is stored in liver and muscle cells as glycogen, the storage form of glucose. When glucose levels fall between meals, glycogen is broken down in a process called **glycogenolysis**, and glucose is released into the bloodstream. Maintaining a stable serum glucose level is simply a matter of storing glucose during times of excess, and returning it to the bloodstream in times of deficiency. The importance of maintaining this delicate balance, however, cannot be overstated. Too much glucose or too little glucose can have lethal consequences.

Following a meal, the pancreas recognizes the rising serum glucose levels and releases insulin. Without insulin, glucose is not able to enter cells of the body. The cells may be surrounded by high amounts of glucose but they are unable to use it until insulin arrives. It may be helpful to visualize insulin as a transporter or "gatekeeper." When present, insulin swings open the gate, transporting glucose inside cells—if there is no insulin, there is no entry. The physiological actions of insulin are summarized as follows:

- Promotes the entry of glucose into cells.
- Provides for the storage of glucose, as glycogen.

- Inhibits the breakdown of fat and glycogen.
- Increases protein synthesis and inhibits **gluconeogenesis**, which is the production of new glucose from noncarbohydrate molecules.

Insulin is produced in beta cells of the pancreas known as islets of Langerhans, whereas alpha cells in the pancreas secrete glucagon. Glucagon maintains stable blood glucose levels between meals and during periods of fasting and has actions that are opposite to those of insulin. It removes glucose from its storage in the liver and sends it to the blood (glycogenolysis), raising serum glucose within minutes.

The level of glucose in the blood regulates the release of both insulin and glucagon. A hypoglycemic state (low serum glucose) stimulates the release of glucagon and inhibits the release of insulin, whereas a hyperglycemic state (high serum glucose) has the opposite effect: It stimulates the release of insulin and inhibits the release of glucagon. The physiological dynamics of insulin and glucagon release are shown in Figure 1.

Additional factors that decrease blood glucose levels are fasting, exercise, and alcohol. Factors that increase blood glucose levels include stress from infection, injury, or surgery, which triggers release of the epinephrine and norepinephrine; large meals or overconsumption of carbohydrates; growth hormone; and corticosteroids.

PharmFACT

According to the Centers for Disease Control and Prevention (CDC, 2010), the incidence of diabetes mellitus in the United States is as follows:

- 1 in every 400 children and adolescents has diabetes.
- 11.3% of all people 20 years or older have diabetes.
- 26.9% of all people 65 years or older have diabetes.
- 35% of all people 20 years or older have prediabetes.

Pathophysiology of Diabetes Mellitus: Types of Diabetes

2 Type 1 diabetes is characterized by insufficient insulin synthesis by the pancreas, whereas type 2 diabetes is characterized by insulin resistance in the target cells.

Diabetes mellitus is a metabolic disorder characterized by an imbalance between insulin availability and insulin need. The

Key Terms

diabetes mellitus

diabetic ketoacidosis (DKA)

fasting plasma glucose (FPG) test

gestational diabetes

gluconeogenesis

glycogenolysis

hemoglobin A1C (HbA1C)

hyperosmolar hyperglycemic state (HHS)

incretins

insulin

insulin resistance

metabolic syndrome

oral glucose tolerance test (OGTT)

polydipsia

polyphagia

polyuria

prediabetes

type 1 diabetes

type 2 diabetes

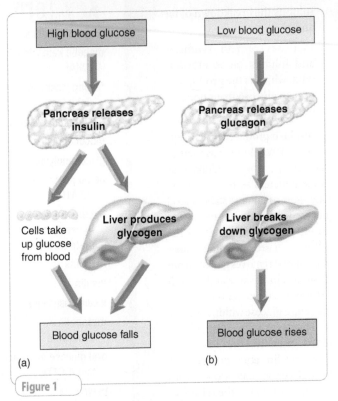

High blood glucose → Pancreas releases insulin → Cells take up glucose from blood / Liver produces glycogen → Blood glucose falls (a)

Low blood glucose → Pancreas releases glucagon → Liver breaks down glycogen → Blood glucose rises (b)

Figure 1

Insulin, glucagon, and blood glucose.

two primary forms of diabetes are called type 1 and type 2. There are significant differences between the two types in terms of pathophysiology and disease management. A third form of the disease occurs during pregnancy and is known as gestational diabetes.

Type 1 diabetes results from an absolute lack of insulin secretion due to destruction of pancreatic beta cells. The destruction of beta cells is believed to result from a combination of autoimmune, genetic, and environmental factors. Type 1 is the less common form of diabetes, accounting for only 5% to 10% of all patients with the disorder. It is seen most frequently among children and young adults, but it may occur at any age.

Because of the lack of sufficient insulin in patients with type 1 diabetes, glucose cannot enter cells and fatty acids are used as the primary energy source. Metabolic by-products of

lipid metabolism known as ketones accumulate in the blood, producing diabetic ketoacidosis (DKA), a dangerous and potentially life-threatening condition (see Section 4).

Patients with type 1 diabetes must receive insulin therapy to survive. In the past, type 1 was called juvenile or insulin-dependent diabetes. While these terms are still in use, they do not accurately reflect the nature of the disease.

Type 2 diabetes is the more common form of the disorder, representing 90% to 95% of people with diabetes. The primary physiological characteristic of type 2 diabetes is hyperglycemia caused by a relative deficiency of insulin. The disorder is characterized by **insulin resistance**, a condition in which cells become unresponsive to insulin due to a defect in insulin receptor function. The pancreas may be producing sufficient amounts of insulin but target cells do not recognize it.

As cells become more resistant to insulin, blood glucose levels rise and the pancreas responds by secreting even more insulin. Eventually, the hypersecretion of insulin leads to beta cell exhaustion, and ultimately to beta cell death. As type 2 diabetes progresses, it becomes a disorder characterized by insufficient insulin levels as well as insulin resistance. The activity of insulin receptors can be increased by exercise, which lowers the level of circulating insulin. In fact, adhering to a healthy diet and regular exercise have been shown to reverse insulin resistance, and to delay or prevent the development of type 2 diabetes.

Eighty percent of persons with type 2 diabetes are overweight, and the degree of obesity directly affects the degree of insulin resistance. In particular, persons with upper body obesity (central obesity) are at increased risk for developing insulin resistance and type 2 diabetes. Although most patients with type 2 diabetes are older, this disease is increasingly being diagnosed in obese adolescents. Risk factors for type 2 diabetes are a family history of diabetes, obesity, and race and ethnicity. African Americans, Native Americans, Hispanic Americans, Asian Americans, and Pacific Islanders are at increased risk for type 2 diabetes (CDC, 2010). Other risk factors are age older than 45 years, a history of elevated fasting serum glucose levels or impaired glucose tolerance, hypertension (HTN), low levels of high-density lipoproteins, triglycerides above 250 mg/dL, and a history of gestational diabetes, delivery of a baby over 9 pounds, or both. Table 1 compares and contrasts type 1 and type 2 diabetes.

TABLE 1 Comparison of Type 1 and Type 2 Diabetes Mellitus

Diabetes Mellitus	Type 1	Type 2
Cause	Destruction of beta cells with lack of insulin	Insulin resistance; insulin deficiency may develop
Incidence	5–10%	90–95%
Age at onset	Children, young adults, usually younger than 35 years	Usually older than 35 years
Symptom onset	Rapid	Gradual
Body weight	Usually underweight	Usually overweight, obese
Symptoms	Polyuria, polydipsia, polyphagia, weight loss	Same (polyuria, polydipsia, polyphagia, weight loss), plus blurred vision, fatigue, recurrent infections
Ketosis	Often present with poor control	Infrequent
Treatment	Insulin replacement, diet, exercise, weight, lipid, and blood pressure control	Oral agents with or without insulin, diet, exercise, weight loss, lipid, and blood pressure control

Most patients with type 2 diabetes do not require insulin administration, at least initially; their condition can be managed with oral antidiabetic agents. Type 2 diabetes was formerly called adult-onset diabetes and non–insulin-dependent diabetes, but these are not accurate descriptions of the disorder because it occurs in children and may require insulin administration.

Gestational diabetes is a condition resulting from glucose intolerance with an onset, or first recognition, during pregnancy. This is a serious disorder that puts both the woman and fetus at risk for complications, and so requires careful management during pregnancy. In addition, women who develop gestational diabetes are at increased risk for developing diabetes 5 to 10 years after delivery. It occurs most frequently in women with a family history of diabetes, a history of stillbirth or spontaneous abortion, a previous large for gestational age baby, women who are obese or of advanced maternal age, women who have had five or more pregnancies, or women who are members of a high-risk population (Hispanic, Native American, Asian, or African American). If careful nutritional management is unable to normalize serum glucose levels, insulin therapy is initiated. Traditionally, oral antidiabetic drugs have not been used for gestational diabetes due to concerns regarding potential teratogenicity; however, the results of research may change that practice in the future.

Symptoms and Diagnosis of Diabetes

3 The classic signs and symptoms of diabetes include polyuria, polydipsia, and polyphagia.

The classic triad of signs and symptoms for either type of diabetes is known as the three "polys": **polyuria**, excessive urine production; **polydipsia**, excessive thirst; and **polyphagia**, excessive appetite.

Glucose is one of the body's most valuable energy molecules, and nondiabetic patients excrete very little. As glucose levels rise in the blood in patients with diabetes, however, the kidneys are unable to reabsorb the large amounts passing through the renal tubules, so glucose is eliminated in the urine (glucosuria). Glucose molecules create increased osmotic pressure in body fluids, pulling water along with it; thus, osmotic diuresis (polyuria) occurs. The glucose increases osmotic pressure in the bloodstream, pulling water out of tissue cells and causing cellular dehydration. This triggers thirst, and causes the person to increase fluid intake (polydipsia). The excess

---

CONNECTIONS

Evidence-Based Practice Oral Antidiabetic Drugs for Gestational Diabetes

Clinical Question

Can oral antidiabetic drugs be used safely and effectively for the treatment of gestational diabetes?

Evidence

Traditionally, oral antidiabetic drugs have not been widely used during pregnancy for the treatment of gestational diabetes due to concerns over teratogenicity. Mirroring the rise in type 2 diabetes in the general population is the occurrence of gestational diabetes, and uncontrolled glucose levels in the mother often lead to complications for both the mother and baby. Insulin injection has been the traditional therapy used in gestational diabetes; however, women may prefer oral antidiabetic drugs. Unlike insulin injections, oral drugs are not required to be taken multiple times per day, they do not require special skills to administer, and adherence to a drug regimen is more likely. Are these oral drugs safe and effective?

Nicholson and Baptiste-Roberts (2011) reviewed available evidence on the use and effectiveness of glyburide and metformin compared to insulin in gestational diabetes, and adverse effects such as postdelivery hypoglycemia in the newborn, fetal weight gain or loss, and congenital abnormalities across all three treatment regimens. Their report was a follow-up review of research based on an earlier analysis conducted for the Agency for Healthcare Research in Quality (AHRQ) in 2008 (Nicholson et al., 2008). Glyburide and metformin were chosen as comparison drugs to insulin in gestational diabetes because they are the most widely prescribed oral antidiabetic drugs in the United States and Europe. The authors noted that while both glyburide and metformin are available for the treatment of type 2 diabetes, neither drug has been approved by the U.S. Food and Drug Administration (FDA) for use in gestational diabetes although several well-controlled studies have been conducted and more studies are continuing. Health care providers in the United States may prescribe the combination based on the analysis by the AHRQ and on the existing, rigorously conducted studies.

Although larger clinical trials are still needed and long-term studies of the effects on babies born to mothers who used glyburide or metformin are also needed, the authors noted that when compared to insulin, both drugs were effective in the treatment of gestational diabetes, and finger-stick and serum glucose levels were similar throughout pregnancy across all three treatment methods. A slight increase was noted in postdelivery hypoglycemia in babies born to mothers taking insulin when compared to metformin, but it was not statistically significant. There were no differences in the number of congenital anomalies noted in any of the treatment groups. However, babies born to mothers taking glyburide were on average 200 g (0.4 lb) heavier than mothers taking metformin.

Implications

While larger studies of the use of glyburide and metformin in gestational diabetes and longitudinal studies of children born to women taking these drugs are still needed, these drugs appear to be as safe and effective as insulin based on the available research. The American Diabetes Association (ADA, 2011a) recommends that to minimize complications to both mother and baby, optimal glucose control in pregnancy should begin preconception, but is especially critical in the first trimester of pregnancy. As more research continues to support the use of glyburide and metformin as safe and effective in gestational diabetes, women may find this goal of optimal glucose control more easily achieved with glyburide and metformin than with insulin.

Critical Thinking Question

How would you respond to the patient with gestational diabetes who asks why she cannot take a pill to control her glucose?

See Answers to Critical Thinking Questions on student resource website.

hunger (polyphagia) occurs primarily with type 1 diabetes, when nutrient stores become too depleted to meet the body's energy needs, and weight is lost. Other signs and symptoms include blurred vision, fatigue, paresthesias, and skin infections. Nocturia, secondary to the polyuria, may occur.

The two primary blood tests for diagnosing diabetes are the **fasting plasma glucose (FPG) test** and the **oral glucose tolerance test (OGTT)**. Testing usually begins with the FPG, obtained following a fast of at least 8 hours. If the FPG results are abnormal (higher than 100 mg/dL), an OGTT is obtained. A loading dose of 75 g of glucose is ingested and the plasma glucose level is obtained 2 hours later. In addition, a random glucose level of greater than 200 mg/dL in the presence of symptoms is diagnostic of diabetes, although a FPG test or OGTT is usually obtained for verification.

Home monitoring of blood glucose is now commonplace, and enables the patient with diabetes to maintain tighter control of glucose levels. Finger-stick testing involves placing a drop of capillary blood on a test strip, which is then read by a glucose meter. Fasting blood glucose levels, as well as preprandial and postprandial testing, may be employed. Another important laboratory test used in the management of diabetes is the glycosylated hemoglobin or **hemoglobin A1C (HbA1C)** test. When glucose levels remain at normal levels, only 4% to 6% of the circulating hemoglobin will have glucose bound to it. Once glucose binds to hemoglobin, it remains bound for the life of the red blood cell, which is an average of 120 days. As serum glucose increases, more glucose becomes bound to hemoglobin. Therefore, the HbA1C provides a measure of glucose control over the 8 to 12 weeks prior to the test. Health care providers recommend that persons with diabetes lower their HbA1C level to 7% or less. In general, every percentage point drop in A1C levels (e.g., from 8.5% to 7.5%) reduces the risk of vascular complications by 40% (CDC, 2010).

Most patients who develop type 2 diabetes go through a period of impaired glucose tolerance referred to as **prediabetes**. In prediabetes, serum glucose levels are elevated but are not high enough to be diagnosed as diabetes. This condition increases the risk for developing diabetes, heart disease, and stroke. Prediabetes may result from impaired fasting glucose, impaired glucose tolerance, or both. Progression from prediabetes to diabetes is not inevitable. Careful management of nutrition, regular exercise, and weight loss (if overweight) may prevent or delay progression to diabetes. Patients with prediabetes should be monitored on an annual basis for the potential development of diabetes and to evaluate the degree of success in managing comorbid conditions such as HTN, hyperlipidemia, and obesity.

A group of abnormalities that tend to occur together has been called insulin resistance syndrome, syndrome X, or the preferred name: **metabolic syndrome**. This syndrome places the patient at increased risk for developing diabetes and vascular complications such as cardiovascular disease, peripheral vascular disease, and stroke. Again, weight loss, exercise, and nutritional management enable people with this syndrome to delay or prevent the progression to type 2 diabetes. The metabolic syndrome is diagnosed by the presence of three or more of the following:

- Central obesity, with waste circumference more than 35 in. for women or more than 40 in. for men
- Serum triglycerides equal to or greater than 150 mg/dL
- High-density lipoprotein (HDL) cholesterol less than 50 mg/dL in women or less than 40 mg/dL in men
- Blood pressure more than 130/85 mm Hg
- Fasting plasma glucose more than 100 mg/dL (Porth, 2011)

Complications of Diabetes Mellitus

4 Acute complications of diabetes include diabetic ketoacidosis, hyperosmolar hyperglycemic state, and hypoglycemia.

The acute complications of uncontrolled or poorly controlled diabetes occur suddenly and require immediate interventions. Diabetic ketoacidosis, hyperosmolar hyperglycemic state (HHS), and hypoglycemia are the three primary acute complications. The chronic complications are discussed in Section 5.

Diabetic ketoacidosis (DKA) is an acute condition that occurs primarily in patients with type 1 diabetes. The three major disturbances that occur with DKA are hyperglycemia, metabolic acidosis, and osmotic diuresis. DKA typically develops over several days with symptoms such as polyuria, polydipsia, nausea, vomiting, and severe fatigue, progressing to stupor and eventual coma. The patient may report having abdominal pain or tenderness, and the breath has a typical fruity smell as the lungs attempt to remove volatile ketoacids. As the acidosis worsens, Kussmaul's respirations may develop, with an increased rate and depth of respirations. Tachycardia and hypotension occur in response to dehydration and fluid depletion.

CONNECTIONS

Treating the Diverse Patient
Weight Gain and Diabetes Risk in Multiethnic Populations

Using a Hawaiian subset of the Multiethnic Cohort Study conducted in California and Hawaii, Morimoto et al. (2011) sought to investigate the effect of weight gain on increasing diabetes risk. It had been previously noted that diabetes in Japanese Americans and Native Hawaiians was twice as high as in Caucasians (Maskarinec et al., 2009a). When comparing BMI at age 21 and when the participants in the cohort study entered the study, a weight gain of between 5 and 10 kg (11 and 22 lb) doubled the risk of diabetes for all participants. With a weight gain of 25 kg (55 lb) or more, the risk increased eightfold. Participants of Japanese and Native Hawaiian descent were more likely to experience adverse effects of weight gain. Previous analysis of the Multiethnic Cohort Study had discovered that the prevalence of type 2 diabetes was significantly higher for all ethnic groups than for Caucasians (Maskarinec et al., 2009b). This latest study highlights the importance of maintaining normal weight throughout adulthood to decrease the risk of diabetes.

DKA may be the first presenting symptoms of a person previously undiagnosed with diabetes. Treatment includes fluid replacement to improve circulating blood volume and tissue perfusion, normalization of blood glucose levels, and correction of electrolyte imbalances and metabolic acidosis. Insulin therapy is begun, usually with an IV loading dose, followed by a continuous low-dose infusion. Serum glucose levels must be lowered gradually because too rapid a drop can cause a fluid shift back into the cells that can lead to cerebral edema. Although DKA is a very serious disorder, the mortality rate for this complication has been reduced to less than 5% with proper treatment.

CONNECTION Checkpoint 69.1

What is the clinical definition of acidosis? What is the drug of choice for reversing metabolic acidosis? *See Answer to Connection Checkpoint 69.1 on student resource website.*

Hyperosmolar hyperglycemic state (HHS) is a serious, acute complication of diabetes that carries a mortality rate of 20% to 40%. HHS is generally seen in persons with type 2 diabetes, and is characterized by extreme hyperglycemia (above 600 mg/dL), hyperosmolarity (above 310 mOsm/L) with dehydration, the absence of ketoacidosis, and central nervous system (CNS) dysfunction. The typical patient is elderly, obese, and has comorbid medical problems, such as heart failure or renal impairment. The elevated serum glucose levels and increased osmolarity produce a large osmotic diuresis with marked dehydration, confusion, and lethargy. Other possible neurologic symptoms are seizures, hemiparesis, abnormal reflexes, aphasia, and visual disturbances. Symptoms can progress to stupor and coma. Tachycardia and hypotension result from fluid depletion and poor tissue perfusion. Acidosis may develop, caused by an accumulation of lactic acid rather than ketoacids.

The onset of HHS is gradual and, because of the neurologic manifestations, may be mistaken for a stroke in older adults. Treatment consists of careful fluid replacement while avoiding cerebral and pulmonary edema, and correction of electrolyte imbalances, particularly potassium. Low-dose insulin is given by continuous IV infusion to slowly lower glucose levels to 250 to 300 mg/dL. Seizure precautions should be instituted, and hemodynamic monitoring should be used in these critically ill patients. The nurse should closely monitor intake and output, blood pressure, heart rate, lung sounds, weight, peripheral pulses, and neurologic status. Finally, the underlying cause of the episode should be investigated and treated as needed.

Hypoglycemia, or abnormally low serum glucose, occurs most often in patients improperly treated with insulin and may occur during therapy with some oral antidiabetic agents. The manifestations of hypoglycemia result from changes in mental status, and by the activation of the sympathetic nervous system. Because the brain relies on a continuous supply of glucose, falling glucose levels may lead to headache, difficulty concentrating, confusion, and behavioral changes, progressing to seizures and coma. The sympathetic nervous system activation results from the body's attempt to increase serum glucose by the release of catecholamines (epinephrine and norepinephrine). These catecholamines cause symptoms that include tachycardia, anxiety, sweating, and the constriction of surface vessels, leading to cool, clammy skin. Acute hypoglycemia is considered a medical emergency, and if prolonged or severe, can lead to brain damage or death.

The symptoms of hypoglycemia may have a very rapid onset. Patients who have had diabetes for an extended time may develop hypoglycemic unawareness, which is the inability to recognize symptoms. Some drugs, such as beta-adrenergic blockers, interfere with the sympathetic symptoms of hypoglycemia, making it more difficult for the patient to recognize the condition and for the body to correct the low glucose levels.

Factors that cause hypoglycemia in patients with diabetes include errors in insulin dosage, failure to eat at regular intervals, increased exercise, medication adjustments, or changes in the insulin injection site. Alcohol consumption can lead to hypoglycemia by decreasing gluconeogenesis. The treatment for hypoglycemia is always glucose, given in a concentrated source of 15 to 20 g. This can be repeated as necessary, while taking care not to overtreat the patient and cause hyperglycemia. If the person is unconscious, or unable to swallow safely, a small amount of glucose gel or spray can be administered to the buccal mucosa. Intravenous (IV) glucose is immediately effective in treating hypoglycemia and glucagon may be administered.

PROTOTYPE DRUG | Glucagon (GlucaGen)

Classification: **Therapeutic:** Antihypoglycemic agent
Pharmacologic: Pancreatic hormone

Therapeutic Effects and Uses: Glucagon is used for the emergency treatment of severe hypoglycemia in patients with diabetes who are unconscious or unable to eat sugar or drink a sweetened beverage. It is also used for radiographic studies to relax the smooth muscle of the GI tract. GlucaGen is obtained through recombinant DNA technology and is identical in structure to human glucagon.

Glucagon can be given intramuscularly (IM), subcutaneously, or IV. Glucagon will raise serum glucose levels in 10 to 20 minutes. Because glucagon raises glucose levels by stimulating breakdown of stored glycogen, it is not effective in patients who experience hypoglycemia due to starvation, because their glycogen stores are depleted.

From 1930 to 1950, massive doses of insulin were administered to agitated psychiatric patients with serious mental illnesses to induce seizures and coma, a procedure called insulin shock therapy. Upon administration of glucose or glucagon, the patient awakened in a more sedated state. Although glucagon is still approved for this purpose, this inhumane practice was discontinued when antipsychotic drugs were discovered in the 1950s.

Mechanism of Action: Glucagon increases glucose levels by increasing glycogenolysis; therefore, its actions are dependent on the presence of adequate liver glycogen stores. Glucagon stimulates the uptake of amino acids, increases their conversion to glucose (gluconeogenesis), and promotes lipolysis in the liver, with the release of fatty acids and glycerol.

Pharmacokinetics:

Route(s)	IM, IV, subcutaneous
Absorption	Easily absorbed IM or subcutaneous
Distribution	Throughout plasma
Primary metabolism	Liver, plasma, and kidneys
Primary excretion	Renal and through the bile
Onset of action	IV: 5–20 min; IM: 30 min; subcutaneous: 30–45 min
Duration of action	1–1.5 h

Adverse Effects: Glucagon is well tolerated. Adverse effects include nausea, vomiting, hypersensitivity reactions, transient changes in blood pressure (either hypotension or HTN), tachycardia, hyperglycemia, and hypokalemia.

Contraindications/Precautions: Glucagon is contraindicated in patients sensitive to protein compounds, in patients with depleted glycogen stores, or in patients with insulinoma or pheochromocytoma. It is used with caution in persons with coronary artery disease because it may affect blood pressure, heart rate, and myocardial oxygen demand.

Drug Interactions: Glucagon increases serum glucose and will antagonize the effects of antidiabetic agents. Beta-adrenergic blockers will inhibit the glucose elevating effect of glucagon, and will also increase the risk of blood pressure or heart rate adverse effects associated with glucagon. **Herbal/Food**: None known.

Pregnancy: Category B.

Treatment of Overdose: An overdose can cause hyperglycemia, which may be treated with insulin, IV fluids, and monitoring of electrolytes.

Nursing Responsibilities:

- Assess the patient's blood glucose level before, during, and after glucagon administration.
- Reconstitute the dry powder of glucagon with the diluent supplied by the manufacturer. Gently roll the vial to mix the drug but do not shake the vial. If glucagon fails to cause a response, IV glucose must be given.
- Administer supplemental oral carbohydrates once consciousness has been achieved to restore glycogen levels and prevent secondary hypoglycemia.
- Instruct the patient on the proper use of the GlucaGen emergency kit.

Lifespan and Diversity Considerations:

- Calculate pediatric dosages carefully. In general, children under the age of 6 require one half the adult dose.

Patient and Family Education:

- Immediately report signs of impending hypoglycemia such as headache, difficulty concentrating, confusion, seizures, palpitations, nervousness, sweating, and cool, clammy skin to the health care provider.
- At the first signs of hypoglycemia, eat sugar or other carbohydrate because this may eliminate the need to administer glucagon. Follow any carbohydrate with a protein source for longer lasting effects.
- Do not mix the GlucaGen solution with the powder until it is ready to be used. Discard any unused portion.
- Wear a medical alert bracelet or jewelry that identifies your medical condition and its treatment.

Drugs Similar to Glucagon (GlucaGen)

There are no drugs similar to glucagon.

5 Serious, chronic complications of diabetes include neuropathy, nephropathy, retinopathy, and vascular disease.

Most patients with type 2 diabetes experience no symptoms of their illness for many years, perhaps even decades. There may be no acute symptoms to motivate the patient to seek medical care. However, while years may pass without symptoms, the effects of uncontrolled blood glucose levels are progressively producing major, irreversible changes on body systems, especially the nervous and circulatory systems.

Teaching patients about the long-term consequences of untreated diabetes can be a major challenge for the nurse. When diagnosed at an asymptomatic stage, it is difficult to convince patients to make radical changes to their lifestyle and to spend money on prescriptions when they do not feel ill. Patients must clearly understand that if they delay treatment until symptoms appear, it will likely be too late to prevent serious, chronic complications. Intensive management of blood glucose levels has been found to dramatically reduce the incidence of long-term complications of diabetes.

Neuropathies are common, affecting an estimated 60% to 70% of persons with diabetes. Diabetic neuropathies affect both the somatic and autonomic nervous systems. Somatic neuropathies include paresthesias, numbness, tingling and pain, motor weakness, and muscle wasting. Autonomic neuropathies include postural hypotension, altered GI functioning including gastroparesis, or gastric atony, diarrhea, altered genitourinary functioning with difficulty voiding or erectile dysfunction, and possible cranial nerve impairment. Intensive management of blood glucose has been shown to reduce the occurrence of neuropathies.

Diabetic nephropathy is the leading cause of end-stage renal disease, which affects patients with both type 1 and type 2 diabetes. Most commonly, the renal glomeruli are damaged, and progressive loss of kidney function leads to eventual renal failure. Comorbid conditions that put the patient at high risk for nephropathy include HTN, poor glucose control, smoking, and hyperlipidemia.

Diabetic retinopathy is the leading cause of acquired blindness in the United States. Twenty years after the onset of diabetes, almost all persons with type 1, and over 60% of those with type 2 diabetes, show some degree of retinopathy (Porth, 2011). Regular eye exams are important for everyone who has diabetes.

Diabetes is a major risk factor for the development of vascular disease, including premature atherosclerosis, which leads to coronary artery disease, cerebrovascular disease, and peripheral vascular disease. Heart disease and stroke account for about 65% of deaths in persons with diabetes. Preventive measures are directed toward reducing risk factors: control of blood pressure, smoking cessation, lowering lipid levels, and optimal glucose control. In addition, antiplatelet agents are often indicated.

Foot ulcers occur in patients with diabetes due to peripheral neuropathies and poor circulation. Neuropathies may impair sensation, so a small area of irritation may go unnoticed. Vascular insufficiency and elevated glucose levels inhibit healing of the ulcer. If the ulcer becomes infected, it is often resistant to treatment, and can ultimately result in the need for amputation. Diabetes is the leading cause of nontraumatic amputations.

Insulin Therapy

6 Insulin is the cornerstone of therapy for patients with type 1 and gestational diabetes.

Because patients with type 1 diabetes are severely deficient in insulin production, insulin replacement therapy is required to survive. Insulin is also required for those with type 2 diabetes who are unable to manage their blood glucose levels with diet, exercise, and oral antidiabetic agents. Among adults with diabetes in the United States, 12% take only insulin, 14% take insulin with oral antidiabetic drugs, 58% take oral antidiabetic drugs only, and 16% take neither insulin nor antidiabetic drugs (CDC, 2010).

The therapeutic goal for patients with type 1 diabetes is to administer insulin as replacement therapy, in normal physiological amounts. Because insulin secretion varies greatly in response to daily activities, pharmacotherapy must be carefully planned in conjunction with proper meal planning and lifestyle habits. The desired outcome of insulin therapy is to prevent the long-term consequences of diabetes by maintaining blood glucose levels strictly within the normal range.

The fundamental principle to remember about insulin therapy is that the right amount of insulin must be available to cells when glucose is present in the blood. Administering insulin when glucose is not available can lead to hypoglycemia and possibly coma. This situation occurs when a patient administers insulin correctly but skips a meal. The insulin is available to cells, but glucose is not. In another example, the patient participates in strenuous exercise. The insulin may have been administered on schedule, and food eaten, but the active muscles quickly use up all the glucose in the blood, and the patient becomes hypoglycemic. Patients with diabetes who engage in competitive sports need to consume food or sports drinks just prior to, and during, the activity to maintain their blood glucose at normal levels. The nurse plays a key role in helping patients plan their meals, activities, and insulin dosages correctly. Figure 2 illustrates the management of type 1 diabetes, and correct timing of the insulin dose with meals.

Many types of insulin are available, differing in their source, time of onset, and peak effect and duration of action. Until the 1980s, the primary source of insulin was beef or pork pancreas. Almost all insulin today, however, is human insulin obtained through recombinant DNA technology because it

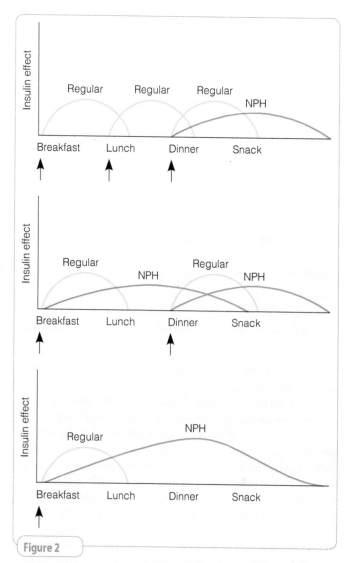

Figure 2

Insulin regimens.

is more effective, causes fewer allergies, and has a lower incidence of resistance. Pharmacologists have modified human insulin to create certain pharmacokinetic advantages, such as a more rapid onset of action (Humalog) or a more prolonged duration of action (Lantus). These modified forms are called insulin *analogs*. The different types of insulins available are listed in Table 2.

Doses of insulin are highly individualized for the precise control of blood glucose levels in each patient. Because the GI tract destroys insulin, it must be given by injection. Some patients require two or more injections daily for proper diabetes management. For ease of administration, two different compatible types of insulin may be mixed, using a standard method, to obtain the desired therapeutic effects. Some of these combinations are marketed in cartridges containing premixed solutions. A long-acting insulin may be taken daily to provide a basal blood level, with supplemental with rapid-acting insulin given shortly before a meal. It is important for nurses and patients to know the time of peak action of any

TABLE 2 Types of Insulin: Actions and Administration

Drug	Action	Onset	Peak	Duration	Administration and Timing	Compatibility
Insulin aspart (NovoLog)	Rapid	10–20 min	1–3 h	3–5 h	Subcutaneous: 5–10 min before meal	Can give with NPH; draw aspart up first, give immediately
Insulin lispro (Humalog)	Rapid	5–15 min	1–1.5 h	3–4 h	Subcutaneous: 15 min before or immediately after a meal	Can give with NPH; draw lispro up first, give immediately
Insulin glulisine (Apidra)	Rapid	15–30 min	1 h	3–4 h	Subcutaneous: 15 min before meal	Can give with NPH; draw glulisine up first, give immediately
Insulin regular (Humulin R, Novolin R)	Short	30–60 min	1–5 h	6–10 h	Subcutaneous: 30–60 min before meal; IV	Can mix with NPH, sterile water, normal saline; do not mix with glargine
Isophane insulin suspension (NPH, Humulin N)	Intermediate	1–2 h	6–14 h	16–24 h	Subcutaneous: Mix (cloudy)	Can mix with aspart, lispro, reg; do not mix with glargine
Insulin detemir (Levemir)	Long	Gradual	6–8 h	To 24 h	Subcutaneous: 1/day or 2/day	Do not mix with any other insulin
Insulin glargine (Lantus)	Long	1.1 h	No peak	To 24 h	Subcutaneous: 1/day, same time each day	Do not mix with any other insulin

insulin, because that is when the risk for hypoglycemic adverse effects is greatest.

All insulin products used clinically are U-100, meaning 1 mL contains 100 units of insulin, and are administered using U-100 syringes. One type of human regular insulin has been formulated in the U-500 strength, but this is available from the manufacturer only, and is reserved for patients who require very large doses of insulin (more than 200 units/day). Insulin preparations are either clear or cloudy. Those that are cloudy require mixing the solution by rolling the vial prior to drawing out the desired dose. Insulins that are clear do not require mixing. Regular insulin is the only type that can be administered by IV injection.

Rapid- or regular-acting insulin can be used in continuous subcutaneous infusion devices, often called insulin pumps. An infusion set, which holds a syringe of the drug, delivers insulin from the pump to a needle anchored in the subcutaneous tissue of the abdomen. The infusion set is replaced every 3 days, at which time the injection site should be moved, preferably to 1 inch away from the old site. The pump is programmed to release small subcutaneous doses of insulin into the abdomen at predetermined intervals, with larger boluses administered manually at mealtime if necessary. Most pumps contain an alarm that reminds patients to take their insulin. They are generally worn on a belt or tucked into a pocket. Figure 3 shows an insulin pump.

The primary adverse effect of insulin therapy is overtreatment; insulin may remove too much glucose from the blood, resulting in hypoglycemia. This may occur when a patient with type 1 diabetes has more insulin in the blood than is needed to balance the amount of circulating blood glucose. Hypoglycemia may occur when the insulin level peaks, during exercise, when the patient receives too much insulin due to a medication error, or if the patient skips a meal. Some of the symptoms of hypoglycemia are the same as those of DKA. Those that differ and help to determine that a patient is hypoglycemic include pale, cool, and moist skin, with blood glucose

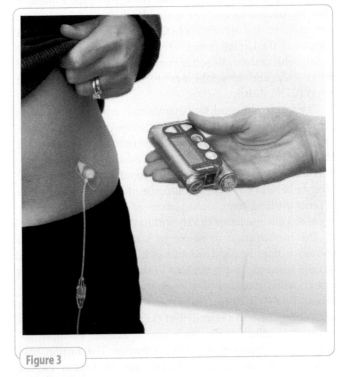

Figure 3

Insulin pump.
Source: © ACE STOCK LIMITED/Alamy

less than 50 mg/dL and a sudden onset of symptoms. Left untreated, severe hypoglycemia may result in death.

Other adverse effects of insulin include injection-site reactions, generalized urticaria, and swollen lymph glands. Some patients will experience Somogyi phenomenon, a rapid decrease in blood glucose, usually during the night, which stimulates the release of hormones that elevate blood glucose (epinephrine, cortisol, and glucagon), resulting in an elevated morning blood glucose level. Administration of insulin above the patient's normal dose may produce a rapid rebound hypoglycemia. The hormone glucagon is administered as a replacement therapy for some patients with diabetes when they are in a hypoglycemic state and have impaired glucagon secretion.

Patients with diabetes who forget their insulin dose face equally serious consequences. Again, remember the fundamental principle of insulin pharmacotherapy: The right amount of insulin must be available to cells when glucose is present in the blood. Without insulin present, glucose from a meal can build up to high levels in the blood, causing hyperglycemia and possible coma. Proper planning and teaching by the nurse is essential to achieve successful outcomes and maximize patient adherence with therapy.

Insulin Adjunct

Pramlintide (Symlin) is an antihyperglycemic drug approved in 2005 that is used along with insulin in persons with type 1 or type 2 diabetes who are not able to achieve glucose control by the use of insulin alone. The drug is a synthetic analog of amylin, a natural hormone released by the beta cells of the pancreas at the same time as insulin. Its natural function is to act synergistically with insulin in glycemic control. The therapeutic actions of pramlintide are to slow gastric emptying time, reduce postprandial glucagon secretion, and increase satiety, thereby leading to reduced calorie intake. Pramlintide is administered subcutaneously immediately prior to each meal, using U-100 insulin syringes. It cannot be mixed with insulin, and must be injected into a different site than insulin. When initiating treatment, rapid- or short-acting insulin doses are usually reduced by 50%. Adverse effects include nausea, vomiting, abdominal pain, headache, dizziness, fatigue, coughing, allergic reaction, or arthralgia. The drug carries a black box warning that severe hypoglycemia may occur during therapy. Hypoglycemia may be prolonged and severe, usually occurring within 3 hours following an injection.

| PROTOTYPE DRUG | Human regular insulin (Humulin R, Novolin R) |

Classification: **Therapeutic:** Antidiabetic agent, pancreatic hormone
Pharmacologic: Short-acting hypoglycemic agent

Therapeutic Effects and Uses: Human regular insulin is used to maintain blood glucose levels within normal limits. The primary effects of human regular insulin are promotion of cellular uptake of glucose, amino acids, and potassium; promotion of protein synthesis, glycogen formation and storage, and fatty acid storage as triglycerides; and conservation of energy stores by promoting the utilization of glucose for energy needs and inhibiting gluconeogenesis. Indications for insulin include the following:

- As monotherapy to lower blood glucose levels in patients with type 1 diabetes
- In combination with oral antidiabetic agents in patients with type 2 diabetes

- For the emergency treatment of DKA or hyperosmolar hyperglycemic state
- For gestational diabetes

Because regular insulin is short acting, it is most often used in combination with intermediate or long-acting insulin to achieve 24-hour glucose control. Nondiabetic indications for insulin include stimulation of growth hormone secretion in the evaluation of growth hormone deficiency and the treatment of hyperkalemia to promote a shift of potassium into cells.

Mechanism of Action: Regular insulin is identical to endogenous insulin. Insulin decreases blood glucose levels by increasing cellular uptake of glucose and stimulating storage of glucose as glycogen; it also inhibits the release of glucagon.

Pharmacokinetics:

Route(s)	Subcutaneous; IV (only regular insulin can be given IV); inhalation
Absorption	Rapidly absorbed following subcutaneous injection; absorption time can vary by site of injection
Distribution	Throughout extracellular fluids
Primary metabolism	Hepatic
Primary excretion	Liver and kidneys
Onset of action	Subcutaneous: 30–60 min; IV: 15 min
Duration of action	6–10 h

Adverse Effects: The most common adverse effect of insulin therapy is hypoglycemia. Rebound hyperglycemia (Somogyi phenomenon) may occur. Irritation at injection sites may occur, including lipohypertrophy, the accumulation of fat in the area of injection. This effect is lessened with rotation of injection sites. Weight gain is a possible adverse effect. Because insulin facilitates the intracellular uptake of potassium, hypokalemia is possible.

Contraindications/Precautions: Beef or pork insulins (which are now rarely used) are contraindicated in persons with hypersensitivity to these animal proteins. Insulin is used with caution in pregnancy, renal impairment or failure, fever, thyroid disease, among the elderly, or in children or infants. Insulin should not be administered to patients with hypoglycemia. Patients with hypokalemia should be monitored carefully because insulin may worsen this condition.

Drug Interactions: Insulin must be used cautiously in conjunction with agents that can produce hypoglycemia, including sulfonylureas, meglitinides, beta-adrenergic blockers, salicylates, anabolic steroids, monamine oxidase inhibitors (MAOIs), and alcohol. Several agents can antagonize the glucose-lowering effects of insulin including dextrothyroxine, corticosteroids, epinephrine or norepinephrine, furosemide, and thiazide diuretics. Angiotensin-converting enzyme (ACE) inhibitors increase insulin sensitivity and may enhance the hypoglycemic effects of insulin. Many other drugs can influence blood glucose and the nurse should consult current drug references when treating patients who take high insulin doses or who have unstable diabetes. **Herbal/Food:** Garlic, chromium, black cohosh, bitter melon, bilberry, and ginseng may potentiate the hypoglycemic effects of insulin. Cocoa and rosemary may have a hyperglycemic effect.

Pregnancy: Insulin glargine is pregnancy category C; other forms of insulin are category B.

Treatment of Overdose: An overdose of insulin can cause profound hypoglycemia, which is treated with a concentrated source of glucose (dextrose), such as D_5W or glucagon, by the parenteral route.

Nursing Responsibilities: Key nursing implications for patients receiving regular insulin are included in the Nursing Practice Application for Patients Receiving Insulin Therapy.

Lifespan and Diversity Considerations:

- Use special caution in administering insulin to the older adult who is at increased risk of hypoglycemia. Monitor dose and food intake.

- Monitor self-administration of insulin in the older adult because normal visual or dexterity changes related to aging may make accurate self-administration of insulin difficult.

Patient and Family Education:

- Always carry a supply of readily available sugar or quick-acting carbohydrate for unexpected episodes of hypoglycemia.

- Wear a medical alert bracelet or jewelry and carry a medical alert card that explains your condition and treatment.

Drugs Similar to Human Regular Insulin (Humulin R, Novolin R)

Many types of insulin are available. They are categorized by their onset of action and duration of action, as given in Table 2. There are also premixed formulations of insulin available, such as human insulin Humulin 70/30. This type contains 70% NPH insulin and 30% regular insulin, so it can be given before a meal to help control postprandial glucose while also providing longer coverage of insulin needs. Other combination insulins include Humalog 75/25, Humulin 50/50, Novolin 70/30, and NovoLog 70/30. The characteristics of selected insulin combinations are shown in Table 3.

Insulin aspart (NovoLog): Insulin aspart is a rapid-onset drug, with a structure very similar to that of endogenous insulin. Insulin aspart has a more rapid onset of action than regular insulin, acting within about 15 minutes when given subcutaneously. Because insulin aspart acts rapidly, injections should be made 5 to 10 minutes before meals. It also has a short duration of action, 3 to 5 hours when compared to regular insulin. Because of its short duration, insulin aspart is usually given in combination with an intermediate or long-acting form of insulin. Insulin aspart is available in 10-mL vials and 3-mL prefilled cartridges.

Insulin detemir (Levemir): Insulin detemir is a long-acting insulin with a slow onset and dose-dependent duration of action. Detemir may be given once or twice a day, depending on the dose; low doses provide shorter durations of action than larger doses, and so dosing is individualized to the patient. At low doses (0.2 units/kg), effects persist about 12 hours. At higher doses (0.4 units/kg), effects last 20 to 24 hours. Because of its slow onset and prolonged duration, insulin detemir is used to provide basal glycemic control. It is not injected before meals to control postprandial hyperglycemia. It cannot be mixed with any other type of insulin and is only given by subcutaneous injection. Insulin detemir is supplied in 10-mL vials, 3-mL cartridges, a 3-mL pen, and a 3-mL InnoLet dosing device. The InnoLet dosing injection device is disposable and has an easy-to-read dial, large push button for injection, and audible clicks that indicate each unit injected.

Insulin glargine (Lantus): Insulin glargine is a newer recombinant insulin analog that exhibits constant, long-duration insulin activity. It has no defined peak effect and provides for the maintenance of steady blood levels; therefore, there is less risk of hypoglycemia with this type of insulin. Insulin glargine allows for once-daily dosing as basal insulin coverage. Although it can be given without regard to meals, it should be given at

TABLE 3 Premixed Insulin Combinations

Drug	Description	Route and Adult Dose (maximum dose where indicated)	Onset (min)	Peak (h)	Duration (h)	Adverse Effects
Humulin 70/30	70% NPH insulin/ 30% regular insulin	IM/subcutaneous: individualized doses	30–60	1.5–16	Up to 36	*Pain and swelling at injection site*
Novolin 70/30	70% NPH insulin/ 30% regular insulin	IM/subcutaneous: individualized doses	30–60	2–12	Up to 36	Hypoglycemia, DKA
Humulin 50/50	50% NPH insulin/ 50% regular insulin	IM/subcutaneous: individualized doses	30–60	2–5.5	Up to 24	
NovoLog Mix 70/30	70% insulin aspart protamine/ 30% insulin aspart	IM/subcutaneous: individualized doses	15–60	1–4	Up to 24	
Humalog Mix 75/25	75% insulin lispro protamine/ 25% insulin lispro	IM/subcutaneous: individualized doses	15–60	1–6.5	Up to 24	

Note: Italics indicate common adverse effects. Underline indicates serious adverse effects.

Lifespan Considerations **Diabetes in the School Setting**

Caring for the school-age child with diabetes in a school setting requires teamwork between the parents or caregiver, school nurse, school staff, the child's health care provider, and most often, the child. For each child, an individual diabetes medical management plan (DMMP) should be established that addresses all aspects of the diabetes care. The ADA (2011b) recommends the following specific instructions be included in each child's DMMP:

- Blood glucose monitoring instructions, including the frequency and circumstances for requiring monitoring. Provision should be made for privacy during testing or insulin administration if the child, parents, or caregiver desires.
- Information on insulin injections if used, to include type(s) of insulin, dose, times for administration, storage, and provider permission for adjustments in insulin dosage if needed.

- Information on meals and snacks, including scheduling, the need for the child to be able to eat prn (as needed) to prevent hypoglycemia, and content and calories of a school lunch.
- Symptoms and treatment for hypoglycemia and hyperglycemia. Specific levels of training should be provided to school personnel based on whether they will administer basic, intermediate, or advanced treatment in caring for the child.
- Information on participation in physical activity.
- Emergency plans for emergency evacuation, shelter-in-place, or school lockdowns.

By establishing a DMMP, routine daily care as well as emergency contingencies can be addressed. When all participants work as a team, a child with diabetes can participate fully and safely in the school setting.

the same time each day to provide steady blood levels. It cannot be mixed with any other type of insulin and is only given by subcutaneous injection. Insulin glargine may also help improve the lipid profiles and A1C levels of type 2 diabetes when added to therapy. Insulin glargine is supplied in 10-mL vials and in 3-mL cartridges.

Insulin glulisine (Apidra): Insulin glulisine has a 10- to 15-minute onset and a short duration of 3 to 5 hours. Owing to its rapid onset, the drug should be administered no sooner than 15 minutes before eating and no later than 20 minutes after starting a meal. Apidra is only given by subcutaneous injection.

Insulin lispro (Humalog): Insulin lispro is a rapid-acting analog of regular insulin, with effects beginning within 15 to 30 minutes of subcutaneous injection. Insulin lispro acts faster than regular insulin but has a shorter duration of action, 5 hours or less. Because of its rapid onset, insulin lispro should be administered immediately before eating, or even after eating. It is meant to help control the rise in blood glucose brought on by a meal, and is normally given concurrently with an intermediate- or long-acting agent that provides a basal coverage of insulin. It is a clear insulin, and does not require mixing prior to injecting. Lispro cannot be given IV. It is often used with insulin infusion pumps.

Isophane insulin (NPH, Humulin N): Isophane insulin is the only intermediate-acting insulin. It has a slower onset of action (1 to 4 hours) than regular insulin and a duration of action up to 18 to 24 hours. It is used to provide a basal level of insulin coverage for between meals and at night. NPH insulin is normally administered 30 minutes before the first meal of the day, but in some instances a second, smaller dose is taken before the evening meal or at bedtime. Many patients are prescribed insulin that is premixed, such as 70% NPH with 30% regular or rapid acting. If the patient is prescribed a premixed insulin solution, it is important that proper instructions be given, especially if the patient will be using additional regular or rapid-acting insulin on a sliding scale. NPH is a cloudy suspension and requires mixing prior to drawing up a dose. NPH can be given with aspart, lispro, or regular insulin, but cannot be

Patient Saftey **Incorrect Insulin Dose**

A patient with diabetes has 30 units of Humulin R (regular) insulin ordered for the morning dose. There are several patients with diabetes on the unit and the nurse has given many doses of insulin that morning. The nurse prepares the insulin but draws up Humalog 30 units instead. The patient begins experiencing symptoms of hypoglycemia within 15 minutes and is treated successfully. What errors occurred and how could they be prevented in the future?

See Answers to Patient Safety Question on student resource website.

mixed with glargine insulin. When mixed with another type of insulin, NPH should be drawn up after the other insulin, and the mixture should be administered immediately. The term NPH stands for Neutral Protamine Hagedom. Hans Christian Hagedom was a scientist who developed the drug in the 1920s.

Antidiabetic Agents for Type 2 Diabetes

7 Antidiabetic drugs from multiple classes are used to treat type 2 diabetes.

The seven primary classes of antidiabetic drugs used to treat type 2 diabetes are differentiated by their chemical structures and their mechanisms of action. Antidiabetic agents prescribed for patients with type 2 diabetes include alpha-glucosidase inhibitors, biguanides, incretin enhancers, meglitinides, sulfonylureas, and thiazolidinediones. An additional group includes miscellaneous drugs from other classes. Therapy with oral antidiabetic agents is not effective in persons with type 1 diabetes.

Treatment goals recommended by the American Association of Clinical Endocrinologists (AACE, 2011) are designed to target an HbA1C level of 6.5% or less with an FPG of less

CONNECTIONS: NURSING PRACTICE APPLICATION

Patients Receiving Insulin Therapy

Assessment	Potential Nursing Diagnoses
Baseline assessment prior to administration: • Understand the reason the drug has been prescribed in order to assess for therapeutic effects and to plan for teaching needs (e.g., new onset of diabetes with hyperglycemia present, change in insulin type or amount, sliding scale coverage, or treatment of hyperkalemia). • Obtain a complete health history including endocrine, cardiovascular, hepatic, or renal disease, pregnancy, or breast-feeding. Obtain a drug history including allergies, current prescription and OTC drugs, herbal preparations, caffeine, nicotine, and alcohol use. Be alert to possible drug interactions. • Obtain a history of current symptoms, duration and severity, and other related signs or symptoms (e.g., paresthesias of hands or feet). Assess feet and lower extremities for possible injury, infection, or ulcerations. • Obtain a dietary history including caloric intake if on an ADA diet, number of meals and snacks per day. Assess fluid intake and type of fluids consumed. • Obtain baseline vital signs, height, and weight. • Evaluate appropriate laboratory findings (e.g., CBC, electrolytes, glucose, A1C level, lipid profile, osmolality, and hepatic and renal function studies). • Assess the patient's ability to receive and understand instructions. Include family and caregivers as needed.	• *Imbalanced Nutrition: Less Than Body Requirements* (type 1 diabetes) • *Imbalanced Nutrition: More Than Body Requirements* (type 2 diabetes) • *Ineffective Health Maintenance* • *Deficient Knowledge* (Drug Therapy) • *Risk for Unstable Blood Glucose* • *Risk for Deficient Fluid Volume* • *Risk for Injury*, related to adverse drug effects • *Risk for Infection*
Assessment throughout administration: • Assess for desired therapeutic effects (e.g., glucose levels remain within normal limits, electrolytes and osmolality remain normal, A1C levels demonstrate adequate control of glucose). • Assess for and report promptly any adverse effects: signs of hypoglycemia (e.g., nausea, paleness, sweating, diaphoresis, tremors, irritability, headache, light-headedness, anxiety, decreased level of consciousness) and hyperglycemia (e.g., flushed, dry skin, polyuria, polyphagia, polydipsia, drowsiness, glycosuria, ketonuria, acetone-breath), lipodystrophy, infection.	

Planning: Patient Goals and Expected Outcomes

The patient will:

• Experience therapeutic effects dependent on the reason the drug is being given (e.g., blood sugar within normal limits).

• Be free from or experience minimal adverse effects.

• Verbalize an understanding of the drug's use, adverse effects, and required precautions.

• Demonstrate proper self-administration of the medication (e.g., dose, timing, and when to notify the provider).

Implementation

Interventions and (Rationales)	Patient-Centered Care
Ensuring therapeutic effects: • Continue assessments as above for therapeutic effects. (Dependent on the severity of hyperglycemia, blood glucose levels should return gradually to normal.)	• Teach the patient to report any return of original symptoms. • Teach the patient the symptoms of hyper- and hypoglycemia to observe for and instruct the patient to check the capillary glucose level routinely and if symptoms are present. Promptly report any noticeable symptoms and concurrent capillary glucose level to the health care provider.
• Administer insulin correctly and per the schedule ordered (e.g., routine dosing with or without additional sliding-scale coverage), plan insulin administration and peak times around mealtimes. Maintaining a steady level of insulin with mealtimes arranged to match peak insulin activity will assist in maintaining a steady blood glucose level.	• Teach the patient or caregiver appropriate administration techniques for all types of insulin used, followed by return demonstration until the patient or caregiver is comfortable with the technique and able to perform correctly. • Teach the patient or caregiver the importance of peak insulin levels and the need to ensure adequate food sources are consumed to avoid hypoglycemia. Provide written materials for future reference whenever possible.
• Ensure dietary needs are met based on the need to lose, gain, or maintain current weight and glucose levels. Consult with the dietitian as needed. Limit or eliminate alcohol use. (Adequate caloric, protein, carbohydrate, and fat amounts support an insulin regimen for glucose control. Activity and lifestyle will also be factored into dietary management. As alcohol is metabolized, it can raise and then precipitously lower blood sugar, raising the risk of hypoglycemia.)	• Review current diet, lifestyle, and activity level with patient. Arrange a dietitian consult based on the need to alter diet or food choices. Teach the patient to limit or eliminate alcohol use. If alcoholic beverages are consumed, limit to one per day, and consume along with a complete meal to ensure that food intake balances alcohol metabolism.

CONNECTIONS: NURSING PRACTICE APPLICATION *(continued)*

Minimizing adverse effects:

- Continue to monitor capillary glucose levels. Hold insulin dose if blood sugar is less than 70 mg/dL or per parameters as ordered, and contact the health care provider for further orders. (Daily glucose levels, especially before meals, will assist in maintaining adequate control of blood glucose and aid in assessing the appropriateness of current insulin types and dosages.)

- Continue to monitor periodic laboratory work: CBC, electrolytes, glucose, A1C level, lipid profile, osmolality, hepatic, and renal function studies. (Periodic monitoring of laboratory work assists in determining glucose control and the need for any change in insulin amounts, and assesses for complications. A1C levels provide a measure of glucose control over several months' time.)

- Assess for symptoms of hypoglycemia, especially around the time of insulin peak activity. If symptoms of hypoglycemia are noted, provide a quick-acting carbohydrate source (e.g., juice or other simple sugar), and then check capillary glucose level. Report to the health care provider if glucose is less than 70 mg/dL or as ordered. If mealtime is not immediate, provide a longer acting protein source to ensure hypoglycemia does not recur. (Hypoglycemia is especially likely to occur around peak insulin activity, especially if food sources are inadequate. Providing a quick-acting carbohydrate source and then checking the capillary glucose level will ensure glucose does not decrease further while locating the glucose testing equipment. When in doubt, treating symptoms for suspected hypoglycemia is safer than allowing further decreases in glucose and possible loss of consciousness with adverse effects. Small additional amounts of carbohydrates will not dramatically increase blood sugar if testing shows a hyperglycemic episode.)

- Monitor blood glucose more frequently during periods of illness or stress. (Insulin needs may increase or decrease during periods of illness or stress. Frequent monitoring during these times helps to prevent hypoglycemia and ensures adequate glucose control.)

- Encourage increased activity and exercise, but monitor blood glucose before and after exercise and begin any new or increased exercise routine gradually. Continue to monitor for hypoglycemia for up to 48 h after exercise. (Exercise assists muscles to use glucose more efficiently and increases insulin receptor sites in the tissues, lowering the blood sugar. Benefits of exercise and lowered blood sugar may continue for up to 48 h, increasing the risk of hypoglycemia during this time. Frequent monitoring helps to prevent hypoglycemia and ensures adequate glucose control.)

- Rotate insulin administration sites weekly. If the patient is hospitalized, use sites that have been less used or are difficult for the patient to reach. Insulin pump subcutaneous catheters should be changed every 2 to 3 days or as recommended by the health care provider. (Rotating injection sites weekly helps to prevent lipodystrophy. Use caution if using a new site, especially if the previous site used by the patient exhibits signs of lipodystrophy. Insulin in an unused site may absorb more quickly than a site with lipodystrophy or tissue changes, resulting in hypoglycemia. Insulin pump subcutaneous catheters should be changed every 2 to 3 days to prevent infections at the site of insertion.)

- Ensure proper storage of insulin to maintain maximum potency. (Unopened insulin may be stored at room temperature, but avoid direct sunlight and excessive heat. Opened insulin vials may be stored at room temperature for up to 1 month. If noticeable change in solution occurs or if precipitate forms, discard the vial.)

Patient understanding of drug therapy:

- Use opportunities during administration of medications and during assessments to discuss the rationale for drug therapy, desired therapeutic outcomes, commonly observed adverse effects, parameters for when to call the health care provider, and any necessary monitoring or precautions. (Using time during nursing care helps to optimize and reinforce key teaching areas.)

- Instruct the patient on blood glucose monitoring the appropriate techniques to obtain capillary blood glucose levels, followed by return demonstration, and when to contact the health care provider (e.g., glucose less than 70 mg/dL). Monitor use and ensure proper functioning of all equipment to be used at home.

- Instruct the patient on the need to return periodically for laboratory work.

- Teach the patient to always carry a quick-acting carbohydrate source in case symptoms of hypoglycemia occur. If unsure whether symptoms indicate hypo- or hyperglycemia, treat as hypoglycemia and then check capillary glucose. If symptoms are not relieved in 10–15 min, or if blood sugar is below 70 mg/dL (or parameters as ordered), immediately notify the health care provider.

- Instruct the patient to check glucose levels more frequently when ill or under stress. Stress may increase insulin needs because the stress response can cause glycogenolysis. Illness, especially associated with anorexia, nausea, or vomiting, may decrease insulin needs. Notify the health care provider if unable to eat normal meals during periods of illness or stress for possible change in insulin dose.

- Teach the patient the benefits of increased activity and exercise and to begin any new routine or increase in exercise gradually. Exercise should occur an hour after a meal or after a 10- or 15-g carbohydrate snack to prevent hypoglycemia. If exercise is prolonged, small frequent carbohydrate snacks can be consumed every 30 min during exercise to maintain blood sugar.
- Instruct the patient to check glucose levels more frequently before, during, and after exercise.

- Instruct the patient on the need to rotate insulin injection sites on a weekly basis to prevent tissue damage or to rotate subcutaneous catheter sites (insulin pumps) every 2 to 3 days.

- Teach the patient methods for proper storage of insulin and for storage during travel.

- The patient, family, or caregiver should be able to state the reason for the drug, appropriate dose and scheduling, what adverse effects to observe for and when to report them, and any special requirements of the medication therapy (e.g., insulin needs during exercise or illness).
- Instruct the patient to carry a wallet identification card and wear medical identification jewelry indicating diabetes.

(continued)

Patient self-administration of drug therapy:

• When administering the medication, instruct the patient, family, or caregiver in the proper self-administration of the drug. (Utilizing time during nurse-administration of these drugs helps to reinforce teaching.)

• The patient, family, or caregiver is able to discuss appropriate dosing and administration needs including:

• Proper preparation of insulin: Rotate vials gently between palms and do not shake; if insulins are mixed, draw up the quickest acting insulin and then the longer acting one if insulins are compatible; insulin glargine or insulin detemir should not be mixed with any other type of insulin; use the appropriate syringe (100 unit) unless small amounts of insulin are ordered, then obtain syringes with smaller volumes to ensure accurate dosing.

• Proper subcutaneous injection techniques: selection and cleansing of the site with rotation every week, injecting at 90-degree angle, and applying a pad to the site after injection but not massaging the site.

• Proper use of all equipment: blood glucose monitoring equipment, insulin pump.

Evaluation of Outcome Criteria

Evaluate the effectiveness of drug therapy by confirming that patient goals and expected outcomes have been met (see "Planning").

than 110 g/dL. In general, all of the antidiabetic agents are similar in their ability to lower HbA1C levels in the short term. There are some differences, however, in long-term control. For example, drugs in the thiazolidinedione class appear to maintain glycemic control for 5 to 6 years, while the sulfonylureas peak at 6 months and slowly decline in efficacy. The adverse effects observed for each class differ: Some cause hypoglycemia, whereas others cause weight gain or GI complaints such as diarrhea. Because there is no perfect drug for type 2 diabetes, choice of therapy is guided by the experiences of the prescriber and the results achieved by the individual patient. A comparison of the oral antidiabetic drugs is presented in Table 4. Doses are listed in Table 5.

Therapy for type 2 diabetes is usually initiated with a single agent. If glycemic control is not achieved with monotherapy, a second agent is added to the therapeutic regimen. Failure to achieve glycemic control with two oral hypoglycemic agents indicates the need for insulin to be added to the regimen.

Several fixed-dose combination products are available for the treatment of people with type 2 diabetes. The main advantage of taking a combination drug is that it is more convenient than taking two separate drugs, and may improve adherence to the therapeutic regimen. Combination products are indicated for patients who fail to adequately control glucose levels with the use of a single drug. Doses for selected combination products are listed in Table 6.

Sulfonylureas

The first oral antidiabetic drug class available, sulfonylureas are divided into first- and second-generation categories. Although drugs from both generations are equally effective at lowering blood glucose, the second-generation drugs exhibit fewer drug–drug interactions.

The sulfonylureas act by stimulating the release of insulin from pancreatic islet cells and by increasing the sensitivity of insulin receptors on target cells. The most common adverse effect is hypoglycemia, which is usually caused by taking too much medication or not eating enough food. Hypoglycemia from these agents may be prolonged and require administration of dextrose to return serum glucose to normal levels. Other adverse effects include weight gain, hypersensitivity reactions, GI distress, and hepatotoxicity. When alcohol is taken with sulfonylureas, some patients experience an uncomfortable disulfiram-like reaction, with flushing, palpitations, and nausea.

TABLE 4 Summary of Oral Antidiabetic Classes

Drug	Action(s)	Nursing Considerations
Alpha-Glucosidase Inhibitors	Interferes with carbohydrate breakdown and absorption; acts locally in GI tract with little systemic absorption.	Common GI effects; hypoglycemia can occur if combined with another oral agent; if this occurs, treat with glucose, not sucrose; take with meals
Biguanides	Decreases production and release of glucose from the liver; increases cellular uptake of glucose; lowers lipid levels; promotes weight loss.	Common GI adverse effects; risk for lactic acidosis (rare); avoid alcohol; low risk for hypoglycemia
Incretin Enhancers	Slows the breakdown of insulin, keeping it circulating in the blood longer; slows the rate of digestion, which increases satiety.	Well tolerated; minor nausea, vomiting, and diarrhea; some weight loss is likely; low risk for hypoglycemia
Meglitinides	Stimulates insulin release.	Can cause hypoglycemia, GI effects; well tolerated; administer shortly before meals
Sulfonylureas	Stimulates insulin release; decreases insulin resistance.	Can cause hypoglycemia, GI disturbances, rash; cross sensitivity with sulfa drugs and thiazide diuretics; possible disulfiram response with alcohol
Thiazolidinedione	Decreases production and release of glucose from the liver; increases insulin sensitivity in fat and muscle tissue.	Can cause fluid retention and worsening of heart failure; therapeutic effects take several weeks to develop

TABLE 5 Antidiabetic Agents for Type 2 Diabetes

Drug	Route and Adult Dose (maximum dose where indicated)	Adverse Effects
Alpha-Glucosidase Inhibitors		
acarbose (Precose)	PO: 25–100 mg tid (max: 300 mg/day)	*Flatulence, diarrhea, abdominal distention*
miglitol (Glyset)	PO: 25–100 mg tid (max: 300 mg/day)	Hypoglycemia (tremors, palpitations, sweating)
Biguanides		
metformin immediate release (Glucophage, Riomet) extended release (Fortamet, Glucophage XR, Glumetza)	PO: 500 mg 2 times/day or 850 mg once daily; increase to 1,000–2,550 mg in two to three divided doses/day (max: 2.55 g/day) Glumetza: 1,000–2,000 mg once daily (max: 2 g/day) Glucophage XR: 500 mg once daily (max 2 g/day) Fortamet: 1,000 mg once daily (max: 2.5 g/day)	*Flatulence, diarrhea, nausea, anorexia, abdominal pain, bitter or metallic taste, decreased vitamin B_{12} levels* Lactic acidosis
Incretin Enhancers (GLP-1 Agonists)		
exenatide (Byetta)	Subcutaneous: 5–10 mcg 2 times/day 60 min prior to meal	*Nausea, vomiting, diarrhea, headache, nervousness*
liraglutide (Victoza)	Subcutaneous: 0.6–1.8 mg once daily	Hypoglycemia (tremors, palpitations, sweating), antibody formation, pancreatitis (exenatide), renal impairment (exenatide)
Incretin Enhancers (DPP-4 Inhibitors)		
linagliptin (Tradjenta)	PO: 5 mg once daily	*Headache, upper respiratory and urinary tract infections*
saxagliptin (Onglyza)	PO: 2.5–5 mg once daily	Hypoglycemia (tremors, palpitations, sweating), anaphylaxis, peripheral edema, exfoliative dermatitis, Stevens–Johnson syndrome
sitagliptin (Januvia)	PO: 100 mg once daily	
Meglitinides		
nateglinide (Starlix)	PO: 60–120 mg tid, 1–30 min prior to meals	*Flulike symptoms, upper respiratory infection, back pain*
repaglinide (Prandin)	PO: 0.5–4 mg bid–qid, 1–30 min prior to meals (max: 16 mg/day)	Hypoglycemia (tremors, palpitations, sweating), anaphylaxis, pancreatitis
Sulfonylureas, First Generation		
chlorpropamide (Diabinese)	PO: 100–500 mg/day (max: 750 mg/day)	*Nausea, heartburn, dizziness, headache, drowsiness*
tolazamide (Tolinase)	PO: 100–500 mg 1–2 times/day (max: 1 g/day)	Hypoglycemia (tremors, palpitations, sweating), cholestatic jaundice, blood dyscrasias
tolbutamide (Orinase)	PO: 250–1,500 mg 1–2 times/day (max: 3 g/day)	
Sulfonylureas, Second Generation		
glimepiride (Amaryl)	PO: 1–4 mg/day (max: 8 mg/day)	*Nausea, heartburn, dizziness, headache, drowsiness*
glipizide (Glucotrol)	PO: 2.5–20 mg 1–2 times/day (max: 40 mg/day)	Hypoglycemia (tremors, palpitations, sweating), cholestatic jaundice, blood dyscrasias
glyburide (DiaBeta, Micronase) glyburide micronized (Glynase)	PO: 1.25–10 mg 1–2 times/day (max: 20 mg/day) PO: 0.75–12 mg 1–2 times/day (max: 12 mg/day)	
Thiazolidinediones		
pioglitazone (Actos)	PO: 15–30 mg/day (max: 45 mg/day)	*Upper respiratory infection, myalgia, headache, edema, weight gain*
rosiglitazone (Avandia)	PO: 4–8 mg 1–2 times/day (max: 8 mg/day)	Hypoglycemia (tremors, palpitations, sweating), hepatotoxicity, bone fractures, heart failure, MI

Note: *Italics* indicate common adverse effects. Underline indicates serious adverse effects.

PROTOTYPE DRUG Glyburide (DiaBeta, Glynase, Micronase)

Classification: **Therapeutic:** Antidiabetic agent
Pharmacologic: Sulfonylurea

Therapeutic Effects and Uses: Approved in 1984, glyburide is a second-generation sulfonylurea used to lower blood glucose levels in patients with type 2 diabetes. Glyburide can be used alone or in combination with another oral hypoglycemic agent. It should be used only if diet and exercise have proven ineffective in controlling the elevated blood glucose levels.

Two types of glyburide are available: the conventional form (DiaBeta, Micronase) and a micronized form (Glynase). Glynase allows for lower doses, compared to the conventional forms. Glucovance is a combination product that contains glyburide and metformin.

TABLE 6 Selected Combination Oral Antidiabetic Agents

Brand Name Drug	Generic Drug Combination	Route and Adult Dose (maximum dose where indicated)
Actoplus Met	pioglitazone/metformin	PO: 15 mg/500–850 mg once or twice daily. Starting dose depends if patient was previously treated with metformin or pioglitazone combination or had an inadequate response with either agent alone (max: 45 mg/2,550 mg daily)
Avandamet	rosiglitazone/metformin	Patients with no prior treatment: PO: 2 mg/500 mg once or twice daily. Previously treated patients: PO: 2–4 mg/500–1,000 mg twice daily (max: 8 mg/2,000 mg daily)
Duetact	pioglitazone/glimepiride	PO: Start with 30 mg/2 mg once daily (max: 45 mg/8 mg daily)
Glucovance	glyburide/metformin	Patients with no prior treatment: PO: 1.25 mg/250 mg once or twice daily Previously treated patients: PO: 2.5 mg/500 mg to 5 mg/500 mg twice daily (max: 20 mg/2,000 mg daily)
Janumet	sitagliptin/metformin	PO: starting dose 50 mg/500 mg twice daily with meals (max: 100 mg/2,000 mg/day)
Metaglip	glipizide/metformin	PO: 2.5 mg/500 mg or 5 mg/500 mg twice daily (max: 20 mg/2,000 mg daily)
PrandiMet	repaglinide/metformin	PO: start with 1 mg/500 mg given twice daily, 15 min before meals (max: 10 mg/2,500 mg daily)

Mechanism of Action: Glyburide stimulates the release of insulin from pancreatic beta cells, and increases the sensitivity of peripheral tissues to insulin. The stimulation of insulin release relies on some residual beta cell functioning; therefore, the drug is not effective for people with type 1 diabetes.

Pharmacokinetics:

Route(s)	Oral (PO)
Absorption	Readily absorbed following PO administration
Distribution	Distributed widely to body tissues, with greatest concentrations in liver, kidneys, and intestines; crosses the placenta
Primary metabolism	Extensive hepatic metabolism
Primary excretion	Equal in urine and feces
Onset of action	15–60 min
Duration of action	Up to 24 h

Adverse Effects: The primary adverse effect of glyburide is hypoglycemia. Patients at increased risk for hypoglycemia include those with renal or hepatic insufficiency, those consuming an improper diet, and patients who are elderly or malnourished. Excessive exercise or alcohol consumption also increases the risk for hypoglycemia. Other adverse effects of therapy include heartburn, nausea, vomiting, diarrhea, pruritus, erythema, urticaria, photosensitivity, and blurred vision. Rare though serious adverse effects include hepatotoxicity, cholestatic jaundice, aplastic anemia, leukopenia, thrombocytopenia, and agranulocytosis.

Contraindications/Precautions: Glyburide is contraindicated in patients with a known sensitivity to sulfa drugs or thiazide diuretics because sulfonylureas are chemically similar to sulfa drugs. It is contraindicated as the primary treatment for type 1 diabetes, diabetic coma, or DKA. The drug is used with caution in patients with renal or hepatic disease because the drug may accumulate to toxic levels. If used during pregnancy, glyburide should be discontinued at least 1 month before delivery because newborns exposed to sulfonylureas may develop severe hypoglycemia lasting several days.

Drug Interactions: Using alcohol with glyburide can cause hypoglycemia or hyperglycemia, and has resulted in a disulfiram-type response, with severe nausea, vomiting, flushing, and palpitations. Drugs that can increase hypoglycemia when taken with glyburide are oral anticoagulants, MAOIs, probenecid, sulfonamides, chloramphenicol, oxyphenbutazone, phenylbutazone, salicylates, and clofibrate. Increased risk of hyperglycemia can occur with use of rifampin and thiazides. **Herbal/Food:** Ginseng, garlic, black cohosh, juniper berries, fenugreek, coriander, or dandelion root can cause hypoglycemia.

Pregnancy: Category C.

Treatment of Overdose: Treatment is the same as for acute hypoglycemia: A concentrated source of glucose is administered.

Nursing Responsibilities: Key nursing implications for patients receiving glyburide are included in the Nursing Practice Application for Patients Receiving Pharmacotherapy for Type 2 Diabetes.

Drugs Similar to Glyburide (DiaBeta, Glynase, Micronase)

First-generation sulfonylureas are typically less potent, require larger doses, have a shorter duration of action, and require more frequent dosing than the second-generation sulfonylureas. Thus, the second-generation agents are more widely prescribed.

First-generation sulfonylureas:

Chlorpropamide (Diabinese): Approved in 1958, chlorpropamide is the longest acting of the first-generation sulfonylureas, with a duration of action of 24 to 72 hours. In addition to treating type 2 diabetes, an unlabeled use is the treatment of neurogenic diabetes insipidus. Rarely, it can produce an antidiuretic effect, with resulting hyponatremia, water intoxication, and edema. Due to the long half-life of the drug (36 hours), hypoglycemia can be severe and prolonged. It is a pregnancy category C drug.

Tolazamide (Tolinase): Approved in 1965, tolazamide is structurally related to tolbutamide, but is five times more potent. It is taken once daily, with breakfast. It can also be used in patients who fail to respond to other sulfonylureas. It is a pregnancy category C drug.

Tolbutamide (Orinase): Tolbutamide is a short-acting sulfonylurea, with a duration of 6 to 12 hours, given once or twice daily after meals. Approved in 1957, it has been used in patients being treated with insulin who have failed to respond to other sulfonylureas. It is a pregnancy category C drug.

Second-generation sulfonylureas:

Glimepiride (Amaryl): A newer agent approved in 1995, glimepiride can be used alone or in combination with insulin for patients with type 2 diabetes. It is most often given once a day with the first meal of the day. Duetact is a combination oral hypoglycemic approved in 2006 that contains glimepiride and pioglitazone. Avandaryl contains both glimepiride and rosiglitazone.

Glipizide (Glucotrol): Approved in 1984, glipizide is available in a standard tablet form, and an extended release (XL) tablet, which should not be crushed or chewed. In addition to treating patients with type 2 diabetes who do not achieve glucose control with diet alone, it can be used for short-term therapy for those who normally can control their glucose levels by diet. Once-a-day dosing is given 30 minutes before the first meal of the day. Metaglip is a combination product approved in 2002 that contains glipizide and metformin.

CONNECTION Checkpoint 69.2

Glyburide combined with alcohol can cause a disulfiram reaction. What causes the symptoms of the disulfiram reaction and what are common symptoms of this reaction? *See Answer to Connection Checkpoint 69.2 on student resource website.*

Biguanides

Metformin (Glucophage) is the only drug in this class. It is a preferred drug for managing type 2 diabetes because of its effectiveness and safety.

PROTOTYPE DRUG | Metformin (Glucophage, Glumetza, Others)

Classification: **Therapeutic:** Antidiabetic agent
Pharmacologic: Biguanide

Therapeutic Effects and Uses: Approved in 1994, metformin lowers blood glucose levels in patients with type 2 diabetes who are unable to control glucose levels by diet and exercise. It can be used alone or in combination with sulfonylureas, alpha-glucosidase inhibitors, or insulin. It is approved for use in children age 10 and older. Several formulations of metformin are available:

- **Regular-release tablets.** Administered once or twice daily, absorption is decreased with food, and the peak plasma level is 2.5 hours.
- **Solution (Riomet).** Administered once or twice daily, absorption is slightly increased with food, and the peak plasma level is 2.3 hours.
- **Sustained release (Fortamet, Glucophage XR, and Glumetza).** These are extended-duration systems where the drug is slowly released from a semipermeable membrane (Fortamet), gel (Glucophage XR), or gastric-retentive technology (Glumetza). Administered once daily, absorption is significantly increased with food, and the peak plasma level is 6 to 8 hours.

Metformin reduces fasting and postprandial glucose levels. Because it does not promote insulin release, it does not cause hypoglycemia, which is a major advantage of the drug. The drug actions do not depend on stimulating insulin release, so it is able to lower glucose levels in patients who no longer secrete insulin. In addition to lowering blood glucose levels, it lowers triglyceride levels, lowers total and low-density lipoprotein (LDL) cholesterol levels, and promotes weight loss.

Metformin is used off-label to treat women with polycystic ovary syndrome. Women with this syndrome have insulin resistance and high serum insulin levels. Metformin reduces insulin resistance, which in turn lowers insulin and androgen levels, thus restoring normal menstrual cycles and ovulation.

Mechanism of Action: Metformin reduces blood glucose levels by multiple mechanisms. The drug reduces gluconeogenesis, thereby suppressing hepatic production of glucose. In addition, the drug decreases the intestinal reabsorption of glucose and increases the cellular uptake of glucose.

Pharmacokinetics:

Route(s)	PO (regular release tablets, solution, and extended release preparations)
Absorption	Approximately 50–60% of a dose reaches systemic circulation; extended release forms are absorbed very slowly
Distribution	Distributed to most tissues; crosses the placenta; secreted in breast milk; not protein bound
Primary metabolism	Not metabolized
Primary excretion	Kidneys
Onset of action	Less than 1 h; peak action: 1–3 h
Duration of action	12 h (regular release); 24 h (extended release)

Adverse Effects: The most common adverse effects that occur in 30% of patients taking metformin are GI related and include nausea, vomiting, abdominal discomfort, metallic taste, diarrhea, anorexia, and moderate weight loss. It may also cause headache, dizziness, agitation, and fatigue. Unlike the sulfonylureas, metformin rarely causes hypoglycemia or weight gain. **Black Box Warning**: Lactic acidosis is a rare, though potentially fatal, adverse effect of metformin therapy. The risk for lactic acidosis is increased in patients with renal insufficiency or any condition that puts them at risk for increased lactic acid production, such as liver disease, severe infection, excessive alcohol intake, shock, or hypoxemia. Another drug in this class, phenformin, was withdrawn from the market in 1977 due to fatal cases of lactic acidosis.

Contraindications/Precautions: Metformin is contraindicated in patients with impaired renal function, because the drug can rise to toxic levels. It is also contraindicated in patients with heart failure, liver failure, history of lactic acidosis, concurrent serious infection, or with any condition that predisposes the patient to hypoxemia. It is contraindicated for 2 days prior to, and 2 days after, receiving IV radiographic contrast. Metformin is used with caution in patients with anemia, diarrhea, vomiting, dehydration, fever, gastroparesis, or GI obstruction; in older adults; and in those with hyperthyroidism, pituitary insufficiency, trauma, or during pregnancy and lactation. Safety in children under age 10 has not been established.

Drug Interactions: Alcohol increases the risk for lactic acidosis, and should be avoided. Captopril, furosemide, and nifedipine may increase the risk for hypoglycemia. Use with IV radiographic contrast may cause lactic acidosis and acute renal failure. The following drugs may decrease renal excretion of metformin: amiloride, cimetidine, digoxin, dofetilide, midodrine, morphine, procainamide, quinidine, ranitidine, triamterene, trimethoprim, and vancomycin. Acarbose may decrease blood levels of metformin. Use with other antidiabetic drugs potentiates hypoglycemic effects. **Herbal/Food**: Metformin decreases the absorption of vitamin B_{12} and folic acid. Garlic and ginseng may increase hypoglycemic effects.

Pregnancy: Category B.

Treatment of Overdose: For overdose or development of lactic acidosis, hemodialysis can be used to correct the acidosis and remove excess metformin.

Nursing Responsibilities: Key nursing implications for patients receiving metformin are included in the Nursing Practice Application for Patients Receiving Pharmacotherapy for Type 2 Diabetes.

Drugs Similar to Metformin (Glucophage, Glumetza, Others)

Metformin is the only biguanide available.

Meglitinides

The meglitinides are a newer class of oral antidiabetic drugs that act by stimulating the release of insulin from pancreatic islet cells in a manner similar to that of the sulfonylureas. Both drugs in this class have short durations of action of 2 to 4 hours. Their efficacy is equal to that of the sulfonylureas, and

they are well tolerated. Hypoglycemia is the most common adverse effect.

PROTOTYPE DRUG | Repaglinide (Prandin)

Classification: **Therapeutic:** Antidiabetic agent
Pharmacologic: Meglitinide

Therapeutic Effects and Uses: Approved in 1997, repaglinide is used to lower blood glucose levels in patients with type 2 diabetes, as an adjunct to diet and exercise. It may be used alone or in combination with metformin or a thiazolidinedione.

Because repaglinide is rapidly absorbed, it should be taken shortly before each meal. It is effective in lowering postprandial glucose levels and in reducing hemoglobin A1C levels, but has little effect on fasting glucose levels. It undergoes almost no renal excretion, and so it can be used in patients with renal insufficiency.

Mechanism of Action: Repaglinide lowers glucose levels by stimulating insulin release from pancreatic beta cells. Patients must have some ability to secrete insulin for the drug to be effective.

Pharmacokinetics:

Route(s)	PO
Absorption	Rapidly absorbed following PO administration
Distribution	98% protein bound
Primary metabolism	Hepatic (CYP3A4)
Primary excretion	90% in feces
Onset of action	15–30 min; peak: 1 h
Duration of action	4 h

Adverse Effects: Repaglinide is generally well tolerated; the most common adverse effect is hypoglycemia. Other adverse effects include nausea, vomiting, diarrhea, and dyspepsia. Headache, paresthesias, upper respiratory infections, sinusitis, rhinitis, or bronchitis may also occur.

Contraindications/Precautions: Repaglinide is contraindicated in persons with type 1 diabetes or DKA. It should be used with caution in patients with hepatic impairment, during pregnancy or lactation, in elderly patients, or in those with systemic infection, surgery, or trauma. Its safety in children has not been established.

Drug Interactions: Drugs that induce hepatic CYP3A4 enzyme such as barbiturates, carbamazepine, rifampin, and pioglitazone may increase repaglinide metabolism and cause hyperglycemia. Drugs that inhibit CYP3A4 such as erythromycin, ketoconazole, and miconazole inhibit repaglinide metabolism and may potentiate hypoglycemia. Gemfibrozil may increase risk for hypoglycemia. Use with isophane insulin may cause myocardial ischemia. **Herbal/Food**: The concurrent intake of grapefruit juice inhibits metabolism and may result in increased repaglinide levels and hypoglycemia. Garlic and ginseng may increase hypoglycemic effects.

Pregnancy: Category C.

Treatment of Overdose: During overdose, provide symptomatic therapy and a concentrated source of glucose for hypoglycemia, preferably by the IV route.

Nursing Responsibilities: Key nursing implications for patients receiving repaglinide are included in the Nursing Practice Application for Patients Receiving Pharmacotherapy for Type 2 Diabetes.

Drugs Similar to Repaglinide (Prandin)

The only other meglitinide is nateglinide.

Nateglinide (Starlix): Approved in 2000, nateglinide has actions and uses similar to those of repaglinide. It is used alone or in combination with metformin for managing glucose levels in persons with type 2 diabetes who have not achieved glycemic control through diet and exercise. It is not effective for type 1 diabetes. Like repaglinide, it is given 5 to 20 minutes before meals. An important difference between these drugs is that nateglinide is primarily renally excreted, and so it should be used with caution in patients with renal impairment. Like repaglinide, nateglinide is well tolerated and hypoglycemia is usually mild. The drug is pregnancy category C.

Thiazolidinediones

The thiazolidinediones (TZDs), or glitazones, reduce blood glucose by decreasing insulin resistance and inhibiting hepatic gluconeogenesis. Optimal lowering of blood glucose may require 3 to 4 months of therapy. The most common adverse effects are fluid retention, headache, and weight gain. Hypoglycemia does not occur with drugs in this class. Because of their tendency to promote fluid retention, thiazolidinediones are contraindicated in patients with serious heart failure or pulmonary edema.

PROTOTYPE DRUG | Rosiglitazone (Avandia)

Classification: **Therapeutic:** Antidiabetic agent
Pharmacologic: Thiazolidinedione

Therapeutic Effects and Uses: Rosiglitazone is used to lower blood glucose levels in persons with type 2 diabetes, as an adjunct to diet and exercise. It can be used as monotherapy or in combination with metformin, a sulfonylurea, or insulin. It is effective in lowering fasting glucose levels and hemoglobin A1C levels. Optimum therapeutic effects take several weeks to occur.

Mechanism of Action: Rosiglitazone lowers blood glucose levels by increasing cellular sensitivity to insulin, thereby reducing insulin resistance. In addition, it decreases gluconeogenesis by the liver.

Pharmacokinetics:

Route(s)	PO
Absorption	Rapidly absorbed
Distribution	Greater than 99% protein bound
Primary metabolism	Hepatic (CYP2C8)
Primary excretion	Primarily renal, with approximately 25% in feces
Onset of action	Within 1 h; peak: 1 h
Duration of action	12–24 h

Adverse Effects: Rosiglitazone is generally well tolerated. The most prominent adverse effect is edema, including macular edema. Anemia, headache, back pain, fatigue, diarrhea, upper respiratory infection, or sinusitis may occur. The drug can also raise serum lipid levels, including HDL cholesterol, triglycerides, and LDL cholesterol. It is recommended that baseline liver function tests be obtained prior to initiating treatment, and then assessed every 3 to 6 months while on this drug. Patients should be informed of the signs of liver damage (nausea, fatigue, dark urine, jaundice) as well as the signs of heart failure (dyspnea, weight gain, edema, fatigue) while taking rosiglitazone. Research has also raised the concern of increased fracture risk among women taking drugs in this class. **Black Box Warning:** Drugs in this class can cause or worsen heart failure due to increased fluid retention. In addition, rosiglitazone may increase the risk of myocardial infarction (MI).

Contraindications/Precautions: Rosiglitazone is contraindicated in persons with severe heart failure, liver disease, or elevated liver enzymes, pregnancy, and lactation. Its safety in children has not been established. Rosiglitazone is contraindicated in persons with type 1 diabetes or DKA.

Drug Interactions: Inducers of hepatic CYP2C8 such as rifampin may decrease the effects of rosiglitazone. Inhibitors of CYP2C8 such as azole antifungal agents, fluvoxamine, gemfibrozil, and trimethoprim may elevate rosiglitazone plasma levels and increase the risk for adverse reactions. Concurrent use of rosiglitazone with insulin can increase edema and the risk for heart failure and myocardial ischemia. Other antidiabetic agents, angiotensin II receptor antagonists, and gemfibrozil can increase the hypoglycemic effects. Use of rosiglitazone with nitrates is not recommended due to the potential for myocardial ischemia. Thiazide diuretics, phenothiazines, and atypical antipsychotic drugs can decrease the hypoglycemic effects of rosiglitazone by increasing blood glucose levels. **Herbal/Food:** Garlic and ginseng can increase the risk for hypoglycemia if used with rosiglitazone. Cocoa and rosemary may decrease the therapeutic effect and have a hyperglycemic effect.

Pregnancy: Category C.

Treatment of Overdose: Standard treatment for hypoglycemia is initiated during overdose, along with symptomatic treatment of edema or fluid overload.

Nursing Responsibilities: Key nursing implications for patients receiving rosiglitazone are included in the Nursing Practice Application for Patients Receiving Pharmacotherapy for Type 2 Diabetes.

Drugs Similar to Rosiglitazone (Avandia)

The only other drug in this class is pioglitazone. Troglitazone (Rezulin) was withdrawn from the market in 2000 because of drug-related deaths due to hepatic failure.

Pioglitazone (Actos): Approved in 1999, pioglitazone has actions and uses similar to those of rosiglitazone. It is rapidly absorbed following PO administration, with peak effects occurring within 7 days of beginning therapy.

Pioglitazone has shown more favorable effects on triglyceride and HDL-cholesterol levels than rosiglitazone, with more benefits seen among women than men (ADA, 2007). Pioglitazone can decrease serum levels of oral contraceptives, and can cause nonovulating premenopausal women to resume ovulation; therefore, a reliable form of contraception is recommended. There is no evidence of liver damage from this drug, but hepatic function should be assessed for a baseline and periodically thereafter as with rosiglitazone. The drug carries the same black box warnings regarding heart failure and myocardial ischemia as rosiglitazone. The drug is pregnancy category C.

Alpha-Glucosidase Inhibitors

The alpha-glucosidase inhibitors act by blocking enzymes in the small intestine responsible for breaking down complex carbohydrates into monosaccharides. Because carbohydrates must be in the monosaccharide form to be absorbed, digestion of glucose is delayed. These agents have minimal adverse effects, with the most common being GI related, such as abdominal cramping, diarrhea, and flatulence. Although alpha-glucosidase inhibitors do not produce hypoglycemia when used alone, hypoglycemia may occur when these agents are combined with insulin or a sulfonylurea.

PROTOTYPE DRUG | Acarbose (Precose)

Classification: **Therapeutic:** Antidiabetic agent
Pharmacologic: Alpha-glucosidase inhibitor

Therapeutic Effects and Uses: Approved in 1995, acarbose lowers blood glucose levels in persons with type 2 diabetes who cannot adequately manage glucose levels by diet and exercise alone. It may be used alone or in combination with a sulfonylurea, metformin, or insulin. By slowing the breakdown and absorption of carbohydrates, the rise in postprandial glucose level is reduced. Hemoglobin A1C level is lowered as well.

Mechanism of Action: Acarbose lowers glucose levels by interfering with carbohydrate absorption from the GI tract. It acts locally in the GI tract to inhibit the enzyme responsible for carbohydrate breakdown.

Pharmacokinetics:

Route(s)	PO
Absorption	Only 2% absorbed (low absorption is desired because the drug acts locally in the GI tract); some metabolites are absorbed
Distribution	Acts locally in the digestive tract
Primary metabolism	Metabolized in the GI tract by intestinal bacteria and digestive enzymes
Primary excretion	Primarily in feces, 30% in urine
Onset of action	Peak: 1 h
Duration of action	2–4 h

Adverse Effects: The most common adverse effects of acarbose are diarrhea, flatulence, abdominal distention, borborygmi, anemia (iron deficiency), urticaria, and erythema. The GI-related effects may diminish as therapy progresses; however, they will worsen if the patient does not adhere to the prescribed diabetic diet. Hypoglycemia may occur if acarbose is combined with other hypoglycemic agents. If hypoglycemia does develop, it must be treated with glucose and not sucrose (table sugar), because the drug inhibits the absorption of sucrose. Acarbose may cause elevation of liver enzymes (plasma transaminases), although liver damage has not been reported, but levels return to normal following drug withdrawal.

Contraindications/Precautions: Acarbose is contraindicated in patients with inflammatory bowel disease, bowel obstruction, colon ulcers, or in those predisposed to bowel obstructions. It is used with caution in patients with GI distress or liver disorders and in pregnancy or lactation. Safety in children has not been established.

Drug Interactions: Use with sulfonylureas may increase the risk for hypoglycemia. Drugs that cause hyperglycemia such as thiazide diuretics, corticosteroids, phenothiazines, estrogens, phenytoin, or isoniazid may decrease the effectiveness of acarbose. **Herbal/Food:** Ginseng, garlic, black cohosh, juniper berries, aloe, or dandelion root can cause hypoglycemia. Cocoa and rosemary have a hyperglycemic effect and may decrease the therapeutic effect of acarbose.

Pregnancy: Category B.

Treatment of Overdose: Unlike the sulfonylureas, overdose with acarbose will not cause hypoglycemia. Abdominal pain, flatulence, and diarrhea are treated symptomatically.

Nursing Responsibilities: Key nursing implications for patients receiving acarbose are included in the Nursing Practice Application for Patients Receiving Pharmacotherapy for Type 2 Diabetes.

Drugs Similar to Acarbose (Precose)

The only other drug in this class is miglitol.

Miglitol (Glyset): Approved in 1996, miglitol is an alpha-glucosidase inhibitor used as monotherapy or in combination with other antidiabetic drugs for the pharmacotherapy of type 2 diabetes. It acts by delaying the conversion of complex carbohydrates to monosaccharides (glucose), thereby lessening the rise in postprandial serum glucose levels. Like acarbose, the drug must be present in the intestine at the same time the carbohydrates are being digested; thus, the drug must be taken with a meal. The adverse effects are similar with the notable exception of not causing increased liver enzymes. Acarbose and miglitol both act locally in the intestine, although miglitol is completely absorbed and has the potential to produce systemic effects. Overdose does not cause hypoglycemia. The drug is pregnancy category B.

CONNECTIONS: NURSING PRACTICE APPLICATION

Patients Receiving Pharmacotherapy for Type 2 Diabetes

Assessment Data	Potential Nursing Diagnoses
Baseline assessment prior to administration: • Understand the reason the drug has been prescribed in order to assess for therapeutic effects and to plan for teaching needs (e.g., new onset of type 2 diabetes with hyperglycemia present, oral agents to be used alone or along with supplemental insulin). • Obtain a complete health history including endocrine, cardiovascular, hepatic, or renal disease, pregnancy, or breast-feeding. Obtain a drug history including allergies, current prescription and OTC drugs, herbal preparations, caffeine, nicotine, and alcohol use. Be alert to possible drug interactions. • Obtain a history of current symptoms, duration and severity, and other related signs or symptoms (e.g., paresthesias of hands or feet). Assess feet and lower extremities for possible ulcerations. • Obtain a dietary history including caloric intake and number of meals and snacks per day. Assess fluid intake and type of fluids consumed. • Obtain baseline vital signs, height, and weight. • Evaluate appropriate laboratory findings (e.g., CBC, electrolytes, glucose, A1C level, lipid profile, hepatic, and renal function studies). • Assess the patient's ability to receive and understand instructions. Include family and caregivers as needed.	• *Imbalanced Nutrition: More than Body Requirements* • *Ineffective Health Maintenance* • *Deficient Knowledge* (Drug Therapy) • *Risk for Unstable Blood Glucose* • *Risk for Injury*, related to adverse drug effects • *Risk for Infection*
Assessment throughout administration: • Assess for desired therapeutic effects (e.g., glucose levels remain within normal limits, A1C levels demonstrate adequate control of glucose). • Continue periodic monitoring of hepatic function studies. • Assess for and report promptly any adverse effects appropriate to the type of oral agent: signs of hypoglycemia (e.g., nausea, paleness, sweating, diaphoresis, tremors, irritability, headache, lightheadedness, anxiety, or decreased level of consciousness) most commonly associated with sulfonylureas and meglitinides, and hyperglycemia (e.g., flushed or dry skin, polyuria, polyphagia, polydipsia, drowsiness, glycosuria, ketonuria, or acetone-breath), gastric upset, diarrhea, infection, edema.	

Planning: Patient Goals and Expected Outcomes

The patient will:

• Experience therapeutic effects dependent on the reason the drug is being given (e.g., blood sugar within normal limits).

• Be free from or experience minimal adverse effects.

• Verbalize an understanding of the drug's use, adverse effects, and required precautions.

• Demonstrate proper self-administration of the medication (e.g., dose, timing, and when to notify the provider).

Implementation

Interventions and (Rationales)	Patient-Centered Care
Ensuring therapeutic effects: • Continue assessments as above for therapeutic effects. (Dependent on the severity of hyperglycemia, supplemental insulin may be needed for blood glucose levels to return gradually to normal.)	• Teach the patient to report any return of original symptoms. • Teach the patient the symptoms of hyper- and hypoglycemia to observe for and to check capillary glucose level routinely and if symptoms are present. Promptly report any noticeable symptoms and concurrent capillary glucose level to the health care provider.
• Ensure dietary needs are met based on the need to lose, gain, or maintain current weight and glucose levels. Consult with the dietitian as needed. Limit or eliminate alcohol use. (Adequate caloric protein, carbohydrate, and fat amounts support the oral hypoglycemic regimen for glucose control. Activity and lifestyle will also be factored into dietary management. As alcohol is metabolized, it can raise and then precipitously lower blood, raising the risk of hypoglycemia. Patients on sulfonylureas should avoid or eliminate alcohol entirely because a disulfiram-like reaction with severe nausea, vomiting, and potential hypotension may result.)	• Review current diet, lifestyle, and activity level with the patient. Arrange a dietitian consult based on the need to alter diet or food choices. Teach the patient to limit or eliminate alcohol use. If alcoholic beverages are consumed, limit to one per day and consume along with a complete meal to ensure food intake balances alcohol metabolism. • Instruct patients on sulfonylureas (e.g., glyburide) to avoid or eliminate alcohol use.
Minimizing adverse effects: • Continue to monitor capillary glucose levels. Check with the health care provider before giving an oral hypoglycemic if blood sugar is less than 70 mg/dL or per the parameters as ordered by the health care provider. (Daily glucose levels, especially before meals, will assist in maintaining adequate control of blood glucose and aid in assessing the appropriateness of current drug therapy.)	• Instruct the patient on appropriate blood glucose monitoring techniques to obtain capillary blood glucose levels, followed by return demonstration, and when to contact the health care provider (e.g., glucose less than 70 mg/dL). Monitor use and ensure proper functioning of all equipment to be used at home.

(continued)

CONNECTIONS: NURSING PRACTICE APPLICATION (continued)

• Continue to monitor periodic laboratory work: CBC, electrolytes, glucose, A1C level, lipid profile, hepatic, and renal function studies. (Periodic monitoring of laboratory work assists in determining glucose control and the need for any change in medication and assesses for complications. A1C levels provide a measure of glucose control over several months' time. Sulfonylureas may cause hepatic toxicity. Biguanides may cause lactic acidosis.)	• Instruct the patient on the need to return periodically for laboratory work. • Teach patients on sulfonylureas to immediately report any nausea, vomiting, yellowing of the skin or sclera, abdominal pain, light or clay-colored stools, or darkening of urine to the health care provider. • Teach patients on biguanides to immediately report any drowsiness, malaise, decreased respiratory rate, or general body aches to the health care provider.
• Assess for symptoms of hypoglycemia. If symptoms are noted, provide a quick-acting carbohydrate source (e.g., juice or other simple sugar), and then check capillary glucose level. Report to the health care provider if glucose is less than 70 mg/dL or as ordered. If mealtime is not immediate, provide a longer acting protein source to ensure hypoglycemia does not recur. (Hypoglycemia is especially likely to occur if the patient is taking sulfonylureas or meglitinides, although it may occur with other types of oral antidiabetic drugs, especially if food sources are inadequate. Providing a quick-acting carbohydrate source and then checking the capillary glucose level will ensure glucose does not decrease further while locating the glucose testing equipment. When in doubt, treating symptoms for suspected <u>hypoglycemia</u> is safer than allowing further decreases in glucose and possible loss of consciousness with adverse effects. Small additional amounts of carbohydrates will not dramatically increase blood sugar if testing shows a hyperglycemic episode.)	• Teach the patient to always carry a quick-acting carbohydrate source in case symptoms of hypoglycemia occur. If unsure whether symptoms indicate hypo- or hyperglycemia, treat as hypoglycemia and then check capillary glucose. If symptoms are not relieved in 10–15 min, or if blood sugar is below 70 mg/dL (or the parameters as ordered), immediately notify the health care provider.
• Monitor blood glucose more frequently during periods of illness or stress. (Blood glucose levels may increase or decrease during periods of illness or stress. Frequent monitoring during these times helps to prevent hypoglycemia and ensures adequate glucose control.)	• Instruct the patient to check glucose levels more frequently when ill or under stress. Stress may increase blood glucose because the stress response can cause glycogenolysis and supplemental insulin may be required if oral antidiabetic drugs do not adequately control the blood sugar. Illness, especially associated with anorexia, nausea, or vomiting, may decrease the need for an oral hypoglycemic drug. Notify the health care provider if unable to eat normal meals during periods of illness or stress for possible change in drug regimen.
• Encourage increased activity and exercise, but monitor blood glucose before and after exercise and begin any new or increased exercise routine gradually. Continue to monitor for hypoglycemia for up to 48 h after exercise. (Exercise assists muscles to use glucose more efficiently and increases insulin receptor sites in the tissues, lowering the blood sugar and assisting with weight control. Benefits of exercise and lowered blood sugar may continue for up to 48 h, increasing the risk of hypoglycemia during this time. Frequent monitoring helps to prevent hypoglycemia and ensures adequate glucose control.)	• Teach the patient the benefits of increased activity and exercise and to begin any new routine or increase in exercise gradually. • Instruct the patient to check glucose levels more frequently before and after exercise.
• Monitor for hypersensitivity and allergic reactions. Continue to monitor the patient throughout therapy. (Anaphylactic reactions are possible although rare. As sensitivity occurs, reactions may continue to develop.)	• Teach the patient to immediately report any itching, rashes, swelling, particularly of the face or tongue, urticaria, flushing, dizziness, syncope, wheezing, throat tightness, or difficulty breathing.
• Assess for pregnancy or the possibility of pregnancy. (Some oral antidiabetic drugs are category C and must be stopped during pregnancy. Due to the increasing metabolic needs of pregnancy, supplemental insulin or switching to insulin coverage may be required for the duration of the pregnancy.)	• Teach female patients of childbearing age to monitor for pregnancy and alert the health care provider if pregnant or if pregnancy is suspected to discuss medication needs.
• Continue to monitor for edema, blood pressure, and lung sounds in patients taking thiazolidinediones. (Drugs such as rosiglitazone may cause edema and worsening of heart failure.)	• Instruct the patient to immediately report any edema of the hands or feet, dyspnea, or excessive fatigue to the health care provider.
• Monitor for hypoglycemia more frequently in patients on concurrent beta-blocker therapy. (Beta blockers antagonize the action of some oral antidiabetic drugs and may mask the symptoms of a hypoglycemic episode, allowing the blood sugar to drop lower before it is perceived.)	• Teach patients on concurrent beta-blocker therapy to monitor capillary blood glucose more frequently and to check blood glucose if minor changes in overall feeling are perceived (e.g., minor agitation or anxiety, slight tremors).
Patient understanding of drug therapy: • Use opportunities during administration of medications and during assessments to discuss the rationale for drug therapy, desired therapeutic outcomes, commonly observed adverse effects, parameters for when to call the health care provider, and any necessary monitoring or precautions. (Using time during nursing care helps to optimize and reinforce key teaching areas.)	• The patient, family, or caregiver should be able to state the reason for the drug, appropriate dose and scheduling, what adverse effects to observe for and when to report them, and any special requirements of medication therapy (e.g., drug needs during exercise or illness). • Instruct the patient to carry a wallet identification card and wear medical identification jewelry indicating diabetes.

Patient self-administration of drug therapy:

- When administering the medication, instruct the patient, family, or caregiver in the proper self-administration of drug. (Utilizing time during nurse-administration of these drugs helps to reinforce teaching.)

- The patient, family, or caregiver is able to discuss appropriate dosing and administration needs, including:
  - Timing of doses: Most oral antidiabetic drugs are taken once or twice a day. For drugs given once a day, take approximately 30 min before the first meal of the day. Alpha-glucosidase inhibitors (e.g., acarbose) should be taken with meals.
  - Insulin requirements: While type 2 diabetics produce some insulin, insulin injections may be required in addition to the oral antidiabetic drug on occasion. This does not necessarily signal a worsening of the disease condition, but may be a temporary need.

Evaluation of Outcome Criteria

Evaluate the effectiveness of drug therapy by confirming that patient goals and expected outcomes have been met (see "Planning").

Incretin Enhancers

8 Incretin therapies offer a different approach to treating type 2 diabetes.

Incretins are hormones released by the mucosa of the small intestine in response to meals. The most important incretin is glucagon-like peptide (GLP-1), which acts rapidly to produce the following effects:

- Increase the amount of insulin secreted by the pancreas.
- Decrease the amount of glucagon secreted by the pancreas.
- Delay gastric emptying (slow glucose absorption).
- Decrease food intake by increasing the level of satiety.

Two groups of drugs have been developed that can influence incretin release. The first activates the GLP-1 receptor, causing essentially the same glucose-lowering actions as the natural hormone. Exenatide (Byetta) and liraglutide are synthetic drugs that mimic the action of incretin. They are both administered by the subcutaneous route, although liraglutide offers the advantage of once-daily dosing.

The second class of drugs that enhance incretin actions are the dipeptidyl peptidase 4 (DPP-4) inhibitors. Linagliptin (Tradjenta), saxagliptin (Onglyza), and sitagliptin (Januvia) prevent the breakdown of incretins, allowing the hormone levels to rise and produce a greater response. These drugs are given orally and are effective at lowering blood glucose with few adverse effects. They work well with other antidiabetic drugs and do not cause hypoglycemia.

PROTOTYPE DRUG	Sitagliptin (Januvia)

Classification: **Therapeutic:** Antidiabetic agent
Pharmacologic: DPP-4 inhibitor, incretin enhancer

Therapeutic Effects and Uses: Approved in 2006, sitagliptin is an oral incretin enhancer that is used to help lower glucose levels in patients with type 2 diabetes who are unable to achieve normal glucose levels with diet and exercise. The drug is used as adjunct therapy along with diet and exercise, and can be administered as monotherapy or in combination with other oral antidiabetic agents. In 2011, the FDA approved Juvisync, a fixed dose combination of sitagliptin with simvastatin. The combination is indicated for patients with type 2 diabetes who also have high serum cholesterol levels.

The actions of sitagliptin are glucose dependent: They occur only in the presence of elevated serum glucose, and so the risk for hypoglycemia is reduced. Sitagliptin has the added benefit of increasing satiety, or the feeling of fullness following a meal, resulting in a lower calorie intake and improved weight control. Sitagliptin lowers both fasting and postprandial glucose levels. Janumet is a fixed-dose combination drug containing sitagliptin and metformin.

Mechanism of Action: Sitagliptin inhibits DPP-4 the enzyme responsible for breaking down incretins. Inhibition of DPP-4 reduces the destruction of incretins. Levels of incretin hormones increase, thus decreasing blood glucose levels in patients with type 2 diabetes.

Pharmacokinetics:

Route(s)	PO
Absorption	Rapidly absorbed
Distribution	Approximately 38% protein bound
Primary metabolism	20% metabolized in the liver by CYP3A4 and CYP2CB
Primary excretion	Renal
Onset of action	30–60 min; peak: 1–4 h
Duration of action	Half-life: 12 h

Adverse Effects: Sitagliptin is well tolerated by most patients and adverse effects are generally not serious. Possible adverse effects include headache, diarrhea, nasopharyngitis, and upper respiratory infection. Allergic skin reactions and anaphylaxis have been reported. As monotherapy, sitagliptin does not cause hypoglycemia; however, when used concurrently with a sulfonylurea or insulin, hypoglycemia may occur.

Contraindications/Precautions: Sitagliptin is contraindicated in type 1 diabetes and DKA. It is used with caution in persons with renal disorders or renal failure, among older adults, or during pregnancy and lactation. Safety for children under age 18 has not been established.

Drug Interactions: Sitagliptin may increase digoxin levels. **Herbal/Food:** Cocoa and rosemary may decrease the therapeutic effect and have a hyperglycemic effect.

Pregnancy: Category C.

Treatment of Overdose: Overdose is treated symptomatically. If used in combination with other glucose-lowering agents and hypoglycemia occurs, a concentrated source of glucose should be administered by the IV route.

Nursing Responsibilities: Key nursing implications for patients receiving sitagliptin are included in the Nursing Practice Application for Patients Receiving Pharmacotherapy for Type 2 Diabetes.

Drugs Similar to Sitagliptin (Januvia)

Other incretin enhancers include the GLP-1 agonists exenatide and liraglutide, and the DPP-4 inhibitors linagliptin and saxaglipton.

Exenatide (Byetta): Exenatide was approved in 2005 for patients with type 2 diabetes who are unable to achieve adequate glycemic control following metformin or sulfonylurea monotherapy. The drug is a synthetic peptide that stimulates the release of insulin from pancreatic beta cells. It mimics the actions of the incretin hormones normally secreted by the intestines, which slow the absorption of glucose. It is effective in lowering fasting and postprandial glucose levels, and causes a consistent, slow weight loss. A major disadvantage of exenatide is that it must be given twice daily by the subcutaneous route, within 60 minutes before the morning and evening meals. It is available as a pen injector. Adverse effects include nausea, vomiting, diarrhea, dyspepsia, anorexia, and gastroesophageal reflux. It can also cause nervousness, dizziness, and diaphoresis. Like sitagliptin, it does not cause hypoglycemia. The drug is pregnancy category C.

Linagliptin (Tradjenta): Approved in 2011, linagliptin is one of the newest of the DPP-4 inhibitors. The drug is well tolerated and has the same actions and adverse effects as sitagliptin. One potential advantage over the other DPP-4 inhibitors is that linagliptin is excreted through the liver rather than the kidneys. This allows the drug to be used in patients with significant renal impairment. The drug is pregnancy category B.

Liraglutide (Victoza): Approved in 2010, liraglutide is an incretin enhancer that acts by the same mechanism as exenatide. Like exenatide, liraglutide is effective at reducing HbA1C levels, as well as decreasing appetite and producing a desirable weight loss. An advantage over exenatide is that it can be given once daily. Both drugs are given by the subcutaneous route. Liraglutide is well tolerated with the most common adverse effects being headache, nausea, diarrhea, and anti-liraglutide antibody formation. Hypoglycemia is not a problem with monotherapy but it may occur if used in combination with other antidiabetic drugs. Pancreatitis has been reported with other incretin enhancers and may also occur in patients taking liraglutide. The drug carries a black box warning about the possibility of rare thyroid tumors. Patients with a personal or family history of thyroid cancer should not take this drug. This drug is pregnancy category C.

Saxagliptin (Onglyza): Saxagliptin is a DPP-4 inhibitor approved in 2009 to improve glycemic control in patients with type 2 diabetes. The drug is well tolerated and has the same actions and adverse effects as sitagliptin. Kombiglyze XR is a fixed-dose combination of saxagliptin and metformin. This drug is pregnancy category B.

Miscellaneous Antidiabetic Agents

A few miscellaneous drugs play minor roles in treating type 2 diabetes. Bromocriptine (Cycloset) is an older drug that was approved for a new indication, treating type 2

Complementary and Alternative Therapies
Chromium for Hyperglycemia

Description: Chromium is a trace mineral naturally found in various foods, including whole-grain cereals, prunes, nuts, and seafood.

History and Claims: The relationship between chromium intake and glucose metabolism was first reported in the 1950s, when chromium-containing brewer's yeast was reported to prevent diabetes in laboratory animals. Since that time, the use of chromium supplements among persons with diabetes has become more common practice. Chromium is thought to increase the number of insulin receptors and improve insulin's ability to bind to receptors, therefore lowering blood glucose levels. This, in theory, would lower insulin requirements in persons with type 1 diabetes.

Standardization: The only approved usage for chromium is 4 mcg/mL (chromic chloride injection, USP), which is indicated for use as a supplement to IV solutions given for total parenteral nutrition.

Evidence: The evidence for the effects of chromium is inconclusive, with some reporting positive and some negative benefits. Nahas and Moher (2009) conducted a meta-analysis of 41 clinical trials and determined that evidence existed for the efficacy of chromium in lowering finger-stick blood glucose and A1C levels at doses of 200 to 1,000 mcg over periods of up to 26 weeks. But the authors cite the need for definitive clinical trials. At low doses, chromium supplements appear to be safe, although patients with diabetes or those with concurrent kidney conditions should monitor their blood glucose levels more frequently because hypoglycemia may occur (National Center for Complementary and Alternative Medicine, 2009). More rigorous, well-controlled studies are needed to fully assess the efficacy and mechanism of action of chromium supplementation as an adjuvant therapy for type 2 diabetes and impaired glucose tolerance.

diabetes, in 2009. Bromocriptine is a dopamine receptor agonist but its mechanism for improving glycemic control is not known. The drug is also approved for acromegaly, Parkinson's disease, and hyperprolactinemia. Common adverse effects include nausea, fatigue, dizziness, vomiting, and headache.

Bile acid sequestrants such as colesevelam (Welchol) are drugs primarily prescribed for reducing low-density lipoprotein cholesterol in patients with hyperlipidemia. The mechanism by which these drugs improve glycemic control is unknown.

UNDERSTANDING THE CHAPTER

Key Concepts Summary

1 Serum glucose is maintained within a narrow range by the hormones insulin and glucagon.

2 Type 1 diabetes is characterized by insufficient insulin synthesis by the pancreas, whereas type 2 diabetes is characterized by insulin resistance in the target cells.

3 The classic signs and symptoms of diabetes include polyuria, polydipsia, and polyphagia.

4 Acute complications of diabetes include diabetic ketoacidosis, hyperosmolar hyperglycemic state, and hypoglycemia.

5 Serious, chronic complications of diabetes include neuropathy, nephropathy, retinopathy, and vascular disease.

6 Insulin is the cornerstone of therapy for patients with type 1 and gestational diabetes.

7 Antidiabetic drugs from multiple classes are used to treat type 2 diabetes.

8 Incretin therapies offer a different approach to treating type 2 diabetes.

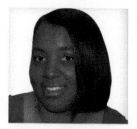

Making the PATIENT *Connection*

Remember the patient "Ellen McIntosh" at the beginning of the chapter? Now read the remainder of the case study. Based on the information presented within this chapter, respond to the critical thinking questions that follow.

Ellen is a 44-year-old woman who works full time as an art teacher in a local high school. She also teaches art courses on the weekends at the local senior center. She visited her health care provider last week for her annual physical exam and to update her TB screening (PPD) for the coming school year. The office called her back this morning with her laboratory reports and requested that she make an appointment to return tomorrow to discuss the results. Her serum glucose level was elevated at 224 mg/dL and she will need further testing to rule out type 2 diabetes.

Ellen has follow-up testing with the results of a fasting serum glucose level returning at 131 mg/dL and a 2-hour 75-g oral glucose test of 242 mg/dL. A diagnosis of new-onset type 2 diabetes is confirmed. Ellen expresses disbelief and tells you, the nurse, "I can't believe it! I watch what I eat; I don't eat a lot of sugar, cookies, or candy. I drink only diet soda. I don't have any of the

symptoms you hear about. And no one in my family has ever had diabetes." A health history and the results of Ellen's recent physical examination confirm overall good health. Her height is 167.6 cm (66 in.) and weight 79.5 kg (175 lb) with a BMI of 28.2 kg/m^2, placing her in the "overweight" category. Vital signs, physical exam, and all other laboratory work are within acceptable limits. Ellen admits that she has been thirstier lately, "But it's summertime and I always drink more when it's hot." She has also been urinating more frequently but attributes that to her increased fluid intake.

Ellen's provider will start her on glyburide (Micronase) and metformin (Glucophage) and will recheck her serum glucose in 1 month. In the meantime, she is to begin capillary blood glucose testing before meals and at bedtime, and to bring her log to the next visit. She is given dietary instructions and you will be providing instruction on her medications.

Critical Thinking Questions

1. Why are two oral antidiabetic drugs prescribed for Ellen?

2. What essential teaching does Ellen need about her glyburide (Micronase) and metformin (Glucophage)?

3. Ellen asks why she is not being started on insulin. Why is insulin not being used at this time?

4. Ellen tells you that she occasionally enjoys a glass of wine with her dinner and wants to know if this is allowed. How will you answer?

See Answers to Critical Thinking Questions on student resource website.

NCLEX-RN® Review

1 A client with type 1 diabetes will use a combination insulin that includes NPH and regular insulins. The nurse is explaining the importance of knowing the peak times for both insulins. Why is this important information for the client to know?

1. The client will be able to estimate the time for the next injection of insulin based on these peaks.
2. The risk of a hypoglycemic reaction is greatest around the peak of insulin activity.
3. It is best to plan activities or exercise around peak insulin times for the best utilization of glucose.
4. Additional insulin may be required at the peak periods to prevent hyperglycemia.

2 Before administering a morning lispro insulin (Humalog) injection, which activity should the nurse perform? Select all that apply.

1. Obtain a morning urine sample for glucose and ketones.
2. Check the client's finger-stick glucose level.
3. Ensure that breakfast trays are present on the unit and the client may eat.
4. Obtain the client's pulse and blood pressure.
5. Assess for symptoms of hypoglycemia.

3 The nurse would consider which of the following assessment findings as adverse effects to metformin therapy?

1. Hypoglycemia
2. Gastrointestinal distress
3. Lactic acidosis
4. Weight loss

4 A client was started on rosiglitazone for type 2 diabetes. He tells the nurse that he has been taking it for 5 days, but his glucose levels are unchanged. What is the nurse's best response?

1. "You should double the dose. That should help."
2. "You need to give the drug more time. It can take several weeks before it becomes fully effective."
3. "You will need to add a second drug since this one has not been effective."
4. "You most likely require insulin now."

5 A young woman calls the clinic and reports that her mother had an insulin reaction, and was found unconscious. The young woman gave her a glucagon injection 20 minutes ago, and her mother woke up, but is still groggy and "does not make sense." What should the nurse tell the daughter?

1. "Let her wake up on her own, then give her something to eat."
2. "Place some hard candies in her mouth."
3. "Just let her sleep. People are sleepy after hypoglycemic episodes."
4. "Give her another injection and call the paramedics."

6 The nurse explains the benefit of using the long-acting insulin glargine (Lantus) over other insulins. What will the nurse tell the client about this insulin?

1. It does not need to be administered by injection.
2. It can be given by intramuscular or subcutaneous injection.
3. It does not require blood glucose monitoring.
4. It has no definite peak but maintains a steady state of insulin in the body.

Additional Case Study

Nicholas Jefferson is 8 years old and has just been diagnosed with type 1 diabetes. After increasing symptoms during the past month, he was hospitalized for continuous nausea, vomiting, and gradually increasing lethargy. His parents report that over the past month or two, Nicholas has had blurry vision and has been thirsty and hungry constantly. He has been eating frequently but does not seem to be gaining any weight. They also tell you that on several occasions, Nicholas has wet the bed, which is very unusual for him. On admission, his serum glucose level is 420 mg/dL with a urine sample positive for glucose and ketones. Nicholas is to remain NPO and will be started on an IV with 0.45 normal saline for fluid replacement, given an IV bolus of insulin, and then started on an insulin drip at 0.5 unit per hour. Finger-stick glucose levels are to be checked every hour with serum blood glucose levels drawn every 4 hours. The IV insulin drip is to be discontinued when Nicholas's blood glucose level is 240 mg/dL and subcutaneous insulin will be started at that time.

1. What type of insulin do you anticipate using for the IV bolus dose and IV drip?
2. Why do you think the insulin IV will be stopped when the blood glucose level is 240 mg/dL and not at the normal level of 70 to 100 mg/dL?
3. What essential teaching will Nicholas and his family need at this time?

See Answers to Additional Case Study on student resource website.

References

American Association of Clinical Endocrinologists. (2011). Medical guidelines for clinical practice for developing a diabetes mellitus comprehensive care plan. *Endocrine Practice, 17*(Suppl. 2), 1–53. Retrieved from https://www.aace.com/sites/default/files/DMGuidelinesCCP.pdf

American Diabetes Association. (2007). *From insulin to incretins: A report from the 67th scientific session of the American Diabetes Association.* Chicago, IL: Author.

American Diabetes Association. (2011a). Standards of medical care in diabetes—2011. *Diabetes Care, 34*(Suppl. 1), S11–S60. doi: 10.2337/dc11-S011

American Diabetes Association. (2011b). Diabetes care in the school and day care setting. *Diabetes Care, 34*(Suppl. 1), S70–S74. doi:10.2337/dc11-S070

Centers for Disease Control and Prevention. (2010). *National diabetes fact sheet, 2011.* Retrieved from http://www.cdc.gov/diabetes/pubs/pdf/ndfs_2011.pdf

Maskarinec, G., Erber, E., Grandinetti, A., Verheus, M., Oum, R., Hopping, B. N., et al. (2009a). Diabetes incidence based on linkages with health plans: The Multiethnic Cohort. *Diabetes, 58*(8), 1732–1738. doi:10.2337/db08-1685

Maskarinec, G., Grandinetti, A., Matsuura, G., Sharma, S., Mau, M., Henderson, B. E., & Kolonel, L. N. (2009b). Diabetes prevalence and body mass index differ by ethnicity: The Multiethnic Cohort. *Ethnicity and Disease, 19*(1), 49–55.

Morimoto, Y., Schembre, S. M., Steinbrecher, A., Erber, E., Pagano, I., Grandinetti, A., et al. (2011). Ethnic differences in weight gain and diabetes risk: The Multiethnic Cohort Study. *Diabetes and Metabolism, 37*(3), 230–236. doi:10.1016/j.diabet.2010.10.005

Nahas, R., & Moher, M. (2009). Complementary and alternative medicine for the treatment of type 2 diabetes. *Canadian Family Physician, 55*(6), 591–596.

National Center for Complementary and Alternative Medicine. (2009). *Get the facts: Diabetes and CAM: A focus on dietary supplements.* Retrieved from http://nccam.nih.gov/health/diabetes/D416_GTF.pdf

Nicholson, W., & Baptiste-Roberts, K. (2011). Oral hypoglycaemic agents in pregnancy: The evidence for effectiveness and safety. *Best Practices and Research Clinical Obstetrics and Gynaecology, 25*(1), 51–63. doi:10.1016/j.bpobgyn.2010.10.018

Nicholoson, W. K., Wilson, L. M., Witkop, C. T., Baptiste-Roberts, K., Bennett, W. L., Bolen, S., et al. (2008). *Therapeutic management, delivery, and postpartum risk assessment and screening in gestational diabetes.* Prepared by the John Hopkins University Evidence-Based Practice Center under Contract No. 290-02-0018. Evidence/Technology Assessment No. 162. (AHRQ Publication No. 08-E004). Retrieved from http://www.ahrq.gov/downloads/pub/evidence/pdf/gestdiabetes/gestdiab.pdf

Porth, C. M. (2011). *Essentials of pathophysiology* (3rd ed.). Philadelphia, PA: Lippincott Williams & Wilkins.

Selected Bibliography

Bennett, W. L., Maruthur, N. M., Singh, S., Segal, J. B., Wilson, L. M., Chatterjee, R., et al. (2011). Comparative effectiveness and safety of medications for type 2 diabetes: An update including new drugs and 2-drug combinations. *Annals of Internal Medicine, 154*(9), 602–613.

LeMone, P., Burke, K., & Bauldoff, G. (2011). *Medical-surgical nursing: Critical thinking in client care* (5th ed.). Upper Saddle River, NJ: Pearson Prentice-Hall.

Meetoo, D., & Allen, G. (2010). Understanding diabetes mellitus and its management: An overview, *Nurse Prescribing, 8*(7), 320–326.

National Diabetes Information Clearinghouse. (2009). *Complementary and alternative medical therapies for diabetes.* Retrieved from http://diabetes.niddk.nih.gov/dm/pubs/alternativetherapies

Powers, A. C., & D'Alessio, D. (2011). Endocrine pancreas and pharmacotherapy of diabetes mellitus and hypoglycemia. In L. L. Brunton, B. A. Chabner, & B. C. Knollman (Eds.), *The pharmacological basis of therapeutics* (12th ed., pp. 1237–1274). New York, NY: McGraw-Hill.

Answers to NCLEX-RN® Review

1 Answer: 2 *Rationale:* Insulin peaks are the times of maximum insulin utilization with the greatest risk of hypoglycemia. Options 1, 3, and 4 are incorrect. Because the risk for hypoglycemia is highest at peak serum insulin levels, exercise or additional insulin may increase the risk further. Insulin schedules for the client are developed by the provider and the client should not self-select a schedule for insulin use. Cognitive Level: Applying; Client Need: Physiological Integrity; Nursing Process: Implementation

2 Answer: 2, 3, 5 Rationale: The blood glucose level should be checked prior to administering any type of insulin. Because lispro is a rapid-acting insulin, the nurse should ensure that a meal is available and that the client will be able to eat shortly after receiving a dose. If signs of hypoglycemia are present, the insulin dose should be held and the client treated for hypoglycemia. The provider should be notified. Options 1 and 4 are incorrect. Urine testing for glucose and ketones does not give exact information, and clients vary on the degree to which glucose and ketones will "spill" into the urine. While a check of the pulse or blood pressure may be included in routine vital signs or to further assess symptoms of hypoglycemia, they do not provide information directly pertinent to the administration of insulin. Cognitive Level: Applying; Client Need: Physiological Integrity; Nursing Process: Implementation

3 Answer: 3 Rationale: A serious adverse effect of metformin is the risk for developing lactic acidosis. Renal insufficiency and failure, excess alcohol use, and IV contrast agents increase the risk for lactic acidosis, and are contraindications to the use of metformin. Options 1, 2, and 4 are incorrect. Hypoglycemia, GI distress, and weight loss are common

adverse effects to most oral antidiabetic drugs and are not specific to metformin. Cognitive Level: Analyzing; Client Need: Physiological Integrity; Nursing Process: Evaluation

4 Answer: 2 Rationale: It can take several weeks for this drug to provide full therapeutic effects, so the appropriate response would be to give it more time to reach effectiveness. Options 1, 3, and 4 are incorrect. It is not within a nurse's scope of practice to prescribe additional drugs or change the dosage. The health care provider should be consulted about any change to the client's drug regimen. Cognitive Level: Applying; Client Need: Health Promotion and Maintenance; Nursing Process: Implementation

5 Answer: 4 Rationale: Glucagon injections can be repeated if one dose is not effective. Hypoglycemia is a medical emergency, and because this woman has not fully recovered, medical attention is needed. Options 1, 2, and 3 are incorrect. The client is still experiencing symptoms of hypoglycemia, and continued treatment is indicated. Because she is still groggy and disoriented, it would not be safe to give this client anything by mouth. Cognitive Level: Applying; Client Need: Physiological Integrity; Nursing Process: Implementation

6 Answer: 4 Rationale: Insulin glargine has no definite peak, so there is a minimal risk for hypoglycemic reaction. Options 1, 2, and 3 are incorrect. Insulin glargine must be given by subcutaneous injection, cannot be given by IM injection, and blood glucose monitoring is required for all clients taking any insulin. Cognitive Level: Applying; Client Need: Physiological Integrity; Nursing Process: Implementation

Review of the Central Nervous System

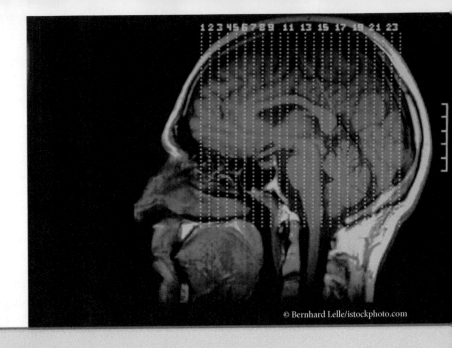

Review of the Central Nervous System

Learning Outcomes

After reading this chapter, the student should be able to:

1. Identify types of conditions for which central nervous system drugs are prescribed.
2. Illustrate the major components of a synapse within the central nervous system.
3. Identify the major neurotransmitters in the central nervous system and their functions.
4. Describe the major structural regions of the brain and their primary functions.
5. Explain the major functional systems of the brain and their primary functions.

Chapter Outline

Scope of Central Nervous System Pharmacology

Neurons and Neurotransmission

Major Structural Components of the Central Nervous System

Functional Systems of the Central Nervous System

The autonomic nervous system (ANS) is the system that provides involuntary control over vital functions of the cardiovascular, digestive, respiratory, and genitourinary systems. The two components of the CNS, the brain and spinal cord, are collectively responsible for interpreting sensory information and formulating appropriate responses. Typical responses may include thinking (deciding if the sensory information is harmful or pleasurable), emotions (anger, depression, euphoria), or movement (running away, pounding a fist, or hugging). The purpose of this chapter is to provide a brief review of concepts of CNS anatomy and physiology that are relevant to neuropharmacology.

PharmFACT

The characteristic loss of cognitive function that occurs during Alzheimer's disease is directly related to a progressive loss of synapses in the cerebral cortex (Itsak, 2010).

Scope of Central Nervous System Pharmacology

1 Medications affect the central nervous system by stimulating or suppressing the firing of specific neurons.

CNS pharmacology is one of the largest and most important divisions in medicine, encompassing 10 chapters in this textbook. Medications may be administered to treat specific neurologic or psychiatric conditions of the CNS. Many drugs cause CNS adverse effects during pharmacotherapy, whereas some are self-administered to produce pleasurable psychoactive effects. At high doses, a large number of drugs affect the brain, and CNS toxicity is a dose-limiting factor in the pharmacotherapy of many diseases.

Of all divisions of pharmacology, CNS drug mechanisms are probably the least understood. For some conditions pharmacologists know that the drug acts on the CNS, but its mechanism of action remains largely unknown. There are two primary reasons for this lack of understanding about how CNS drugs produce their effects: the uniqueness of the human brain and the complexity of the disorders affecting it.

The human brain is truly unique, with no other species having the same complexity. It is not known if animals experience the same types of mental disorders as humans, and measurement of hallucinations, euphoria, or depression is difficult, if not impossible, in most species. If a drug does induce changes in animal behavior such as depression or anxiety, it is not known whether these data apply to humans because of the enormous differences in brain physiology as well as human social networks that can profoundly influence mental health conditions. Pharmacologists are certainly able to measure changes in brain activity or in the amounts of neurotransmitters in specific regions of the brain, but these do not adequately explain complex changes in thinking, mood, or behavior. Without good animal models, pharmacologists must rely largely on empirical observations—evidence derived from giving the drugs to patients and determining what works rather than how it works.

Also complicating the study of CNS pharmacology is that mental disorders themselves are incompletely understood. The physiological basis for conditions such as schizophrenia, major depression, bipolar disorder, panic attacks, or post-traumatic stress disorder is not well established. There is great patient variability in symptoms and disease progression with these conditions, and social factors play important roles. Without a complete understanding of the etiology and pathophysiology of mental disorders, pharmacotherapy of these conditions and the development of new drug therapies for CNS disorders will remain challenging.

The next nine chapters present the major classes of drugs whose pharmacotherapeutic goal is to modify the activity of some portion of the CNS. In a few cases, these drugs affect the function of very specific regions of the brain. Most CNS drugs, however, are nonspecific and affect multiple brain regions.

In simplest terms, CNS drugs have two basic actions: They either stimulate (activation) or suppress (inhibition) the firing of neurons. In some cases, CNS drugs may have both actions: activation of some neurons and inhibition of others. The pharmacologic effects of a CNS drug observed in a patient are the result of precisely which neurons are changed, and how many are affected. As a result of neuron modification, the following beneficial effects of CNS drugs are observed.

- Reduction in anxiety
- Improved sleep patterns
- Elevated mood
- Management of psychotic symptoms
- Slowing the progression of chronic degenerative diseases of the brain
- Termination and prevention of seizures
- Reduction in muscle spasms and spasticity
- Reduction of hyperactivity and mania
- Reduction in pain
- Induction of anesthesia

CONNECTION Checkpoint 21.1

What are the two divisions of the peripheral nervous system and what are their primary functions? See Answer to Connection Checkpoint 21.1 on student resource website.

Key Terms

acetylcholine (Ach)

basal nuclei

dopamine

extrapyramidal system

gamma aminobutyric acid (GABA)

glutamate

limbic system

neuron

norepinephrine (NE)

reticular activating system (RAS)

serotonin

synapses

Neurons and Neurotransmission

2 Neurons in the central nervous system communicate with each other and with body tissues, using neurotransmitters.

The **neuron** is the primary functional cell in all portions of the nervous system. The function of the 100 billion neurons making up the nervous system is to communicate messages through conduction of an action potential. In the CNS, the vast majority of neurons are communicating with other neurons. These neuronal pathways or circuits are extremely complex and provide the basis for the higher level functions of the brain such as thinking, memory, and intelligence. Although a single neuron in the CNS serves no practical function, the interconnections among 100 billion neurons are a major part of what distinguishes the human brain from that of all other species.

Communication between neurons in the brain, as well as that between the brain and other organs, is provided through **synapses**. Synapses are junctions between two neurons, or between a neuron and a muscle.

Synapses within the CNS operate by the same basic principles as those in the ANS. An action potential from the presynaptic neuron releases a neurotransmitter that moves across the synaptic cleft to activate receptors on the postsynaptic neuron, as illustrated in Figure 1a. In some cases, the neuron may be excitatory, enhancing neural transmission (Figure 1b). In other cases the impulse *inhibits* a neurotransmitter from being released, or it causes the release of an inhibitory neurotransmitter that suppresses neuronal conduction (Figure 1c). All interconnections in the CNS depend on synaptic transmission of the action potential from one neuron to another neuron, or to multiple neurons.

In the ANS only two neurotransmitters account for nearly all synaptic transmission: **acetylcholine (Ach)** and **norepinephrine (NE)**. Although these two chemicals also are found in the CNS, more than 30 additional substances have been identified as neurotransmitters in the brain, making the study of neuronal communication in this organ very complex. Some neurotransmitters such as glutamate are primarily stimulatory, whereas others such as gamma aminobutyric acid (GABA) inhibit neuronal activity. NE can activate or inhibit neuronal activity, depending on its location in the brain. A summary of relevant brain neurotransmitters is shown in Table 1.

Adrenergic synapses: Adrenergic synapses utilize NE as the neurotransmitter. Adrenergic synapses in the CNS are abundant in the hypothalamus, the limbic system, and the reticular activating system (RAS). NE activates parts of the brain to heighten alertness and is prominent during waking hours. Adrenergic neurons likely play a role in mood disorders such as depression and anxiety. Drugs used to modify adrenergic synapses in the CNS include caffeine, amphetamines, and tricyclic antidepressants.

Cholinergic synapses: Cholinergic synapses utilize Ach as the neurotransmitter. In the brain, these synapses are most often

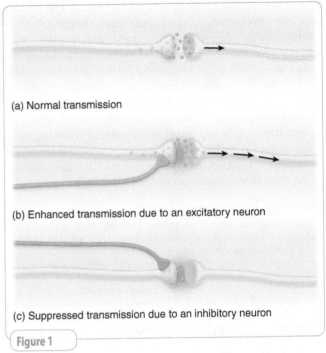

(a) Normal transmission

(b) Enhanced transmission due to an excitatory neuron

(c) Suppressed transmission due to an inhibitory neuron

Figure 1

Modification of neural transmission in the central nervous system: (a) normal transmission; (b) enhanced transmission; (c) suppressed transmission.

stimulatory. Cholinergic synapses are abundant in the motor cortex and basal ganglia but are uncommon in other areas. Cholinergic synapses are especially important in the pathophysiology of Parkinson's disease and Alzheimer's disease. Ach is also a major neurotransmitter in the ANS.

Dopaminergic synapses: These synapses utilize dopamine as the neurotransmitter. **Dopamine** is a chemical precursor in the synthesis of NE and, like epinephrine and NE, is classified chemically as a catecholamine. Dopaminergic synapses are generally excitatory and affect arousal and wakefulness. However, two major receptor subtypes exist: D1 is stimulatory, and D2 is inhibitory. Cocaine and amphetamines produce their stimulatory actions by affecting dopamine receptors; marijuana is also thought to exert some of its psychoactive effects by increasing dopaminergic activity. Dopamine receptors are important in the pharmacotherapy of psychosis and Parkinson's disease.

Endorphins and enkephalins: Endorphins and enkephalins are small peptides secreted by neurons in the hypothalamus, pituitary, limbic system, and spinal cord. The receptor for these molecules is the opioid receptor, which is involved in pain transmission. Endorphins and enkephalins are sometimes called natural opiates because they produce effects very similar to those of morphine and other opioid drugs. Drugs used to modify the types of synapses in the CNS include opioids such as codeine and morphine.

Gamma aminobutyric acid synapses: These synapses utilize **gamma aminobutyric acid (GABA)** as a neurotransmitter. GABA synapses are the second most common type in the CNS, accounting for 30% to 40% of all brain synapses. GABA is the

TABLE 1 Selected Central Nervous System Neurotransmitters and Their Functions

Neurotransmitter	Abundance	Effect	Clinical Significance
Acetylcholine (Ach)	Widely distributed in the CNS; a major transmitter in the ANS	CNS: May be excitatory or inhibitory; controls voluntary skeletal muscle movement. ANS: Activates the parasympathetic nervous system	Myasthenia gravis, Alzheimer's disease
Dopamine	Basal ganglia and limbic system	Usually excitatory; locomotion, attention, learning, and the reinforcing effects of abused drugs	Parkinson's disease; psychoses; motivation, pleasure
Endorphins and enkephalins	Widely distributed in the CNS and peripheral nervous system (PNS)	Usually inhibitory; reduction of pain	Opioids bind to endorphin receptors
Gamma aminobutyric acid (GABA)	Widely distributed in the CNS	Most common inhibitory CNS neurotransmitter	Seizure and anxiety disorders
Glutamate	Widely distributed in the CNS	Most common excitatory CNS neurotransmitter	Memory
Norepinephrine (NE)	Widely distributed in the CNS; a major transmitter in the ANS	CNS: May be excitatory or inhibitory ANS: Activates the sympathetic nervous system	Depression, memory, panic attacks
Serotonin	Common in the brainstem but also found in the limbic system	Usually inhibitory	Anxiety, bipolar disorder, and depression

primary inhibitory neurotransmitter in the CNS and is found throughout the brain, with greatest abundance in the basal ganglia and hypothalamus. Several GABA receptor subtypes have been identified. GABA receptors are the primary site of action for several classes of drugs, including the benzodiazepines and barbiturates.

Glutamate synapses: Glutamate synapses utilize the amino acid **glutamate** (glutamic acid) as a neurotransmitter. Glutamate is the most common neurotransmitter in the CNS, and its synapses are always excitatory in nature. It is found in nearly all regions of the brain. Several glutamate receptor subtypes have been identified, with the N-methyl-D-aspartate (NMDA) receptor being particularly important to memory and learning. In addition to glutamate, zinc, magnesium, glycine, and even phencyclidine (a hallucinogen) bind to the NMDA receptor, thus modulating neuronal activity. High amounts of glutamate can cause neuron death and may be the mechanism responsible for certain types of neurotoxicity.

Serotonergic synapses: Serotonergic synapses utilize **serotonin**, also known as 5-hydroxytryptamine (5-HT), as a neurotransmitter. Although some serotonergic synapses are located in the CNS, 98% of the serotonergic receptors are found outside the CNS in platelets, mast cells, and other peripheral cells. Serotonergic receptors are found throughout the limbic system of the brain, often in close association with adrenergic synapses. Serotonin is used by the body to synthesize the hormone melatonin in the pineal gland. Low serotonin levels in the CNS are associated with anxiety and impulsive behavior, including suicidal ideation. Serotonergic receptors play an important role in the mechanism of action of antidepressant drugs.

CONNECTION Checkpoint 21.2

The neurotransmitter dopamine is also available as a drug. What are the indications for dopamine therapy? *See Answer to Connection Checkpoint 21.2 on student resource website.*

PharmFACT

Conduction of nerve impulses in large-diameter myelinated neurons can reach speeds up to 268 miles/h (120 m/s) (Silverthorn, 2010).

Major Structural Components of the Central Nervous System

3 The central nervous system is divided into several major structural components.

The brain consists of dozens of structural divisions that serve common functions. Identification of the many anatomic components in the CNS is complex and beyond the scope of this text. This section focuses on regions of the CNS that have applications to neuropharmacology. For a more complete discussion of CNS anatomy, the student should consult anatomy and physiology textbooks. Basic brain structures are illustrated in Figure 2.

Cerebrum: The cerebrum is the "thinking" part of the brain responsible for perception, speech, conscious motor movement, movement of skeletal muscles, memory, and smell. It is the largest part of the brain, by weight, and the most advanced. Portions of the cerebrum are organized for specialized functions. For example, the occipital lobe is associated with vision and the frontal lobes are concerned with reasoning and

LATERAL VIEW OF THE CNS

ANATOMY OF THE BRAIN

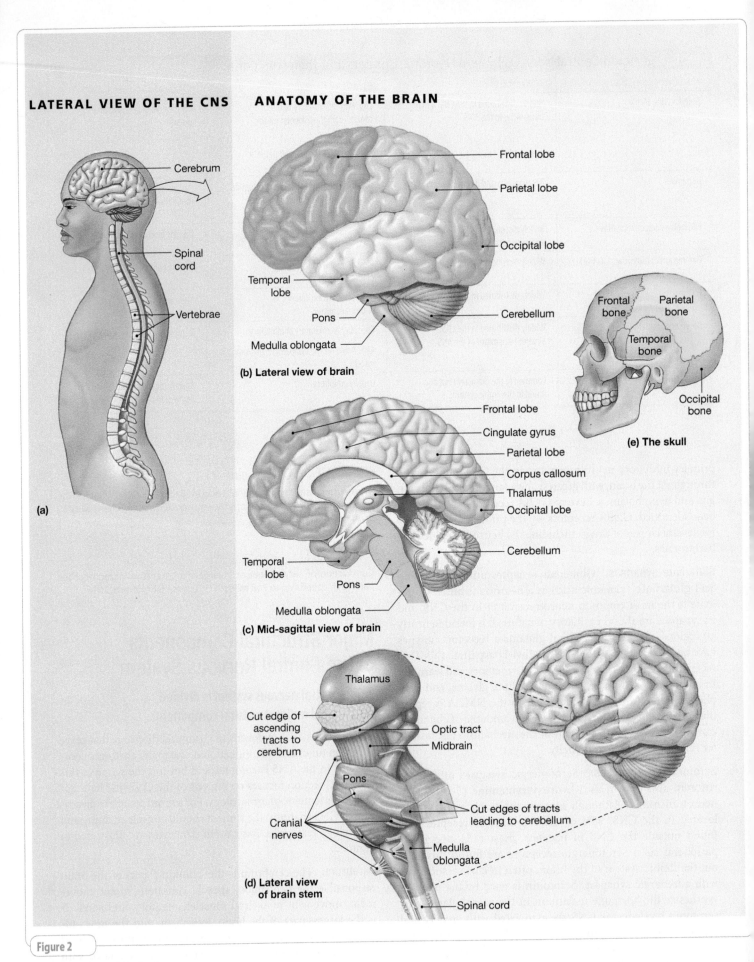

(a)

Cerebrum

Spinal cord

Vertebrae

(b) Lateral view of brain

Frontal lobe

Parietal lobe

Occipital lobe

Temporal lobe

Pons

Medulla oblongata

Cerebellum

(c) Mid-sagittal view of brain

Frontal lobe

Cingulate gyrus

Parietal lobe

Corpus callosum

Thalamus

Occipital lobe

Cerebellum

Temporal lobe

Pons

Medulla oblongata

(e) The skull

Frontal bone

Parietal bone

Temporal bone

Occipital bone

(d) Lateral view of brain stem

Thalamus

Cut edge of ascending tracts to cerebrum

Optic tract

Midbrain

Pons

Cut edges of tracts leading to cerebrum

Cranial nerves

Medulla oblongata

Spinal cord

Figure 2

Basic anatomy of the brain.

Source: From SILVERTHORN, DEE UNGLAUB, HUMAN PHYSIOLOGY, 2nd Ed., © 2001. Reprinted and Electronically reproduced by permission of Pearson Education, Inc., Upper Saddle River, New Jersey

planning. Other areas are specific to language, hearing, motor, or sensory functions.

Disorders of the cerebrum may be focal or generalized. Focal abnormalities, often the result of a stroke, occur in specific regions and may affect a single brain function such as vision, hearing, or movement of a particular limb. Generalized disorders of the cerebrum affect widespread areas or multiple regions and can produce drowsiness, coma, hallucinations, depression, or generalized anxiety.

Thalamus: The thalamus is the major relay center in the brain that sends sensory information such as sounds, sights, pain, touch, and temperature to the cerebral cortex for analysis. To reach the cerebrum, all sensory information must travel through the thalamus. Portions of the thalamus comprise the limbic system, an area that controls mood and motivation. Abnormalities of the thalamus have been associated with diverse mood disorders such as obsessive-compulsive disorder, bipolar disorder, anxiety, and panic disorder.

Hypothalamus: The hypothalamus is the major visceral control center in the body. Regulation of hunger, thirst, water balance, and body temperature are functions of this region. The hypothalamus is also part of the limbic system, which is associated with emotional balance. Some neurons in the hypothalamus connect to the brainstem to affect vital centers such as heart rate, respiratory rate, blood pressure, and pupil size. These responses are associated with the fight-or-flight response of the ANS. Disorders of the hypothalamus may affect some or all of these essential functions.

CONNECTION Checkpoint 21.3

Describe the symptoms of the fight-or-flight response. *See Answer to Connection Checkpoint 21.3 on student resource website.*

Cerebellum: The cerebellum controls muscle movement, balance, posture, and tone. It is involved in learning fine motor skills that make muscular movements smooth and continuous. The cerebellum receives sensory information, including vision, position, equilibrium, and touch, and calculates the strength and extent of muscle movement needed to maintain posture and coordinate complex tasks such as walking, driving, or playing a musical instrument. Injury or disease in this region results in uncoordinated, jerky body movements.

Brainstem: The brainstem, consisting of the medulla oblongata, pons, and midbrain, connects the spinal cord to the brain. Because of its critical location, it serves as the major relay center for messages traveling to and from the brain. In addition, it contains major reflex and control centers involving breathing, heart rate, vision, swallowing, coughing, and vomiting. Injury to the brainstem can be fatal if vital centers are disrupted. The brainstem contains clusters of scattered neurons known as the reticular formation, which help maintain alertness.

Spinal cord: The spinal cord is essentially a conduction pathway to and from the brain. Disruptions of these pathways will

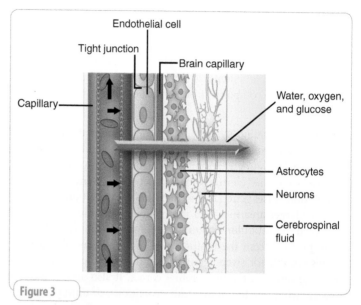

Figure 3

Blood–brain barrier.

prevent transmission of nerve impulses and cause loss of sensory (paresthesia) or motor (paralysis) function.

Blood–brain barrier: The brain must receive a continuous supply of oxygen and glucose; interruptions for even brief periods may cause loss of consciousness. At the same time it needs large quantities of nutrients, the brain must also protect itself from pathogens or toxins that may have entered the blood. Capillaries in most regions of the brain are not as porous as those in other organs; the endothelial cells form tight junctions, creating a seal or barrier to many substances. This is important to pharmacology because CNS drugs must have the capability of penetrating the blood–brain barrier to produce their effects. The blood–brain barrier is illustrated in Figure 3.

Functional Systems of the Central Nervous System

4 Several functional divisions of the central nervous system are important to pharmacotherapy.

Functional brain systems are clusters of neurons that work together to perform a common function. These clusters are physically located far apart in the CNS but form a communication network to act as a coordinated unit. Some CNS drugs produce their effects by modifying the functions of these systems.

Limbic system: The **limbic system** is a group of structures deep in the brain that are responsible for emotional expression, learning, and memory. Emotional states associated with this system include anxiety, fear, anger, aggression, remorse, depression, sexual drive, and euphoria. Signals routed through the limbic system ultimately connect with the hypothalamus (see Section 3). Through its connection with the hypothalamus, autonomic actions such as rapid heart rate, high blood pressure, or peptic ulcers are associated with intense emotional states.

The limbic system also communicates with the cerebrum, which allows people to think and reflect on their emotional states. The connection to the cerebrum allows one to use logic to "override" emotional reactions that might be inappropriate or harmful. Parts of the limbic system also allow one to remember emotional responses. The components of the limbic system are illustrated in Figure 4.

Reticular activating system: The reticular formation, a network of neurons found along the entire length of the brainstem, is shown in Figure 5. Stimulation of the reticular formation causes heightened alertness and arousal of the brain as a whole. Inhibition causes general drowsiness and the induction of sleep.

The larger area in which the reticular formation is found is called the **reticular activating system (RAS)**. This structure projects from the brainstem to the thalamus. The RAS is responsible for sleeping and wakefulness and performs an alerting function for the cerebral cortex. It also acts as a filter, allowing one to ignore weak, repetitious, or unimportant sensory stimuli and to focus attention on individual tasks by transmitting information to higher brain centers. This is important in busy, noisy environments when a person must concentrate on a specific task, such as studying or reading. In any given situation, as much as 99% of all sensory information may be filtered and never reach consciousness.

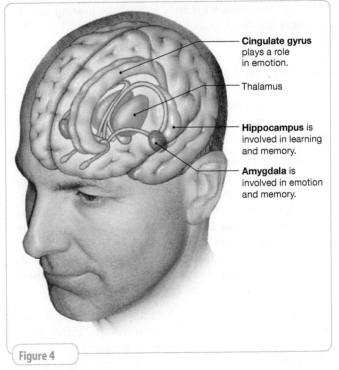

Figure 4

Limbic system.
Source: From SILVERSTHORN, DEE UNGLAUB, HUMAN PHYSIOLOGY: AN INTEGRATED APPROACH, 4th Ed., © 2007. Reprinted and Electronically reproduced by permission of Pearson Education, Inc., Upper Saddle River, New Jersey.

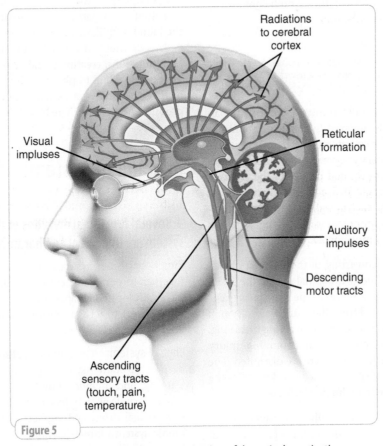

Figure 5

With input from sensory neurons, activation of the reticular activating system causes arousal of the cerebral cortex, thus maintaining the awake-and-alert state.

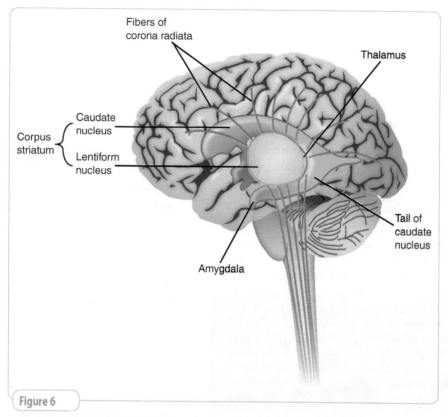

Fibers of
corona radiata

Thalamus

Corpus
striatum

Caudate
nucleus

Lentiform
nucleus

Tail of
caudate
nucleus

Amygdala

Figure 6

The basal ganglia are clusters of gray matter that control learned movement
and are involved with the subconscious control of skeletal muscle tone.

The RAS has particular importance to pharmacology because many drugs act by decreasing neuronal activity in this system to cause drowsiness or sleep. Examples include alcohol and sedative–hypnotics. Lysergic acid diethylamide (LSD) interferes with portions of the RAS, causing unusual sensory experiences such as seeing odors or hearing colors.

Basal nuclei: The **basal nuclei**, also called basal ganglia are a cluster of neurons in the brain that help regulate the initiation and termination of skeletal muscle movement. They also help initiate and terminate certain cognitive functions such as memory, learning, planning, and attention. Connections between the basal ganglia and the limbic system are thought to be associated with psychoses, attention deficit/hyperactivity disorder, and obsessive-compulsive disorder. Reduced dopaminergic transmission through the basal ganglia is the most common etiology for Parkinson's disease. The basal ganglia are illustrated in Figure 6.

Extrapyramidal system: Messages controlling the voluntary movement of skeletal muscle originate in the cerebrum and travel down the CNS in tracts or pathways. The two motor pathways, traveling through the brain, brainstem, and spinal cord, are called pyramidal (direct) and extrapyramidal (indirect). The pyramidal tracts are voluntary tracts involved with the movement of skeletal muscles. The **extrapyramidal system** controls locomotion, complex muscular movements, and posture. The extrapyramidal system has particular importance to pharmacology because it is adversely affected by certain medications, especially the conventional antipsychotic agents. Adverse extrapyramidal symptoms include jerking motions, muscular spasms of the head, face, and neck, and akathisia, an inability to remain at rest. Some extrapyramidal symptoms resemble those of Parkinson's disease.

PharmFACT

Some of the postsynaptic neurons connect with and receive information from as many as 150,000 presynaptic neurons (Silverthorn, 2010).

UNDERSTANDING THE CHAPTER

Key Concepts Summary

1 Medications affect the central nervous system by stimulating or suppressing the firing of specific neurons.

2 Neurons in the central nervous system communicate with each other and with body tissues, using neurotransmitters.

3 The central nervous system is divided into several major structural components.

4 Several functional divisions of the central nervous system are important to pharmacotherapy.

Pearson Nursing Student Resources

Find additional review materials at nursing.pearsonhighered.com

Prepare for success with additional NCLEX®-style practice questions, interactive assignments and activities, web links, animations, videos, and more!

References

Itsak, A. T. (2010). Late onset Alzheimer's disease in older people. *Clinical Interventions in Aging, 5,* 307–311. doi:10.2147/CIA. S11718

Silverthorn, D. U. (2010). *Human physiology: An integrated approach* (5th ed.). San Francisco, CA: Benjamin Cummings.

Selected Bibliography

Krogh, D. (2011). *Biology: A guide to the natural world* (5th ed.). San Francisco, CA: Benjamin Cummings.

Marieb, E. N., & Hoehn, K. (2010). *Human anatomy and physiology* (8th ed.). San Francisco, CA: Benjamin Cummings.

Martini, F. H., Nath, J. L., & Bartholomew, E. F. (2012). *Fundamentals of human anatomy and physiology* (9th ed.). San Francisco, CA: Benjamin Cummings.

Westfall, T. C., & Westfall, D. P. (2011). Neurotransmission: The autonomic and somatic motor nervous systems. In L. L. Brunton, B. A. Chabner, & B. C. Knollman (Eds.), *The pharmacological basis of therapeutics* (12th ed., pp. 171–218). New York, NY: McGraw-Hill.

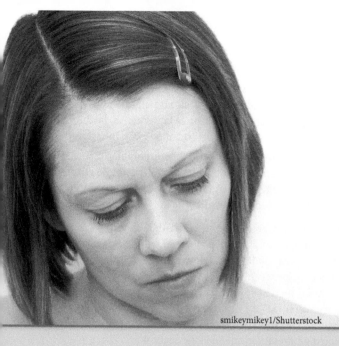

"For the past 4 to 5 weeks my wife, Jane, has been having problems. She doesn't get up to see that the children are off to school, dinner is not started when I get home from work at 6:00 p.m., no housework or laundry has been done, she is frequently still in pajamas with her hair uncombed, and obviously has not showered or brushed her teeth. Her friends say that Jane has not returned their calls in weeks now."

"Charlie Albright," Jane's husband

smikeymikey1/Shutterstock

Pharmacotherapy of Mood Disorders

Chapter Outline

Types of Mood Disorders

Major Depressive Disorder

Pathophysiology of Depression

Assessment of Depression

Nonpharmacologic Therapies for Depression

Pharmacotherapy of Depression

Tricyclic Antidepressants

PROTOTYPE **Imipramine (Tofranil)**

Selective Serotonin Reuptake Inhibitors

PROTOTYPE **Fluoxetine (Prozac, Sarafem)**

Atypical Antidepressants

PROTOTYPE **Venlafaxine (Effexor)**

Monoamine Oxidase Inhibitors

PROTOTYPE **Phenelzine (Nardil)**

Bipolar Disorder

Drugs for Bipolar Disorder

PROTOTYPE **Lithium Carbonate (Eskalith, Lithobid)**

Learning Outcomes

After reading this chapter, the student should be able to:

1. Compare and contrast the major categories of mood disorders and their symptoms.

2. Explain the pathophysiology of major depression and bipolar disorder.

3. Discuss the nurse's role in the assessment of patients with mood disorders.

4. Identify the relationship between suicide and depression.

5. Describe the nurse's role in the pharmacologic and nonpharmacologic management of mood disorders.

6. For each of the classes shown in the chapter outline, identify the prototype and representative drugs and explain the mechanism(s) of drug action, primary indications, contraindications, significant drug interactions, pregnancy category, and important adverse effects.

7. Apply the nursing process to care for patients receiving pharmacotherapy for mood disorders.

From Chapter 23 of *Pharmacology: Connections to Nursing Practice*, Second Edition. Michael Patrick Adams, Carol Quam Urban. Copyright © 2013 by Pearson Education, Inc. All rights reserved.

Key Terms

antidepressants

atypical antidepressants

bipolar disorder

depression

electroconvulsive therapy (ECT)

hypomania

major depressive disorder

mania

monoamine oxidase inhibitors (MAOIs)

mood disorder

mood stabilizers

phototherapy

postpartum onset depression

seasonal affective disorder

serotonin

serotonin syndrome (SES)

suicide

tricyclic antidepressants (TCAs)

tyramine

Inappropriate or unusually intense emotions are among the leading mental health disorders. Although mood changes are a normal part of life, when they become prolonged and severe and impair functioning within the family, work environment, or interpersonal relationships, a patient may be diagnosed as having a mood disorder. The purpose of this chapter is to explain the role of pharmacotherapy in treating the two primary categories of mood disorders: major depression and bipolar disorder.

PharmFACT

Clinical depression affects more than 19 million Americans each year. Depression affects people of all ethnic groups, income levels, ages, and cultural backgrounds (Dryden-Edwards, n.d.).

Types of Mood Disorders

1 The two primary types of mood disorders are depression and bipolar disorder.

Mood disorders form a cluster of mental health conditions that occur frequently in the population. They affect all cultures and people of all ages, from children to older adults. Mood disorders are a major cause of disability and can significantly strain social relationships. They are a leading cause of absenteeism and diminished productivity in the workplace.

Defining and diagnosing mood disorders is sometimes difficult; the line between normal emotion and a mood disorder is often unclear. Because health care providers see patients for such brief periods, they must rely on patient self-reports or caregiver information, both of which are often unreliable. As a working definition, a **mood disorder** is a change in emotion that impairs the patient's ability to effectively deal with normal activities of daily living.

The American Psychiatric Association's *Diagnostic and Statistical Manual of Mental Disorders*, Fourth Edition, Text Revision *(DSM-IV-TR)*, provides the criteria for a wide variety of mental illnesses. According to this manual, mood disorders may be classified as follows:

- **Major depressive disorder.** When people use the word *depression*, they are most often referring to major depressive disorder.
- **Dysthymic disorder.** This is mild, chronic depression that persists for at least 2 continuous years.
- **Bipolar disorder.** Formerly called manic depression, the patient alternates between intense excitement (mania) and major depressive disorder.

- **Manic and hypomanic episodes.** Includes mania symptoms that last for at least 1 week and significantly impact social functioning. Hypomania is less intense, lasting only 4 days and has less impact on social or work functioning.
- **Cyclothymic disorder.** A mild form of bipolar disorder in which the patient alternates between hypomania and mild depression. Largely undiagnosed, 33% of these patients will eventually develop bipolar disorder.

Mood disorders often coexist with other conditions. For example, about 50% of patients diagnosed with major depression also meet the criteria for an anxiety disorder. Of those patients with mood disorder 25% to 40% have a comorbid substance abuse condition. Those with chronic medical conditions such as hypertension (HTN) or arthritis have a higher incidence of depression. The most serious of the comorbid conditions is completed or attempted suicide (see Section 5).

Major Depressive Disorder

2 Major depressive disorder is characterized by a depressed mood, with accompanying symptoms, that lasts at least 2 weeks.

Depression is a disorder characterized by a sad or despondent mood that becomes out of proportion to actual life events. Depression can manifest as an extremely diverse set of symptoms, including lack of energy, sleep disturbances, abnormal eating patterns, or feelings of despair, guilt, and hopelessness. Depression is the most common mental health disorder, affecting approximately 10% to 20% of the population. Although women between the ages of 25 and 45 are more likely to have a depressive disorder than any other group, depression in men more frequently results in suicide. Many persons who are depressed never seek or receive care for their depression.

The *DSM-IV-TR* describes **major depressive disorder** as a depressed mood lasting for a minimum of 2 weeks that is present for most of the day, every day, or almost every day. In addition, at least five of the symptoms shown in Table 1 must be present. Depressed moods caused by general medical conditions or by substances such as alcohol or other central nervous system (CNS) depressants do not warrant a diagnosis of major depressive disorder. For the purposes of this text, the terms *depression* and *major depressive disorder* are considered interchangeable unless otherwise specified.

The *DSM-IV-TR* also states that the current mood of the patient who is depressed must represent a change from previous functioning. For example, some people who might appear depressed to a health care provider may be exhibiting the exact same functioning level that they have exhibited their entire lives; these people would not fit the *DSM-IV-TR* classification of depression.

Once a diagnosis of a mood disorder is made, additional details about the condition may be provided by the health care provider in the form of "specifiers." The use of specifiers gives mental health professionals additional information about the disorder and its treatment. Specifiers are best thought of as subcategories of major depressive disorder and bipolar disorder. Some of the specifiers used with depression include with or without

TABLE 1 Symptoms of Depression

CNS Symptoms	Behavioral Symptoms	General Symptoms
Feelings of despair, lack of self-worth, guilt, and misery	Staying in bed most of the day and night	Extremely tired; without energy
Obsessed with death; expresses desire to die or to commit suicide	Neglecting usual household chores	Vague physical symptoms (GI pain, joint or muscle pain, or headaches)
Delusions or hallucinations	Not going to work, or unable to function effectively at work	Physiological depression (constipation, sleep disorders, or decreased heart rate)
	Abnormal eating patterns (eating too much or not enough)	
	Lack of interest in personal appearance or sex	
	Avoiding psychosocial and interpersonal interactions	

psychotic features, single episode or recurrent, melancholic features, atypical features, and catatonic features. Two additional important specifiers are postpartum onset and seasonal onset.

Up to 80% of women experience brief "baby blues" or **postpartum onset depression** during the first 2 weeks after the birth of a baby. About 10% of new mothers will experience major depression within the first 6 months postdelivery, which is related to the dramatic hormonal shifts that occur during that period. Along with the hormonal changes, additional situational stresses such as changing responsibilities at work and at home, single parenthood, and caring for children and for aging parents may contribute to the onset of symptoms. Because of the potentially serious consequences of postpartum onset depression, some states mandate that all new mothers receive information about these mood disorders prior to their discharge after giving birth. All levels of health care providers in obstetricians' offices, pediatric outpatient settings, and family medicine centers are encouraged to conduct routine screening for symptoms of perinatal mood disorders.

During the dark winter months, some patients experience a type of depression known as **seasonal affective disorder**. Seasonal affective disorder is more common in areas such as Alaska, where the days are very short during the winter months and there is little natural sunlight. This type of depression is associated with a reduced release of the hormone melatonin from the pineal gland. The condition is generally self-limiting and resolves when spring arrives. Exposing patients on a regular basis to specific wavelengths of light may relieve this type of depression and prevent future episodes.

PharmFACT

The lifetime risk for major depression for women is 20% to 30%, and for men 7% to 12%. Overall, 25% of patients who have had a major depressive episode will have chronic, recurrent depression (Ikezu & Gendelman, 2008).

Pathophysiology of Depression

3 The pathophysiology of depression has biologic, genetic, and environmental components.

Depression is one of the oldest known mental health conditions and one of the most frequently diagnosed. Despite this, the etiology of depression is not well understood. Several theories have been proposed to explain the causes of depression and why some people are predisposed to developing the disease. The etiology and pathogenesis are likely influenced by multiple, complex variables.

Research attempting to identify the biologic causes of depression has focused on the levels and function of neurotransmitters in the limbic system of the brain. The limbic system is the region that regulates emotions. Major depression has been associated with abnormally low levels of neurotransmitters such as norepinephrine, serotonin, and dopamine in the limbic system. Although it is well known that some of the antidepressant medications act by increasing the levels of these neurotransmitters, scientists are many years from discovering what role each specific neurotransmitter plays in the development of major depressive disorder. Does having depression deplete the brain of these neurotransmitters, or does a loss of neurotransmitters cause depression? The answers remain elusive.

Certain hormonal abnormalities are associated with depression, suggesting that the endocrine system also plays an important physiological role in the pathogenesis of the disease. About half of depressed persons have abnormally high serum cortisol levels. Cortisol mobilizes the body for stress situations and is thought to reduce serotonin levels in the brain, bringing about symptoms of depression. Hypothyroidism is also strongly linked to depression. In some patients, therapy with thyroid hormone (T_3) results in a marked improvement in depression symptoms.

It is well established that depression has a genetic component. Major depression is 1.5 to 3 times more common in persons who have a first-degree relative (parent or sibling) with depression compared to the general population. In identical twins, when one twin is diagnosed with depression, the other twin has a 50% probability of acquiring the disorder. This relationship holds true whether the twins were raised together or separately. Even fraternal twins have a 19% chance of developing depression when the other twin is diagnosed, which is a percentage higher than that of the general population.

Environmental causes of depression include prolonged stress at work or at home, loss of a loved one, and other traumatic life events. Various childhood events have been associated with an increased risk of adult depression, including sexual or physical abuse, and death of, separation from, or mental illness of a parent.

CONNECTION Checkpoint 23.1

What are the connections between the limbic system, the hypothalamus, and the cerebrum, and how can these connections be used to explain symptoms of depression? *See Answer to Connection Checkpoint 23.1 on student resource website.*

Assessment of Depression

4 Assessment and diagnosis of depression are a collaborative effort among health care providers.

The majority of people who are depressed are not found in psychiatric hospitals but in mainstream everyday settings. For proper diagnosis and treatment to occur, the recognition of depression must be a collaborative effort among health care providers. Because people who are depressed are present in multiple settings and in all areas of practice, every nurse should be proficient in the assessment and nursing care of patients afflicted with this disorder.

The first step in implementing appropriate treatment for depression is a complete medical examination, because the diagnosis of depression begins by ruling out other medical conditions. Certain drugs such as corticosteroids, beta blockers, levodopa, antipsychotic agents, oral contraceptives, and CNS depressants can cause symptoms of clinical depression, and the health care provider must rule out this possibility. Depression may be mimicked by a variety of medical and neurologic disorders, ranging from B-vitamin deficiencies to thyroid gland malfunction to early Alzheimer's disease. If medical causes for the depression are discovered, proper treatment of the underlying disorder may be enough to resolve symptoms of depression. If causes for the depression cannot be identified, a psychiatrist or psychologist may be consulted to perform a comprehensive psychological evaluation to confirm the diagnosis.

Because they are comorbid with depression in a significant number of patients, inquiries should be made about alcohol and drug use and any thoughts about suicide. The initial exam should also include questions about any family history of depressive illness. If other family members have been treated, the nurse should document what therapies they may have received and which were effective. The manifestation of depression that is most obvious to those surrounding a depressed person is a change in attitude toward usual daily activities. The patient loses interest in work, school, or other hobbies or activities that he or she previously enjoyed.

Severe depressive illness, particularly that which is recurrent, will require both medication and psychotherapy to achieve optimum outcomes. Daily outpatient visits to a treatment facility may be necessary when beginning treatment, then tapered to a less frequent schedule as improvement is noted. Some patients, especially those at high risk for suicide, will require an initial period of hospitalization where continuous monitoring is provided.

Depression remains greatly underdiagnosed among older adults despite the fact that as many as 6 million Americans over the age of 65 have this disorder. Of this group, only about 10% receive treatment. Too often elderly patients are reluctant to admit to depression, seeing this as a sign of weakness or an inability to continue to care for themselves. Depression in the older adult may be manifested as difficulty making decisions and as a growing reluctance to leave the home. Feelings of despair, lack of self-worth, and guilt are common. In some cases the person may overuse alcohol or combine alcohol with other CNS depressants, resulting in further depression.

Some people incorrectly believe that the symptoms of depression are a normal part of aging and therefore need no special attention. Factors that contribute to depression in the older adult include loss of spouse or children; the need to move from a long-term residence to a smaller home or in with other family or to assisted living; loss of friends and other support

---

CONNECTIONS

Treating the Diverse Patient

Cultural Influences and Treatment of Depression

Depression (and other mental illness) is universal in all cultures. However, the symptoms, willingness to talk about the disease, and a person's decision to follow a health care provider's recommendation for treatment are not universal. Age, gender, and other factors play a role. Because a stigma is attached to mental illness, assuming there are cultural patterns of depression may prevent health care providers from fully understanding their patient's symptoms unless the patient openly recognizes or admits a relationship between physical symptoms and emotional or mental distress. Mood disorders such as depression may not be viewed as mental health problems but as social or moral ones. An example is a person who makes others uncomfortable by a personal expression of depression. And for many patients in all cultures, it may be considered more acceptable to discuss physical symptoms, but not emotional or mental ones with a health care provider. *Somatization* or the experience of physical symptoms in response to emotional or mental distress, may be a possible reason behind health-seeking behaviors. Unless the provider probes beyond the reported symptoms, depression may go unrecognized.

Nurses have the opportunity to help patients gain optimum health care treatment for undiagnosed depression through the nurse–patient relationship. Through taking a health history, a nurse can indicate a willingness and interest in understanding a patient's explanation for illness. This also helps the nurse to understand the patient's priorities and the cultural importance placed on such symptoms. By recognizing that physical complaints such as excessive fatigue, pain, GI disorders, and lack of concentration may be symptoms of depression, a nurse can ask the patient for help in understanding the cultural meaning of those symptoms to the patient. This holistic approach of listening and validating the patient's experience of illness strengthens the nurse–patient relationship while assessing the extent of impact on the patient's life. By avoiding stereotypes related to culture, nurses can help to increase the opportunity for patients with depression to gain appropriate, culturally sensitive care that works within their own culture and beliefs.

systems; being unmarried; living alone; having multiple health challenges; the expense of polypharmacy; decreased finances; and worry about end-of-life issues.

5 The majority of patients who attempt suicide have major depression.

Suicide is defined as the intentional act of ending one's life. The Centers for Disease Control and Prevention (CDC, 2007) lists suicide as the 11th cause of death in the United States; almost 30,000 people every year take their own lives. Suicide is the third leading cause of death, behind accidents and homicide, among Americans between the ages of 15 and 24. No age group, income level, educational level, race, religion, or other demographic group is exempt from it. About 90% of all persons who turn to suicide, whether successful or not, have a diagnosed mental health or substance abuse disorder (National Institute of Mental Health [NIMH], n.d). Comorbid conditions include mood disorders, psychoses, personality disorder, anxiety disorders, severe insomnia, chronic alcohol or substance use, chronic disabling or painful disease, and family history, especially in the same-sex parent.

The majority of persons who commit suicide have been diagnosed with major depression. Unfortunately, depending on the drug and the individual patient's response, 6 or more weeks of antidepressant pharmacotherapy may be required before the patient begins to feel less depressed. Suicide may occur early in treatment during the period when a patient is being stabilized on the antidepressant. Some theories have proposed that antidepressant medications actually increase the risk of suicide. This prompted the U.S. Food and Drug Administration (FDA) to issue a black box warning in 2004 indicating that antidepressant medications are associated with an increased risk of suicidal thinking and behavior in children and adolescents. This black box warning was expanded in 2007 to include patients 18 to 24 years of age.

A recent study of more than 100,000 patients on antidepressant drugs disputed this theory; the patterns of suicide attempts before and after starting antidepressant therapy were the same (Simon & Savarino, 2007). The highest risk of suicide was in the month before pharmacotherapy, and attempts declined after pharmacotherapy was initiated. Another recent study of patients in the Veterans Administration (VA) system came to similar conclusions; the highest rate of suicide was in depressed patients without pharmacotherapy, and the suicide rate significantly declined in those receiving antidepressants (Gibbons et al., 2007). The relationship between antidepressants and suicide will likely be a continuing topic of research.

So what interventions can the nurse implement to reduce the potential for suicidal behavior during antidepressant therapy? Careful monitoring of the patient is the simplest yet most important intervention. Weekly and even daily patient contact may be necessary until the antidepressant begins to effectively elevate mood, which would typically be 4 to 12 weeks. A patient who has had a previous suicide attempt is at higher risk and must be more carefully monitored. If a person verbalizes about committing suicide, the talk must be taken seriously. It is a myth that a person who talks about suicide will not actually act. The person may be so depressed that suicide seems like the only option, and talking about it to a friend or nurse may be a last attempt at getting help or having someone intercede. The nurse must judiciously monitor all prescribed drugs because suicidal patients often take overdoses of their medications. Therapy with multiple CNS depressants such as for pain, anxiety, insomnia, and depression is strongly discouraged because these agents produce additive sedation. Worsening symptoms of depression must be reported immediately because these may indicate that the drug is not working or that the patient is not compliant with pharmacotherapy. Switching to a different antidepressant or even hospitalization may be necessary.

Nonpharmacologic Therapies for Depression

6 Depression is sometimes treated with nonpharmacologic therapies.

Although pharmacotherapy is the standard treatment for patients with serious depression, other therapies may be beneficial for patients with mild to moderate depression or for those whose condition is refractory to conventional treatment. Indeed, psychotherapy is often the treatment of choice when the patient is willing to participate and the depressive state is mild to moderate in severity. Other nonpharmacologic therapies for depression are shown in Table 2.

Counseling therapies help patients gain insight into and resolve mental health issues through verbal "give-and-take" with the therapist. Behavioral therapies help patients learn how to obtain more satisfaction and rewards through their own actions and how to unlearn the behavioral patterns that contribute to or result from their depression. Interpersonal therapy focuses on a patient's disturbed personal relationships that both cause and exacerbate the depression. Cognitive–behavioral therapies help patients change negative styles of thought and behavior that are often associated with their depression. Psychodynamic therapies focus on resolving the patients' internal conflicts by looking at the influence of past experiences on current behavior and how behavior is influenced by emotional factors. These therapies are sometimes postponed until the acute depressive symptoms have improved.

Light therapy or **phototherapy** is a type of therapy especially useful for people with seasonal affective disorder. Phototherapy uses artificial lighting approximately 5 to 20 times brighter than normal indoor lighting while the patient sits with eyes open about 3 feet away from and at eye level with the light source. Normal activities can be pursued during the treatment, which can be conducted in the patient's home.

As illness and other factors limit the ability of older adults to function in their normal routines, the risk of depression rises, especially if the need for health care in the home or in a health care setting becomes a necessity. Not all depression is overt and symptoms such as trouble sleeping, fatigue, changes in appetite, or forgetfulness may be diagnosed as "normal" processes of aging while a possible cause, underlying depression, is not diagnosed or treated. As in younger patients, accurate

TABLE 2 Nonpharmacologic Therapies for Major Depression

Type	Definition
Cognitive–behavioral therapy	Therapy that helps patients change the negative styles of thought and behavior that are often associated with their depression.
Electroconvulsive therapy (ECT)	The induction of a brief convulsion by passing an electric current through the brain as therapy for affective disorders, especially in patients who have not responded to pharmacotherapy.
Interpersonal therapy	Therapy focusing on the patient's disturbed personal relationships that both cause and exacerbate the depression.
Light therapy or phototherapy	Therapy that uses artificial lighting that is 5 to 20 times brighter than usual indoor lighting; it is used to simulate natural sunlight in areas where there is little natural sunlight for several months of the year, such as Alaska and other areas near the North Pole.
Psychodynamic therapy	Therapy focusing on resolving a patient's internal conflicts.
Repetitive transcranial magnetic stimulation (rTMS) therapy	An effective somatic therapy, experimental in the United States, that involves a device that administers a train of multiple stimuli per second. The device is a metal coil that is placed on or near the patient's head, allowing the magnetic field to pass through the skull and into specific targeted areas of the brain.
Vagus nerve stimulation (VNS)	Somatic therapy that involves placing a small generator into the patient's chest; it is attached to an electrode with ends wrapped around the left vagus nerve on the patient's neck; the generator is programmed for frequency and intensity of stimulus. The electrical current stimulates the vagus nerve.

CONNECTIONS

Lifespan Considerations
Depression and Suicide Risk in Older Adults

While depression and suicide risk may seem like health issues affecting the younger populations of adolescence or young or middle adulthood, the rate of suicide linked to depression is actually higher in the over-age-65 population than in younger age groups. According to NIMH (2010), the rate of suicide was 12.7 out of 100,000 people for young adults ages 20 to 24, while the rate for adults older than age 65 was 14.3 of every 100,000 and for non-Hispanic white males over 85, the number was 47 out of every 100,000.

diagnosis is key and the nurse can be alert to vague symptoms that may signify the development of depression, especially if changes in health or routines have led to a decreased ability in functioning for the older adult. Treatments such as selective serotonin reuptake inhibitors (SSRIs) and psychotherapy have been shown both to improve symptoms of depression in older adults and to increase their quality of life with improved social, mental, and physical functioning (Unutzer, 2007).

In patients with serious and life-threatening mood disorders that are unresponsive to pharmacotherapy and psychotherapy, **electroconvulsive therapy (ECT)** continues to be a useful treatment. ECT induces a brief convulsion (grand mal seizure) by passing an electric current into the brain through electrodes applied to one or both temples. The patient is anesthetized and given a muscle relaxant prior to the treatment and therefore is unaware of the convulsion as it is occurring. Although ECT has been found to be safe, there are still deaths (1 in 10,000 patients) and other serious complications related to seizure activity and anesthesia caused by ECT. Typically, 6 to 12 treatments are needed to relieve depression: in severe, refractory cases ECT may be continued over a period of years. Adverse effects of ECT include transient short-term memory loss and confusion

immediately after the procedure. If the patient is aware of these before beginning treatment, there is much less anxiety when one or both of them occur.

Repetitive transcranial magnetic stimulation (rTMS) is an emerging therapy for major depression. rTMS is a noninvasive procedure that passes a high electric current through a wire stimulation coil placed on or close to a specific area of the head. Treatments are generally administered daily; the length of treatment varies according to patient response. In contrast with ECT, rTMS has minimal effects on memory, does not require general anesthesia, and produces its effects without a generalized seizure. The major concern with this type of therapy is the possibility of inducing seizures. Further research is needed to confirm its effectiveness at relieving depression.

Another somatic therapy currently under investigation is vagus nerve stimulation (VNS). VNS involves the surgical implantation of a small generator, about 3 to 4 inches in diameter, into the patient's chest. An electrode is threaded through the subcutaneous tissue from the generator to the vagus nerve on the left side of the patient's neck. The left vagus connects to the brainstem and deep brain structures thought to be involved in epilepsy and some psychiatric disorders. Stimulating these fibers affects the concentration of the neurotransmitter gamma aminobutyric acid (GABA) and other neurotransmitters in that area. Once implanted, the generator is programmed via computer to adjust both the intensity and frequency of the stimulus according to the patient's needs. VNS is approved in the United States for treating epilepsy, and for the adjunctive treatment of chronic depression for adult patients who are experiencing a major depressive episode and have not had an adequate response to multiple antidepressant medications. Adverse effects have been mild and mostly involve hoarseness, which is thought to be secondary to the vagal stimulation.

PharmFACT

Approximately 22% of female and 12% of male students in grades 9 through 12 seriously consider suicide each year. Over 8% state that they actually attempted suicide. Among people ages 15 to 24, suicide accounts for 13% of all deaths annually (CDC, 2007).

Pharmacotherapy of Depression

7 The mechanism of action of antidepressants involves modulation of neurotransmitter levels in the brain.

Antidepressants are drugs used to enhance, elevate, or stabilize mood. In the treatment of depression they are used to treat all symptoms of major depressive disorder as well as the depressive phases of bipolar disorder. They are ineffective against the manic phases of bipolar disorder, and other drugs must be used to control those symptoms (see Section 12).

The antidepressants act by restoring normal neurotransmitter balances in specific regions of the brain. Depending on the medication, the primary neurotransmitters affected are norepinephrine, serotonin, and, to a lesser degree, dopamine. The two basic mechanisms of action of antidepressants are blocking the enzymatic breakdown of norepinephrine and slowing the reuptake of serotonin into neurons. Although antidepressants may not be able to completely restore chemical balance, they help to manage depressive symptoms while the patient develops effective strategies for coping.

In addition to elevating mood, changing the neurotransmitter balance has a number of other effects on the brain. Some of the antidepressants have become major drugs in the treatment of anxiety disorders such as phobia, obsessive–compulsive behavior, panic disorder, and generalized anxiety disorder. Certain antidepressants are also beneficial as adjuvant analgesics in the pharmacotherapy of pain. Antidepressants are beneficial in treating depression that is often associated with painful, chronic conditions such as fibromyalgia or muscle spasticity.

Once patients begin to "feel better" they sometimes want to discontinue drug therapy due to the expense of the medication or because they are experiencing uncomfortable adverse effects. Nurses must be aware that many patients taking antidepressants stop taking their medication without notifying their health care provider. Unfortunately, about half of these patients will relapse within 6 months of discontinuing antidepressant therapy; the percentage increases to 85% after 3 years. It is important to teach patients that antidepressant therapy may extend for many years and that adherence to the health care provider's instructions is essential for the long-term maintenance of mental health. In general, antidepressant therapy should continue for a minimum of 6 months after the depressive symptoms resolve.

When administered at therapeutic doses, all antidepressants have similar effectiveness; therefore, the choice of drug is not usually based on this factor. The treatment of depression, however, is highly individualized and patients who are unresponsive to one class of medications may respond favorably to drugs from a different class. In fact, patients may respond differently to drugs within the *same* class. Furthermore, the spectrum of adverse effects differs among the classes, and patients may find that drugs from one class are more tolerable than another. Overall, about 65% of patients will respond favorably to antidepressant pharmacotherapy. Success rates improve to 85% when psychotherapy or alternative or adjunctive medicine is used along with antidepressant medications. The four primary classes of antidepressants, shown in Table 3, are as follows:

- Tricyclic antidepressants (TCAs)
- Selective serotonin reuptake inhibitors (SSRIs)
- Atypical antidepressants
- Monoamine oxidase inhibitors (MAOIs).

Tricyclic Antidepressants

8 Tricyclic antidepressants have been the mainstay for the treatment of depression but have many adverse effects.

The **tricyclic antidepressants (TCAs)** have been available in the United States for more than 50 years, and they are still prescribed for some patients with major depressive disorder. Imipramine (Tofranil), the prototype drug for this class, was the first TCA available. This group of medications is named after its molecular structure, which has a nucleus that consists of three rings. This arrangement is very similar to the structure of the phenothiazine antipsychotics. Thus these two classes of drugs share similar adverse effects.

The TCAs act by blocking the reuptake transport of the neurotransmitters norepinephrine and serotonin, as shown in Figure 1. This blockade results in more neurotransmitters being available in the synaptic space, leading to a more intensified action. Some TCAs such as desipramine, maprotiline, and protriptyline are specific to blocking the reuptake of norepinephrine, whereas the other drugs in this class affect both norepinephrine and serotonin. In general, all TCAs have similar effectiveness and exhibit the same types of adverse effects.

The advantages of TCAs are that they are inexpensive and their effectiveness in treating depression has been well

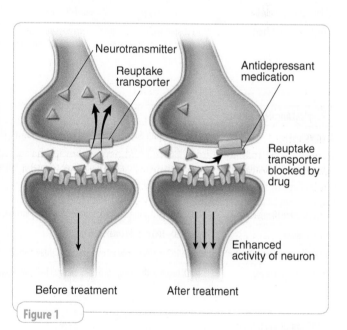

Figure 1

Mechanisms of action of antidepressants: (a) In adrenergic and serotonergic neurons the activity of the neurotransmitter is terminated by reuptake. (b) Tricyclic antidepressants and SSRIs produce their effects by inhibiting the reuptake of neurotransmitters. The neurotransmitter accumulates in the synaptic cleft and activates more receptors, thus causing an enhanced effect at the synapse.

439

TABLE 3 Antidepressant Drugs

Drug	Route and Adult Dose (maximum dose where indicated)	Adverse Effects
Tricyclic Antidepressants (TCAs)		
amitriptyline (Elavil)	PO: 75–100 mg/day (max: 300 mg/day)	*Drowsiness, sedation, dizziness, orthostatic hypotension, dry mouth, constipation, urinary retention, constipation, blurred vision, mydriasis, tachycardia* <u>Bone marrow depression, seizures, dysrhythmias, heart block, MI, hepatitis, acute renal failure</u>
clomipramine (Anafranil)	PO: 25 mg once daily (max: 250 mg/day)	
desipramine (Norpramin)	PO: 75–100 mg/day; may increase to 150–300 mg/day	
doxepin (Sinequan)	PO: 75–150 mg/day at bedtime (max: 300 mg/day)	
imipramine (Tofranil)	PO: 75–150 mg/day (max: 300 mg/day)	
	IM: 50–100 mg/day in divided doses	
maprotiline (Ludiomil)	PO: 25 mg tid (max: 225 mg/day)	
nortriptyline (Aventyl, Pamelor)	PO: 25 mg tid or qid (max: 150 mg/day)	
protriptyline (Vivactil)	PO: 15–40 mg/day in 3–4 divided doses (max: 60 mg/day)	
trimipramine (Surmontil)	PO: 75–100 mg/day in divided doses (max: 300 mg/day)	
Selective Serotonin Reuptake Inhibitors (SSRIs)		
citalopram (Celexa)	PO: start at 20 mg once daily; may increase to 40 mg after 1 week (max: 60 mg/day)	*Nausea, vomiting, dry mouth, insomnia, somnolence, headache, nervousness, anxiety, diarrhea, dizziness, anorexia, fatigue, sexual dysfunction, weight changes* <u>Stevens–Johnson syndrome (SJS), serotonin syndrome, suicidal ideation in children and young adults</u>
escitalopram (Lexapro)	PO: 10 mg once daily; may increase to 20 mg after 1 week (max: 20 mg/day)	
fluoxetine (Prozac)	PO: 20 mg/day in the a.m., may increase by 20 mg/day at weekly intervals (max: 80 mg/day); when stable may switch to 90-mg sustained release capsule once weekly (max: 90 mg/week)	
fluvoxamine (Luvox)	PO: start with 50 mg/day and increase every 4–7 days as needed (max: 300 mg/day)	
paroxetine (Paxil, Pexeva)	PO (immediate release): start with 20 mg once daily and increase by 10 mg each week as needed (max: 60 mg/day for immediate release form)	
	PO (sustained release): 25 mg daily and increase by 12.5-mg intervals (max: 62.5 mg/day)	
sertraline (Zoloft)	PO: start with 50 mg once daily and increase at weekly intervals as needed (max: 200 mg/day)	
Serotonin–Norepinephrine Reuptake Inhibitors (SNRIs)		
desvenlafaxine (Pristiq)	PO: 50 mg once daily (max: 100 mg/day)	*Nausea, dry mouth, constipation, sweating, agitation, somnolence, decreased appetite, changes in weight (loss or gain), increased blood glucose level (duloxetine)* <u>Suicidal ideation, hepatotoxicity, syncope, neuroleptic malignant syndrome, abnormal bleeding, HTN (desvenlafaxine, venlafaxine), seizures</u>
duloxetine (Cymbalta)	PO: 40–60 mg/day in 1–2 divided doses (max: 60 mg/day)	
venlafaxine (Effexor)	PO: start with 75 mg/day and increase slowly at 4–7-day intervals as needed (max: 375 mg/day for regular release; 225 mg/day for extended release)	
Atypical Antidepressants		
amoxapine	PO: start with 50 mg bid–tid and increase to 100 mg bid–tid by the end of the first week (max: 400 mg/day)	*Insomnia, nausea, dry mouth, constipation, increased blood pressure and heart rate, dizziness, sweating, agitation, blurred vision, headache, dizziness, tremor, vomiting, drowsiness, somnolence, increased appetite, orthostatic hypotension* <u>SJS, seizures, vaginal, uterine, or anal hemorrhage, suicidal ideation, priapism, neuroleptic malignant syndrome (amoxapine), parkinsonism (amoxapine), elevated hepatic enzymes (mirtazapine), bone marrow suppression (mirtazapine), liver failure (nefazodone)</u>
bupropion (Wellbutrin, Zyban)	PO: start with 100 mg bid (immediate release) or 150 mg once daily (extended release) and increase gradually as needed (max: 450 mg/day for immediate release, 400 mg/day for extended release, or 300 mg/day for Zyban)	
mirtazapine (Remeron)	PO: 15 mg/day in a single dose at bedtime; may increase every 1–2 weeks (max: 45 mg/day)	
nefazodone	PO: 50–100 mg bid (max: 600 mg/day)	
trazodone (Desyrel, Oleptro)	PO: 150 mg/day; may increase by 50 mg/day every 3–4 days (max: 375 mg/day)	
vilazodone (Viibryd)	PO: begin with 10 mg once daily and gradually increase to 40 mg once daily with food	
MAO Inhibitors (MAOIs)		
isocarboxazid (Marplan)	PO: 10–30 mg/day (max: 30 mg/day)	*Drowsiness, insomnia, orthostatic hypotension, blurred vision, nausea, constipation, anorexia, dry mouth, urinary retention, sexual dysfunction, overactivity* <u>Hypertensive crisis, circulatory collapse, dysrhythmias</u>
phenelzine (Nardil)	PO: 15 mg tid rapidly increase to at least 60 mg/day tid or qid (max: 90 mg/day)	
selegiline (Emsam)	Transdermal: one patch (6 mg)/day	
tranylcypromine (Parnate)	PO: 30 mg/day; may increase by 10 mg/day at 3-week intervals (max: 60 mg/day)	

Note: Italics indicate common adverse effects. <u>Underline</u> indicates serious adverse effects.

established for many decades. They are rapidly absorbed when given orally (PO) and widely distributed throughout the body. Frequent adverse effects, however, have limited their use. Many health care providers prefer to prescribe drugs in the SSRI class because they are better tolerated by most patients.

Blockade of muscarinic receptors by TCAs is responsible for causing a high incidence of anticholinergic adverse effects with symptoms such as dry mouth, blurred vision, constipation, urinary retention, and tachycardia. Orthostatic hypotension is frequently reported and may be serious enough to cause injury due to falls. One of the most serious adverse effects is the ability of TCAs and some of their metabolites to accumulate in cardiac tissue and depress the myocardium. They can cause life-threatening cardiac dysrhythmias, especially if the patient receives an overdose.

A few of the TCAs have central effects that cause sedation, which can usually be managed by taking the drugs at bedtime. Sedation is worsened by the concurrent use of other CNS depressants such as alcohol. Confusion, dizziness, and fatigue are other possible dose-limiting effects of TCAs. At high doses some cause seizures.

Compared to other classes of antidepressants, TCAs exhibit a relatively high incidence of sexual dysfunction, including impotence and delayed ejaculation in men, and breast enlargement and impaired orgasm in women. Weight gain is possible. In addition, some patients quickly change mood from depression to hypomania or mania and may begin to display symptoms of bipolar disorder. These patients require a dosage adjustment or a change to a different antidepressant.

Tolerance and psychological dependence are usually not major problems when using TCAs. Therapy may often be conducted for years without requiring a dosage adjustment. Unlike many CNS depressants, antidepressants such as the TCAs are not drugs of abuse. Patients on high doses for prolonged periods, however, may exhibit a mild withdrawal syndrome on discontinuation and experience symptoms such as irritability, nausea, sleep impairment, muscle aches, and fatigue. To avoid unpleasant symptoms, and to ensure that depression does not quickly return, these drugs are usually withdrawn gradually.

CONNECTION Checkpoint 23.2

Anticholinergic effects are common with TCAs and some other antidepressants. Name the prototype anticholinergic drug. If anticholinergic effects become prominent in a patient, what class of drugs can be used to counteract the cardiovascular adverse effects? *See Answer to Connection Checkpoint 23.2 on student resource website.*

| PROTOTYPE DRUG | Imipramine (Tofranil) |

Classification: **Therapeutic:** Tricyclic antidepressant
Pharmacologic: Norepinephrine reuptake inhibitor

Therapeutic Effects and Uses: Approved in 1959, imipramine is an older drug that is effective in treating major depressive disorder. Like other TCAs, it is given PO and is well absorbed from the GI tract. Although very effective, a drawback to the use of imipramine is that it takes 2 to 6 weeks to achieve full therapeutic effect. During the initial weeks of therapy when

blood levels of imipramine have not yet produced their full therapeutic effects, suicide risks may increase, especially in children and adolescents. Although it is not a preferred therapy for the disorder, imipramine is one of only two drugs approved for nocturnal enuresis, or bedwetting, in children. The urge to urinate is diminished by the anticholinergic (urinary retention) effects of the drug.

Like other TCAs, imipramine has a number of off-label indications. These include the adjuvant treatment of cancer or neuropathic pain, overactive bladder, attention deficit/hyperactivity disorder (ADHD), insomnia and bulimia. The active metabolite of imipramine is desipramine, which is marketed separately as Norpramin.

Mechanism of Action: Imipramine blocks the reuptake of norepinephrine and serotonin into presynaptic nerve terminals. This results in an increased action of both neurotransmitters in neurons. Imipramine also blocks acetylcholine receptors, which is likely responsible for its effectiveness in treating enuresis.

Pharmacokinetics:

Route(s)	PO, IM (rare)
Absorption	Well absorbed from the GI tract and muscle
Distribution	Widely distributed; crosses the placenta; secreted in breast milk; 85–95% bound to plasma protein
Primary metabolism	Hepatic; metabolized to the active metabolite desipramine
Primary excretion	Renal; small amounts in bile and feces
Onset of action	1–2 h for peak serum level; mood elevation requires 2–3 weeks
Duration of action	Not known

Adverse Effects: Frequent adverse reactions with imipramine include orthostatic hypotension (the most common adverse effect), dizziness, confusion, drowsiness, diarrhea, dry mouth, increased appetite, jaundice, urinary retention, rash, pruritus, and photosensitivity. Serious adverse reactions include seizures, hepatitis, acute renal failure, paralytic ileus, leukopenia, agranulocytosis, thrombocytopenia, or eosinophilia. Serious adverse reactions occur with acute doses when imipramine accumulates in cardiac tissue; dysrhythmias, heart failure, or myocardial infarction (MI) can occur. **Black Box Warning:** Antidepressants increase the risk of suicidal thinking and behavior in children, adolescents, and young adults. Patients of all ages should be monitored and observed closely during therapy for clinical worsening, suicidality, or unusual changes in behavior.

Contraindications/Precautions: Imipramine should not be used by patients with seizure disorders because it lowers the seizure threshold. It must be used with caution in persons with suicidal tendencies, urinary retention, prostatic hyperplasia, cardiac or hepatic disease, increased intraocular pressure, or hyperthyroidism. Use in patients with Parkinson's disease will induce or worsen parkinsonism symptoms. Patients with cardiac disease such as heart failure, QT prolongation, or history of MI should be carefully monitored during therapy; use in patients recovering from MI has resulted in sudden death. Imipramine should not be used during pregnancy or lactation.

Drug Interactions: Like other TCAs, imipramine is metabolized by hepatic P450 enzymes and is highly protein bound; thus there is a high potential for drug–drug interactions. Increased sedation can occur when imipramine is given concurrently with alcohol, barbiturates, benzodiazepines, direct-acting sympathomimetics, and other CNS depressants. Drug interactions causing decreased effects of imipramine include oral contraceptives, clonidine, carbamazepine, and indirect-acting sympathomimetics. Concurrent use with thyroid hormone may induce dysrhythmias. Imipramine should not be given concurrently with other drugs that prolong the QT interval, such as the Class IA antidysrhythmics, because of the potential for serious cardiac toxicity. Phenothiazines and TCAs are structurally very similar and concurrent use will likely cause additive anticholinergic adverse effects. Concurrent use of MAOIs must be avoided because this combination may cause hypertensive crisis, seizures, or hyperpyretic crisis. SSRIs must not be used concurrently; this can cause increased toxicity of TCAs. **Herbal/Food:** Several commonly used herbal products may lead to increased imipramine effects, including kava, hops, lavender, valerian, skullcap, and chamomile. An increased anticholinergic effect can occur with the use of belladonna, jimsonweed, or henbane. Serotonin syndrome may occur with the use of St. John's wort.

Pregnancy: Category C.

Treatment of Overdose: Overdoses with TCAs may be life threatening with symptoms that include mixed mania and depression followed by coma. Medical management includes treating possible seizures, hypotension, and dysrhythmias.

Nursing Responsibilities: Key nursing implications for patients receiving imipramine are included in the Nursing Practice Application for Patients Receiving Antidepressant Therapy.

Lifespan and Diversity Considerations:

- Use special caution when administering this drug to the older adult who is at increased risk of falls. Provide assistance with ambulation as needed if dizziness or blurred vision occur.
- Monitor the older adult for urinary retention, dry mouth, and other anticholinergic effects.

Patient and Family Education:

- The full therapeutic effects of the medication will take 2 to 6 weeks or more to appear. Monitor the patient more closely during the early stages of therapy because suicide risk may increase during this time.
- Make position changes slowly when moving from a lying to a standing position to prevent dizziness and possible fainting.

- Do not take any other prescription or nonprescription drugs, dietary supplements, or herbal products without approval of the health care provider.
- Maintain all recommended follow-up appointments with mental health professionals.
- Immediately notify the health care provider of any known or suspected pregnancy. Oral contraceptives may be less effective, so barrier contraception must be used.
- Anticholinergic effects such as dry mouth may occur. Some simple ways to decrease symptoms are to increase fluids, suck on sugarless hard candy, chew sugarless gum, or take frequent sips of water.
- The drug should not be withdrawn abruptly but must be tapered off. Notify the health care provider if the patient suddenly stops taking the drug.

Drugs Similar to Imipramine (Tofranil)

Nine TCAs are available. Desipramine is an active metabolite of imipramine, and the two drugs have the same actions and adverse effects, as previously described.

Amitriptyline (Elavil) and nortriptyline (Aventyl, Pamelor): Amitriptyline has been available by the PO route since 1961 for the therapy of major depression. It has been used for a large number of off-label indications, including neuropathic pain syndromes such as fibromyalgia, and nocturnal enuresis, social anxiety disorder, ADHD, migraines, persistent hiccups, insomnia, and bulimia. It produces more sedation than most other TCAs and is thus taken at bedtime. It is metabolized in the liver to nortriptyline, which is marketed as a separate drug. Both amitriptyline and nortriptyline produce significant anticholinergic adverse effects. Like other TCAs, cardiac toxicity is a concern at high doses. These drugs are pregnancy category D.

Clomipramine (Anafranil): Approved in 1991, the only FDA-approved indication for clomipramine is obsessive–compulsive disorder (OCD). Depression is an off-label indication. Other off-label uses are premature ejaculation and childhood autism. The drug produces significant anticholinergic effects and orthostatic hypotension; thus it is not a first-line drug for depression. This drug is pregnancy category C.

Doxepin (Sinequan): Approved in 1969 to treat major depression, doxepin is also FDA approved to treat insomnia (Silenor) and anxiety. Doses used to treat depression (75–150 mg/day) are much higher than those used for insomnia (3–6 mg). When given PO, the most common adverse effects are sedation, nausea, and upper respiratory tract infection. A topical form of doxepin (Zonalon) is available for pruritus associated with atopic dermatitis. Because doxepin is absorbed through the skin, topical applications can result in systemic adverse effects. This drug is pregnancy category C.

Maprotiline (Ludiomil): Maprotiline does not have a tricyclic chemical structure but it is included with the TCAs because it has very similar therapeutic and adverse effects. It was approved to treat depression in 1980. Off-label indications include ADHD and enuresis. It has the same adverse effects as other drugs in this class and offers no specific advantages over other TCAs. This drug is pregnancy category D.

Protriptyline (Vivactil): Protriptyline is an oral antidepressant that was approved in 1967. It has the same adverse effects as other TCAs except that it tends to produce CNS stimulation rather than sedation. It is the only TCA that has respiratory stimulant activity. These respiratory effects have led to its occasional off-label use for treating chronic obstructive pulmonary disease or sleep apnea. This drug is pregnancy category C.

Trimipramine (Surmontil): Trimipramine was approved in 1979 for major depression. Off-label indications include anxiety, schizophrenia, and rheumatoid arthritis. Drowsiness is a serious problem; however, the incidence of anticholinergic effects is one of the lowest of any drug in its class. It offers no major benefits over other TCAs. This drug is pregnancy category C.

Selective Serotonin Reuptake Inhibitors
9 Selective serotonin reuptake inhibitors are the drugs of choice for treating depression due to their low incidence of serious adverse effects.

Serotonin is a natural neurotransmitter in the CNS that is found in high concentrations in certain neurons in the hypothalamus, limbic system, medulla, and spinal cord. It is essential for several body activities, including the cycling between NREM and REM sleep, pain perception, and emotions. Lack of adequate serotonin in the limbic regions of the CNS can lead to depression. The actions of serotonin are terminated when it is metabolized to a less active substance by the enzyme monoamine oxidase (MAO). This mechanism is illustrated in Figure 2. In the scientific literature, serotonin is commonly referred to by its chemical name, 5-hydroxytryptamine (5-HT).

In the 1970s, it became increasingly clear that serotonin had a more substantial role in depression than once thought. Clinicians knew that the TCAs altered the sensitivity of serotonin to certain receptors in the brain, but they did not know how this chemical change connected to symptoms of depression. Ongoing efforts to find antidepressants with fewer adverse effects than TCAs and monoamine oxidase

inhibitors (MAOIs) led to the development of the selective serotonin reuptake inhibitors (SSRIs), which were first introduced in 1987. Whereas the TCAs inhibit the reuptake of both norepinephrine and serotonin into presynaptic nerve terminals, the SSRIs selectively target serotonin. Increased levels of serotonin in the synaptic spaces induce complex neurotransmitter changes in presynaptic and postsynaptic neurons in the brain. Essentially, presynaptic receptors become less sensitive, and postsynaptic receptors become more sensitive.

SSRIs are as effective in treating depression as the TCAs but exhibit fewer significant adverse effects. Sympathomimetic effects (increased heart rate and HTN) and anticholinergic effects (dry mouth, blurred vision, urinary retention, and constipation) are less common with this drug class. Sedation occurs less frequently, and cardiotoxicity is not observed. The greater safety profile of the SSRIs has led to their becoming drugs of choice for depression.

One of the most common adverse effects of SSRIs relates to sexual dysfunction. Up to 70% of both men and women can experience decreased libido and lack of ability to reach orgasm. In men, delayed ejaculation and impotence may occur. For patients who are sexually active, these adverse effects may be serious enough to cause nonadherence with pharmacotherapy, and a different antidepressant may be indicated. The SSRIs can cause weight gain, which may also lead to discontinuation. Other common adverse effects include nausea, headache, nervousness, and insomnia.

All drugs in the SSRI class have equal effectiveness and similar adverse effects. In general, SSRIs produce elevations in mood more quickly than TCAs, which can be a major advantage when treating serious depression disorders. Like the TCAs, the SSRIs are used for a wide variety of other mental health disorders, including OCD, social anxiety disorder, panic disorder, generalized anxiety disorder, PTSD, and premenstrual dysphoric disorder. They are one of the most widely prescribed drug classes in the United States.

Serotonin syndrome (SES) is a serious medical condition that can occur when a patient is taking multiple medications that affect the metabolism, synthesis, or reuptake of serotonin, causing this neurotransmitter to accumulate in neurons in the CNS. These drugs include SSRIs, MAOIs, TCAs, lithium, St. John's wort, opioids, and triptans. SES sometimes occurs as a result of

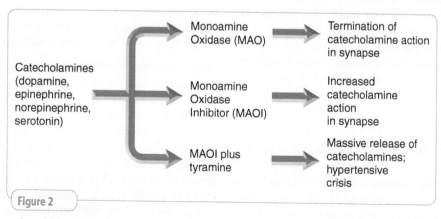

Figure 2

Catecholamines and monoamine oxidase.

illicit drug use because amphetamines, cocaine, MDMA or ecstasy, and opioids also affect serotonin levels. Symptoms of SES include mental status changes (confusion, anxiety, restlessness), HTN, tremors, sweating, hyperpyrexia, and ataxia. Symptoms can begin as early as 2 hours after taking the first dose or as late as several weeks after initiating pharmacotherapy. Conservative treatment is to discontinue the drugs responsible for causing the syndrome and to provide supportive care; the condition usually resolves in 24 hours. In severe cases, mechanical ventilation and administration of muscle relaxants such as benzodiazepines may be necessary. If left untreated, death may occur.

PROTOTYPE DRUG | Fluoxetine (Prozac, Sarafem)

Classification: **Therapeutic:** Antidepressant, antianxiety agent
Pharmacologic: Selective serotonin reuptake inhibitor (SSRI)

Therapeutic Effects and Uses: Approved in 1987, fluoxetine was the first SSRI marketed to treat major depressive disorder in the United States. Fluoxetine was subsequently approved to treat bulimia nervosa, the first medication ever approved for this condition. It is the only SSRI approved for the treatment of pediatric depression. It is approved for the treatment of OCD in both adults and children and for panic disorder. Fluoxetine is available as tablets, capsules, oral solution, and delayed release capsules. Sarafem is a formulation of fluoxetine specifically marketed for premenstrual dysphoric disorder in a pulvule—a gelatin-based capsule. It is taken daily or for just the 2 weeks prior to an expected menses. Prozac Weekly is a capsule containing enteric-coated granules. Patients who have stabilized on daily fluoxetine can be switched to Prozac Weekly, which offers the convenience of once-a-week dosing. Symbyax is a fixed-dose combination of fluoxetine and olanzapine that is indicated for bipolar disorder. Olanzapine, an antipsychotic agent, is marketed by itself as Zyprexa for schizophrenia and the manic phase of bipolar disorder.

Fluoxetine is used off-label to treat many other disorders involving multiple body systems. Off-label indications include anorexia nervosa, obesity, alcohol dependence in patients with alcoholism, fibromyalgia, autism, refractory orthostatic hypotension, premature ejaculation, premenstrual dysphoric disorder, and menopausal hot flashes. Although patients gradually begin to feel less depressed after about 2 weeks of therapy, optimal response may take 8 weeks or longer.

Fluoxetine is extensively metabolized in the liver to norfluoxetine, which has about the same pharmacologic activity as the parent drug. Fluoxetine and norfluoxetine have long half-lives; it takes 30 to 60 days after discontinuing the drug for them to be eliminated by the body. This duration is even more prolonged in patients with liver disease.

Mechanism of Action: As with other serotonin reuptake inhibitors, fluoxetine blocks the uptake of the neurotransmitter serotonin (but not norepinephrine) at the neuronal presynaptic membrane. This increases the amount of neurotransmitter available at the postsynaptic receptor sites, thus enhancing the actions of serotonin.

Pharmacokinetics:

Route	PO
Absorption	Readily absorbed
Distribution	Widely distributed, including the cerebrospinal fluid; likely crosses the placenta; secreted in breast milk; 94% bound to plasma protein
Primary metabolism	Metabolized in the liver to norfluoxetine, an active metabolite
Primary excretion	Renal, small amounts in feces
Onset of action	Peak plasma level: 6–8 h
Duration of action	Half-life: 2–3 days

Adverse Effects: Fluoxetine is better tolerated than drugs from either the TCA or the MAOI classes. The most common adverse effects are nausea and vomiting, which diminish as therapy progresses. Other common GI effects include diarrhea, anorexia, cramping, and flatulence. Fluoxetine does not cause sedation; in fact, insomnia may occur in as many as 25% of patients receiving the drug. Fluoxetine also does not cause the serious cardiotoxicity, orthostatic hypotension, or anticholinergic effects seen with the TCAs. Fluctuations in weight are common. Significant anorexia and weight loss occur in 10% to 15% of patients, whereas others experience a weight gain of as much as 20 pounds or more. Patients may experience various types of sexual dysfunction, including delayed ejaculation, impotence, anorgasmia, decreased libido, and priapism. The drug may induce seizures in patients with preexisting seizure disorders or during overdoses. Other adverse effects include cramping, constipation, poor concentration, diarrhea, hot flashes, palpitations, and nervousness. Serotonin syndrome can occur. Pediatric patients may experience personality disorders or hyperkinesia. **Black Box Warning:** Antidepressants increase the risk of suicidal thinking and behavior in children, adolescents, and young adults. Patients of all ages should be monitored and observed closely during therapy for clinical worsening, suicidality, or unusual changes in behavior.

Abrupt withdrawal of fluoxetine or other SSRIs can result in a withdrawal syndrome; the patient may experience dizziness, headache, tremor, anxiety, dysphoria, and sensory disturbances. These symptoms usually begin 1 to 7 days after the last dose and may continue for 1 to 3 weeks. Because fluoxetine has an extended half-life and serum levels diminish gradually, withdrawal symptoms are generally less serious than those of the shorter acting SSRIs. Tapering the dose over 2 weeks or longer can prevent withdrawal symptoms.

Contraindications/Precautions: Hypersensitivity to fluoxetine is a contraindication to using the drug. The drug should not be administered to patients with bipolar disorder because it may precipitate a manic episode. It must be used cautiously in persons with cardiac dysfunction, diabetes, or seizure disorders. Children or young adults with a history of attempted suicide should not receive fluoxetine. There are no known age-related precautions for use in the elderly, but children may experience more behavioral adverse effects such as restlessness and insomnia.

Caution must be used when fluoxetine is administered late in pregnancy. The neonate may exhibit symptoms of withdrawal, including irritability, respiratory distress, tremors, abnormal crying, and, possibly, seizures. With supportive care, symptoms of withdrawal in the neonate will disappear in a few days. In most cases, the benefits of treating pregnant women who have major depression with fluoxetine are greater than the potential risks to the neonate.

Drug Interactions: Fluoxetine inhibits multiple CYP450 isozymes and has the potential to interact with many other drugs and herbal products. Drugs that are metabolized by CYP450 may build to toxic levels due to their impaired metabolism. Some drugs affected by diminished metabolism include TCAs, phenothiazines, most atypical antipsychotics, certain antidysrhythmics, and benzodiazepines. Excessive sedation may occur if fluoxetine is given concurrently with other CNS depressants, including opioids, sedative–hypnotics, or alcohol. Taken concurrently with or within 14 days of MAOIs can result in serotonin syndrome or neuroleptic malignant syndrome (NMS). Concurrent use with warfarin, aspirin, or other nonsteroidal anti-inflammatory drugs (NSAIDs) may increase the risk of bleeding. Fluoxetine may cause an increased risk of toxicity to phenytoin, digoxin, or carbamazepine. Concurrent use with certain antipsychotic agents may lead to increased extrapyramidal symptoms such as akathisia, dystonia, tardive dyskinesia, and pseudoparkinsonism. Fluoxetine can increase the half-life of diazepam. Caution must also be used if the patient is taking lithium because fluoxetine may increase plasma levels of the drug. **Herbal/Food:** Increased CNS effects may occur if fluoxetine is given concurrently with lavender, kava, or hops. There is an increased risk of serotonin syndrome with the concurrent use of St. John's wort. Increased anticholinergic effects may result from the use of jimsonweed or corkwood. Because grapefruit juice may cause elevated serum levels of fluoxetine, it should be avoided during therapy.

Pregnancy: Category C.

Treatment of Overdose: Overdose can result in seizures, somnolence, and, rarely, death. Supportive treatment is indicated, including gastric lavage and activated charcoal.

Nursing Responsibilities: Key nursing implications for patients receiving fluoxetine are included in the Nursing Practice Application for Patients Receiving Antidepressant Therapy.

Lifespan and Diversity Considerations:

- Monitor daily weights in children and in the older adult to assess for weight loss and proper nutrition.

- Use special caution when administering this drug to the older adult who is at increased risk of falls. Provide assistance with ambulation as needed if dizziness occurs.

- Monitor hepatic and renal function laboratory values more frequently with the older adult because normal physiological changes related to aging may affect the drug's metabolism and excretion.

- Because SSRIs are metabolized through the P450 system pathways, monitor ethnically diverse populations more frequently to ensure optimal therapeutic effects and minimize adverse effects.

Patient and Family Education:

- Do not take any other prescription or nonprescription drugs, dietary supplements, grapefruit or grapefruit juice, or herbal products without approval of the health care provider.

- The full therapeutic effects of the medication will take 2 to 6 weeks or more to appear. Monitor the patient more closely during the early stages of therapy because suicide risk may increase during this time.

- If unpleasant adverse effects occur, contact the health care provider but continue taking the medication until adjustments can be made.

- Immediately notify the health care provider of any known or suspected pregnancy.

- Take the last dose before 4 p.m. to prevent insomnia.

- Immediately report any of the following to the health care provider: suicidal thoughts, palpitations, major changes in sexual function, excessive weight gain, or excessive drowsiness.

Drugs Similar to Fluoxetine (Prozac, Sarafem)

Other SSRIs include citalopram, escitalopram, fluvoxamine, paroxetine, and sertraline.

Citalopram (Celexa): Citalopram was approved by the FDA in 1998 for the treatment of major depressive disorder in adults. All of its antianxiety uses are off-label. These include all five major antianxiety categories: generalized anxiety disorder, social anxiety disorder, OCD, panic disorder, and post-traumatic stress disorder (PTSD). Other off-label uses include schizophrenia, premenstrual dysphoric disorder, and menopausal hot flashes. Citalopram is available as regular tablets, as oral disintegrating tablets, or as an oral solution. It is almost identical structurally to escitalopram but is very different from other SSRIs. Older adults are more susceptible to the anticholinergic effects of citalopram than to other SSRIs. There are fewer drug interactions than with fluoxetine. All other actions and adverse effects are the same as those of fluoxetine and escitalopram. This drug is pregnancy category C.

Escitalopram (Lexapro): Escitalopram was approved in 2002 to treat major depressive disorder in adults and in pediatric patients ages 12 to 17 years. Since its approval, it has become one of the most frequently prescribed drugs in the United States. Escitalopram is also FDA approved for the treatment of generalized anxiety disorder and is used off-label to treat seasonal affective disorder and panic attacks. It is nearly identical structurally to citalopram although it is more potent; 20 mg of escitalopram is bioequivalent to 40 mg of citalopram. It is available as a tablet or solution. Escitalopram has the same spectrum of adverse effects as fluoxetine and other SSRIs. It appears to elevate mood relatively quickly, in 1 to 2 weeks. Its safety and effectiveness in children have not been established. This drug is pregnancy category C.

Fluvoxamine (Luvox): Approved in 1994, fluvoxamine is available as oral tablets. Fluvoxamine is FDA approved as a treatment for OCD, although it is also used off-label to treat depression, anxiety disorders in children, generalized anxiety disorder, PTSD, bulimia nervosa, and panic disorder. In 2007, the FDA approved an extended release capsule of Luvox (Luvox CR) for the treatment of OCD and social anxiety disorder. Adverse reactions are the same as with fluoxetine except that fluvoxamine causes sedation rather than CNS excitement. This drug is pregnancy category C.

Paroxetine (Paxil, Pexeva): Approved in 1992, paroxetine is available as oral tablets, oral suspension, or controlled release tablets (Paxil CR). It is approved to treat major depression, OCD, social anxiety disorder, panic disorder, generalized anxiety disorder, PTSD, and premenstrual dysphoric disorder. Off-label indications include hot flashes and premature ejaculation. Adverse effects are mild, dose dependent, and similar to those of other SSRIs. These effects usually diminish or disappear completely in time. A lower starting dosage is recommended for older adults. Precautions are similar to those for other SSRIs except that paroxetine is a pregnancy category D drug.

Sertraline (Zoloft): Approved in 1991, sertraline is one of the most frequently prescribed SSRIs. It is available as tablets or as an oral concentrate that must be diluted before use. Approved indications include major depressive disorder, OCD, PTSD, social anxiety disorder, or premenstrual dysphoric disorder. Contraindications and precautions are the same as with escitalopram. The main difference between sertraline and fluoxetine is that sertraline blocks the uptake of dopamine in addition to blocking the uptake of serotonin. Adverse effects, uses, and drug interactions are the same as those of fluoxetine. The oral concentrate contains 12% alcohol, which is contraindicated in patients taking disulfiram (Antabuse). This drug is pregnancy category C.

Atypical Antidepressants

10 Atypical antidepressants are alternatives to the selective serotonin reuptake inhibitors that are prescribed for depression and anxiety disorders.

Atypical antidepressants are a diverse class of newer drugs that act by mechanisms other than those of the SSRIs, TCAs, and MAOIs. In effect, this is a "miscellaneous" class of drugs because they have very little in common with each other except their ability to alleviate symptoms of depression. They act by preventing the reuptake of specific neurotransmitters in the CNS or by blocking neurotransmitter receptors. Mechanisms include the following:

- Serotonin–norepinephrine reuptake inhibitors (SNRIs): desvenlafaxine (Pristiq), venlafaxine (Effexor), and duloxetine (Cymbalta)
- Norepinephrine and dopamine reuptake inhibitors (NDRIs): bupropion (Wellbutrin)
- Norepinephrine reuptake inhibitors (NRIs): reboxetine (Edronax, Vestra)
- Combined reuptake inhibitor and receptor blocker: trazodone (Desyrel), nefazodone, and mirtazapine (Remeron).

As a group, the atypical antidepressants have similar pharmacologic actions to the SSRIs and exhibit fewer adverse effects than the TCAs and MAOIs. Each drug in the class has certain specific adverse effects, as described next. Like other antidepressants some are used for indications other than depression, such as neuropathic pain and anxiety disorders. Although some are quite effective, they are generally not superior to other, well-established antidepressants.

PROTOTYPE DRUG | **Venlafaxine (Effexor)**

Classification: **Therapeutic:** Atypical antidepressant
Pharmacologic: Serotonin–norepinephrine reuptake inhibitor (SNRI)

Therapeutic Effects and Uses: Venlafaxine is an atypical antidepressant approved by the FDA in 1993 to treat major depression. Later, its approved indications were extended to include panic disorder, generalized anxiety disorder, and social anxiety disorder. It has been used off-label to treat a large number of other conditions, including neuropathic pain, premenstrual dysphoric disorder, menopausal hot flashes, migraines, OCD, and fibromyalgia. Venlafaxine XR is an extended release capsule that permits once-daily dosing. It is metabolized to an active metabolite in the liver. Venlafaxine has pharmacologic effects, drug interactions, and adverse effects very similar to those of the SSRIs.

Like other antidepressants, there is little potential for psychological dependence with venlafaxine—it is not a drug of abuse. Abrupt discontinuation, however, can cause mild to moderate withdrawal symptoms similar in nature to those resulting from SSRI withdrawal. Gradual tapering of the dose is a means of preventing withdrawal symptoms.

Mechanism of Action: Venlafaxine inhibits the presynaptic neuronal reuptake of both norepinephrine and serotonin in the CNS.

Pharmacokinetics:

Route(s)	PO
Absorption	92% absorbed from the GI tract
Distribution	Widely distributed; crosses the placenta; secreted in breast milk; 27% bound to plasma protein
Primary metabolism	Metabolized in the liver to desmethylvenlafaxine, an active metabolite; substantial first-pass effect
Primary excretion	Renal
Onset of action	Peak serum level: 5.5 h but the antidepressant action may take 2–3 weeks
Duration of action	Half-life: 5–7 h (9–11 h for the active metabolite)

Adverse Effects: The most common adverse effect of venlafaxine is nausea, which can occur in 37% of patients. Tolerance may develop to the nausea as therapy progresses. The nausea, combined with anorexia, sometimes leads to weight loss. Pediatric patients taking venlafaxine have been shown to have a decrease in overall height as well as weight. Venlafaxine has structural similarities to amphetamines and can cause CNS stimulation, nervousness, and insomnia. Other patients, however, exhibit sedative effects from the drug. Other CNS adverse effects include headache, emotional lability, dizziness, and asthenia. Sustained elevations, 10 to 15 mmHg, of blood pressure may occur. Types of sexual dysfunction seen with venlafaxine include impotence, abnormal ejaculation, and delayed or absent orgasm in women. Rare, life-threatening adverse reactions include rectal, vaginal, or uterine hemorrhage. **Black Box Warning**: Antidepressants increase the risk of suicidal thinking and behavior in children, adolescents, and young adults. Patients of all ages should be monitored and observed closely during therapy for clinical worsening, suicidality, or unusual changes in behavior.

Contraindications/Precautions: Venlafaxine is contraindicated if the patient has hypersensitivity to venlafaxine or an SSRI, if a MAOI is being used concurrently, or during lactation. Caution must be used when administered to patients with cardiac, hepatic, or renal impairment; recent MI; seizure disorder; anorexia; or suicidal ideation. Venlafaxine is not administered to patients with bipolar disorder or with a history of mania because it can trigger manic episodes. Safety in children under age 18 has not been established. Patients with hepatic impairment may require as much as a 50% reduction in dose. Venlafaxine should be discontinued by tapering doses gradually because abrupt discontinuation can result in uncomfortable withdrawal symptoms such as nervousness, headache, agitation, fatigue, drowsiness, tremor, and sweating.

Drug Interactions: Venlafaxine is primarily metabolized by the hepatic CYP2D6 isozyme; drugs that inhibit CYP2D6 may cause venlafaxine serum levels to rise. Serotonin syndrome may occur if venlafaxine is given concurrently with SSRIs, MAOIs, lithium, or other drugs that act by increasing serotonin levels. If switching from venlafaxine to an MAOI, venlafaxine must be withdrawn at least 7 days before beginning the MAOI. Alcohol, opioids, sedatives, hypnotics, or antihistamines can cause additive CNS depression. Cimetidine, haloperidol, fluoxetine, sertraline, or phenothiazine can lead to increased toxicity. **Herbal/Food**: No food interactions have been reported, but there are several possible interactions with herbal products. St. John's wort and SAM-e may increase the risk of SES. CNS depression may occur with concurrent use of chamomile, kava, hops, lavender, valerian, or skullcap. Jimsonweed or corkwood may cause increased anticholinergic effects. Yohimbe may increase the risk for HTN.

Pregnancy: Category C.

Treatment of Overdose: Overdoses are generally not fatal but can cause serious symptoms such as CNS depression, seizures, altered level of consciousness, hypotension, and dysrhythmias. General measures include inducing emesis and administering activated charcoal and gastric lavage. The ECG must be monitored and antiseizure drugs administered as necessary.

Nursing Responsibilities, Lifespan and Diversity Considerations, and Patient and Family Education: These are the same as for the SSRIs.

Drugs Similar to Venlafaxine (Effexor)

Other atypical antidepressants include amoxapine, bupropion, desvenlafaxine, duloxetine, mirtazapine, nefazodone, trazodone, and vilazodone.

Amoxapine (Asendin): Approved in 1980, amoxapine is chemically related to older TCAs and phenothiazines. The drug exhibits potentially serious adverse effects, which limit its use to patients who have major depression with psychotic symptoms. Adverse effects resemble those of TCAs (blood dyscrasias, orthostatic hypotension, sedation, anticholinergic effects, sexual dysfunction, and cardiac toxicity) and phenothiazines (neuroleptic malignant syndrome and parkinsonism symptoms). There is cross hypersensitivity between amoxapine and TCAs. Amoxapine must be used cautiously in those with suicidal ideation. This drug is pregnancy category C.

Bupropion (Wellbutrin, Zyban): Approved in 1985, bupropion has a chemical structure similar to that of amphetamine and unrelated to other antidepressants. It is approved to treat major depression as well as being the first approved therapy for persistent seasonal affective disorder. Bupropion is also marketed as Zyban for the management of nicotine withdrawal during smoking cessation. Off-label uses include neuropathic pain and ADHD.

The naming of bupropion has resulted in medication errors. It is available as immediate release tablets (100 mg, 3 times daily), and as extended release formulations, Wellbutrin SR (150 mg, twice daily) and Wellbutrin XL (300 mg, once daily). In pharmacology, the terms sustained release (SR) and extended release (XL or XR) are usually used interchangeably, but this is not the case for bupropion. Further confusing the naming is that the U. S. Pharmacopeia requires that all generic versions of prolonged-release medications be labeled "extended release." In 2008 a new salt form, bupropion hydrobromide (Aplenzin), was approved as a once-daily tablet (348 mg, once daily) for depression. Caution must be used when dispensing bupropion to be certain the correct salt and dosing schedule is used.

Bupropion not only inhibits the reuptake of serotonin, but it may also affect the activity of norepinephrine and dopamine. Like amphetamine, bupropion has stimulant actions and suppresses the appetite. It does not cause weight gain or sexual dysfunction, which makes it appealing to women who are experiencing hypoactive sexual disorder. It is sometimes used to counteract the sexual dysfunction that occurs in patients taking SSRIs. Antidepressant action begins in 1 to 3 weeks and is equal to that of the TCAs. Because bupropion has a greater potential for causing seizures than other antidepressants, it should be used with caution in patients with seizure disorders. The risk for seizures is dose dependent and increases for patients drinking alcohol or taking other drugs that lower the seizure threshold. Seizures have been reported in infants receiving breast milk from mothers taking bupropion. Common adverse reactions include CNS stimulation (agitation, insomnia, and restlessness), weight loss, headache, dry mouth, constipation, and GI upset. About 20% of patients taking this drug will develop tremors. It is an alternative to SSRIs in those persons who cannot tolerate their adverse effects. This drug is pregnancy category C.

Desvenlafaxine: Desvenlafaxine (Pristiq) is a SNRI approved in 2008 for the treatment of major depressive disorder. It is available as an extended release tablet that is taken once daily. Common adverse effects include nausea, dizziness, excessive sweating, constipation, somnolence, anxiety, male function disorders, and decreased appetite. Because this drug can raise blood pressure, preexisting HTN should be corrected before starting therapy. Desvenlafaxine should be discontinued gradually to prevent the appearance of withdrawal symptoms. This drug is pregnancy category C.

Duloxetine (Cymbalta): Like venlafaxine, duloxetine is an atypical antidepressant that is classified as an SNRI. First approved for major depression in 2004, it has since received FDA approval to treat neuropathic pain in people with diabetes, fibromyalgia, and generalized anxiety disorder. Stress urinary incontinence is an off-label indication. Abnormal vision is the most frequently reported adverse effect, and nausea is a common reason for discontinuation of therapy. Other adverse events include photosensitivity, bruising, anorexia, thrombophlebitis, constipation, diarrhea, dry mouth, insomnia, and anxiety. No life-threatening adverse effects have been identified. Postmarketing incidences of liver injury suggest that the drug should be used with great caution in patients with preexisting hepatic impairment or in alcoholics. Caution must be exercised when administered to persons with mania, seizures, HTN, cardiac, renal or hepatic disease, the elderly, children, or lactating women. When discontinuing therapy, the dose should be tapered slowly to prevent withdrawal symptoms. Patients may begin feeling the antidepressant effects of duloxetine within 2 weeks of beginning treatment. This drug is pregnancy category C.

Mirtazapine (Remeron): Classified as a tetracyclic compound, this drug was approved in 1996 for major depression in adults. It blocks presynaptic serotonin and norepinephrine receptors, thereby enhancing release of these neurotransmitters from nerve terminals. Unlike the TCAs, it has few anticholinergic actions. It does carry a higher risk of seizure activity in patients with no previous seizure history. Serious adverse reactions include acute renal failure, hepatitis, jaundice, thrombocytopenia, leukopenia, eosinophilia, or agranulocytosis. Other adverse reactions include dizziness, orthostatic hypotension, ECG changes, sedation (which may be a positive effect in those having insomnia secondary to depression), tachycardia, HTN, or extrapyramidal symptoms in the elderly. Mirtazapine should not be used in patients with hypersensitivity to TCAs, seizure disorders, prostatic hypertrophy, serious hepatic or renal impairment, or those who are recovering from MI. Mirtazapine usually elevates mood within 2 to 4 weeks after the initiation of therapy. This drug is pregnancy category C.

Nefazodone: Chemically similar to trazodone, nefazodone causes minimal cardiovascular effects, fewer anticholinergic effects, less sedation, and less sexual dysfunction than some of the other antidepressants. The most common adverse effects are xerostomia, drowsiness, nausea, vomiting, dizziness, and constipation. Although approved only for major depression, off-label indications include anxiety, panic attacks, premenstrual dysphoric disorder, PTSD, and social anxiety disorder. Nefazodone acts by blocking serotonin receptors and inhibiting serotonin reuptake. It also has some blocking effect on norepinephrine reuptake. Originally approved in 1994, a brand name form of the drug, Serzone, was removed from the market in 2004 due to a possibility of liver damage; generic nefazodone is still available. A black box warning indicates that the drug should not be used in patients with acute liver impairment, and that hepatic laboratory values should be regularly monitored during therapy. The drug should be withdrawn if the patient develops signs of hepatic injury such as increased serum AST or serum ALT levels greater than three times normal. This drug is pregnancy category C.

Trazodone (Desyrel, Oleptro): Approved in 1981, trazodone works by producing a moderate, selective blockade of serotonin reuptake. It is not very effective when used alone as an antidepressant, but its sedative properties are especially useful in patients who have antidepressant-induced insomnia. In fact, trazodone is most frequently used off-label as a sleep aid, rather than as an antidepressant. Other off-label indications include generalized anxiety disorder, panic disorder, and as an adjuvant to reduce cravings for alcohol in patients with alcohol dependency. It causes little cardiac toxicity and few anticholinergic effects so it may be useful for older adults and other persons for whom either of these may be intolerable. Common adverse effects include orthostatic hypotension, nausea, sedation, and dry mouth. Reported sexual effects include priapism, anorgasmia, and ejaculation dysfunctions. Overdose with trazodone is considered to be safer than overdose from MAOIs or TCAs, and there have been no reports of death from trazodone use alone. However, death can occur from overdose when the patient combines trazodone with other CNS depressants. In 2010, the FDA approved Oleptro, a controlled release form of trazodone that is taken once daily. This drug is pregnancy category C.

Vilazodone (Viibryd): Approved in 2011, vilazodone is one of the newest drugs for treating major depressive disorder in adults. The drug acts by blocking serotonin reuptake and by demonstrating partial agonist action at serotonin receptors. It appears to have equivalent effectiveness to other drugs in this class. One advantage of vilazodone is that clinical improvement is noted after 7 days of therapy, compared to the 4 to 6 weeks required for some of the other antidepressants. In addition, the drug has only minor adverse effects with GI-related symptoms being the most common. Like other antidepressants, the drug carries a black box warning about possible increased suicidality in adolescents and young adults. This drug is pregnancy category C.

CONNECTION Checkpoint 23.3

Atypical antidepressants are sometimes used to treat anxiety when other agents are not effective. What class of drugs is the traditional choice for the short-term therapy of generalized anxiety disorder? *See Answer to Connection Checkpoint 23.3 on student resource website.*

Monoamine Oxidase Inhibitors

11 Monoamine oxidase inhibitors are effective antidepressants but are seldom used due to potentially serious adverse effects.

MAO is a key enzyme located in the liver, intestinal wall, and adrenergic neurons. It is responsible for inactivating monoamines: substances that contain one $-NH_2$ (amine) group. Not only does MAO inactivate natural monoamines such as norepinephrine, dopamine, and serotonin, but it also acts on those present in food and drugs. The **monoamine oxidase inhibitors (MAOIs)** are antidepressants that block the actions of MAO.

In adrenergic neurons, MAOIs slow the destruction of norepinephrine, dopamine, and serotonin. This creates higher levels of these neurotransmitters and enhances their activity in the brain. Through mechanisms incompletely understood, this increase in neurotransmitters creates an antidepressant action.

Although they are as effective in treating depression as the SSRIs or TCAs, serious adverse reactions limit their use. Because of their low safety margin, these drugs are reserved for patients with refractory depression that has not responded to TCAs, atypical antidepressants, or SSRIs. They are rarely used in clinical practice.

A serious adverse reaction with MAOIs is their ability to cause a hypertensive crisis if combined with foods that contain **tyramine**. Widely found in nature, tyramine is a type of monoamine that is formed by the metabolism of tyrosine, an amino acid. When a patient is taking an MAOI, the drug blocks the breakdown of dietary tyramine, causing it to accumulate to high levels. In turn, tyramine causes the release of norepinephrine stored in adrenergic neurons. Rapid vasoconstriction occurs with a potential rise of blood pressure of 30 mmHg or more. Table 4 contains a list of tyramine-rich foods that must be avoided by patients taking MAOIs. Products containing tyramine are sometimes marketed as dietary supplements to increase fat loss from the body. There is no valid scientific evidence to support this claim, and these supplements must be strictly avoided by patients taking MAOIs.

PROTOTYPE DRUG | Phenelzine (Nardil)

Classification: Therapeutic: Antidepressant
Pharmacologic: Monoamine oxidase inhibitor

Therapeutic Effects and Uses: An older drug approved in 1959, phenelzine was once widely used to treat major depression. It has also been used off-label to treat OCD, panic disorder, and social anxiety disorder and for migraine prophylaxis. Although very effective in treating these disorders, phenelzine interacts with tyramine in foods and with many other drugs to produce potentially serious interactions.

TABLE 4 Foods High in Tyramine

Category of Food	Specific Foods
Meats	Beef or chicken liver, pate
	Hot dogs, bologna
	Pepperoni, salami, sausage
Dairy products	Aged cheese
	Sour cream
	Yogurt
Fruits	Avocados
	Bananas, in large amounts
	Canned figs
	Papaya products, including meat tenderizers
	Raisins
Vegetables	Pods of fava beans
	Fermented soybeans, soybean paste
Fish	Dried or cured fish
	Fermented, smoked, aged fish
	Pickled or kippered herring
Alcohol	Beer
	Wine, especially red wine
Miscellaneous	Protein dietary supplements
	Soups (may contain protein extract)
	Shrimp paste
	Soy sauce
	Yeast, brewer's or extracts

Like other antidepressants, phenelzine may take up to 4 to 8 weeks to produce a maximum antidepressant response. This drug is changed to active metabolites in the liver.

Mechanism of Action: Phenelzine produces its effects by binding irreversibly to MAO. This intensifies the actions of endogenous epinephrine, norepinephrine, serotonin, and dopamine

Complementary and Alternative Therapies
St. John's Wort for Depression

Description: St. John's wort (*Hypericum perforatum*) is an herb found throughout Great Britain, Asia, Europe, and North America.

History and Claims: The herb gets its name from a legend that red spots once appeared on its leaves on the anniversary of St. John's beheading. The word *wort* is a British term for "plant." Use of the plant dates to ancient Greece, and Native Americans used the herb as an antiseptic or anti-inflammatory agent. Modern uses have focused on the antidepressant properties of the herb.

Standardization: The active agents in St. John's wort are believed to be hyperforin and hypericin. There is no standard dosage; however, some manufacturers are beginning to report dose by the percentage of hypericin in the extract. For example, one commonly used dose is 300 mg tid of St. John's wort standardized to 0.3% hypericin. Some studies use 5% hyperforin.

Evidence: Scientists once thought that St. John's wort produced its effects via the same mechanism as MAOIs, by increasing the levels of serotonin, norepinephrine, and dopamine in the brain. More recent evidence suggests that it may selectively inhibit serotonin reuptake. The National Center for Complementary and Alternative Medicine (2010) cites evidence that St. John's wort may be useful for short-term treatment of mild to moderate depression. St. John's wort induces hepatic P450 enzymes and has been reported to interact with many medications, including oral contraceptives, warfarin, digoxin, and cyclosporine. It should not be taken concurrently with antidepressant medications.

An active ingredient in St. John's wort is a photoactive compound that when exposed to light produces substances that can damage myelin. Patients have reported feeling stinging pain on the hands after sun exposure while taking the herbal remedy. Patients who take this herb should be advised to apply sunscreen or to wear protective clothing when outdoors.

A review of the literature concluded that St. John's wort is more effective than a placebo in treating major depression and that it is safer than conventional antidepressant medications (Linde, Berner & Kriston, 2008).

in the CNS. Increased concentrations of these neurotransmitters result in elevated mood.

Pharmacokinetics:

Route(s)	PO
Absorption	Well absorbed
Distribution	Widely distributed; crosses the placenta
Primary metabolism	Hepatic
Primary excretion	Renal
Onset of action	Peak level: 2–4 h (antidepressant action takes 2–8 weeks)
Duration of action	Half-life: 11 h

Adverse Effects: The most serious adverse effect of phenelzine is hypertensive crisis precipitated by foods containing tyramine, which can induce fatal intracranial bleeding. Dizziness and orthostatic hypotension are common during therapy. Other frequent adverse reactions include drowsiness, sexual dysfunction, and anorexia. Life-threatening adverse reactions include dysrhythmias and a syndrome of inappropriate antidiuretic hormone-like symptoms. **Black Box Warning**: Antidepressants increase the risk of suicidal thinking and behavior in children, adolescents, and young adults. Patients of all ages should be monitored and observed closely during therapy for clinical worsening, suicidality, or unusual changes in behavior.

Contraindications/Precautions: Patients with schizophrenia, cardiovascular or cerebrovascular disease, hepatic or renal impairment, or pheochromocytoma should not take phenelzine. Caution should be used when prescribing phenelzine to a person with epilepsy, severe or frequent headaches, HTN, dysrhythmias, or suicidal tendencies.

Drug Interactions: Phenelzine interacts with many other drugs. The nurse should consult a current drug guide for a comprehensive list of drug–drug interactions. Other CNS depressants, including alcohol, may lead to additive CNS depression. Concurrent administration with buspirone may increase blood pressure. Use with opioid analgesics may lead to immediate excitation, severe HTN or hypotension, and, occasionally, severe respiratory distress, vascular collapse, seizures, coma, and death. CNS stimulants and sympathomimetics may increase the cardiac stimulant and vasopressor effects of phenelzine. SES may occur if phenelzine is administered with other drugs such as SSRIs, lithium, or dextromethorphan that potentiate the actions of serotonin. **Herbal/Food**: Patients who are taking phenelzine or any MAOI must avoid tyramine-containing foods (see Table 4) because these foods may precipitate a hypertensive crisis. Medications containing caffeine, including OTC products, should be avoided because they may increase the risk of HTN and dysrhythmias. An increased sympathomimetic effect may occur when phenelzine is combined with capsicum peppers or large amounts of green tea. Ginkgo, nutmeg, and yohimbe use can result in increased effects. Ginseng use can lead to irritability, hallucinations, mania, and increased tension headaches. Decreased effects can occur with the use of valerian. Serotonin syndrome may occur with the use of St. John's wort.

Pregnancy: Category C.

Treatment of Overdose: Overdosage with phenelzine is serious and can result in death if untreated. Symptoms may include either CNS stimulation (seizures) or depression (coma). Induction of gastric lavage with activated charcoal may be beneficial. Electrolytes and vital signs must be monitored and the appropriate intervention administered to keep values within normal ranges.

Nursing Responsibilities:

- Obtain a comprehensive health history, including cardiovascular, hepatic, and renal disease as well as previous episodes of major depression. Obtain baseline vital signs and weight.

- Obtain a complete drug history, including drugs used to treat depression currently or in the past, and length of time since the patient has taken the last dose. Assess all prescription and nonprescription drugs taken for possible interactions.

- Monitor caffeine intake. Excessive amounts of caffeine can potentiate hypertensive reactions.

- Monitor the patient closely in the first few weeks of therapy while the drug takes full effect. Assist with ambulation if dizziness from orthostatic hypotension occurs during early weeks of therapy. Monitor for early signs of hypertensive crisis: stiff neck, occipital headache, tachycardia, nausea and vomiting, sweating, and skin flushing, and report immediately.

Lifespan and Diversity Considerations:

- Use special caution when administering this drug to the older adult who is at increased risk of falls. Provide assistance with ambulation as needed if drowsiness, dizziness, or blurred vision occur.

- Monitor hepatic and renal function laboratory values more frequently with the older adult because normal physiological changes related to aging may affect the drug's metabolism and excretion.

- Evaluate culturally specific diets for high-tyramine foods and assist the patient and family with menu choices or substitutes.

Patient and Family Education:

- Provide explicit instruction on foods and beverages that must be avoided while taking MAOIs Assist with menu choices and substitutions. Thaw foods in refrigerator or microwave and consume foods within 48 hours of purchase because tyramine content may increase with aging.

- Avoid caffeine intake including coffee, tea, chocolate, or cola beverages because these may affect blood pressure.

- Do not take any other prescription or nonprescription drugs, dietary supplements, or herbal products without approval of the health care provider.

- The full therapeutic effects of MAOIs may take 2 to 6 weeks or more to appear.

- Report headache, palpitations, neck stiffness, dizziness, insomnia, changes in urinary pattern or color of urine, change in muscle strength, or constriction in the chest or throat to the health care provider immediately.

- Avoid alcohol and other CNS depressants.

- Wear or carry medical identification stating that you are taking an MAOI.
- If sedation occurs take the medication at bedtime.
- Make position changes slowly when moving from a lying to a standing position to prevent dizziness and possible fainting.

Drugs Similar to Phenelzine (Nardil)

The other MAOIs that are available include isocarboxazid, selegiline, and tranylcypromine.

Isocarboxazid (Marplan): Like phenelzine, isocarboxazid was initially approved by the FDA for depression in the 1950s.

CONNECTIONS: NURSING PRACTICE APPLICATION

Patients Receiving Antidepressant Therapy

Assessment	Potential Nursing Diagnoses
Baseline assessment prior to administration: • Understand the reason the drug has been prescribed in order to assess for therapeutic effects. • Obtain a complete health history including hepatic, renal, urologic, cardiovascular, or neurologic disease, current mental status, narrow-angle glaucoma status, and pregnancy or breast-feeding status. Obtain a drug history including allergies, current prescription and OTC drugs, and herbal preparations. Be alert to possible drug interactions. • Obtain a history of depression or mood disorder, including a family history of same and severity. Use objective screening tools when possible (e.g., Beck Depression Inventory or Geriatric Depression Scale). • Obtain baseline vital signs and weight. • Evaluate appropriate laboratory findings (e.g., CBC, electrolytes, glucose, hepatic and renal function studies). • Assess the patient's ability to receive and understand instructions. Include the family and caregivers as needed.	• *Ineffective Coping* • *Powerlessness* • *Anxiety* • *Disturbed Thought Processes* • *Disturbed Sleep Pattern* • *Self-Care Deficit (Bathing, Dressing, Feeding)* • *Imbalanced Nutrition: More or Less Than Body Requirements* • *Complicated Grieving* • *Social Isolation* • *Impaired Social Interaction* • *Interrupted Family Processes* • *Urinary Retention*, related to anticholinergic side effects of drug therapy • *Noncompliance*, related to adverse drug effects of decreased sexual libido or weight gain • *Deficient Knowledge (Drug Therapy)* • *Risk for Self-Directed Violence* • *Risk for Self-Mutilation* • *Risk for Suicide* • *Risk for Injury*
Assessment throughout administration: • Assess for desired therapeutic effects (e.g., increased mood, lessening depression, increased activity level, return to normal ADLs, appetite, and sleep patterns). • Continue periodic monitoring of CBC, electrolytes, glucose, and hepatic and renal function studies. • Assess vital signs and weight periodically or as symptoms warrant. • Assess for and promptly report adverse effects: dizziness or lightheadedness, drowsiness, confusion, agitation, suicidal ideations, palpitations, tachycardia, blurred or double vision, skin rashes, bruising or bleeding, abdominal pain, jaundice, change in color of stool, flank pain, or hematuria.	

Planning: Patient Goals and Expected Outcomes

The patient will:
- Experience therapeutic effects dependent on the reason the drug is being given (e.g., increased mood, lessened depression).
- Be free from or experience minimal adverse effects.
- Verbalize an understanding of the drug's use, adverse effects, and required precautions.
- Demonstrate proper self-administration of the medication (e.g., dose, timing, and when to notify the provider).

Implementation

Interventions and (Rationales)	Patient-Centered Care
Ensuring therapeutic effects: • Continue assessments as above for therapeutic effects. (Drugs used for depression may take 2 to 8 weeks before full effects are realized. Use objective measures, e.g., Beck Depression Inventory, when possible to help quantify therapeutic results. For outpatient therapy, prescriptions may be limited to 7 days' supply of medication. Have patient sign "No Harm/No Suicide" contract as appropriate.)	• Teach the patient that full effects may not occur for a prolonged period of time, but that some improvement should be noticeable after beginning therapy. • Encourage the patient to keep all appointments with the therapist and to discuss ongoing symptoms of depression, reporting any suicidal ideations immediately.

(continued)

CONNECTIONS: NURSING PRACTICE APPLICATION *(continued)*

Minimizing adverse effects:

- Continue to monitor vital signs, mental status, coordination, and balance periodically. Ensure patient safety; monitor ambulation until the effects of the drug are known. Be particularly cautious with the older adult who is at increased risk for falls. (Antidepressant drugs may cause drowsiness and dizziness, hypotension, or impaired mental and physical abilities, increasing the risk of falls.)

- Teach the patient to rise from lying or sitting to standing slowly to avoid dizziness or falls.
- Instruct the patient to call for assistance prior to getting out of bed or attempting to walk alone, and to avoid driving or other activities requiring mental alertness or physical coordination until the effects of the drug are known.

- Continue to monitor CBC, electrolytes, and renal and hepatic function. (Some antidepressant drugs may cause hepatotoxicity as an adverse effect.)

- Instruct the patient on the need to return periodically for laboratory work.
- Teach the patient to promptly report any abdominal pain, particularly in the upper quadrants, changes in stool color, yellowing of sclera or skin, or darkened urine.

- Assess for changes in level of consciousness, disorientation or confusion, or agitation. (Neurologic changes may indicate under- or overmedication, exacerbation of other psychiatric illness, or adverse drug effects.)

- Instruct the patient or caregivers to report increasing lethargy, disorientation, confusion, changes in behavior or mood, agitation or aggression, slurred speech, or ataxia immediately.

- Assess for changes in visual acuity, blurred vision, loss of peripheral vision, seeing rainbow halos around lights, or acute eye pain, especially if accompanied by nausea and vomiting, and report immediately. (Increased intraocular pressure in patients with narrow-angle glaucoma may occur in patients taking TCAs.)

- Instruct the patient to report any visual changes or eye pain immediately.

- Monitor cardiovascular status. (Early signs of SES include rapid increases in blood pressure and pulse.)

- Instruct the patient to report severe headache, dizziness, paresthesia, palpitations, tachycardia, chest pain, nausea, vomiting, diaphoresis, or fever immediately.

- Assess for bruising, bleeding, or signs of infection. (TCAs may cause blood dyscrasias and increased chances of bleeding or infection.)

- Teach the patient to report any signs of increased bruising, bleeding, or infections (e.g., sore throat, fever, or skin rash) promptly.

- Assess for dry mouth, blurred vision, urinary retention, and sexual dysfunction. (Anticholinergic-like effects and sexual dysfunction, including loss of libido and impotence, are common antidepressant adverse effects. Tolerance to anticholinergic effects usually develops in 2 to 4 weeks.)

- Teach the patient to use ice chips, frequent sips of water, chewing gum, or hard candy to alleviate dry mouth, and to avoid alcohol-based mouthwashes, which may increase dryness.
- Use of "dry eye" drops and resting the eyes periodically may help decrease dry eye feeling. Teach the patient to report any feelings of scratchiness or eye pain immediately.
- Instruct the patient to report difficulty with urination, hesitancy, or dysuria promptly.
- Encourage the patient to discuss concerns about sexual functioning and refer to the health care provider if concerns affect medication adherence.

- Continue weekly weights and report gain or loss above 2 kg (5 lb). (Weight gain may be a reason for nonadherence with drug therapy. Adolescents and older adults may be at risk for anorexia and weight loss.)

- Have the patient weigh self weekly and report significant weight gain or loss to the provider.

- Avoid abrupt discontinuation of therapy. (Profound depression, seizures, or withdrawal symptoms may occur with abrupt discontinuation.)

- Instruct the patient to take the drug exactly as prescribed and to not discontinue it abruptly.

Patient understanding of drug therapy:

- Use opportunities during administration of medications and during assessments to discuss the rationale for drug therapy, desired therapeutic outcomes, commonly observed adverse effects, parameters for when to call the health care provider, and any necessary monitoring or precautions. (Using time during nursing care helps to optimize and reinforce key teaching areas.)

- The patient should be able to state the reason for the drug, appropriate dose, scheduling, and what adverse effects to observe for and when to report them.

Patient self-administration of drug therapy:

- When administering the medication, instruct the patient, family, or caregiver in proper self-administration of the drug, e.g., take the drug as prescribed and do not substitute brands. (Utilizing time during nurse-administration of these drugs helps to reinforce teaching.)

- Teach the patient to take the medication:
- Exactly as ordered and the same manufacturer's brand each time the prescription is filled. (Switching brands may result in differing pharmacokinetics and alterations in therapeutic effect.)
- Take a missed dose as soon as it is noticed but do not take double or extra doses to "catch up."
- Take with food to decrease GI upset.
- If medication causes drowsiness, take at bedtime.
- Do not abruptly discontinue the medication.

Evaluation of Outcome Criteria

Evaluate the effectiveness of drug therapy by confirming that patient goals and expected outcomes have been met (see "Planning").

Off-label indications include refractory panic disorder and social anxiety disorder. It is only used when other therapies have failed to produce satisfactory outcomes. The drug has the same precautions and potential interactions as phenelzine, including the possibility of a hypertensive crisis occurring when taken with tyramine-containing products. This drug is pregnancy category C.

Selegiline (Emsam): Approved in 2006 for major depression, selegiline is a transdermal patch that delivers a controlled amount of the MAOI over 24 hours. Absorption across the skin bypasses MAO in the intestine; thus there is less risk of a hypertensive crisis when eating foods containing tyramine. The drug is also indicated for the treatment of Parkinson's disease by capsule (Eldepryl) or orally disintegrating tablets (Zelapar). The various forms of this drug should not be administered concurrently due to the risk of hypertensive crisis caused by drug overdose. Common adverse effects include skin irritation at the site of the patch application, headache, sleep disorders, diarrhea, and dry mouth. This drug is pregnancy category C.

Tranylcypromine (Parnate): Tranylcypromine was approved in 1961 for the therapy of depression. Off-label indications include refractory panic disorder and social anxiety disorder. The drug binds reversibly to MAO. This results in a more rapid onset of antidepressant action than phenelzine or isocarboxazid and a more rapid return to normal MAO levels after the drug is discontinued. However, it has the same precautions and potential interactions as phenelzine and is rarely used due to its adverse effects. This drug is pregnancy category C.

Bipolar Disorder

12 Bipolar disorder is a serious psychiatric disorder characterized by extreme mood swings from depression to euphoria.

Bipolar disorder, once known as manic-depression, is a common and serious psychiatric disorder. Suicide risk is high and many patients stop taking their medication during the course of pharmacotherapy. The etiology of the disorder is unknown, and symptoms may persist throughout the patient's life span.

Mania is characterized by symptoms that are generally the opposite of depressive symptoms. The excessive CNS stimulation that is characteristic of mania can be recognized by the following symptoms:

- Inflated self-esteem or grandiosity; the belief that one's ideas are far superior to anyone else's
- Decreased need for sleep or food
- Distractibility; racing thoughts with attention too easily drawn to irrelevant external stimuli
- Increased psychomotor or goal-directed activity (either socially, at work or school, or sexually)
- Excessive pursuit of pleasurable activities without consideration of the negative consequences, such as shopping sprees, sexual indiscretions, or unsound business investments

- Increased talkativeness or pressure to keep talking
- With severe disease, delusions, paranoia, hallucinations, and bizarre behavior.

To be diagnosed with bipolar disorder, these symptoms must persist for at least 1 week and evidence of impaired functioning must be present. Suicide is a major risk in patients who have bipolar disorder; up to 50% of these patients attempt suicide, and 10% to 20% succeed in taking their lives. **Hypomania** is characterized by the same symptoms, but they are less severe and do not cause impaired functioning. In some cases, patients may experience a mixed episode where depression and mania are experienced simultaneously.

Although the pathophysiology of bipolar disorder is incompletely understood, mania and hypomania likely result from abnormal functioning of neurotransmitters in the brain. Mania may involve an excess of excitatory neurotransmitters (such as glutamate or norepinephrine) or a deficiency of inhibitory neurotransmitters (such as GABA). It is important to distinguish bipolar disorder from drug abuse, severe anxiety disorders, schizophrenia, dementia, or electrolyte disturbances, which can all produce symptoms similar to those of bipolar disorder.

Nonpharmacologic interventions play important roles in the treatment of patients with bipolar disorder. Lack of sleep, excessive stress, and poor nutrition are triggers for manic episodes and should be addressed in the plan of care. Support groups and psychotherapy are helpful for many patients. ECT is very effective at treating acute manic and depressive episodes.

Pharmacotherapy of bipolar disorder is highly individualized. For patients with mild symptoms that cause only slight functional disruption, monotherapy with low doses of a mood stabilizer is indicated. More severely affected patients usually require combination therapy with a mood stabilizer plus an atypical antipsychotic. If the patient is on antidepressant medications, these are usually discontinued because they can worsen mania or hypomania. Caution must be used in female patients of childbearing potential because some agents used for bipolar disorder cause fetal malformations.

Like the treatment of major depression, nonadherence with drug therapy is a serious problem in patients with bipolar disorder. As many as 50% of patients discontinue their medication during the first year of therapy. Lack of awareness is the single most common reason for nonadherence; mania is simply not viewed as abnormal by the person experiencing it. In fact, people with mania are often able to work tirelessly on projects and accomplish many work- and home-related tasks. Surprisingly, the second most common reason for nonadherence is the presence of a comorbid substance abuse disorder, usually alcoholism. Psychotherapy and family support may be necessary to achieve proper adherence.

Drugs for Bipolar Disorder

13 Lithium is the conventional therapy for the treatment of bipolar disorder.

Drugs for bipolar disorder are called **mood stabilizers**, because they have the ability to moderate extreme shifts in emotion and relieve symptoms of mania and depression during acute

TABLE 5 Drugs for Bipolar Disorder

Drug	Route and Adult Dose (maximum dose where indicated)	Adverse Effects
lithium carbonate (Eskalith, Lithobid)	PO: initially 600 mg tid or 900 mg sustained release bid or 30 mL (48 mEq) of solution tid Maintenance: 300 mg tid or qid or 15–20 mL (24–32 mEq) in two to four divided doses (max: 2.4 g/day)	*Headache, lethargy, fatigue, recent memory loss, nausea, vomiting, anorexia, abdominal pain, diarrhea, dry mouth, muscle weakness, nephrogenic diabetes insipidus, fine hand tremors, reversible leukocytosis* <u>Peripheral circulatory collapse</u>
Antiseizure Drugs		
carbamazepine (Tegretol)	PO: 200 mg bid, gradually increased to 800–1,200 mg/day in three to four divided doses	*Dizziness, ataxia, somnolence, headache, nausea, diplopia, blurred vision, sedation, drowsiness, nausea, vomiting, prolonged bleeding time, transient leukopenia* <u>Heart block, aplastic anemia, agranulocytosis, respiratory depression, exfoliative dermatitis, SJS, toxic epidermal necrolysis, deep coma, death (with overdose), liver failure, pancreatitis, bone marrow depression</u>
lamotrigine (Lamictal)	PO: 50 mg/day for 2 weeks, then 50 mg bid for 2 weeks; may increase gradually up to 300–500 mg/day in two divided doses (max: 700 mg/day)	
valproic acid (Depakene)	PO: 250 mg tid (max: 60 mg/kg/day)	
Atypical Antipsychotic Drugs		
aripiprazole (Abilify)	PO: 30 mg daily; may decrease to 15 mg (max: 30 mg daily)	*Tachycardia, sedation, dizziness, headache, lightheadedness, somnolence, anxiety, nervousness, agitation, hostility, insomnia, nausea, vomiting, transient fever, constipation, akathisia, parkinsonism* <u>Agranulocytosis, neuroleptic malignant syndrome (risperidone, rare), risk of stroke in elderly with dementia-related psychosis (aripiprazole)</u>
olanzapine (Zyprexa)	PO: start with 10 mg once daily; may increase or decrease in 5 mg/day increments	
quetiapine (Seroquel)	PO: start with 25 mg bid and increase by 25–50 mg bid to tid to target dose of 300–400 mg/day divided bid or tid (max: 800 mg/day)	
risperidone (Risperdal)	PO: start with 2–3 mg daily, may increase dose at intervals of 1 mg/day (max: 6 mg/day)	
ziprasidone (Geodon)	PO: 40 mg bid with food, may increase every 2 days up to 80 mg bid	

Note: Italics indicate common adverse effects. <u>Underline</u> indicates serious adverse effects.

episodes. The traditional treatment for bipolar disorder is lithium carbonate (Eskalith), a mood stabilizer prescribed as monotherapy or in combination with other drugs. In recent years, valproic acid (Depakene) has begun to replace lithium as the first-line therapy for bipolar disorder due to its improved safety profile. Valproic acid and other miscellaneous drugs for bipolar disorder are discussed in Section 14. Drugs used to treat bipolar disorder are shown in Table 5.

PROTOTYPE DRUG	Lithium Carbonate (Eskalith, Lithobid)

Classification: **Therapeutic:** Antimanic, agent for bipolar disorder
Pharmacologic: Alkali metal ion salt

Therapeutic Effects and Uses: Lithium was approved for use in 1970. Its benefit in treating bipolar disorder has been established since the 1950s, but its therapeutic safety has not been proved. Lithium is a simple inorganic element that is found in the same group as sodium and potassium. It is available for PO administration, as tablets, syrup, and controlled release and slow release tablets. Onset of action may take 1 to 3 weeks. Dosing is highly individualized and is based on serum drug levels and clinical response. Lithium has a short half-life and must be taken in multiple doses each day.

Lithium is an effective drug for controlling the acute manic episodes characteristic of bipolar disorder and in preventing the recurrence of mania or depression. In the patient with mania, lithium decreases euphoria, hyperactivity, and other symptoms without causing sedation. Previously lithium was used for all patients with mania; at the present time it is used primarily for those patients with classic euphoric mania. Lithium, rather than valproic acid, appears to be more effective in reducing suicide risk in persons diagnosed with bipolar disorder. Lithium may also be used for off-label indications, including alcoholism, bulimia, neutropenia, schizophrenia, prevention of vascular headaches, and hyperthyroidism.

Mechanism of Action: The precise mechanism of action of lithium is not known. It likely acts by changing neurotransmitter balance in specific brain regions. Lithium increases the synthesis of serotonin.

Pharmacokinetics:

Route(s)	PO
Absorption	Completely absorbed
Distribution	Distributed to all tissues and body fluids; crosses the blood–brain barrier and placenta; secreted in breast milk; not bound to plasma protein
Primary metabolism	Not metabolized
Primary excretion	Renal
Onset of action	Peak levels: 4–12 h (tablets) or 15–60 minutes (solutions)
Duration of action	Unknown

Adverse Effects: Many possible adverse effects are associated with the use of lithium. These are sometimes divided into those that occur at the initiation of therapy and those that occur with long-term therapy. Initial adverse effects are muscle weakness, lethargy, nausea, vomiting, polyuria, nocturia, headache, dizziness, drowsiness, tremors, and confusion. Many of the initial adverse effects are transient or may be easily managed. Long-term therapy can produce serious toxicity, including kidney impairment (proteinuria, albuminuria, or glycosuria), dysrhythmias, circulatory collapse, and leukocytosis. Lithium interferes with the synthesis of thyroid hormone and can cause hypothyroidism and goiter. **Black Box Warning**: Toxicity from lithium is closely related to serum concentrations and may occur at doses close to therapeutic levels. Facilities should be available to provide prompt and accurate serum concentration data. Serum lithium levels are monitored regularly during therapy and should be maintained within the narrow range of 0.8 to 1.4 mEq/L at the start of therapy and 0.4 to 1 mEq/L during maintenance therapy.

Contraindications/Precautions: Contraindications to the use of lithium include serious cardiovascular or renal impairment and severe dehydration or sodium depletion. Older adults and debilitated patients must be carefully monitored. Caution must be used when the drug is given to patients with cardiovascular disease, thyroid disease, history of a seizure disorder, diabetes, urinary retention, or a systemic infection. Lithium produces an increased incidence of congenital defects, especially those involving the heart, and is normally not used during pregnancy. Its use should be discouraged during lactation.

Drug Interactions: There are many potential drug interactions, some of which can be serious. Diuretics can increase the risk of lithium toxicity by promoting sodium loss; the body replaces lost sodium with lithium, which is also a salt. NSAIDs and thiazide diuretics can increase lithium levels by increasing the renal reabsorption of lithium. Lithium may cause an increased hypothyroid effect of antithyroid drugs or drugs containing iodine. Concurrent administration with haloperidol may cause increased neurotoxicity. SES may result if lithium is administered with other drugs, such as SSRIs or dextromethorphan, or MAOIs that potentiate the actions of serotonin. **Herbal/Food**: An increased lithium effect may occur with the use of dandelion, goldenrod, juniper, parsley, nettle, or horsetail. Black or green tea, cola nut, or plantain may lead to a decreased lithium effect. Significant changes in sodium intake from foods will alter lithium excretion.

Pregnancy: Category D.

Treatment of Overdose: Overdose of lithium is treated with supportive measures such as emesis or lavage, maintaining airway and respiratory function, and dialysis, if lithium intoxication is severe.

Nursing Responsibilities:
- Obtain a complete health history and history of depression and mania symptoms. Obtain a medication history, particularly other medications used for depression or bipolar disorder.
- Assess baseline vital signs, weight, and laboratory studies, especially serum sodium, CBC, hepatic, and renal values. Monitor drug levels, weight, CBC, electrolytes, and

urinalysis for protein, albumin, and glucose periodically during therapy.
- Provide supportive environment during the early phase of treatment until mood has stabilized.
- Report thirst, dizziness, lethargy or confusion, muscle weakness, or polyuria to the provider immediately after the early period of therapy as possible toxic effects.

Lifespan and Diversity Considerations:
- Carefully assess the older adult for signs of sodium imbalance or dehydration and for therapeutic and adverse effects. Monitor the older adult frequently because lithium toxicity may occur at lower therapeutic levels than in a younger patient.
- Monitor ethnically diverse patients closely for signs of lithium toxicity. Evaluate normal diet routines for high-sodium content foods or beverages that may affect the therapeutic range of the drug.

Patient and Family Education:
- The full therapeutic effects of lithium may take 2 to 3 weeks or more to appear. Monitor the patient more closely during the early stages of therapy.
- Return regularly for laboratory work. Weigh self weekly and report a gain or loss of 1 kg (2.2 lb) in a day or 2 kg (5 lb) in a week.
- Maintain a normal-sodium diet and fluid intake without unusual or dramatic increases or decreases, which can affect drug level. Be cautious with exercising or on hot days because excessive sweating will lead to water and sodium loss. Avoid caffeine and alcohol.
- Report excessive thirst, urination, dizziness, muscle weakness, tachycardia, palpitations, or confusion promptly to the health care provider.
- Do not abruptly discontinue the drug. If discontinuation of the drug is desired, it should be discussed with the health care provider and alternative therapy considered.

Drugs Similar to Lithium Carbonate (Eskalith, Lithobid)

There are no drugs similar to lithium carbonate.

14 Antiseizure and atypical antipsychotic agents are used to control symptoms of bipolar disorder.

Although lithium is well established as an effective treatment for bipolar disorder, pharmacologists have searched for safer alternatives. Several drugs have been found to be effective for this disorder and have received FDA approval. A number of others are prescribed off-label for bipolar disorder. All of these agents have additional primary indications. The other classes include antiseizure agents, atypical antipsychotics, and antidepressants.

Antiseizure agents: The antiseizure drugs for bipolar disorder are classified as mood stabilizers. These agents have pharmacologic actions similar to lithium: relieving symptoms and preventing the recurrence of mania and depression.

Valproic acid (Depakene) and divalproex sodium (Depakote ER) are FDA approved for mood stabilization and mania suppression. Valproic acid has replaced lithium as the drug of choice for many patients because it has far fewer adverse effects, a higher therapeutic index, and a more rapid onset of action. The only area in which it does not compare favorably with lithium is in the ability to prevent suicide. Valproic acid is well tolerated in most patients but can occasionally cause serious toxicity. Rare cases of thrombocytopenia, pancreatitis, and liver failure have occurred and signs of any of these adverse events require immediate withdrawal of the drug. As with lithium, valproic acid is teratogenic and should not be used during pregnancy. It is secreted in breast milk and therefore should not be used during lactation.

Carbamazepine (Tegretol) was one of the initial drugs studied as a lithium alternative, but it was not until 2005 that it was approved for that indication. It reduces the symptoms of both manic and depressive phases of bipolar disorder and can reduce recurrence of the condition. It is preferred over lithium for patients who have mixed mania or rapid-cycling bipolar disorder. Neurologic adverse effects such as vertigo, headache, unsteadiness, and ataxia are common during early therapy but usually subside with continued use. Oral contraceptives may be less effective, and pregnant women should not take carbamazepine because this drug is pregnancy category D. Increased CNS toxicity can result if carbamazepine is used concurrently with lithium. Carbamazepine is one of the most frequently prescribed antiseizure drugs.

Approved for treating bipolar disorder in 2003, the antiepileptic drug lamotrigine (Lamictal) is indicated for long-term maintenance therapy to prevent or delay relapses. It may be used alone or in combination with other mood stabilizers. The drug is well tolerated by most patients, with the most common adverse events being drowsiness, dizziness, ataxia, headache, diplopia, blurred vision, nausea, vomiting, and rash. Because

rare cases of Stevens–Johnson syndrome (SJS) have been documented, any appearance of rash calls for discontinuation of the drug. To minimize the risk of serious skin rashes, the dose of lamotrigine is increased gradually. Lamotrigine is a pregnancy category C drug and should be used cautiously in lactating women.

Other antiseizure drugs have been used off-label for bipolar disorder but they do not appear to be more effective than existing medications. These include oxcarbazepine (Trileptal), gabapentin (Neurontin), and topiramate (Topamax). Clonazepam (Klonopin) and lorazepam (Ativan) are benzodiazepines used for seizures that have been used off-label for bipolar disorder in combination with other agents.

Atypical antipsychotics: Antipsychotic drugs are used to control acute symptoms during episodes of mania and as long-term mood stabilizers. They benefit patients with or without psychotic symptoms. These agents are usually used in combination with lithium or valproic acid, but they are also effective if used as monotherapy. The atypical antipsychotics are preferred over the conventional antipsychotics because of a much lower incidence of extrapyramidal adverse effects. Five atypical antipsychotics have been approved for use in treating bipolar disorder: aripiprazole (Abilify), olanzapine (Zyprexa), quetiapine (Seroquel), risperidone (Risperdal), and ziprasidone (Geodon). All of these drugs are effective against manic episodes, but only olanzapine is approved for long-term maintenance therapy.

Antidepressants: Antidepressants may be used to treat the depressed stage of bipolar disorder. These agents must be used with caution because they have a tendency to cause hypomania or mania in depressed patients with bipolar disorder. Because of this potentially serious adverse effect in patients with bipolar disorder, antidepressants are administered concurrently with a mood stabilizer. The antidepressants of choice for treating patients with bipolar disorder are the SSRIs, venlafaxine (Effexor), and bupropion (Wellbutrin). The antidepressant medications are discussed earlier in this chapter.

UNDERSTANDING THE CHAPTER

Key Concepts Summary

1 The two primary types of mood disorders are depression and bipolar disorder.

2 Major depressive disorder is characterized by a depressed mood, with accompanying symptoms, that lasts at least 2 weeks.

3 The pathophysiology of depression has biologic, genetic, and environmental components.

4 Assessment and diagnosis of depression are a collaborative effort among health care providers.

5 The majority of patients who attempt suicide have major depression.

6 Depression is sometimes treated with nonpharmacologic therapies.

7 The mechanism of action of antidepressants involves modulation of neurotransmitter levels in the brain.

8 Tricyclic antidepressants have been the mainstay for the treatment of depression but have many adverse effects.

9 Selective serotonin reuptake inhibitors are the drugs of choice for treating depression due to their low incidence of serious adverse effects.

10 Atypical antidepressants are alternatives to the selective serotonin reuptake inhibitors that are prescribed for depression and anxiety disorders.

11 Monoamine oxidase inhibitors are effective antidepressants but are seldom used due to potentially serious adverse effects.

12 Bipolar disorder is a serious psychiatric disorder characterized by extreme mood swings from depression to euphoria.

13 Lithium is the conventional therapy for the treatment of bipolar disorder.

14 Antiseizure and atypical antipsychotic agents are used to control symptoms of bipolar disorder.

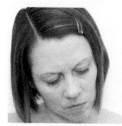

Making the PATIENT *Connection*

Remember the patient "Jane Albright" at the beginning of the chapter? Now read the remainder of the case study. Based on the information presented within this chapter, respond to the critical thinking questions that follow.

Jane is a 42-year-old mother of three young children. Before the children were born she was employed as a corporate attorney, but she and her husband decided prior to the birth of their first child that she would stay at home until the children completed high school. They are financially stable. Jane has been a soccer coach, Boy Scout leader, president of the ladies' group at her church, and involved in various other community organizations. Within the past month, she has not participated in any of her previous activities and she has not explained why. Jane is in good physical health and had her annual physical exam the previous month. She takes no routine medications or herbal products.

Critical Thinking Questions

1. What first step must Charlie take to aid his wife with her depression?

2. When Jane is evaluated by a mental health professional, they begin talking about how antidepressant drug therapy works. Provide a brief explanation of antidepressant therapy.

3. How can a nurse determine if a therapeutic effect from the antidepressant medication is being achieved with Jane?

See Answers to Critical Thinking Questions on student resource website.

NCLEX-RN® Review

1 A health care provider has ordered imipramine (Tofranil) for each of these clients. A nurse would question the order for the client with:

1. Seizure disorders.
2. Depression.
3. Enuresis.
4. Neuropathic pain.

2 The nurse determines that the client understands an important principle in self-administration of fluoxetine (Prozac) when the client makes which statement?

1. "I should not decrease my sodium or water intake."
2. "This drug can be taken concurrently with a monoamine oxidase inhibitor."
3. "It may take up to 1 month to reach full therapeutic effects."
4. "There are no problems associated with concurrent use of other central nervous system depressants."

3 The nurse is monitoring the client for early lithium carbonate (Eskalith) toxicity. Which symptoms, if manifested by the client, would indicate that toxicity may be developing? Select all that apply.

1. Persistent gastrointestinal upset
2. Confusion
3. Polyuria
4. Convulsions
5. Ataxia

4 Which statement made by the client who is taking lithium carbonate (Eskalith) indicates that further teaching is necessary?

1. "I will be sure to remain on a low-sodium diet."
2. "I will have blood levels drawn every 2 to 3 months, even when I have no symptoms."
3. "Lithium has a narrow margin of safety, so toxicity is a very real concern."
4. "I will not be able to breast-feed my baby."

5 The client who has been taking venlafaxine (Effexor) for 2 weeks calls the nurse to report that there is no improvement in the depression. The nurse's best response is:

1. "Call your health care provider and see if he or she will change the order to a different medication."

2. "Are you sure that you are taking it as it is ordered? Perhaps you should consider increasing the dosage gradually."

3. "The medication may take up to 3 weeks or longer to be effective. Continue taking the medication as ordered."

4. "Add an over-the-counter antianxiety agent to your daily medications."

6 A 17-year-old client is started on fluoxetine (Prozac) for treatment of depression. When teaching the client and his family, what would the nurse include? Select all that apply.

1. Report any sedation to the provider and exercise caution with activities requiring mental alertness.

2. Fluctuations in weight may be managed with a healthy diet and adequate amounts of exercise.

3. Report any thoughts of suicide to the provider immediately, especially during early initiation of the drug.

4. The drug may be safely stopped if unpleasant side effects occur and reported to the provider at the next scheduled visit.

5. The drug may cause excessive thirst but dramatic increase in fluid intake should be avoided.

Additional Case Study

Andrew Phillips, age 17, was diagnosed with bipolar illness with acute mania at age 15. He was stabilized with lithium for the manic periods and is also taking valproic acid. This fall, he played football and is looking forward to playing baseball this spring and summer. Although they have a close relationship, his parents have concerns about his dietary habits and postgame festivities, especially now that he is driving and they are not available to monitor the situation.

1. Considering Andrew's activities and eating habits, what risks are possible and what assessments would the nurse make to ensure Andrew's lithium dosage remains effective and within a therapeutic range?

2. What suggestions could the nurse make that would help Andrew participate fully in his sports interests and post-game festivities?

3. What strategies might the nurse suggest for helping Andrew's parents participate in his activities and care?

See Answers to Additional Case Study on student resource website.

Pearson Nursing Student Resources

Find additional review materials at nursing.pearsonhighered.com

Prepare for success with additional NCLEX®-style practice questions, interactive assignments and activities, web links, animations, videos, and more!

References

American Psychiatric Association. (2000). *Diagnostic and statistical manual of mental disorders* (4th ed., Text revision). Washington, DC: Author.

Centers for Disease Control and Prevention (CDC). (2007). *Suicide facts at a glance.* Retrieved from http://www.cdc.gov/ncipc/dvp/Suicide/SuicideDataSheet.pdf

Dryden-Edwards, R. (n.d.). *Depression.* Retrieved from http://www.emedicinehealth.com/depression/article_em.htm

Gibbons, R. D., Brown, C. H., Hur, K., Marcus, S. M., Bhaumik, D. K., & Mann, J. J. (2007). Relationship between antidepressants and suicide attempts: An analysis of the Veterans Health Administration data sets. *American Journal of Psychiatry, 164,* 1044–1049. doi:10.1176/appi.ajp.164.7.1044

Ikezu, T., & Gendelman, H. E. (2008). *Neuroimmune pharmacology.* New York, NY: Springer.

Linde, K., Berner, M. M., & Kriston, L. (2008). St. John's wort for major depression. *Cochrane Database of Systematic Reviews, 8*(4), CD000448.

National Center for Complementary and Alternative Medicine. (2010). *Herbs at a glance: St. John's wort.* Retrieved from http://nccam.nih.gov/health/stjohnswort/ataglance.htm

National Institute of Mental Health (NIMH). (2010) *Suicide in the U.S.: Statistics and prevention.* Retrieved from http://www.nimh.nih.gov/health/publications/suicide-in-the-us-statistics-and-prevention/index.shtml

Simon, G. E., & Savarino, J. (2007). Suicide attempts among patients starting depression treatment with medications or psychotherapy. *American Journal of Psychiatry, 164,* 1029–1034. doi:10.1176/appi.ajp.164.7.1029

Unutzer, J. (2007). Clinical practice: Late-life depression. *New England Journal of Medicine, 29,* 2269–2276. doi:10.1056/NEJMcp073754

U.S. Food and Drug Administration. (2004). *FDA launches a multi-pronged strategy to strengthen safeguards for children treated with antidepressant medications* (FDA Publication No. P04-97). Washington, DC: U.S. Government Printing Office.

Selected Bibliography

Barbui, C., Esposito, E., & Cipriani, A. (2009). Selective serotonin reuptake inhibitors and risk of suicide: A systematic review of observational studies. *Canadian Medi-cal Association Journal, 180*(3), 291–297. doi:10.1503/cmaj.081514

Juckett, G., & Rudolph-Watson, L. (2010). Recognizing mental illness in culture-bound syndromes. *American Family Physician, 81*(2), 209–210.

Maskill, V., Crowe, M., Luty, S., & Joyce, P. (2010). Two sides of the same coin: Caring for a person with bipolar disorder. *Journal of Psychiatric and Mental Health Nursing, 17,* 535–542. doi:10.1111/j.1365-2850.2010.01555.x

Nardi, D. (2007). Depression in school-aged children: Assessment and early interventions. *Journal of Psychosocial Nursing and Mental Health Services, 45*(3), 48–53.

Price, L. H., Tyrka, A. R., Henry, C., Demotes-Mainard, J., Leboyer, M., El-Mallakh, R. S., et al. (2007). Adjunctive antidepressant treatment for bipolar depression. *New England Journal of Medicine, 357,* 614–615. doi:10.1056/NEJMc071459

Sherrod, T., Quinlan-Colwell, A., Lattimore, T. B., Shatell, M. M., & Kennedy-Malone, L. (2010). Older adults with bipolar disorder: Guidelines for primary care providers. *Journal of Gerontological Nursing, 36*(5), 20–27. doi:10.3928/00989134-20100108-05

U.S. Food and Drug Administration Center for Drug Evaluation and Research. (2006). *Clinical review: Relationship between antidepressant drugs and suicidality in adults.* Retrieved from http://www.fda.gov/ohrms/dockets/ac/06/briefing/2006-4272b1-01-FDA.pdf

VanLieshout, R. J., & MacQueen, G. M. (2010). Efficacy and acceptability of mood stabilizers in the treatment of acute bipolar depression: Systematic review. *British Journal of Psychiatry 196,* 266–273. doi:10.1192/bjp.bp.108.057612

Answers to NCLEX-RN® Review

1 Answer: 1   Rationale: Imipramine should not be used by clients with seizure disorders because it lowers the seizure threshold. Options 2, 3, and 4 are incorrect. Imipramine is a drug that is effective in treating depression, and is one of only two drugs approved for enuresis (bedwetting) in children. Like other TCAs, imipramine has a number of off-label indications. These include the adjuvant treatment of cancer or neuropathic pain. Cognitive Level: Applying; Client Need: Physiological Integrity; Nursing Process: Implementation

2 Answer: 3   Rationale: Full therapeutic effects of fluoxetine may take up to 1 month. Options 1, 2, and 4 are incorrect. Normal water and sodium intake do not affect fluoxetine. The client cannot take an MAOI or other CNS depressant concurrently. The use of other drugs or CNS depressants such as alcohol could increase the risk of adverse effects or increased depression. Cognitive Level: Analyzing; Client Need: Physiological Integrity; Nursing Process: Evaluation

3 Answer: 1, 2   Rationale: Persistent GI upset and confusion are signs of elevated lithium levels between 1.5 and 2.0, which signify early toxicity. Options 3, 4, and 5 are incorrect. Polyuria is an adverse effect that may occur in early therapy, but is not associated with early toxicity. Convulsions may occur at serum levels above 2.5, but not in early stages of toxicity. Ataxia is also not a sign of early lithium toxicity. Cognitive Level: Analyzing; Client Need: Physiological Integrity; Nursing Process: Evaluation

4 Answer: 1   Rationale: The client taking lithium must be conscious of maintaining normal sodium intake. Because lithium is a salt, if sodium intake is low the body will replace the sodium with lithium, leading to lithium toxicity. Options 2, 3, and 4 are incorrect. The client taking lithium must have regular blood studies and toxicity is a very real concern; hence the necessity for routine blood studies. Women should refrain from breast-feeding while taking lithium. Cognitive Level: Analyzing; Client Need: Physiological Integrity; Nursing Process: Evaluation

5 Answer: 3   Rationale: A typical antidepressant such as venlafaxine may take up to 3 weeks or longer to reach full therapeutic effect, so the client must continue taking the medication as ordered so that therapeutic drug levels can be reached and maintained. Options 1, 2, and 4 are incorrect. It is not within a nurse's scope of practice to suggest changes in medication routine without consulting the prescriber, and these comments are not helpful to maintaining a therapeutic nurse–client relationship. Cognitive Level: Analyzing; Client Need: Health Promotion and Maintenance; Nursing Process: Evaluation

6 Answer: 2, 3   Rationale: Fluoxetine causes weight loss in some clients, while other clients experience weight gain or fluctuations in weight. A healthy diet and adequate exercise will help maintain normal weight while on this drug. While rare, an increased risk of suicide has been noted in clients up to age 24, and the client should be carefully monitored, especially during the early initiation of therapy. Options 1, 4, and 5 are incorrect. Fluoxetine may cause insomnia but not sedation. Abrupt withdrawal of fluoxetine may lead to withdrawal symptoms. If the drug needs to be discontinued, gradually tapering the dose is recommended. Fluoxetine is not known to cause excessive thirst. Cognitive Level: Analyzing; Client Need: Physiological Integrity; Nursing Process: Evaluation

Review of the Gastrointestinal System

From Chapter 61 of *Pharmacology: Connections to Nursing Practice*, Second Edition. Michael Patrick Adams, Carol Quam Urban. Copyright ©
2013 by Pearson Education, Inc. All rights reserved.

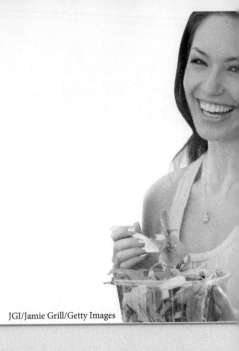

Review of the Gastrointestinal System

Learning Outcomes

After reading this chapter, the student should be able to:

1. Describe the major anatomic structures of the digestive system.
2. Outline the steps in the process of digestion.
3. Describe the primary functions of the stomach.
4. Analyze how the anatomic structures of the small intestine promote the absorption of nutrients and drugs.
5. Describe the primary structures and functions of the large intestine.
6. Describe the functions of the liver and their relevance to drug therapy.
7. Explain the hepatic portal system and its importance to drug therapy.
8. Explain the nervous control of digestion.
9. Explain the enzymatic breakdown of nutrients by the digestive system.

Chapter Outline

Overview of the Digestive System

Physiology of the Upper Gastrointestinal Tract

Physiology of the Lower Gastrointestinal Tract

Physiology of the Accessory Organs of Digestion

Regulation of Digestive Processes

Nutrient Categories and Metabolism

Very little of the food we eat is directly available to body cells. Food must be broken down, absorbed, and chemically modified before it is in a form that is useful to cells. The digestive system performs these, and more, functions. This chapter focuses on the aspects of digestion and physiology that are applicable to pharmacotherapy. For a complete review of the digestive system, the student should refer to an anatomy and physiology textbook.

Overview of the Digestive System

1 The function of the digestive system is to extract nutrients from food so that they may be used to fuel the metabolic processes in the body.

The **digestive system** consists of two basic anatomic divisions: the alimentary canal and the accessory organs. The **alimentary canal**, or gastrointestinal (GI) tract, is a long, continuous, hollow tube that extends from the mouth to the anus. The **accessory organs of digestion** include the salivary glands, liver, gallbladder, and pancreas. The major structures of the digestive system are illustrated in Figure 1.

The overall function of the digestive system is to extract nutrients from food so that they may be used to fuel the metabolic processes in the body. Because food is a complex substance, multiple steps are necessary before cells can use its components. These steps are ingestion, propulsion, digestion, absorption, and defecation.

Key Terms

absorption
accessory organs of digestion
alimentary canal
chief cells
chyme
defecation
digestion
digestive system
enteric nervous system (ENS)
enteroendocrine cells
enterohepatic recirculation
first-pass effect
hepatic portal system
ingestion
parietal cells
peristalsis

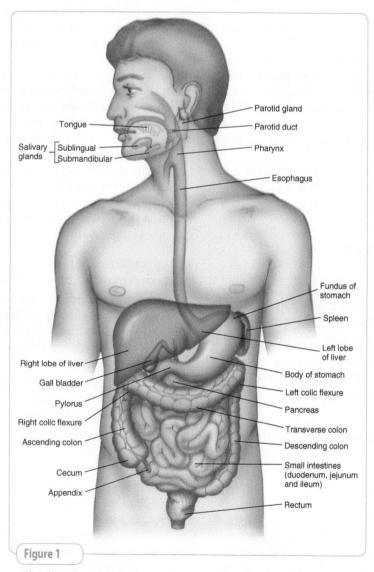

Parotid gland
Tongue
Parotid duct
Salivary glands — Sublingual
Submandibular
Pharynx
Esophagus
Fundus of stomach
Spleen
Left lobe of liver
Right lobe of liver
Gall bladder
Body of stomach
Pylorus
Left colic flexure
Pancreas
Right colic flexure
Transverse colon
Ascending colon
Descending colon
Cecum
Small intestines (duodenum, jejunum and ileum)
Appendix
Rectum

Figure 1

The digestive system.

Ingestion is taking food into the body by mouth. In some patients, ingestion bypasses the mouth and delivers nutrients directly into the stomach or small intestine via a feeding tube.

Substances are propelled along the GI tract by **peristalsis**, which is the rhythmic contractions of layers of smooth muscle. The speed at which substances move through the GI tract is critical to the absorption of drugs, nutrients, and water, and for the removal of wastes. If peristalsis is too fast, substances will not have sufficient contact with the GI mucosa to be absorbed. In addition, the large intestine will not have enough time to absorb water, and diarrhea may result. Abnormally slow transit may result in constipation or even obstructions in the small or large intestine.

Digestion is the mechanical and chemical breakdown of food into a form that may be absorbed into the systemic circulation. To chemically break down ingested food, a large number of enzymes and other substances are required. Digestive enzymes are secreted by the salivary glands, stomach, small intestine, and pancreas. The liver makes bile, which is stored in the gallbladder until it is needed for lipid digestion.

Absorption is the movement of nutrients and other substances from the alimentary canal to the circulation. The inner lining of the alimentary canal, called the mucosa layer, provides a surface area for the various acids, bases, and enzymes to break down food. In many parts of the alimentary canal, the mucosa is folded and contains deep grooves and pits. The small intestine is lined with tiny projections called villi and microvilli that provide a huge surface area for the absorption of nutrients and medications.

Not all components of ingested food are useful to the human body or can be digested. The elimination of indigestible substances from the body is called **defecation**.

Physiology of the Upper Gastrointestinal Tract

2 The upper gastrointestinal tract is responsible for mechanical and chemical digestion.

The upper GI tract consists of the mouth, pharynx, esophagus, and stomach. From a pharmacologic perspective, the most important regions of the upper GI tract are the buccal and sublingual areas of the mouth and the stomach.

PharmFACT

Most people believe that obese people have larger stomachs. However, people who are naturally thin have the same size as or even larger stomachs than people who have problems with weight control. Weight has nothing to do with the size of the stomach (Bouchez, 2008).

The epithelial mucosa of the buccal and sublingual regions is very thin, being only 40 to 50 cells in thickness. The mucosal layer, along with the salivary glands, secretes mucus, which lubricates and moistens the oral cavity. The mucus also serves as a liquid medium for drug administration inside the mouth. The oral mucosa in the sublingual region is relatively permeable, and drugs are rapidly absorbed. The buccal region is less permeable, and drug absorption is slower. The buccal region, however, has less salivary flow and drugs can be retained longer, making it better suited for sustained release delivery systems. For example, Striant is a buccal form of testosterone that is designed to release the drug over an 8- to 12-hour period.

The pharynx and esophagus serve as passageways for ingested food and liquids. Obstruction of these areas, or a loss of the swallowing reflex, precludes the administration of oral drugs. Little absorption occurs across the pharyngeal or esophageal mucosa because drugs travel quickly through these regions of the alimentary canal.

Food passes from the esophagus to the stomach by traveling through the lower esophageal (cardiac) sphincter. This ring of smooth muscle usually prevents the stomach contents from moving backward, a condition known as gastroesophageal reflux. The stomach has both mechanical and chemical functions. The muscular squeezing of the stomach churns and mixes the food, breaking it down mechanically to a semi-solid known as **chyme**. Strong peristaltic contractions push the chyme toward the pylorus, where it encounters a second ring of smooth muscle called the pyloric sphincter. Located at the entrance to the small intestine, this sphincter regulates the flow of substances leaving the stomach. Chyme moves in "spurts" through the sphincter into the small intestine. Large pieces of food are refluxed back into the body of the stomach, where they are subjected to more churning to reduce them in size to about 2 mm so that they may pass through the sphincter.

The stomach also secretes substances that promote the processes of chemical digestion. Gastric glands extending deep into the mucosa of the stomach contain several cell types that are critical to digestion and that are important to the pharmacotherapy of digestive disorders:

- **Chief cells** secrete pepsinogen, an inactive form of the enzyme pepsin that chemically breaks down proteins.
- **Parietal cells** secrete 1 to 3 liters of hydrochloric acid each day. This strong acid helps to break down food, activates pepsinogen, and kills microbes that may have been ingested. Parietal cells also secrete intrinsic factor, which is essential for the absorption of vitamin B_{12}.
- **Enteroendocrine cells** secrete hormones that modify the digestive processes. In the stomach, the most important secretion is gastrin, which stimulates acid production.

The combined secretion of the chief and parietal cells, known as gastric juice, is the most acidic fluid in the body, having a pH of 1.5 to 3.5. A number of natural defenses protect the stomach mucosa against this extremely acidic fluid. Certain cells that line the surface of the stomach secrete a thick, mucous layer and bicarbonate ion to neutralize the acid. These form such an effective protective layer that the pH at the mucosal surface is nearly neutral. On reaching the duodenum, the stomach contents are further neutralized by bicarbonate from pancreatic and biliary secretions.

The pharmacologic importance of the stomach lies in its capacity to absorb drugs. For most oral drugs, the stomach is not the primary site of absorption because the drug does not stay long in the organ. Stomach acidity (pH 1 to 2) can either assist in the absorption process or destroy the drug entirely. Drugs that are weak acids tend to be absorbed in the stomach. Protein drugs are destroyed by pepsin in the stomach before they are absorbed or have a chance to reach the small intestine.

CONNECTION Checkpoint 61.1

Nitroglycerin is the most frequently prescribed sublingual medication. What is the primary indication for nitroglycerin and what is the onset of action time of the drug when it is given by the sublingual route? *See Answer to Connection Checkpoint 61.1 on student resource website.*

Physiology of the Lower Gastrointestinal Tract

3 The small intestine is the longest portion of the alimentary canal and is the primary organ for absorption.

The lower GI tract consists of the small and large intestines. With its many folds and finger-like projections of villi and microvilli, the small intestine is highly specialized for absorption. The lining of each villus is composed of a single layer of epithelial cells and contains blood capillaries, as illustrated in Figure 2. Essentially, only a single cell separates a nutrient or drug molecule from the intestinal lumen of the body's circulatory system.

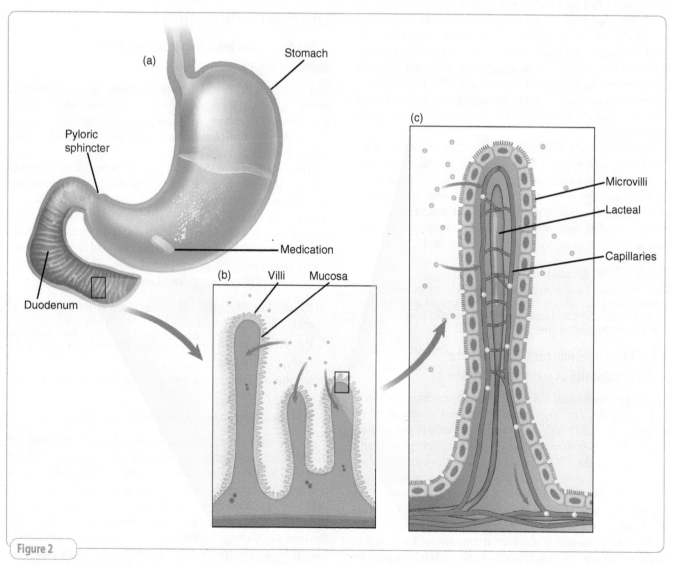

Figure 2

Villi and microvilli of the small intestine: (a) Tablet dissolves in the stomach. (b) Medication reaches the villi of the duodenum. (c) Drug molecules are absorbed into the microvilli capillaries.

The first 10 inches of the small intestine, known as the duodenum, is the site where chyme mixes with bile from the gallbladder and digestive enzymes from the pancreas. Bile and pancreatic juice enter through an opening in the duodenum known as the duodenal papilla. The duodenum is sometimes considered part of the upper GI tract because of its proximity to the stomach. The most common disorder of the duodenum is called peptic ulcer.

PharmFACT

Energy drinks are consumed by 30% to 50% of children, adolescents, and young adults (Seifert, Schaechter, Hershorin, & Lipshultz, 2011). Because these drinks are classified as nutritional supplements, they avoid the limit of 71 mg of caffeine per 12 fluid ounces that the U.S. Food and Drug Administration has set for soda. Energy drinks contain as much as 75 to 400 mg of caffeine per container, and sometimes contain even more caffeine (not included on the label) coming from additives such as guarana, kola nut, yerba mate, and cocoa.

The remainder of the small intestine consists of the jejunum and ileum. Because of its length and enormous absorptive surface, the first 1 to 2 meters of the jejunum is the site of the majority of nutrient and drug absorption. As the jejunum becomes the ileum, the diameter of the intestinal lumen diminishes and the villi become fewer in number. The terminal ileum is a primary site for the absorption of vitamin B_{12}, long-chain fatty acids, and fat-soluble vitamins. The ileum empties its contents into the large intestine through the ileocecal valve. Travel time for chyme through the entire small intestine varies from 3 to 6 hours.

The mucosa of the small intestine secretes intestinal juice, which is a mixture of mucus, digestive enzymes, and hormones. The mucus has an alkaline pH, which neutralizes the acidity from the stomach. The small intestine also secretes cholecystokinin, a hormone that promotes pancreatic enzyme secretion and secretin, which stimulates bicarbonate production to make the small intestine more alkaline.

CONNECTION Checkpoint 61.2

Many oral drugs have enteric coatings. What is the purpose of the enteric coating and why are these drugs not to be split or crushed? *See Answer to Connection Checkpoint 61.2 on student resource website.*

4 The large intestine contains host flora and is a major site of water reabsorption.

The large intestine, or colon, receives chyme from the ileum in a fluid state. The large intestine does not secrete digestive enzymes nor does it have enteroendocrine cells to secrete hormones. With few exceptions, little reabsorption of nutrients occurs during the 12- to 24-hour journey through the colon. The large intestine does secrete a large amount of mucus, which helps lubricate the fecal matter. The major functions of the colon are to reabsorb water and electrolytes from the waste material and excrete the remaining fecal material from the body.

The colon harbors a substantial amount of bacteria and fungi, called the host flora, which serve a useful purpose by synthesizing B-complex vitamins and vitamin K. Disruption of the normal host flora can lead to diarrhea.

From a pharmacologic perspective, the large intestine may be the site of therapeutic or adverse drug effects. A large number of drugs cause either diarrhea or constipation. These effects are usually self-limiting and can be prevented or managed through nursing interventions. When bowel patterns are significantly disrupted, drugs may be given to slow the activity (antidiarrheals) or increase the activity (laxatives) of the large intestine.

Of additional pharmacologic importance are the drugs given by the rectal route. The mucosa of the rectum provides an excellent and rapid absorptive surface for drugs. It is a route of particular importance in children and in patients who are unable to take oral medications due to nausea, vomiting, or other pathology that prevents oral administration. The onset of action is usually slower than the oral route, and drug action is limited by the length of time that the patient can retain the drug without defecation.

Physiology of the Accessory Organs of Digestion

5 The liver is the most important accessory digestive organ.

The accessory organs of digestion include the teeth, tongue, salivary glands, pancreas, gallbladder, and liver. Of these, the pancreas and liver have the most pharmacologic importance. The endocrine functions of the pancreas, which include the secretion of insulin and glucagon.

The liver is one of the most important organs in pharmacology. Along with the kidneys, any drug that reaches the circulation, regardless of its route of administration, will pass through the liver. The overall function of the liver is to filter and process the nutrients and drugs delivered to it. Substances may be stored, chemically altered, or removed from the blood before they reach the general circulation. The following are some of the primary functions of the liver:

- **Regulation.** Stabilizes the serum levels of glucose, triglycerides, and cholesterol
- **Protection.** Removes toxic substances and waste products such as ammonia
- **Synthesis.** Synthesizes bile, plasma proteins, and certain clotting factors
- **Storage.** Stores iron and fat-soluble vitamins

When most drugs reach the liver, they are metabolized to less toxic substances that are more easily excreted by the kidney. The cytochrome P450 enzyme system in liver cells is especially active at metabolizing drugs. In a few cases, the liver changes the drug to a more active form. It is important to note that the handling of drugs and toxic substances by the liver can damage hepatocytes and impair their functions. This is especially true if the hepatocytes are chronically exposed to harmful substances such as alcohol. Hepatic impairment is a relatively common adverse effect of certain drugs.

Whereas drug-induced hepatic impairment is often transient and asymptomatic, some drugs can cause severe, permanent, and even fatal liver damage.

PharmFACT

Acetaminophen (Tylenol) overdose is the leading cause of acute liver failure in the United States. Normal doses of the drug can cause acetaminophen poisoning in malnourished patients or those with chronic alcohol abuse (Farrell, 2010).

The unique structure of the vascular system serving the liver is important to digestion as well as pharmacology. The liver receives both oxygenated and deoxygenated blood. The **hepatic portal system**, shown in Figure 3, is a network of venous vessels that collects blood draining from the stomach, small intestine, and most of the large intestine. This blood is extremely rich in nutrients because it contains substances absorbed during digestion. It is important to know that this blood is delivered to the liver via the hepatic portal vein before it reaches the arterial circulation. The liver then can remove, store, excrete, or perform metabolic functions on these substances before they are sent into the inferior vena cava to reach other organs.

The hepatic portal system serves as an important homeostatic mechanism, allowing a relatively stable composition of blood to circulate through the body. In terms of drug therapy, nearly all oral medications enter the hepatic portal vein for processing by the liver before they reach their target tissue. In some cases, the liver removes a substantial percentage of the drug before it reaches the inferior vena cava, a phenomenon called the **first-pass effect**. Drugs that have a significant first-pass effect may be given by other routes, such as intramuscular, intravenous, subcutaneous, or topical. Although a drug will still eventually reach the liver by these routes, it will have an opportunity to also reach its target tissue. Note that the venous systems serving the head and the lower rectum are not parts of the hepatic portal system. Thus, drugs that are given by the buccal, sublingual, or rectal routes bypass the first-pass effect of the liver.

As the liver makes bile, the bile is sent to the gallbladder where it is stored. When lipids enter the small intestine, the gallbladder contracts and sends its contents into the duodenum. The bile salts emulsify the lipids, making them easier to digest enzymatically. When bile salts reach the terminal portion of the ileum, 95% are reabsorbed back into the hepatic portal circulation by a process called **enterohepatic recirculation**. This process has direct implications to pharmacotherapy. Certain drugs, including digoxin (Lanoxin), morphine, and estrogens, are eliminated in the bile and are reabsorbed by enterohepatic recirculation. Enterohepatic recirculation recycles the drug multiple times and can significantly extend a drug's half-life. Interactions can occur if one drug interferes with the enterohepatic recycling of another drug. Preventing

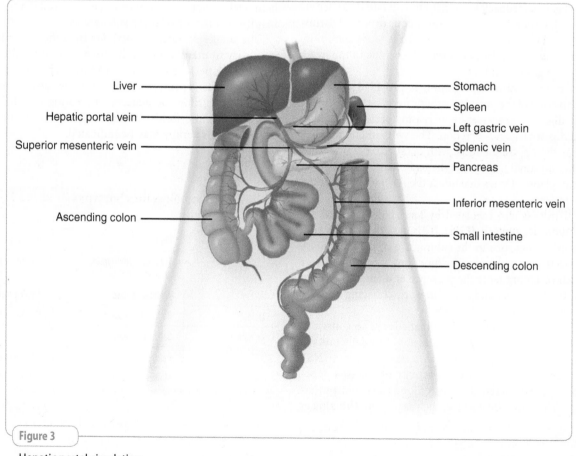

Liver — Stomach
Hepatic portal vein — Spleen
— Left gastric vein
Superior mesenteric vein — Splenic vein
— Pancreas
— Inferior mesenteric vein
Ascending colon — Small intestine
— Descending colon

Figure 3

Hepatic portal circulation.

this recycling can speed the elimination of a drug and reduce its therapeutic effectiveness. An example of such an interaction is when cholestyramine (Questran) interferes with the recycling of lorazepam (Ativan) and increases the clearance of lorazepam from the body.

The pancreas is an essential accessory digestive organ, secreting about a quart of pancreatic fluid into the duodenum each day. This fluid is alkaline (pH 7.5 to 8.8) and contains digestive enzymes to chemically break down carbohydrates, lipids, proteins, and nucleic acids. From a pharmacologic perspective, the pancreas is relatively protected from drugs and there are only a few therapies for pancreatic digestive disorders.

CONNECTION Checkpoint 61.3

The tricyclic antidepressant imipramine is a substrate for the CYP2D6 enzyme, and the selective serotonin reuptake inhibitor (SSRI) fluoxetine is a potent inhibitor of this enzyme. Predict the type of drug interaction that will occur to a patient stabilized on imipramine therapy when fluoxetine is added to the regimen. *See Answer to Connection Checkpoint 61.3 on student resource website.*

Regulation of Digestive Processes

6 Digestion is regulated by numerous hormonal and nervous factors.

Digestion is controlled through a large number of hormonal and nervous factors that influence the speed of peristalsis and the amount of saliva, mucus, acid, and enzyme secretions. Various negative feedback loops help to regulate these activities so that digestion is a smooth, continuous process. Disruption of normal homeostatic mechanisms can cause cramping, due to excessive peristalsis, or peptic ulcers, due to the overproduction of gastric acid.

The nervous control of digestion is provided at several levels. Activation of the parasympathetic nervous system stimulates the digestive processes by increasing peristalsis, salivation, and digestive gland secretion. The sympathetic nervous system has the opposite effects, with beta$_2$-adrenergic receptors in the intestinal wall and alpha$_1$-adrenergic receptors in the salivary glands. Drugs that affect the ANS often affect the digestive processes.

The GI tract is also regulated by local reflexes called the **enteric nervous system (ENS)**. This system consists of a vast network of neurons in the submucosa of the alimentary canal that has sensory and motor functions. Chemoreceptors and stretch receptors sense the presence and amount of food in the GI tract and respond accordingly by changing motility without sending signals to the ANS.

The GI tract functions at an automatic level; no conscious thought is required as the system goes about its daily tasks of secretion and digestion. The central nervous system (CNS), however, can greatly influence the activity of digestive functions. For example, merely thinking of food can evoke powerful images. These may be positive, such as perhaps thinking of a steak sizzling on the grill or bread baking in the oven, and increase salivation and peristalsis. Images may also be negative and evoke feelings of nausea and vomiting at the sight of food. Mental health conditions such as depression, anxiety, excessive stress, or bipolar disorder can affect the appetite and digestive processes.

Nutrient Categories and Metabolism

7 The chemical breakdown of food is accomplished by digestive enzymes.

The three basic nutrients are carbohydrates, lipids, and proteins. In food these nutrients are large molecules that cannot be absorbed across the mucosa of the alimentary canal. Chemical digestion must break down these complex food molecules into simpler substances so that they can be absorbed and used by the body for metabolic processes.

The breakdown of complex carbohydrates, lipids, and proteins requires digestive enzymes to be delivered when food is present at various parts of the alimentary canal, primarily the stomach and small intestine. These enzymes and their locations are listed in Table 1. Secretion of digestive enzymes is regulated by hormones and the nervous system, as described in Section 6. Patients who secrete insufficient quantities of digestive enzymes may be administered these substances as drugs.

In addition to the three basic nutrients, the body requires a host of other vitamins and minerals for proper metabolism. Deficiency symptoms will be observed if a patient has insufficient intake of these substances.

The intake of various nutrients in sufficient amounts is necessary to maintain good health and to allow the body to heal during periods of illness or injury. The intake of sufficient amounts of proteins, carbohydrates, fats, vitamins, and minerals can often be achieved by eating a well-balanced diet of foods and fluids. When this does not occur, enteral or parenteral therapy may be indicated.

TABLE 1 Major Digestive Enzymes

Nutrient	Enzyme	Source
Proteins and polypeptides	Pepsin	Gastric glands
	Trypsin, chymotrypsin, carboxypeptidase	Pancreatic juice
	Aminopeptidase	Small intestine
Lipids	Pancreatic lipase	Pancreatic juice
Carbohydrates and starches	Salivary amylase	Saliva
	Pancreatic amylase	Pancreatic juice
	Maltase, sucrase, lactase	Small intestine

UNDERSTANDING ᴛʜᴇ CHAPTER

Key Concepts Summary

1 The function of the digestive system is to extract nutrients from food so that they may be used to fuel the metabolic processes in the body.

2 The upper gastrointestinal tract is responsible for mechanical and chemical digestion.

3 The small intestine is the longest portion of the alimentary canal and is the primary organ for absorption.

4 The large intestine contains host flora and is a major site of water reabsorption.

5 The liver is the most important accessory digestive organ.

6 Digestion is regulated by numerous hormonal and nervous factors.

7 The chemical breakdown of food is accomplished by digestive enzymes.

Pearson Nursing Student Resources

Find additional review materials at
nursing.pearsonhighered.com
Prepare for success with additional NCLEX®-style practice questions, interactive assignments and activities, web links, animations, videos, and more!

References

Bouchez, C. (2008). *9 surprising facts about your stomach*. Retrieved from http://www.webmd.com/digestive-disorders/features/nine-surprising-facts-about-your-stomach

Farrell, S. E. (2010). *Toxicity: Acetaminophen*. Retrieved from http://emedicine.medscape.com/article/820200-overview

Seifert, S. M., Schaechter, J. L., Hershorin, E. R., & Lipshultz, S. E. (2011). Health effects of energy drinks on children, adolescents, and young adults. *Pediatrics, 127*(3), 511–528. doi:10.1542/peds.2009-3592

Zelman, M., Tompary, E., Raymond, J., Holdaway, P., & Mulvihill, M. L. (2010). *Human diseases: A systemic approach* (7th ed., p. 201). Upper Saddle River, NJ: Pearson.

Martini, F. H., Nath, J. L., & Bartholomew, E. F. (2012). *Fundamentals of human anatomy and physiology* (9th ed.). San Francisco, CA: Benjamin Cummings.

Silverthorn, D. U. (2012). *Human physiology: An integrated approach* (5th ed.). San Francisco, CA: Benjamin Cummings.

Selected Bibliography

Krogh, D. (2011). *Biology: A guide to the natural world* (5th ed.). San Francisco, CA: Benjamin Cummings.

Pharmacotherapy of Peptic Ulcer Disease

From Chapter 62 of *Pharmacology: Connections to Nursing Practice*, Second Edition. Michael Patrick Adams, Carol Quam Urban. Copyright ©
2013 by Pearson Education, Inc. All rights reserved.

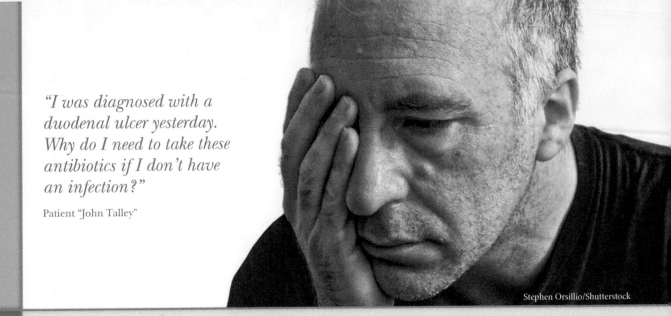

Stephen Orsillio/Shutterstock

"I was diagnosed with a duodenal ulcer yesterday. Why do I need to take these antibiotics if I don't have an infection?"

Patient "John Talley"

Pharmacotherapy of Peptic Ulcer Disease

Learning Outcomes

After reading this chapter, the student should be able to:

1. Explain the physiological regulation of gastric acid secretion.

2. Describe factors that suppress and those that promote the formation of peptic ulcers.

3. Compare and contrast duodenal ulcers and gastric ulcers.

4. Identify the etiology, signs, and symptoms of peptic ulcer disease and gastroesophageal reflux disease.

5. Outline the treatment goals for the pharmacotherapy of peptic ulcer disease and gastroesophageal reflux disease.

6. Identify the classification of drugs used to treat peptic ulcer disease and gastroesophageal reflux disease.

7. Explain the pharmacologic strategies for eradicating *Helicobacter pylori*.

8. Describe the nurse's role in the pharmacologic management of patients with peptic ulcer disease and gastroesophageal reflux disease.

9. For each of the classes shown in the chapter outline, identify the prototype and representative drugs and explain the mechanism(s) of drug action, primary indications, contraindications, significant drug interactions, pregnancy category, and important adverse effects.

10. Apply the nursing process to care for patients who are receiving pharmacotherapy for peptic ulcer disease and gastroesophageal reflux disease.

Acid-related diseases of the upper gastrointestinal (GI) tract are some of the most common medical conditions. Drugs for these disorders are available over the counter (OTC), and many patients attempt self-treatment before seeking assistance from their health care provider. Signs and symptoms of acid-related conditions of the upper GI tract, however, may indicate more serious disease. This chapter examines the pharmacotherapy of two common disorders of the upper digestive system: peptic ulcer disease (PUD) and gastroesophageal reflux disease (GERD).

Physiology of the Upper Gastrointestinal Tract

1 The stomach secretes acid, enzymes, and hormones that are essential to digestive physiology.

The upper GI tract consists of the mouth, pharynx, esophagus, and stomach. The duodenum, the first 10 inches of the small intestine, is sometimes considered part of the upper GI tract because of its proximity to the stomach.

Gastric glands in the stomach contain several cell types that are critical to digestion and important to the pharmacotherapy of digestive disorders. Chief cells secrete the enzyme pepsinogen, which is then activated to become **pepsin**, which is the digestive enzyme that breaks down proteins from food. Parietal cells secrete gastric (hydrochloric) acid in the stomach, which provides a strongly acidic environment that promotes the conversion of pepsinogen to pepsin, helps to break down food, and kills microbes that may have been ingested. Parietal cells also secrete intrinsic factor, which is essential for the absorption of vitamin B_{12}. Parietal cells are targets for the classes of drugs that reduce acid secretion. The cell types present in gastric glands are shown in Figure 1.

Parietal cells receive messages from several sources, which tell them to increase or decrease acid production. These cells contain receptors for the hormone gastrin, histamine (H_2), and the neurotransmitter acetylcholine, which are the three principal physiological stimuli that regulate acid secretion from the proton pump, or H^+, K^+-ATPase, located on the surface of parietal cells.

Ingestion of food and distention of the stomach stimulate the secretion of the hormone gastrin into the bloodstream. The target cells for gastrin are enteroendocrine cells in the gastric glands. When gastrin binds to their cell surface, the enteroendocrine cells produce and secrete histamine. Histamine then binds to the H_2 receptor on the parietal cell to stimulate acid secretion. In addition to promoting acid secretion, gastrin signals the chief cells to secrete pepsin, promotes the production of pancreatic enzymes, and increases gastric blood flow.

Like most hormones, gastrin is regulated by a negative feedback loop. As the stomach contents reach pH 3 or lower, the hormone **somatostatin** is released by cells in the stomach, small intestine, and pancreas. This hormone suppresses the secretion of gastrin, thus lowering acid secretion. Interestingly, somatostatin is also released by the anterior pituitary gland and is known as growth hormone-inhibiting hormone.

However, the nervous system secretion and actions are independent of its digestive actions.

Cells lining the surface of the stomach mucosa secrete a thick mucous layer that provides a continuous, protective physical barrier against acid and pepsin. Bicarbonate ion is also secreted by the epithelial cells in the stomach and serves to neutralize gastric acid on the mucosal surface. The mucus and bicarbonate ion form such an effective protective layer that the pH at the mucosal surface is nearly neutral. Once the stomach contents reach the duodenum, they are further neutralized by the bicarbonate ion from pancreatic and biliary secretions.

Another protective substance is the hormone **prostaglandin E_2**. This hormone stimulates the secretion of mucus and bicarbonate, promotes repair of damaged gastric mucosal cells, and increases blood flow to the mucosa to help maintain optimal mucosal conditions. Several frequently prescribed drugs, including corticosteroids and nonsteroidal anti-inflammatory drugs (NSAIDs), cause peptic ulcers because they are prostaglandin antagonists. The natural defenses of the stomach are shown in Figure 2.

Etiology and Pathogenesis of Peptic Ulcer Disease

2 Peptic ulcer disease is associated with a number of etiologic risk factors.

A **peptic ulcer** is a lesion or erosion located in either the stomach (gastric) or small intestine (duodenal) mucosa that is usually associated with acute inflammation. PUD was an uncommon condition until the 19th century. Thus it is considered to be a "disease of civilization." Although PUD occurs most often in middle age, it may occur at any time, including infancy and childhood. A significant family history is present in at least half of children with PUD.

PUD occurs when there is an imbalance of protective factors versus aggravating factors: The levels of protective mucus and bicarbonate ion secretions are unable to protect against the aggravating factors of pepsin and gastric acid. Complications of PUD include bleeding, perforation, penetration, and GI obstruction due to scarring. The incidence of PUD is associated with the following risk factors:

- Infection with the bacterium *Helicobacter pylori* (*H. pylori*)
- Close family history of PUD

Key Terms

adhesins

antacids

antiflatulent

Barrett's esophagus

gastroesophageal reflux disease (GERD)

H^+, K^+-ATPase

H_2-receptor antagonists

milk-alkali syndrome

pepsin

peptic ulcer

prostaglandin E_2

proton pump inhibitors (PPIs)

somatostatin

Zollinger-Ellison Syndrome (ZES)

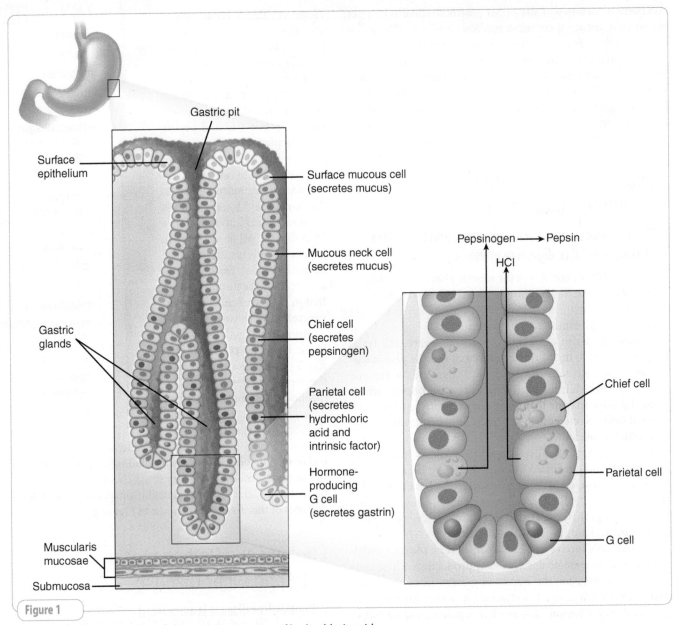

Figure 1

The stomach lining: gastric glands and the secretion of hydrochloric acid.

- Use of drugs, particularly corticosteroids, NSAIDs, and platelet inhibitors such as aspirin and clopidogrel

- Blood group O (the antigen may be a target of *H. pylori* attachment)

- Smoking tobacco (increases gastric acid secretion and reduces bicarbonate production)

- Consumption of beverages and foods that contain excessive caffeine

- Excessive psychological stress

PharmFACT

Approximately 4.5 million Americans are affected by PUD, and about 10% of Americans will experience an ulcer in their lifetime (Anand, 2011).

For many decades, it was thought that mental and physiological stress, smoking, and spicy foods were the primary causes of PUD. It was theorized that bacteria could not survive the acidic environment of the stomach, thus the hypothesis that an infectious agent could be the cause of PUD was not accepted. In the 1980s, however, researchers discovered an association between the gram-negative bacterium *H. pylori* and PUD. Over time, the hypothesis was accepted, and treatment of PUD as an infectious disease was aggressively promoted by the Centers for Disease Control and Prevention (CDC). The pharmacotherapy of *H. pylori* is described in Section 8.

Many causes of PUD are not related to *H. pylori* infection. For example, drug therapy with NSAIDs is likely responsible for almost half of peptic ulcer cases. Gastric and duodenal ulcers occur in about 20% of patients using NSAIDs on a regular basis, with 4% experiencing serious bleeding.

NSAIDs promote ulcer formation and inflammation both topically and systemically. Topically, NSAIDs cause direct cellular damage to GI mucosal cells. Systemically NSAIDs

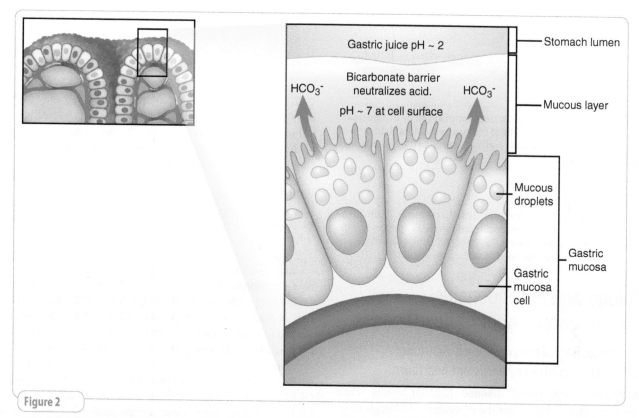

Figure 2

Natural defenses against stomach acid.

interfere with prostaglandin synthesis via the enzyme cyclo-oxygenase (COX) in the stomach, which normally aids in the production of mucus and bicarbonate. NSAIDs decrease gastric blood flow and slow cellular repair. NSAIDs are also weak acids that are nonionized in gastric acid and able to diffuse across the mucous barrier into the gastric epithelial cells, which leads to further cellular damage.

Risk factors for NSAID-induced PUD include long-term use of NSAIDs, advanced age, history of ulcers, concomitant use of corticosteroids or anticoagulants, or alcohol and cigarette smoking. In addition, *H. pylori* infection and NSAIDs act synergistically to promote ulcers. The combination poses a 3.5-fold greater risk of ulcers than either factor alone.

The characteristic symptom of duodenal ulcer is a gnawing or burning, upper abdominal pain that occurs 1 to 3 hours after a meal. The pain is usually worse when the stomach is empty and often disappears with ingestion of food. This is because the presence of food closes the pyloric sphincter and allows the acid to remain in the stomach, rather than to come into contact with the duodenal ulcer. Night-time pain may awaken the patient. If the erosion progresses deeper into the mucosa, bleeding occurs and may be evident as either bright red blood in vomit or black, tarry stools. Many duodenal ulcers heal spontaneously, although scar tissue remains, predisposing the mucosa to future ulceration, and they frequently recur after months of remission. Perforation and hemorrhage are sometimes the first signs of a duodenal ulcer in infants. Many patients with PUD are asymptomatic.

Gastric ulcers are less common than the duodenal type and have different symptoms. Pain is often relieved with food; however, in some patients the pain is exacerbated with eating.

Anorexia, weight loss, and vomiting are more common with gastric ulcers. Remissions may be infrequent or absent. Medical follow-up of gastric ulcers should continue for several years because a small percentage of the erosions become cancerous. The most severe ulcers may penetrate the wall of the stomach and cause death. Whereas duodenal ulcers most frequently occur in males in the 30- to 50-year age group, gastric ulcers are more common in women over age 60. NSAID-related ulcers are more likely to produce gastric ulcers, whereas *H. pylori*–associated ulcers are more likely to be duodenal.

Patients who are experiencing physiological stress resulting from severe trauma, surgery, burns, illness, or shock may experience stress ulcers. Stress ulcers are typically asymptomatic initially, and about 25% of patients present with painless upper GI bleeding. Vasoconstriction secondary to sympathetic nervous system involvement causes decreased blood flow to the small intestine, which may play a role in the development of stress ulcers. Patients who are placed on mechanical ventilation and other seriously ill patients are sometimes administered prophylactic antiulcer drugs to prevent complications due to PUD.

Zollinger-Ellison Syndrome (ZES) is a less common cause of PUD. It is caused by a tumor that secretes the hormone gastrin. Because gastrin is the hormonal signal for increasing hydrochloric acid secretion, the huge amounts of acid easily overcome the protective defenses, leading to multiple gastric and duodenal ulcers. Peptic ulcers are persistent, difficult to treat, and slow to heal. Symptoms of ZES are the same as those of PUD. The acid also irritates the GI tract, resulting in diarrhea. Treatment involves aggressive acid suppression with drugs.

Ulceration in the distal small intestine is known as Crohn's disease, and erosions in the large intestine are called ulcerative colitis. These diseases, together are categorized as inflammatory bowel disease (IBD).

PharmFACT

Zollinger-Ellison syndrome is most frequently caused by a tumor (gastrinoma) located in the islet cells of the pancreas. More than 50% of these gastrinomas are malignant and metastasize to the lymph nodes or liver (MedlinePlus, 2011).

CONNECTION Checkpoint 62.1

Although surgery is often indicated for ZES, chemotherapy with doxorubicin (Adriamycin) plus streptozocin (Zanosar) is a common combination. What are the drug classes for these two antineoplastics? *See Answer to Connection Checkpoint 62.1 on student resource website.*

Etiology and Pathogenesis of Gastroesophageal Reflux Disease

3 Gastroesophageal reflux disease is a chronic condition characterized by persistent heartburn.

Gastroesophageal reflux disease (GERD) results when acidic stomach contents enter the esophagus. Although most often considered a disease of people older than age 40, GERD can also occur in infants. The prevalence of the disease is increasing among both children and adults.

In adults, the cause of GERD is usually transient weakening or relaxation of the lower esophageal sphincter (LES), a specialized muscle segment at the end of the esophagus. The sphincter may no longer close tightly, allowing movement of gastric contents upward into the esophagus when the stomach contracts. The acidic gastric contents cause an intense burning (heartburn) and, in some cases, injury to the esophagus. In addition, the pathogenesis of GERD involves decreased salivary secretions and diminished esophageal motility. The pathophysiology of GERD is shown in Pharmacotherapy Illustrated 1.

Symptoms of GERD include heartburn, dysphagia, dyspepsia, chest pain, nausea, and belching. Symptoms worsen following large meals, exercise, or when in a reclining or recumbent position. There is growing evidence that patients with GERD may also present with symptoms such as chronic cough, wheezing, bronchitis, sore throat, or hoarseness. GERD is a chronic condition with alternating periods of exacerbation and remission.

A large number of substances and conditions can worsen GERD symptoms. These include caffeine, alcohol, citrus fruits, tomato-based products, onions, carbonated beverages, spicy food, chocolate, smoking, pregnancy, and obesity. Certain medications may also contribute to or worsen GERD. They include nitrates, benzodiazepines, anticholinergics, beta blockers, alpha blockers, estrogen, progesterone, iron, calcium channel blockers, NSAIDs, tricyclic antidepressants, opioids, levodopa, bisphosphonates, and some chemotherapy agents.

Left untreated, GERD can lead to complications such as esophagitis, esophageal ulcers, or strictures. Approximately 10% of patients diagnosed with GERD will develop **Barrett's esophagus**, a condition that is associated with an increased risk of esophageal cancer. Warning signs and symptoms of GERD that suggest a more complicated disease may include unexplained weight loss, early satiety, anemia, vomiting, initial onset of symptoms after age 50, and prolonged anorexia or dysphagia. Patients who are experiencing these symptoms should notify their health care provider.

PharmFACT

Twenty-five to forty percent of adults in the United States have GERD. Males are two to three times more likely to have the condition than females (Patti, 2011).

If GERD is associated with obesity, losing weight may eliminate the symptoms. Other lifestyle changes that can improve GERD symptoms include elevating the head of the bed, avoiding fatty or acidic foods, eating smaller meals at least 3 hours before sleep, and eliminating tobacco and alcohol use. Because patients often self-treat this disorder with OTC drugs, a good medication history may give clues to the presence of GERD. Also, patients should be informed that some medications can provoke GERD, and reviewing their medication history may prove helpful. Because drugs provide only symptomatic relief, surgery may become necessary to eliminate the cause of persistent GERD.

An emerging theory suggests that GERD may be a premalignant condition and that chronic acid suppression leads to an increase in esophageal malignancy. This theory is not universally accepted, however, and acid suppression currently remains the mainstay in the treatment of GERD. The presence of GERD does not warrant testing for *H. pylori* infection. Large studies have shown that neither the presence nor absence of *H. pylori* has any influence on the development of GERD.

Pharmacotherapy of Peptic Ulcer Disease and Gastroesophageal Reflux Disease

4 Peptic ulcer disease and gastroesophageal reflux disease are best treated with a combination of pharmacotherapy and lifestyle changes.

Before initiating pharmacotherapy, patients are usually advised to change lifestyle factors that may be contributing to the severity of PUD or GERD. For example, eliminating tobacco and alcohol use and reducing stress often allow healing of the ulcer and cause it to go into remission. Avoiding certain foods and beverages can lessen the severity of symptoms. For patients with GERD, losing weight may alleviate symptoms of the disorder.

The goals of PUD pharmacotherapy are to provide immediate relief from symptoms, promote healing of the ulcer, prevent complications, and prevent future recurrence of the disease. Eradication of *H. pylori* and discontinuing NSAIDs or other ulcer-promoting medications when possible are key factors.

PHARMACOTHERAPY ILLUSTRATED 1

Treatment of Gastroesophageal Reflux Disease (GERD)

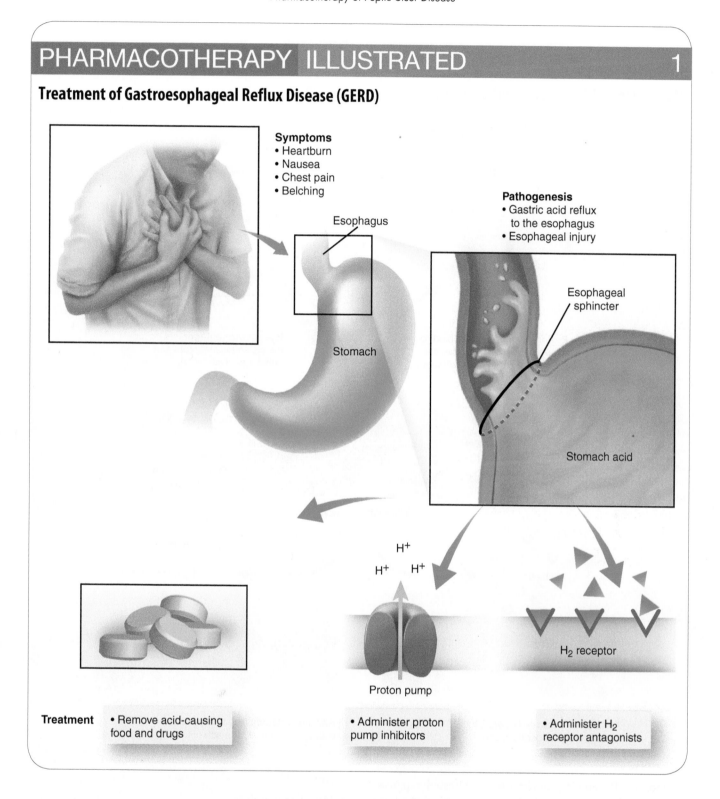

Symptoms
- Heartburn
- Nausea
- Chest pain
- Belching

Pathogenesis
- Gastric acid reflux to the esophagus
- Esophageal injury

Esophagus

Stomach

Esophageal sphincter

Stomach acid

H^+
H^+ H^+

Proton pump

H_2 receptor

Treatment
- Remove acid-causing food and drugs
- Administer proton pump inhibitors
- Administer H_2 receptor antagonists

For patients who are taking NSAIDs, the initial approach to PUD is to switch to an alternative medication, such as acetaminophen or another analgesic. This is not always possible, however, because NSAIDs are the drugs of choice for treating chronic arthritis and other disorders associated with pain and inflammation. Those with a history of PUD should be advised to avoid NSAIDs in the future to prevent ulcer recurrences. If discontinuation of the NSAID is not possible, concurrent antiulcer drugs are indicated. Platelet inhibitors such as aspirin or clopidogrel should be used cautiously in patients at risk for ulcer complications.

For PUD patients with *H. pylori* infection, elimination of the bacteria using anti-infective therapy is the primary goal of pharmacotherapy. If the treatment includes only antiulcer drugs without eradicating *H. pylori*, a very high recurrence rate of PUD is observed. It has also been found that eradicating *H. pylori* infection prophylactically decreases the incidence of peptic ulcers in patients who subsequently take NSAIDs.

PHARMACOTHERAPY ILLUSTRATED 2

Mechanisms of Action of Antiulcer Drugs

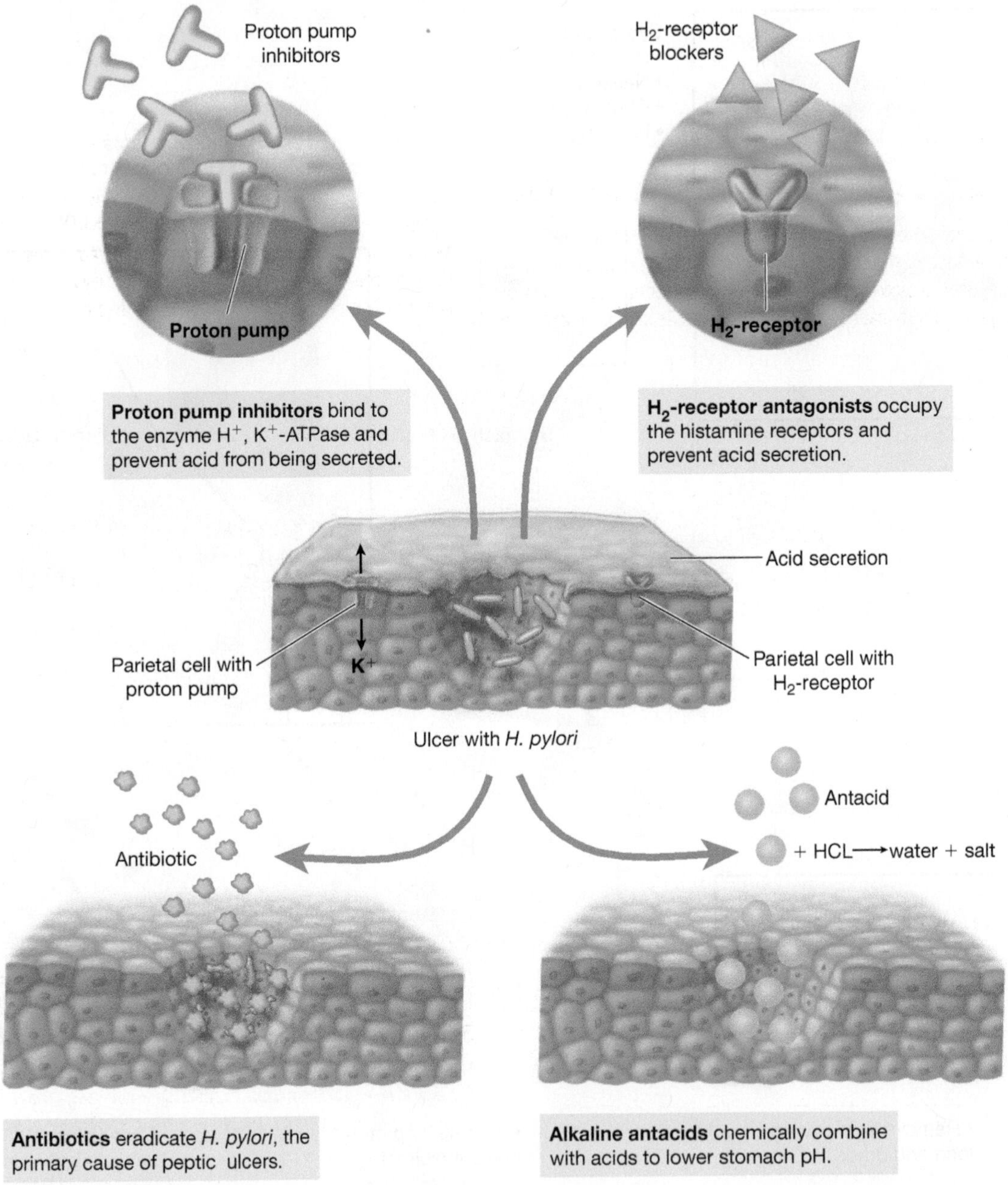

Proton pump inhibitors

Proton pump

Proton pump inhibitors bind to the enzyme H⁺, K⁺-ATPase and prevent acid from being secreted.

H₂-receptor blockers

H₂-receptor

H₂-receptor antagonists occupy the histamine receptors and prevent acid secretion.

Acid secretion

Parietal cell with proton pump

K⁺

Parietal cell with H₂-receptor

Ulcer with *H. pylori*

Antibiotic

Antibiotics eradicate *H. pylori*, the primary cause of peptic ulcers.

Antacid

+ HCL ⟶ water + salt

Alkaline antacids chemically combine with acids to lower stomach pH.

Once NSAIDs and *H. pylori* have been addressed, suppressing or neutralizing gastric acid is the aim of the pharmacologic treatment of both PUD and GERD. A wide variety of both prescription and OTC drugs are available to suppress acid secretion. The mechanisms of action of the major drug classes for PUD are shown in Pharmacotherapy Illustrated 2. These drugs fall into three primary classes and one miscellaneous group:

- Proton pump inhibitors
- H₂-receptor antagonists
- Antacids
- Miscellaneous drugs

Because medications used in treating GERD and PUD suppress acid, it should be kept in mind that certain nutrients and drugs need an acidic environment for complete absorption. For example, long-term acid suppression could lead to a deficiency in folic acid, iron, and vitamin B₁₂. Also, the effects of certain drugs such as fluconazole, tetracyclines, and indomethacin may be decreased because these drugs require an acidic environment for complete absorption.

Complementary and Alternative Therapies

Ginger's Effect on the Gastrointestinal Tract

Description: Originally from Asia, ginger (*Zingiber officinalis*) is now cultivated in most tropical regions of the world. The active ingredients of ginger, and those that create its spicy flavor and pungent odor, are located in its roots or rhizomes. It has both culinary and medicinal uses.

History and Claims: The use of ginger for medicinal purposes dates to antiquity in India and China, and it is found in many ancient pharmacopeias. Its claimed uses are many and diverse, including antiemetic, antithrombotic, diuretic, anti-inflammatory, promotion of gastric secretions, promotion of blood glucose, and stimulation of peripheral circulation.

Standardization: Like most herbs, ginger contains multiple substances that may contribute to its pharmacologic activity. It is sometimes standardized according to its active substances, known as gingerols and shogaols. It is sold in pharmacies as dried ginger root powder and is readily available at most grocery stores for home cooking. A typical dose is 250 mg of dried root two to four times per day.

Evidence: Ginger is one of the best studied herbs, and it appears to be useful for a number of digestive-related conditions. Perhaps its widest use is for treating nausea, including that caused by motion sickness, pregnancy morning sickness, chemotherapy, and postoperative procedures. It has been shown to stimulate appetite, promote gastric secretions, and increase peristalsis. Newer research has shown that ginger may inhibit the effects of *H. pylori* and may help heal peptic ulcers. Its effects appear to stem from direct action on the GI tract, rather than on the CNS. Ginger has no toxicity when used at recommended doses. Adverse effects include abdominal discomfort and diarrhea. Overdoses may lead to CNS depression, inhibition of platelet aggregation, and cardiotonic effects.

Pharmacotherapy with Proton Pump Inhibitors

5 Proton pump inhibitors block gastric acid secretion and are the drugs of choice in the therapy of peptic ulcer disease and gastroesophageal reflux disease.

The **proton pump inhibitors (PPIs)** act by blocking H^+, K^+-ATPase, the enzyme that is responsible for secreting hydrochloric acid in the stomach. PPIs are indicated for treatment of gastric and duodenal ulcers for 4 to 8 weeks, treatment of GERD, maintenance therapy to prevent recurrence, and treatment of ZES. Omeprazole is available OTC. These agents are listed in Table 1.

PPIs reduce acid secretion in the stomach by binding irreversibly to the H^+, K^+-ATPase enzyme at the surface of the parietal cell, thereby blocking the final step in acid production. This enzyme acts as a pump to release acid (also called H^+, or protons) onto the surface of the GI mucosa. The PPIs reduce acid secretion to a greater extent than the H_2-receptor antagonists and have a longer duration of action. About 95% of the acid production is blocked, making the PPIs the most efficient agents available for treating acid-related disease.

Because the proton pump is activated by food intake, the PPI should be taken 20 to 30 minutes before the first major meal of the day. This allows the peak serum drug levels to coincide with the time at which the proton pumps are activated. PPIs are formulated in a delayed release formation because the drug would be destroyed in the acidic environment of the stomach.

Although the PPIs have a short serum half-life (about 1.5 hours), they continue to suppress acid for about 24 hours because the inactivation of the proton pump is irreversible. Because not all of the proton pumps are inactivated with the first dose, several days of PPI therapy are needed to achieve maximal acid inhibition. Beneficial effects continue for 3 to 5 days after the drugs have been discontinued. The PPIs are highly protein bound, metabolized in the liver, and excreted in the urine (80%) and feces (20%). Doses do not need to be adjusted for patients with renal insufficiency because there is negligible renal clearance.

All agents in this class have similar effectiveness and adverse effects. The incidence of adverse effects with PPIs is very low, with headache, abdominal pain, diarrhea, nausea, and vomiting being the most commonly reported ones. Rashes and blood dyscrasias are rare. Rebound hypersecretion of acid does not appear to occur after the drugs are discontinued. PPIs can mask an *H. pylori* infection because of the marked reduction in the bacterial load that they initiate. Long-term therapy with PPIs increases the risk for osteoporosis-related fractures, perhaps due to their interference with calcium absorption. Some health care providers recommend calcium supplements during therapy to prevent these types of fractures.

TABLE 1 Proton Pump Inhibitors

Drug	Route and Adult Dose (maximum dose where indicated)	Adverse Effects
esomeprazole (Nexium)	PO: 20–40 mg daily or bid for up to 8 weeks IV: 20–40 mg daily for up to 10 days	*Diarrhea, nausea, rash, abdominal pain*
lansoprazole (Prevacid)	PO: 15–30 mg daily for 4–8 weeks IV: 30 mg over 30 min daily for up to 7 days	Increased risk for osteoporosis-related fractures of the hip, wrist, or spine
omeprazole (Prilosec)	PO: 20–60 mg daily or bid	
pantoprazole (Protonix)	PO: 40 mg daily or bid IV: 40 mg IV daily for up to 7 days	
rabeprazole (AcipHex)	PO: 20–60 mg once daily	

Note: Italics indicate common adverse effects. Underline indicates serious adverse effects.

479

Evidence-Based Practice

Use of Proton Pump Inhibitors and Increased Risk of Infections

Clinical Question

The acidic environment of the stomach is known to be a natural barrier to infection caused by ingested bacteria and it plays a role in the destruction of respiratory pathogens. The long-term effects of decreasing the acidity of the gastric fluid are uncertain. Because PPIs decrease the acidity, is there an association between PPI use and GI or respiratory infections?

Evidence

An increased risk of enteric bacterial infection (such as salmonella) has been demonstrated to exist in patients taking PPIs (Canani & Terrin, 2010). Evidence also suggests a link between PPI use and an increased risk of respiratory infections, including pneumonia. These effects are related to the decrease in gastric acidity and the protective mechanism against respiratory bacteria that it provides. Bacterial overgrowth may be of concern in patients who take PPIs and subsequently develop *Clostridium difficile*–associated diarrhea (CDAD). This infection has been associated previously with prior antibiotic use or immunosuppression. Recently, an increased risk for the development of *C. difficile* colitis

or pseudomembranous colitis (PMC) in hospitalized patients who are receiving PPIs has been noted (O'Keefe, 2010). The use of PPIs, as well as other gastric acid inhibitors such as H_2-antagonists, has been shown to increase the risk of community-acquired pneumonia, particularly in children.

Implications

In patients who are receiving PPIs, the nurse should frequently assess for the development of severe diarrhea, especially that which is watery and contains mucus, blood, or pus. Respiratory symptoms such as cough, congestion, adventitious breath sounds, and dyspnea, especially when associated with fever, should also be assessed and reported.

Critical Thinking Question

What categories of patients may be at increased risk for developing infections associated with PPI use?

See Answers to Critical Thinking Questions on student resource website.

PPIs heal more than 90% of duodenal ulcers within 4 weeks and about 90% of gastric ulcers in 6 to 8 weeks. GERD may require 8 to 12 weeks of therapy for symptoms to diminish, and long-term maintenance therapy may be needed. PPIs are best suited for the long-term prevention of heartburn rather than the treatment of acute symptoms. In patients with PUD who must take NSAIDs for a chronic pain or inflammatory condition, PPIs taken once daily are effective in reducing the incidence of ulcers.

PROTOTYPE DRUG	Omeprazole (Prilosec)

Classification: **Therapeutic:** Antiulcer drug
Pharmacologic: Proton pump inhibitor

Therapeutic Effects and Uses: Omeprazole was the first PPI to be approved in 1989 for PUD and is available by prescription and OTC. By prescription it is approved for the short-term, 4- to 8-week therapy of active peptic ulcers. OTC, it is indicated for the relief of heartburn. Most patients are symptom free after 2 weeks of therapy. It is used for longer periods in patients who have ZES. It is combined with antibiotics in regimens for eliminating *H. pylori*. Omeprazole may be prescribed off-label to prevent PUD in patients taking NSAIDs.

Although omeprazole can take 2 hours to reach therapeutic levels, its effects last up to 72 hours. Omeprazole is available only in oral (PO) form in the United States and is approved for pediatric use in children ages 2 years and older. Zegerid is a combination drug that contains omeprazole and the antacid sodium bicarbonate.

Mechanism of Action: Omeprazole reduces acid secretion in the stomach by binding irreversibly to the enzyme H^+,K^+-ATPase. It inhibits the final pathway involved in acid secretion and effectively inhibits the active proton pumps.

Pharmacokinetics:

Route(s)	PO
Absorption	Rapidly absorbed; food does not influence bioavailability
Distribution	Bioavailability after oral dosing: 50–60%; crosses the placenta; secreted in breast milk; 95% bound to plasma protein
Primary metabolism	Hepatic; significant first-pass effect
Primary excretion	Renal
Onset of action	0.5–3.5 h
Duration of action	3–4 days; half-life: 0.5–1.5 h

Adverse Effects: PPIs are generally well-tolerated drugs. The most common adverse effects are minor and include headache, nausea, diarrhea, rash, and abdominal pain. Although rare, blood disorders may occur, causing unusual fatigue and weakness. Long-term studies have been conducted on the possible effects of omeprazole on cardiovascular events and gastric tumors. None of the studies has shown any significant increase in cardiovascular adverse effects or gastric cancer.

Contraindications/Precautions: The only contraindication is hypersensitivity to the drug. It is not recommended for children under 2 years of age. Patients with hepatic impairment should be treated with caution. The drug should be avoided or used with caution in pregnant or lactating patients.

Drug Interactions: Clinically significant interactions with PPIs are rare. Omeprazole has been shown to both inhibit and induce certain hepatic P450 enzyme systems, although clinically significant interactions are rare. Concurrent use with other drugs using the P450 system, including warfarin, carbamazepine, diazepam, and phenytoin, may inhibit or delay metabolism and cause increased blood levels of these drugs. Concurrent use of omeprazole and clopidogrel (Plavix) reduces the conversion of clopidogrel to its active metabolite, thus reducing its effectiveness. Thus concurrent use with warfarin may increase the likelihood of bleeding. Coadministration of omeprazole and clarithromycin has been shown to increase plasma levels of both omeprazole and clarithromycin.

PPIs increase gastric pH and have the potential to affect the bioavailability of medications that depend on a lower pH for absorption (e.g., iron salts, digoxin, ampicillin, ketoconazole, atazanavir). Because an acidic environment promotes mineral absorption, mineral deficiencies could occur with long-term PPI use. Decreased vitamin B_{12} absorption may occur because an acid is optimal for vitamin B_{12} absorption. **Herbal/Food**: Ginkgo and St. John's wort may decrease the plasma concentration of omeprazole.

Pregnancy: Category C.

Treatment for Overdose: Overdose is uncommon and is treated symptomatically.

Nursing Responsibilities: Key nursing implications for patients receiving omeprazole are included in the Nursing Practice Application for Patients Receiving Proton Pump Inhibitor Therapy.

Lifespan and Diversity Considerations:

- Monitor hepatic function laboratory values more frequently in the older adult because normal physiological changes related to aging may affect the drug's metabolism and serum drug levels.

- Carefully monitor for diarrhea, especially in the child or older adult. Cases of CDAD and PMC have been reported with PPI use, greatly increasing the risk of fluid and electrolyte imbalances and the risk for severe bowel effects in all patients, but especially in these populations.

Patient and Family Education:

- Take this medication 30 minutes before meals, preferably before breakfast.

- Do not crush, break, or chew the tablets or capsules. If taking lansoprazole, the granules from the capsule may be sprinkled into soft foods such as applesauce. Afterward, drink a full glass of water to ensure that all medication is ingested.

- Immediately report severe or persistent diarrhea accompanied by fever to the health care provider. Do not attempt to treat diarrhea with OTC products.

- Do not take clopidogrel (Plavix) with omeprazole unless directed by the health care provider. The combination may increase the risk of adverse effects due to possible reduced effectiveness of the clopidogrel.

- Do not breast-feed while taking this drug without the approval of the health care provider.

Drugs Similar to Omeprazole (Prilosec)

The other PPIs include esomeprazole, lansoprazole, pantoprazole, and rabeprazole.

Esomeprazole (Nexium): Approved in 2001, this drug is very similar in structure, effectiveness, and safety to omeprazole. Its effects may last longer than those of omeprazole. It is available by the PO and intravenous (IV) routes. Adverse effects include headache, diarrhea, and nausea. Similar to other PPIs, esomeprazole is available as once-daily dosing for uncomplicated PUD and GERD and twice-daily dosing for complicated conditions such as ZES. It is approved by the U.S. Food and Drug Administration (FDA) for the prophylaxis of ulcers in patients who are taking NSAIDs. Esomeprazole capsules can be opened and the pellets mixed with soft foods and swallowed without chewing. With all PPIs there is a risk of pneumonia due to the elevation in gastric pH. Esomeprazole is pregnancy category B.

Lansoprazole (Prevacid) and dexlansoprazole (Dexilant): Approved in 1995, lansoprazole has a similar effectiveness and safety profile to omeprazole and is available by both the PO and IV routes. Its antisecretory effects can last up to 24 hours. Similar to other PPIs, its adverse effects include headache, diarrhea, and nausea. As with other PPIs, lansoprazole offers once-daily dosing for uncomplicated PUD and GERD and twice-daily dosing for ZES. With lansoprazole, as with other PPIs, there is a risk of pneumonia due to the elevation in gastric pH. This drug is eliminated from the body by the biliary system.

For patients who have difficulty swallowing capsules, lansoprazole is available in an oral liquid suspension or the capsule can be easily opened and its contents mixed with soft food and swallowed. Lansoprazole is available as a PO disintegrating tablet (Prevacid SoluTab) that is placed under the tongue and disintegrates within 1 minute. Dexlansoprazole (Dexilant) is a stereoisomer of lansoprazole that has identical effects to its parent drug. Lansoprazole is pregnancy category B.

Pantoprazole (Protonix): Approved in 2000, pantoprazole has a similar efficacy and safety profile to omeprazole and is available intravenously. Adverse effects include headache, diarrhea, and nausea. Because pantoprazole does not inhibit CYP450 enzymes, it is not likely to affect the metabolism of other drugs.

As with the other PPIs, pantoprazole offers once-daily dosing for uncomplicated PUD and GERD and twice-daily dosing for ZES. With all PPIs, there is a risk of pneumonia due to the elevation in gastric pH. Pantoprazole may be prescribed off-label to prevent ulcers in patients taking NSAIDs. Pantoprazole is pregnancy category B.

Rabeprazole (AcipHex): Although rabeprazole is similar to omeprazole, it causes reversible inhibition of the proton pump; thus its effects are of shorter duration. Approved in 1999, rabeprazole is available by the PO route. The tablets should be swallowed whole and not crushed or chewed. Like other PPIs rabeprazole accentuates the eradication of *H. pylori* when used with appropriate antibiotics. Although rabeprazole is metabolized by the hepatic CYP450 drug-metabolizing system, there are no significant clinical drug interactions. Adverse effects are mild and transient and include headache, diarrhea, nausea, malaise, dizziness, and rash. Rabeprazole is pregnancy category B.

Lifespan Considerations
Use of Proton Pump Inhibitors in the Older Adult

According to Madanick (2011), recent studies suggest a link between PPIs and an increased risk for osteoporosis due to malabsorption of calcium and other nutrients. Long-term use has also been considered as a possible cause of iron and vitamin B_{12} deficiencies. Because age-related changes in the gastric acid levels of older adults may also explain these conditions, the links are inconclusive. Risk reduction strategies to avoid long-term complications such as osteoporosis or iron and vitamin B_{12} deficiencies in the older adult include increasing the intake of calcium and magnesium, reducing the intake of sodas and other nonnutrient beverages, increasing weight-bearing exercise to a minimum of three times weekly, and increasing intake of iron and vitamin B_{12}-rich foods such as meats, fish, fortified cereals, and green leafy vegetables. Laboratory and radiologic studies such as a DEXA scan may indicate the need for more aggressive therapies such as the bisphosphonates for bone building and iron or vitamin B_{12} supplementation.

Pharmacotherapy with H_2-Receptor Antagonists

6 The H_2-receptor antagonists suppress gastric acid secretion and are widely prescribed for treating peptic ulcer disease and gastroesophageal reflux disease.

The discovery of the **H_2-receptor antagonists**, or H_2 blockers, in the 1970s marked a major breakthrough in the treatment of PUD. Since then they have become available OTC and are used extensively in the treatment of mild to moderate hyperacidity disorders of the GI tract. H_2-receptor antagonists are indicated for treatment of PUD and GERD to promote healing and prevent recurrence. Duodenal ulcers usually heal in 6 to 8 weeks, and gastric ulcers may require up to 12 weeks of therapy. All of the H_2-receptor antagonists are available OTC for the short-term (2 weeks) treatment of heartburn. These agents are listed in Table 2.

Histamine has two types of receptors: H_1 and H_2. Activation of the H_1 receptors produces the classic symptoms of inflammation and allergy, whereas the H_2 receptors, which are located on the parietal cells in the stomach, promote gastric acid secretion when activated. The H_2-receptor antagonists effectively reduce both fasting and food-stimulated secretion, and are also helpful in decreasing nocturnal acid secretion, which is largely dependent on histamine.

Pharmacokinetic properties of drugs in this class include rapid absorption from the small intestine, which is not affected by food, and a 30-minute onset of action. These drugs undergo hepatic metabolism and renal excretion and their half-lives range from 1 to 4 hours. Although there are no known harmful effects on the fetus, these agents cross the placenta and are secreted in breast milk. All drugs in this class have similar safety profiles: Their adverse effects are minor and rarely cause discontinuation of therapy. Patients who are receiving higher doses, those with renal or hepatic disease, or older adults may experience confusion, restlessness, hallucinations, or depression. With moderate to severe kidney disease, doses of H_2-receptor antagonists should be cut in half to avoid toxicity. Antacids should not be taken at the same time as H_2-receptor antagonists because absorption is diminished.

TABLE 2 H_2-Receptor Antagonists

Drug	Route and Adult Dose (maximum dose where indicated)	Adverse Effects
cimetidine (Tagamet)	Active ulcers: PO: 300 mg every 6 h or 800 mg at bedtime or 400 mg bid with food; IV: 300 mg every 6 h (over a minimum of 5 min) or 37.5 mg/h by continuous infusion GERD: 400 mg every 6 h or 800 mg bid for 12 weeks	*Diarrhea, constipation, headache, fatigue, nausea, gynecomastia* Rare: hepatitis, blood dyscrasias, anaphylaxis, dysrhythmias, skin reactions, galactorrhea, confusion, or psychoses
famotidine (Pepcid)	Active ulcers: PO: 40 mg/day for 4–8 weeks, then 20 mg at bedtime GERD: PO: 20 mg bid for 6 weeks IV: 20 mg every 12 h	*Headache, nausea, dry mouth* Rare: musculoskeletal pain, tachycardia, blood dyscrasia, blurred vision
nizatidine (Axid)	Active ulcers: PO: 150 mg bid or 300 mg at bedtime GERD: PO: 150 mg bid IV: 20 mg every 12 h	
ranitidine (Zantac)	PO: 150 mg bid or 300 mg once daily after the evening meal IV/IM: 50 mg every 6–8 h by intermittent bolus or infusion	

Note: Italics indicate common adverse effects. Underline indicates serious adverse effects.

CONNECTIONS: NURSING PRACTICE APPLICATION

Patients Receiving Proton Pump Inhibitor Therapy

Assessment	Potential Nursing Diagnoses
Baseline assessment prior to administration: • Understand the reason the drug has been prescribed in order to assess for therapeutic effects. • Obtain a complete health history including GI, hepatic, renal, respiratory, or cardiovascular disease, pregnancy, or breast-feeding. Obtain a drug history including allergies, current prescription and OTC drugs, herbal preparations, caffeine, nicotine, and alcohol use. Be alert to possible drug interactions. • Obtain a history of past and current symptoms, noting any correlations between onset and presence of any pain related to meals, sleep, positioning, or other medications. Also note what measures have been successful to relieve the pain (e.g., eating). • Obtain baseline vital signs and weight. • Evaluate appropriate laboratory findings (e.g., CBC, platelets, electrolytes, hepatic, or renal function studies). • Assess the patient's ability to receive and understand instructions. Include family and caregivers as needed.	• *Acute Pain* • *Altered Nutrition: Less Than Body Requirements* • *Ineffective Health Maintenance* • *Deficient Knowledge* (Drug Therapy)
Assessment throughout administration: • Assess for desired therapeutic effects (e.g., diminishing gastric area pain, lessened bloating or belching). • Continue periodic monitoring of CBC, electrolytes, hepatic, and renal function laboratory values. Testing for *H. pylori* may be needed if symptoms fail to resolve. • Assess for adverse effects: nausea, vomiting, diarrhea, headache, drowsiness, or dizziness. Immediately report severe abdominal pain, vomiting, coffee-ground emesis, hematemesis, blood in stool, or tarry stools.	

Planning: Patient Goals and Expected Outcomes

The patient will:
- Experience therapeutic effects dependent on the reason the drug is being given (e.g., diminished or absent gastric pain, absence of related symptoms such as bloating or belching).
- Be free from or experience minimal adverse effects.
- Verbalize an understanding of the drug's use, adverse effects, and required precautions.
- Demonstrate proper self-administration of the medication (e.g., dose, timing, and when to notify the provider).

Implementation

Interventions and (Rationales)	Patient-Centered Care
Ensuring therapeutic effects: • Follow appropriate administration guidelines. (For best results, PPIs should be taken before meals, usually in the morning for single, daily-dose drugs.)	• Teach the patient to take the drug following appropriate guidelines and not to crush, open, or chew tablets unless directed to do so by the health care provider or label directions.
• Encourage appropriate lifestyle changes: lowered fat intake, eliminating alcohol intake, smoking cessation, increasing intake of yogurt and *acidophilus*-containing foods. As needed, have the patient keep a food diary noting correlations between discomfort or pain and meals or activities. (Smoking and alcohol use are known to increase gastric acid and irritation and should be eliminated. Correlating symptoms with dietary intake or activities may help to eliminate a triggering factor. Overall healthy lifestyle changes will support and minimize the need for drug therapy.)	• Encourage the patient to adopt a healthy lifestyle of low-fat food choices, increased exercise, and elimination of alcohol consumption and smoking. Provide for dietitian consultation or information on smoking cessation programs as needed.
Minimizing adverse effects: • Continue to monitor for the presence of gastric area pain. Continued discomfort or pain should be reported. (Continued symptoms may indicate ineffectiveness of the current drug therapy, or the need to test for *H. pylori*.)	• Teach the patient that while some easing of discomfort may be noticed after beginning drug therapy, full effects may take several days to weeks or longer. Consistent drug therapy will provide the best results. If gastric discomfort or pain continue or worsen after several weeks of therapy, the health care provider should be notified.
• Monitor for any severe abdominal pain, vomiting, coffee-ground emesis or hematemesis, blood in stool, or tarry stools, and report immediately. (PPIs decrease gastric acidity, making the gastric environment less favorable for ulcer development, but they do not heal existing ulcers. Severe abdominal pain or blood in emesis or stools may indicate a worsening of the disease or a more serious condition and should be reported immediately.)	• Teach the patient that severe abdominal pain or any blood in emesis or stools should be reported immediately to the health care provider.

(continued)

CONNECTIONS: NURSING PRACTICE APPLICATION (continued)

• Continue to monitor periodic electrolyte levels. (PPIs have been associated with a possible increase in osteopenia and osteoporosis. Calcium supplements or other preventive drug therapy may be needed.)	• Instruct the patient on the need to return periodically for laboratory work.
• Monitor respiratory status and for fever, congestion, adventitious breath sounds such as crackles or wheezing, and dyspnea. Immediately report adventitious sounds or dyspnea accompanied by fever to the provider. (PPIs raise the gastric pH and impact the body's normal defense mechanisms against respiratory pathogens. Antibacterial therapy may be needed if respiratory infections develop.)	• Teach the patient to report symptoms of respiratory infection and report lung congestion or dyspnea accompanied by fever to the health care provider.
• Monitor for severe diarrhea, especially if mucus, blood, or pus is present. (Severe diarrhea may indicate the presence of CDAD, or PMC. PPIs and other drugs that raise gastric pH have been associated with an increased risk for CDAD.	• Instruct the patient to immediately report any diarrhea that increases in frequency or amount or that contains mucus, blood, or pus. • Instruct the patient to consult the health care provider before taking any antidiarrheal drugs, which cause the retention of harmful bacteria. • Teach the patient to increase intake of dairy products containing live active cultures, such as yogurt, kefir, or buttermilk, to help restore normal intestinal flora.
• Monitor for the effectiveness of other drugs taken along with the PPI. (PPIs, H_2 blockers, and antacids may significantly impair the effects of other drugs [e.g., clopidogrel].)	• Instruct the patient to immediately report any unusual symptoms related to other drugs used (e.g., increased risk of GI bleeding or bruising, or increased angina if clopidogrel is taken concurrently).
Patient understanding of drug therapy: • Use opportunities during administration of medications and during assessments to discuss the rationale for drug therapy, desired therapeutic outcomes, commonly observed adverse effects, parameters for when to call the health care provider, and any necessary monitoring or precautions. (Using time during nursing care helps to optimize and reinforce key teaching areas.)	• The patient, family, or caregiver should be able to state the reason for the drug, appropriate dose and scheduling, what adverse effects to observe for and when to report them, and the anticipated length of medication therapy.
Patient self-administration of drug therapy: • When administering the medication, instruct the patient, family, or caregiver in proper self-administration of drug, e.g., during the evening meal. (Utilizing time during nurse-administration of these drugs helps to reinforce teaching.)	• Teach the patient to take the drug following appropriate guidelines as follows: • Take it 30 min before meals. If once-daily dosing is ordered, take the drug in the morning before breakfast. Antacids may be used concurrently. • Do not continue taking the drug beyond 3 to 4 months unless directed by the health care provider.

Evaluation of Outcome Criteria

Evaluate the effectiveness of drug therapy by confirming that patient goals and expected outcomes have been met (see "Planning").

PROTOTYPE DRUG | Ranitidine (Zantac)

Classification: **Therapeutic:** Antiulcer drug
Pharmacologic: H_2-receptor antagonist

Therapeutic Effects and Uses: Approved in 1983, ranitidine has a higher potency than cimetidine, which allows it to be administered once daily, usually at bedtime. Adequate healing of the ulcer takes 4 to 8 weeks, although those at high risk for PUD may continue on drug maintenance for prolonged periods to prevent recurrence. Gastric ulcers heal more slowly than duodenal ulcers and thus require longer therapy. IV and intramuscular (IM) forms are available for the treatment of acute stress-induced bleeding ulcers. Tritec is a combination drug with ranitidine and bismuth citrate. An OTC preparation of ranitidine was approved in 1995.

Ranitidine is indicated for duodenal ulcers, gastric ulcers, hypersecretory conditions, heartburn, and GERD. In some cases, it is used off-label to prevent PUD in those who are taking medications known to cause peptic ulcers. It is not effective as monotherapy for the elimination of *H. pylori*. Ranitidine is available in a dissolving tablet form (EFFERdose) for treating GERD in children and infants older than 1 month of age.

Mechanism of Action: Ranitidine acts by blocking H_2 receptors on the parietal cells in the stomach to decrease acid production. Both daytime and nocturnal basal gastric acids are suppressed.

Pharmacokinetics:

Route(s)	PO, IV, IM (rare)
Absorption	Rapid absorption following PO administration; all three routes achieve comparable blood levels.
Distribution	PO bioavailability is approximately 50%; very little enters the central nervous system (CNS); crosses the placenta; secreted in breast milk; 15% bound to plasma protein
Primary metabolism	Hepatic
Primary excretion	Renal (mostly unchanged)
Onset of action	30–60 min; peak effect: 1–3 h
Duration of action	6–12 h; half-life: 2–3 h

Adverse Effects: Adverse effects are uncommon and transient. Although rare, blood dyscrasias, especially neutropenia and thrombocytopenia, have been reported; thus, periodic blood counts should be performed. Confusion may occur rarely and is usually in the elderly or with IV dosing. High doses may result in gynecomastia, impotence, or loss of libido in men, although these effects are more common with cimetidine.

Contraindications/Precautions: Contraindications include hypersensitivity to H_2-receptor antagonists, acute porphyria, and OTC administration in children younger than 12 years of age. The drug should be used with caution in patients with renal impairment; dosages should be reduced.

Drug Interactions: Because ranitidine has much less affinity for CYP450 enzymes, it is less likely to participate in drug–drug interactions than cimetidine. Ranitidine may reduce the absorption of cefpodoxime, ketoconazole, and itraconazole because of the increase in gastric pH induced by H_2-receptor antagonists. Concurrent use can increase the effects of alcohol, sulfonylureas, salicylates, and warfarin. Antacids should not be given within 1 hour of H_2-receptor antagonists because their effectiveness may be decreased due to reduced absorption. Smoking decreases the effectiveness of ranitidine. **Herbal/Food:** Absorption of vitamin B_{12} depends on an acidic environment, so deficiency may occur. Iron is also better absorbed in an acidic environment.

Pregnancy: Category B.

Treatment of Overdose: Overdose is uncommon and is treated symptomatically.

Nursing Responsibilities: Key nursing implications for patients receiving ranitidine are included in the Nursing Practice Application for Patients Receiving H_2-Receptor Antagonist and Antacid Therapy.

Lifespan and Diversity Considerations:

- Monitor hepatic and renal function laboratory values more frequently in the older adult because normal physiological changes related to aging may affect the drug's metabolism or excretion.

- Carefully monitor for diarrhea, especially in children and older adults. Cases of CDAD and PMC have been reported with drugs used to treat hyperacidity, greatly increasing the risks of fluid and electrolyte imbalances and severe bowel effects in all patients, but especially in these populations.

- Monitor for increased agitation or confusion in the older adult, particularly if IV doses are administered.

Patient and Family Education:

- Take H_2-receptor antagonists with or immediately after meals.

- Immediately report severe or persistent diarrhea accompanied by fever to the health care provider. Do not attempt to treat diarrhea with OTC products.

- Do not breast-feed while taking this drug without approval of the health care provider.

- Immediately notify the health care provider of any known or suspected pregnancy.

Drugs Similar to Ranitidine (Zantac)

Other H_2-receptor antagonists include cimetidine, famotidine, and nizatidine.

Cimetidine (Tagamet): The first of the H_2 blockers that was approved in 1977, cimetidine is used less frequently than other drugs in this class because (1) it inhibits hepatic drug-metabolizing enzymes and exhibits numerous drug–drug interactions; (2) it has a high incidence of adverse effects; and (3) it must be taken up to four times a day. Because cimetidine interacts with CYP450 enzymes, it may delay the metabolism of other drugs metabolized in the liver, including warfarin, phenytoin, diazepam, and theophylline. Cimetidine also may cause gynecomastia or impotence, because it binds to androgen receptors, causing antiandrogenic effects. Cimetidine crosses the blood–brain barrier and therefore is more likely to cause CNS depression and confusion than the other H_2-receptor antagonists. A low-dose OTC preparation is available. Routes of administration include PO, IM, and IV. This drug is pregnancy category B.

Famotidine (Pepcid): Approved by the FDA in 1986, famotidine has indications, actions, and adverse effects that are almost identical to those of ranitidine. Famotidine does not inhibit CYP450 enzymes; therefore, it exhibits fewer drug–drug interactions than cimetidine. Famotidine is the most potent of the H_2-receptor antagonists. It is available OTC and may be given by the PO or IV routes. This drug is pregnancy category B.

Nizatidine (Axid): Although thought to have a similar safety and adverse effect profile to ranitidine and famotidine, nizatidine is not metabolized by the liver CYP450 enzyme system and therefore causes fewer drug interactions. Adverse effects are infrequent and transient. Nizatidine is indicated for up to 8 weeks of PUD therapy (12 weeks for GERD) and is available as PO capsules or a PO solution. Prescription nizatidine was approved in 1988. An OTC preparation was approved in 1995. This drug is pregnancy category B.

CONNECTION Checkpoint 62.2

How is the excretion of drugs affected when they are metabolized through the hepatic CYP450 system? *See Answer to Connection Checkpoint 62.2 on student resource website.*

Pharmacotherapy with Antacids

7 Antacids are alkaline substances that neutralize stomach acid to treat symptoms of heartburn.

Prior to the development of H_2-receptor antagonists and PPIs, antacids were the mainstay of peptic ulcer and GERD pharmacotherapy. Indeed, many patients still use these inexpensive and readily available OTC drugs. Antacids may provide temporary relief from heartburn or indigestion, but they are no longer recommended as the primary drug class for acid-related disorders. Although antacids relieve symptoms of heartburn, they do not promote ulcer healing or help to eliminate *H. pylori*. These agents are listed in Table 3.

TABLE 3 Antacids

Drug	Route and Adult Dose (maximum dose where indicated)	Adverse Effects
aluminum hydroxide (AlternaGEL, Others)	PO: 600 mg tid–qid	*Constipation, nausea* Fecal impaction, hypophosphatemia with chronic use
calcium carbonate (Titralac, Tums)	PO: 1–2 g bid–tid	*Constipation, flatulence* Fecal impaction, metabolic alkalosis, hypercalcemia, renal calculi
calcium carbonate with magnesium hydroxide (Mylanta Supreme, Rolaids)	PO: 2–4 capsules or tablets prn (max: 12 tablets/day)	
magnesium hydroxide (Milk of Magnesia)	PO: 5–15 mL or 2–4 tablets as needed up to 4 times daily	*Diarrhea, nausea, vomiting, abdominal cramping* Hypermagnesemia (patients with renal disease), dysrhythmias (when given parenterally)
magnesium trisilicate and aluminum hydroxide (Gaviscon)	PO: 2–4 tablets prn (max: 16 tablets/day)	
magnesium hydroxide and aluminum hydroxide with simethicone (Mylanta, Maalox Plus, Others)	PO: 10–20 mL prn (max: 120 mL/day) or 2–4 tablets prn (max: 24 tablets/day)	
magaldrate (Riopan)	PO: 540–1,080 mg/day (5–10 mL suspension or 1–2 tablets) (max: 20 tablets or 100 mL/day)	
sodium bicarbonate (Alka-Seltzer, baking soda)	PO: 325 mg–2 g 1 to 4 times/day	*Abdominal distention, belching* Metabolic alkalosis, fluid retention, edema, hypernatremia

Note: Italics indicate common adverse effects. <u>Underline</u> indicates serious adverse effects.

Antacids are inorganic compounds containing aluminum, magnesium, sodium, or calcium that neutralize gastric acid and inactivate pepsin. They are also thought to stimulate prostaglandin production in the mucosa and increase LES tone, which reduces gastroesophageal reflux. These drugs do not protect the stomach by coating the stomach wall. To be considered therapeutic, the dose of antacids should increase the gastric pH to a minimum of 3.5.

Self-medication with antacids is safe when taken in doses as directed on the labels. Although antacids act within 10 to 15 minutes, their duration of action is only 2 hours; thus, they must be taken often during the day. Combinations of aluminum hydroxide and magnesium hydroxide, the most common types, are capable of rapidly neutralizing stomach acid.

All the antacids are equally effective at neutralizing acid and reducing symptoms of heartburn when given in therapeutic doses. Each type has certain disadvantages that may preclude their use:

- **Sodium.** Antacids that contain sodium should not be taken by patients on sodium-restricted diets or by those with hypertension (HTN), heart failure, or renal impairment because they may promote fluid retention.

- **Magnesium.** Absorption of magnesium from high doses of magnesium-containing antacids can cause symptoms of hypermagnesemia (fatigue, hypotension, and dysrhythmias). Magnesium also acts as a laxative when it reaches the large intestine.

- **Calcium.** Antacids that contain calcium can cause constipation and may cause or aggravate kidney stones. When absorbed, hypercalcemia is possible, and renal failure may occur at very high doses. Administering calcium carbonate antacids with milk or any items with vitamin D can cause **milk-alkali syndrome** to occur. Early symptoms are the same as those of hypercalcemia and include headache, urinary frequency, anorexia, nausea,

and fatigue. Milk-alkali syndrome may result in permanent renal damage if the drug is continued at high doses.

- **Aluminum.** Aluminum antacids are not absorbed to any great extent but they can cause constipation. The constipation effect is balanced when aluminum is combined with magnesium salts. Aluminum carbonate and aluminum hydroxide may interfere with dietary phosphate absorption to cause hypophosphatemia.

- **Bicarbonate.** Being a base, antacids that contain bicarbonate may provoke metabolic alkalosis (e.g., fatigue, mental status changes, muscle twitching, depressed respiratory rate) in patients at risk. Bicarbonate combines with gastric acid to form carbon dioxide, which causes bloating and belching.

Drug interactions with antacids occur by several mechanisms. Because antacids increase stomach pH, they affect the solubility and absorption of many oral drugs. Drugs that are weak acids are nonionized in the acidic environment of the stomach and are thus readily absorbed. If an antacid is given concurrently with a weak acid, the pH of the stomach will rise and result in a more ionized drug that is less readily absorbed. On the other hand, a drug that is a weak base is absorbed in a more alkaline medium. In other words, when taken with antacids, acidic drugs may have less therapeutic effect, and basic drugs may exhibit a greater effect. Examples of acidic drugs include NSAIDs, sulfonylureas, salicylates, warfarin, barbiturates, isoniazid, and digoxin. Basic drugs include morphine sulfate, antihistamines, tricyclic antidepressants, amphetamines, and quinidine.

Enteric-coated or delayed release drugs are designed to dissolve when they reach the alkaline environment in the small intestine. By raising the pH of the stomach, antacids may "fool" enteric-coated tablets into dissolving early and releasing their contents into the stomach. The drug may either irritate the stomach lining, causing nausea or vomiting, or be inactivated.

Drug interactions may also occur if the antacid physically binds to other drugs. For example, certain antacids form chemical complexes with tetracyclines, preventing the antibiotic from being absorbed. Digoxin is another drug whose absorption is affected by binding to antacids.

A third mechanism of drug interaction is due to the effects of antacids on urine pH. Making the urine pH more alkaline increases the excretion of acidic drugs such as aspirin and inhibits the excretion of basic drugs such as amphetamines.

Because antacids are widely used OTC by patients for self-treatment, nurses must emphasize that these drugs be used only as directed on the label due to the potential for adverse effects. To decrease the potential for antacid–drug interactions, nurses should advise that other medications be taken at least 1 hour before or 2 hours after giving an antacid.

CONNECTIONS: NURSING PRACTICE APPLICATION

Patients Receiving H$_2$-Receptor Antagonist and Antacid Therapy

Assessment	Potential Nursing Diagnoses
Baseline assessment prior to administration: • Understand the reason the drug has been prescribed in order to assess for therapeutic effects. • Obtain a complete health history including GI, hepatic, renal, respiratory, or cardiovascular disease, pregnancy, or breast-feeding. Obtain a drug history including allergies, current prescription and OTC drugs, herbal preparations, caffeine, nicotine, and alcohol use. Be alert to possible drug interactions. • Obtain a history of past and current symptoms, noting any correlations between onset and presence of any pain related to meals, sleep, positioning, or other medications. Also note what measures have been successful to relieve the pain (e.g., eating). • Obtain baseline vital signs and weight. • Evaluate appropriate laboratory findings (e.g., CBC, platelets, electrolytes, hepatic, or renal function studies). • Assess the patient's ability to receive and understand instructions. Include family and caregivers as needed.	• *Acute Pain* • *Altered Nutrition: Less Than Body Requirements* • *Constipation* or *Diarrhea*, related to adverse drug effects • *Deficient Knowledge* (Drug Therapy) • *Risk for Ineffective Health Maintenance*
Assessment throughout administration: • Assess for desired therapeutic effects (e.g., diminishing gastric area pain, lessened bloating or belching). • Continue periodic monitoring of CBC, electrolytes, hepatic, and renal function laboratory values. Testing for *H. pylori* may be needed if symptoms fail to resolve. • Assess for adverse effects: nausea, vomiting, diarrhea, headache, drowsiness, or dizziness. Immediately report severe abdominal pain, vomiting, coffee-ground emesis, hematemesis, blood in stool, or tarry stools.	

Planning: Patient Goals and Expected Outcomes

The patient will:
• Experience therapeutic effects dependent on the reason the drug is being given (e.g., diminished or absent gastric pain, absence of related symptoms such as bloating or belching).
• Be free from or experience minimal adverse effects.
• Verbalize an understanding of the drug's use, adverse effects, and required precautions.
• Demonstrate proper self-administration of the medication (e.g., dose, timing, and when to notify the provider).

Implementation

Interventions and (Rationales)	Patient-Centered Care
Ensuring therapeutic effects: • Follow appropriate administration guidelines. (For best results, most H$_2$-receptor blockers should be taken with or immediately after meals. Antacids should be taken 2 h before or after meals with a full glass of water.)	• Teach the patient to take the drug following appropriate guidelines and not to crush, open, or chew tablets unless directed to do so by the health care provider or label directions.
• Encourage appropriate lifestyle changes: lowering fat intake, eliminating alcohol intake, stopping smoking, and increasing intake of yogurt and *acidophilus*-containing foods. As needed, have the patient keep a food diary noting correlations between discomfort or pain and meals or activities. (Smoking and alcohol use are known to increase gastric acid and irritation and should be eliminated. Correlating symptoms with dietary intake or activities may help eliminate a triggering factor. Overall healthy lifestyle changes will support and minimize the need for drug therapy.)	• Encourage the patient to adopt a healthy lifestyle of low-fat food choices, increased exercise, and elimination of alcohol consumption and smoking. Provide for dietitian consultation or information on smoking cessation programs as needed.

CONNECTIONS: NURSING PRACTICE APPLICATION (continued)

Minimizing adverse effects:

- Continue to monitor for the presence of gastric area pain. Continued discomfort or pain should be reported. (Continued symptoms may indicate ineffectiveness of the current drug therapy, or the need to test for *H. pylori*.)

- Teach the patient that while some easing of discomfort may be noticed after beginning drug therapy, full effects may take several days to weeks or longer. Consistent drug therapy will provide the best results. If gastric discomfort or pain continue or worsen after several weeks of therapy, the health care provider should be notified.

- Monitor for any severe abdominal pain, vomiting, coffee-ground emesis, hematemesis, blood in stool, or tarry stools and report immediately. (H$_2$-receptor antagonists and antacids decrease gastric acidity, making the gastric environment less favorable for ulcer development, but they do not heal existing ulcers. Severe abdominal pain or blood in emesis or stools may indicate a worsening of disease or a more serious condition and should be reported immediately.)

- Teach the patient that severe abdominal pain or blood in emesis or stools should be reported immediately to the health care provider.

- Continue to monitor periodic hepatic and renal function tests and CBC, platelets, and electrolyte levels. (Abnormal liver function tests may indicate drug-induced adverse hepatic effects. Decreased RBC, WBC, or platelets have been noted with long-term H$_2$-receptor antagonist therapy, and decreases should be reported to the health care provider. Excessive use of antacids may affect electrolyte levels.)

- Instruct the patient on the need to return periodically for laboratory work.

- Ensure patient safety, especially in the older adult. Observe for light-headedness or dizziness. Monitor ambulation until the effects of the drug are known. (Drowsiness or dizziness from H$_2$-receptor blockers may occur and increases the risk of injury and falls, particularly in the older adult. Continued dizziness or drowsiness may require a change in drug therapy.)

- Instruct the patient to call for assistance prior to getting out of bed or attempting to walk alone, and to avoid driving or other activities requiring mental alertness or physical coordination until the effects of the drug are known.

- Monitor respiratory status and for fever, congestion, adventitious breath sounds such as crackles or wheezing, and dyspnea. Immediately report adventitious sounds or dyspnea accompanied by fever to the health care provider. (Drugs used to treat hyperacidic conditions such as H$_2$-receptor antagonists and antacids raise the gastric pH and impact the body's normal defense mechanisms against respiratory pathogens. Antibacterial therapy may be needed if respiratory infections develop.)

- Teach the patient to report symptoms of respiratory infection and report lung congestion or dyspnea accompanied by fever to the health care provider.

- Monitor for severe diarrhea, especially if mucus, blood, or pus is present. (Severe diarrhea may indicate the presence of CDAD or PMC. H$_2$ blockers and other drugs that raise gastric pH have been associated with an increased risk for CDAD.)

- Instruct the patient to immediately report diarrhea that increases in frequency or amount or that contains mucus, blood, or pus.
- Instruct the patient to consult the health care provider before taking any antidiarrheal drugs because they cause the retention of harmful bacteria.
- Teach the patient to increase intake of dairy products containing live active cultures, such as yogurt, kefir, or buttermilk, to help restore normal intestinal flora.

- Monitor for the effectiveness of other drugs taken along with the H$_2$-receptor antagonist or antacid. (H$_2$-receptor antagonists and antacids may significantly impair the effects of other drugs. In rare instances, effects may be enhanced [e.g., pseudoephedrine (Sudafed)].)

- Instruct the patient to immediately report any unusual symptoms related to other drugs taken concurrently.

Patient understanding of drug therapy:

- Use opportunities during administration of medications and during assessments to discuss the rationale for drug therapy, desired therapeutic outcomes, commonly observed adverse effects, parameters for when to call the health care provider, and any necessary monitoring or precautions. (Using time during nursing care helps to optimize and reinforce key teaching areas.)

- The patient, family, or caregiver should be able to state the reason for the drug, the appropriate dose and scheduling, the adverse effects to observe for and when to report them, and the anticipated length of medication therapy.

Patient self-administration of drug therapy:

- When administering the medication, instruct the patient, family, or caregiver in proper self-administration of drug, e.g., during the evening meal. (Utilizing time during nurse-administration of these drugs helps to reinforce teaching.)

- Teach the patient to take the drug following appropriate guidelines as follows:
  - **H$_2$-receptor blockers:** Take the drug with or immediately after meals unless otherwise instructed. Do not take concurrently with antacids unless using a combination product (e.g., famotidine with calcium and magnesium-based antacids as Pepcid-Complete). Exceeding the recommended dose increases the risk of adverse effects such as dizziness or drowsiness.
  - **Antacids:** Take 2 h before or after meals with a full glass of water. Do not take other medications concurrently unless available as a combination product or directed to do so by the health care provider. If relief is not achieved after several weeks of therapy, consult the health care provider for additional treatment recommendations.

Evaluation of Outcome Criteria

Evaluate the effectiveness of drug therapy by confirming that patient goals and expected outcomes have been met (see "Planning").

Treating the Diverse Patient

Public Health Implications of *H. Pylori* Infection

H. pylori occurs worldwide and has a noted association with an increased risk of gastric cancer, particularly in genetically susceptible subgroups. *H. pylori* is also associated with gastritis and PUD. Infection with the bacteria usually occurs in infancy or childhood, years before symptoms of gastric effects may appear. Ford and Axon (2010) reviewed literature published between April 2009 and March 2010 and discovered that many studies confirmed what was already known: an association between *H. pylori* and gastric cancer, the existence of multiple possible routes of transmission (e.g., fecal–oral, respiratory droplet), and populations particularly at risk for the infection (e.g., disease prevalence of 48% to 78% noted in studies in South American populations). However, they also discovered that no reports addressed public health measures to eradicate the disease. Because gastric cancer is a significant cause of death worldwide, public health measures such as adequate sanitation, drinking water, and nutrition may decrease the risk of transmission and improve the general health of those infected with the disease. Vaccine development is currently being researched, and Agarwal and Agarwal (2008) have proposed that a vaccine may offer a better strategy for worldwide eradication of *H. pylori* that traditional treatment measures with multidrug regimens have failed to attain.

Chewable tablets and liquid formulations of antacids are available. A few products combine antacids and H_2-receptor antagonists into a single tablet. For example, Pepcid Complete contains calcium carbonate, magnesium hydroxide, and famotidine. Simethicone is sometimes added to antacid preparations because it reduces gas bubbles that cause bloating and discomfort. For example, Mylanta contains simethicone, aluminum hydroxide, and magnesium hydroxide. Simethicone is classified as an **antiflatulent** because it reduces gas. It also is available by itself in OTC products such as Gas-X and Mylanta Gas. Some manufacturers advertise their calcium-based antacid products as mineral supplements.

PROTOTYPE DRUG	Aluminum Hydroxide (AlternaGEL, Others)

Classification: **Therapeutic:** Antiheartburn agent
Pharmacologic: Antacid

Therapeutic Effects and Uses: Aluminum hydroxide is an inorganic agent used alone or in combination with other antacids such as magnesium hydroxide. Combining aluminum compounds with magnesium (Gaviscon, Maalox, Mylanta) increases their effectiveness and reduces the potential for constipation. Unlike calcium-based antacids that can be absorbed and cause systemic effects, aluminum compounds are minimally absorbed. Their primary action is to neutralize stomach acid by raising the pH of the stomach contents. Unlike H_2-receptor antagonists and PPIs, aluminum antacids do not reduce the volume of acid secretion. They are most effectively used in combination with other antiulcer agents for the symptomatic relief of heartburn due to PUD or GERD. A second aluminum salt, aluminum carbonate (Basaljel), is also available to treat heartburn.

Mechanism of Action: Aluminum hydroxide combines with gastric (hydrochloric) acid to produce aluminum chloride and water. This raises the pH of the stomach contents and inactivates pepsin.

Pharmacokinetics:

Route(s)	PO
Absorption	17–30% absorbed
Distribution	Widely distributed
Primary metabolism	Hepatic
Primary excretion	Renal
Onset of action	20–40 min
Duration of action	2 h when taken with food; 3 h when taken 1 h after meals

Adverse Effects: Aluminum antacids frequently cause constipation. At high doses aluminum products bind with phosphate in the GI tract and long-term use can result in phosphate depletion. Those at risk include people who are malnourished, those who have alcoholism, and those with renal disease. The antacids are often combined with magnesium compounds, which counteract the constipation commonly experienced with aluminum antacids.

Contraindications/Precautions: Prolonged use in patients with low serum phosphate levels should be avoided. This drug should not be used in patients with suspected bowel obstruction.

Drug Interactions: Aluminum compounds should not be taken with other medications because they may interfere with their absorption. Concurrent use decreases the absorption of cimetidine, ciprofloxacin and other fluoroquinolones, digoxin, isoniazid, chloroquine, NSAIDs, iron salts, phenytoin, tetracycline, and thyroxine. Use with sodium polystyrene sulfonate may cause systemic alkalosis. Use of anticholinergic drugs can increase the effects of antacids. **Herbal/Food:** Aluminum antacids may inhibit the absorption of dietary iron.

Pregnancy: Category C.

Treatment of Overdose: There is no specific treatment for overdose.

Nursing Responsibilities: Key nursing implications for patients receiving aluminum hydroxide are included in the Nursing Practice Application for Patients Receiving H_2-Receptor Antagonist and Antacid Therapy.

Lifespan and Diversity Considerations:

- Monitor bowel function more frequently in the older adult because normal physiological changes related to aging may increase the risk for severe constipation.

Patient and Family Education:

- Do not take antacids with magnesium if you have kidney disease.
- Do not take antacids with sodium if you have heart failure, HTN, or are on a sodium-restricted diet.

Drugs Similar to Aluminum Hydroxide (AlternaGEL, Others)

All aluminum salts have similar effects to those of aluminum hydroxide.

Pharmacotherapy of *Helicobacter pylori* Infection

8 The gram-negative bacterium *H. pylori* is associated with approximately 70% of patients with peptic ulcer disease.

It is estimated that 60% to 80% of patients with duodenal ulcers are infected with *H. pylori* and that the majority of patients with gastric ulcers have the bacterium. Research has shown that the eradication of *H. pylori* decreases the recurrence of PUD. Risk factors for *H. pylori* include residing in a developing country, domestic crowding, unclean water, and exposure to the gastric contents of an infected individual. It is the only known microorganism that has been found to survive the hostile conditions in the stomach.

H. pylori has adapted well to the acidic environment in the stomach. It has devised ways to neutralize the high acidity surrounding it and make chemicals called **adhesins** that allow the organism to penetrate the GI mucosa and alter the epithelial cell structure, which initiates inflammation. The inflammatory and immune responses lead to the chronic production of inflammatory cells, including lymphocytes, plasma cells, and macrophages. This response then leads to the formation of immunoglobulin G antibodies and increased production of cytokines, including interleukins and tumor necrosis factor, all of which contribute to the inflammation of the gastric mucosa. Increased gastrin secretion and decreased bicarbonate production also play a role in ulcer formation caused by *H. pylori*.

Another mechanism involves ammonia. *H. pylori* produces large amounts of urease, an enzyme that breaks down urea to ammonia and carbon monoxide. Ammonia neutralizes the acid around the bacterium and allows *H. pylori* to survive in the acidic environment of the stomach. Unfortunately, the ammonia is toxic to mucosal cells and erodes the mucous barrier. *H. pylori* then finds its home in the submucosal layer of the stomach, producing damage to the gastric and duodenal mucosae, which allows pepsin and gastric acid to further damage the mucosae. There may also be a genetic predisposition that determines one's susceptibility to *H. pylori* infection.

Perforated, bleeding, or refractory ulcers are usually tested for the presence of *H. pylori*. The most reliable means of diagnosis is by obtaining a culture during endoscopy. Less invasive means include checking for antibodies to *H. pylori* in a blood sample or by using a breath test to check for urease, which is given off by the bacterium.

Prior to the identification of the link between *H. pylori* and ulcers, PUD was treated with acid-reducing drugs. Although this therapy was successful at treating symptoms, the majority of patients experienced relapses. This is because the acid-reducing drugs have little effect on *H. pylori*, which can remain active for life if not treated appropriately. Thus for infected patients, elimination of this bacterium is the prime pharmacologic objective.

Eradication of the organism allows ulcers to heal more rapidly and remain in remission longer, often permanently.

A combination of antibiotics is used concurrently to eradicate *H. pylori* and help decrease antibiotic resistance. A PPI or bismuth compound is usually included in the regimen. Once eliminated from the stomach, reinfection with *H. pylori* is uncommon. Those with peptic ulcer who are not infected with *H. pylori* should not receive antibiotics because it has been shown that these patients have a worse outcome if they receive *H. pylori* treatment. Thus, patients should be tested for *H. pylori* before initiating treatment for infection. Example regimens used to eradicate *H. pylori* include the following:

- **Initial regimen.** Omeprazole, clarithromycin (Biaxin), and amoxicillin (Amoxil, Others)
- **Alternative regimens.**
  - Omeprazole (or other PPI), clarithromycin (Biaxin), and metronidazole (Flagyl), or
  - Omeprazole (or other PPI), bismuth subsalicylate (Pepto-Bismol), metronidazole (Flagyl), and tetracycline

Although technically not antibiotics, bismuth compounds inhibit bacterial growth by disrupting their cell wall and preventing *H. pylori* from adhering to the gastric mucosa. The PPI further suppresses *H. pylori*, and the increased pH that results from PPI administration creates a hostile environment for *H. pylori*, thus enhancing the effectiveness of the antibiotics.

H. pylori therapy generally continues for 7 to 14 days. Should resistance occur, rifabutin (Mycobutin) and fluoroquinolones have been and can be used as part of the regimen. Drug regimens continue to evolve as antibiotic resistance patterns change. The American College of Gastroenterology publishes periodic guidelines offering different pharmacologic strategies.

Indiscriminate use of antibiotics can lead to antibiotic resistance; thus treatment should be reserved for patients who would benefit from the regimen. Patient adherence is vital to successful

CONNECTIONS

Lifespan Considerations

Peptic Ulcer Disease and Gastroesophageal Reflux Disease in Children

Antacids, H_2-receptor antagonists, and PPIs are widely used in children in the treatment of GERD. Although rare, PUD does occur in children and these drugs are also used, although in smaller doses than in adults. They are frequently used in critically ill children to prevent GI bleeding. The dosing of PPIs in children is higher per kilogram than for adults. Dietary alterations, including a change in feeding technique, are often included in the treatment. Thickening feedings with cereal has been shown to improve GERD symptoms in infants. A 2-week trial of soy and milk products may be diagnostic and therapeutic in those infants suspected of having intolerance to these foods. Older children are advised to avoid the same aggravating factors as adults, which include chocolate, mints, tomatoes, and caffeinated beverages, and to lose weight if applicable.

eradication of *H. pylori*. Patients should be instructed on the importance of completing the drug regimen, because discontinuing the anti-infectives too soon may result in reinfection. Interestingly, following treatment for eradication of *H. pylori* infection, certain other conditions such as idiopathic thrombocytopenic purpura (ITP), a blood disorder, have been alleviated.

CONNECTION Checkpoint 62.3

Explain why antibiotic resistance has become a major public health problem throughout the world. *See Answer to Connection Checkpoint 62.3 on student resource website.*

Miscellaneous Drugs Used for Peptic Ulcer Disease and Gastroesophageal Reflux Disease

9 **Several miscellaneous drugs, including sucralfate, bismuth subsalicylate, and misoprostol, are beneficial in treating peptic ulcer disease.**

A few additional drugs are used in the pharmacotherapy of PUD and GERD. These agents act by mechanisms other than the ones described for PPIs, H_2-receptor blockers, or antacids.

Sucralfate: Sucralfate (Carafate) is a PO medication that consists of sucrose (a sugar) plus aluminum hydroxide (an antacid). This drug stimulates mucus, bicarbonate, and prostaglandin secretion, all of which enhance mucosal defenses. Sucralfate also acts locally to produce a thick protective barrier that coats and binds to the ulcer, protecting it against further erosion from acid and pepsin to promote healing. It does not affect the secretion of gastric acid. It is intended for short-term therapy (up to 8 weeks). It is sometimes used in critically ill patients to prevent bleeding from stress-related gastritis. Sucralfate is not effective in preventing NSAID-related ulcers.

Other than constipation, the adverse effects of sucralfate are minimal because little of the drug is absorbed from the GI tract. Because sucralfate requires an acid medium to work effectively, concurrent use of antacids, H_2-receptor antagonists, and PPIs will reduce its effectiveness. Sucralfate may bind to other drugs and decrease their absorption, especially digoxin, warfarin, the quinolones and tetracyclines, and phenytoin. Antacids and other medications should be taken 2 hours before or after a dose of sucralfate. A major disadvantage of sucralfate is that it must be taken four times daily.

Bismuth compounds: In the United States the only bismuth compound available is bismuth subsalicylate (Kaopectate, Pepto-Bismol), a nonprescription formula containing both bismuth and salicylate. Bismuth subsalicylate stimulates mucosal bicarbonate and prostaglandin production and inhibits *H. pylori* from adhering to the ulcerated tissue. It has been shown to have local antimicrobial actions to *H. pylori* by causing cell wall death to the bacterium. Bismuth is often included as a component of a multidrug regimen containing tetracycline and metronidazole (Pylera, Helidac) to eradicate *H. pylori* infection. As monotherapy, it is approved to treat dyspepsia, heartburn, and diarrhea.

Therapeutic doses of bismuth produce no significant adverse effects. This drug can cause stools to turn black, which is a normal side effect. In stomach acid bismuth subsalicylate is converted to salicylic acid, which is absorbed. Patients who are taking other salicylates, such as aspirin, may experience adverse effects such as tinnitus, headache, nausea, vomiting, or dizziness. In addition, it is not recommended for use in pediatric patients under the age of 19 because of the increased risk of Reyes' syndrome associated with salicylate use. A "Children's Pepto" is available that contains the antacid calcium carbonate but no salicylates.

Misoprostol: Misoprostol (Cytotec) is a synthetic form of prostaglandin E_2 that stimulates the production of protective mucus and inhibits gastric acid secretion. Normally, the stomach synthesizes a number of prostaglandins, which suppress acid, promote bicarbonate secretion, and maintain blood flow to the gastric mucosa. The primary use of misoprostol is for the prevention of gastric ulcers in patients who are taking high doses of NSAIDs or corticosteroids. It has a serum half-life of less than 30 minutes and is administered three to four times per day. No reduction is needed in patients with renal insufficiency although the drug is excreted in the urine.

Diarrhea and abdominal cramping are relatively common with misoprostol. Classified as a pregnancy category X drug, misoprostol is absolutely contraindicated during pregnancy. This drug is combined with mifepristone for pregnancy termination. The use of misoprostol as an antiulcer agent is not widespread because of the availability of other drugs that are as effective and better tolerated.

Metoclopramide: Approved in 1985, metoclopramide (Reglan) is occasionally used for the short-term (4 to 12 weeks) therapy of symptomatic, documented GERD or PUD in patients who fail to respond to first-line agents. It is more commonly prescribed to treat nausea and vomiting associated with surgery or cancer chemotherapy. Metoclopramide is available by the PO, IM, or IV routes. It causes muscles in the upper intestine to contract, resulting in faster emptying of the stomach. It also decreases esophageal relaxation and blocks food from entering the esophagus, which is of benefit in patients with GERD.

CNS adverse effects such as drowsiness, fatigue, confusion, and insomnia may occur in a significant number of patients. Although uncommon, symptoms of parkinsonism such as bradykinesia, akathisia, and tardive dyskinesia may occur. Due to the potential for significant adverse effects and the development of PPIs and H_2-receptor antagonists, metoclopramide is used infrequently. This drug is pregnancy category B.

Anticholinergic drugs: Anticholinergic drugs such as atropine were used to treat peptic ulcers prior to the discovery of safer and more effective drugs. Pirenzepine (Gastrozepine) is a cholinergic blocker (muscarinic) available in Canada that inhibits gastric acid secretion. Although the action of pirenzepine is somewhat selective to the stomach, other anticholinergic effects such as dry mouth and constipation are possible. Anticholinergics are now rarely used for PUD owing to the availability of safer, more effective drugs.

UNDERSTANDING THE CHAPTER

Key Concepts Summary

1 The stomach secretes acid, enzymes, and hormones that are essential to digestive physiology.

2 Peptic ulcer disease is associated with a number of etiologic risk factors.

3 Gastroesophageal reflux disease is a chronic condition characterized by persistent heartburn.

4 Peptic ulcer disease and gastroesophageal reflux disease are best treated with a combination of pharmacotherapy and lifestyle changes.

5 Proton pump inhibitors block gastric acid secretion and are the drugs of choice in the therapy of peptic ulcer disease and gastroesophageal reflux disease.

6 The H_2-receptor antagonists suppress gastric acid secretion and are widely prescribed for treating peptic ulcer disease and gastroesophageal reflux disease.

7 Antacids are alkaline substances that neutralize stomach acid to treat symptoms of heartburn.

8 The gram-negative bacterium *H. pylori* is associated with approximately 70% of patients with peptic ulcer disease.

9 Several miscellaneous drugs, including sucralfate, bismuth subsalicylate, and misoprostol, are beneficial in treating peptic ulcer disease.

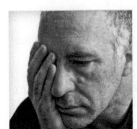

Making the PATIENT *Connection*

Remember the patient "John Talley" at the beginning of the chapter? Now read the remainder of the case study. Based on the information presented within this chapter, respond to the critical thinking questions that follow.

John Talley is a 51-year-old man who is employed as a truck driver. He has been taking NSAIDs for a shoulder injury and assumed that this was the cause of his ulcers. He is a one-pack-per-day smoker and consumes alcohol. His medical history includes HTN for which he takes a combination diuretic and ACE inhibitor. Because of worsening symptoms, an endoscopy was performed, which confirmed the presence of *H. pylori*. He is worried about using antibiotics because he has been allergic to penicillin in the past.

Critical Thinking Questions

1. Based on the scenario above, what risk factors for PUD does John have?

2. How would you as the nurse describe the recommended treatment for *H. pylori*–induced PUD to him?

3. Why would you be concerned about this patient using NSAIDs with a history of HTN?

See Answers to Critical Thinking Questions on student resource website.

NCLEX-RN® Review

1 The client has developed severe diarrhea following 4 days of self-administered antacid preparation. The nurse suspects that the diarrhea may be caused by which type of antacid?

1. Aluminum compounds
2. Magnesium compounds
3. Calcium compounds
4. Sodium compounds

2 Omeprazole (Prilosec) is prescribed for a client with gastroesophageal reflux disease. The nurse would monitor a reduction in which symptom to determine if the drug therapy is effective? Select all that apply.

1. Dysphagia
2. Dyspepsia
3. Appetite
4. Nausea
5. Belching

3 The nurse is scheduling the client's daily medication. When would be the most appropriate time for the client to receive proton pump inhibitors?

1. At night
2. After fasting at least 2 hours
3. About ½ hour before a meal
4. About 2 to 3 hours after eating

4 A client who has duodenal ulcers is receiving long-term therapy with ranitidine (Zantac). The nurse includes in the care plan that the client should be monitored for which adverse effects?

1. Photophobia and skin irritations
2. Neutropenia and thrombocytopenia
3. Dyspnea and productive coughing
4. Urinary hesitation and fluid retention

5 The prescriber orders sucralfate (Carafate) for a client with peptic ulcer disease. The nurse should question the order if the client is concurrently taking:

1. Proton pump inhibitors.
2. Calcium salt antacids.
3. H_2-receptor antagonists.
4. Aluminum salt antacids.

6 The nurse who is caring for a client with gastroesophageal reflux disease should question the order for which drug?

1. H_2-receptor antagonists
2. Proton pump inhibitors
3. Antibiotics
4. Antacids

Additional Case Study

Sara Gaggi is a 51-year-old overweight white female with HTN who presents for an evaluation of heartburn that has been increasing in both intensity and frequency during the past 18 months. She reports epigastric burning after eating. It is worse after eating spicy foods or drinking red wine. She is occasionally awakened at night with symptoms. OTC antacids and H_2-receptor antagonists relieved her symptoms initially, but lately they have provided only minimal relief. Her only routine medication is amlodipine, a calcium channel blocker for her high blood pressure. Because the symptoms are increasing and her current therapy is not relieving her symptoms, an endoscopy was performed, which revealed the presence of GERD.

1. How would you describe to Sara the dangers of self-medicating GERD symptoms with OTC medications?

2. What three risk factors in this case predispose Sara for the development of GERD?

3. What medications will her health care provider likely prescribe?

See Answers to Additional Case Study on student resource website.

Pearson Nursing Student Resources

Find additional review materials at nursing.pearsonhighered.com

Prepare for success with additional NCLEX®-style practice questions, interactive assignments and activities, web links, animations, videos, and more!

References

Agarwal, K., & Agarwal, S. (2008). *Helicobacter pylori* vaccine: From past to future. *Mayo Clinic Proceedings, 83*(2), 169–175. doi:10.4065/83.2.169

Anand, B. S. (2011). *Peptic ulcer disease.* Retrieved from http://emedicine.medscape.com/article/181753-overview#a0101

Canani, B., & Terrin, G., (2010). Gastric acidity inhibitors and the risk of intestinal infections. *Current Opinions in Gastroenterology, 26*(1), 31–35. doi:10.1097/MOG.0b013e328333d781

Ford, A. C., & Axon, A. T. R. (2010). Epidemiology of *Helicobacter pylori* infection and public health implications. *Helicobacter, 15*(suppl. 1), 1–6. doi:10.1111/j.1523-5378.2010.00779.x

Madanick, R. D. (2011). Proton pump inhibitor side effects and drug interactions: Much ado about nothing? *Cleveland Clinic Journal of Medicine, 78*(1), 39–49. doi:10.3949/ccjm.77a.10087

Medline Plus. (2011). *Zollinger-Ellison syndrome.* Retrieved at http://www.nlm.nih.gov/medlineplus/ency/article/000325.htm

O'Keefe, S. J. D. (2010). Tube feeding, microbiota, and *Clostridium difficile* infection. *World Journal of Gastroenterology, 16*(2), 139–142. doi:10.3748/wjg.v16.i2.139

Patti, M. G. (2011). *Gastroesophageal reflux disease.* Retrieved from http://emedicine.medscape.com/article/176595-overview

Selected Bibliography

Malfertheiner, P., Chan, F. K., & McColl, K. (2009). Peptic ulcer disease. *The Lancet, 374*(9699), 1449–1461. doi:10.1016/S0140-6736(09)60938-7

National Center for Complementary and Alternative Medicine. (2010). *Herbs at a glance: Ginger.* Retrieved from http://nccam.nih.gov/health/ginger

Podein, R. (2007). Peptic ulcer disease. In D. Rakel (Ed.), *Integrative medicine* (2nd ed., pp. 279–289). Philadelphia, PA: Elsevier.

Answers to NCLEX-RN® Review

1 Answer: 2 **Rationale:** Magnesium compounds, especially in higher doses, often cause diarrhea. Options 1, 3, and 4 are incorrect. Aluminum compounds and calcium compounds may cause constipation. Sodium compounds may cause flatulence. Cognitive Level: Applying; Client Need: Physiological Integrity; Nursing Process: Evaluation

2 Answer: 1, 2, 4, 5 Rationale: Symptoms of GERD include dysphagia, dyspepsia, nausea, belching, heartburn, and chest pain. Option 3 is incorrect. The nurse would not expect a decrease in the client's appetite due to this medication. Cognitive Level: Applying; Client Need: Physiological Integrity; Nursing Process: Evaluation

3 Answer: 3 Rationale: The proton pump is activated by food intake. Thus, administering it about 20 to 30 min before the first major meal of the day allows peak serum levels to coincide with when the maximum levels of pumps are activated, allowing maximum efficiency of the PPI. Options 1, 2, and 4 are incorrect. The proton pumps are less active at night, in the fasting state, or between meals. Cognitive Level: Applying; Client Need: Physiological Integrity; Nursing Process: Planning

4 Answer: 2 Rationale: Blood dyscrasias have been reported, especially neutropenia and thrombocytopenia, with long-term use. Periodic blood counts should be performed. Options 1, 3, and 4 are incorrect. Ranitidine does not cause photophobia and skin irritations. Dyspnea and productive cough are not expected adverse effects for this medication. Ranitidine is not known to cause these symptoms. Cognitive Level: Applying; Client Need: Physiological Integrity; Nursing Process: Planning

5 Answer: 4 Rationale: Concurrent use of aluminum salts and sucralfate poses a risk for aluminum toxicity. Options 1, 2, and 3 are incorrect. There is no risk of aluminum toxicity with PPIs, other antacids, or H_2-receptor antagonists. Cognitive Level: Applying; Client Need: Physiological Integrity; Nursing Process: Implementation

6 Answer: 3 Rationale: Antibiotics have no role in the treatment of GERD although certain antibiotics are used in treating PUD to eradicate the *H. pylori* organism. Options 1, 2, and 4 are incorrect. H_2-receptor antagonists and PPIs are used routinely to relieve symptoms of GERD. OTC antacids provide intermittent relief for mild cases. Cognitive Level: Applying; Client Need: Physiological Integrity; Nursing Process: Implementation

Glossary

Glossary

A

Abortifacients drugs used to induce abortion

Absence seizures seizures with a loss or reduction of normal activity, including staring and transient loss of responsiveness

Absorption the process by which drug molecules move from their site of administration to the blood; movement of nutrients and other substances from the alimentary canal to the circulation

Accessory organs of digestion include the salivary glands, liver, gallbladder, and pancreas

Acetylation a general biochemical process that adds a two-carbon chain to a drug molecule, which usually renders the drug less effective

Acetylcholine (Ach) primary neurotransmitter of the autonomic nervous system

Acetylcholinesterase (AchE) enzyme that resides in the synaptic cleft and catalyzes the destruction of Ach

Acetylcholinesterase (AchE) inhibitors indirect-acting cholinergic agonists that are nonselective and affect all Ach synapses

Acidosis condition of having too much acid in the blood; plasma pH below 7.35

Acne vulgaris disorder of the hair follicles and sebaceous glands characterized by small inflamed bumps that appear on the surface of the skin

Acquired immunodeficiency syndrome (AIDS) infection caused by the human immunodeficiency virus (HIV)

Acquired resistance ability of an organism to become unresponsive over time to the effects of an anti-infective

Acromegaly excessive growth hormone disorder in which bones become deformed

Action potentials electrical impulses that carry the signal that instructs the cardiac muscle cells to contract

Activated partial thromboplastin time (aPTT) laboratory test used to measure blood coagulation

Active immunity resistance resulting from a previous exposure to an antigen

Acute dystonia occurs during early pharmacotherapy with antipsychotics and involves severe muscle spasms, particularly of the back, neck, tongue, and face

Acute gouty arthritis condition in which uric acid crystals accumulate in the joints of the big toes, ankles, wrists, fingers, knees, or elbows, resulting in extremely painful and red, inflamed tissue

Acute retroviral syndrome symptoms during the initial phase of HIV infection

Adaptive defenses defenses that are specific to certain threats; the immune response

Addiction the continued use of a substance despite serious health and social consequences

Addison's disease hyposecretion of glucocorticoids and mineralocorticoids by the adrenal cortex

Additive effect type of drug interaction in which two agents combine to produce a summation response

Adherence taking medications in the manner prescribed by the health care provider, or in the case of OTC drugs, following the instructions on the label or as provided by the prescriber; also called compliance

Adhesins chemicals produced by *H. pylori* that allow the organism to penetrate the GI mucosa and cause inflammation

Adipocytes fat cells

Adjuvant analgesics drugs that have indications other than pain but are used to enhance analgesia

Adjuvant chemotherapy administration of antineoplastic drugs *after* surgery or radiation therapy

Adrenal atrophy condition in which the adrenal cortex shrinks and stops secreting endogenous corticosteroids due to lack of stimulation by adrenocorticotropic hormone (ACTH)

Adrenal crisis condition that occurs when corticosteroid medication is abruptly withdrawn

Adrenergic receptors at the ends of postganglionic sympathetic neurons

Adrenergic agonists agents that activate adrenergic receptors in the sympathetic nervous system; also known as sympathomimetics

Adrenergic antagonists drugs that block norepinephrine from reaching its receptors

Adrenocortical insufficiency lack of adequate corticosteroid secretion by the adrenal cortex

Adrenocorticotropic hormone (ACTH) hormone secreted by the anterior pituitary that stimulates the release of glucocorticoids by the adrenal cortex

Adverse drug effect an undesirable and potentially harmful action caused by the administration of medication

Adverse event reporting system (AERS) voluntary program that encourages health care providers and consumers to report suspected adverse effects directly to the FDA or the product manufacturer

Aerobic pertaining to an oxygen environment

Aerosol suspension of minute liquid droplets or fine solid particles in a gas

Affinity the ability of some tissues to attract, accumulate, and store drugs in high concentrations relative to other tissues

Afterload pressure in the aorta that must be overcome for blood to be ejected from the left ventricle

Agonist drug that activates a receptor and produces the same type of response as the endogenous substance

Agoraphobia an extreme avoidance of closed places where a panic attack might occur such as airplanes, public meetings, or elevators

Akathisia inability to rest or relax; constantly moving

Alimentary canal a long, continuous, hollow tube that extends from the mouth to the anus; the GI tract

Alkalosis plasma pH above 7.45

Alkylating agents agents that kill cancer cells by altering the shape of the DNA double helix and preventing the DNA from duplicating during cell division

Allergen anything that is recognized as foreign by the body's defense system; also called antigen

Allergic rhinitis inflammation of the nasal mucosa due to exposure to allergens

Allopathy refers to conventional Western medicine that is focused on treating symptoms of the patient without addressing the underlying causes

Alopecia hair loss

Alpha-adrenergic antagonists drugs that block alpha-adrenergic receptors in the sympathetic nervous system

Alzheimer's disease (AD) neurodegenerative disease that involves a chronic progressive loss of cognitive function

Amide local anesthetic that has the same mechanism of action as esters but has less effect on myocardial contraction and lower allergic reaction

Amygdala a key part of the limbic system that helps determine the emotional significance of the conscious or unconscious signals received from the cerebral cortex

Anabolic effects testosterone hormone's ability to accelerate the growth of RBCs, muscle, bone, and neural tissues

Anabolic steroids testosterone-like substances with hormonal activity that are commonly abused by athletes

Anaerobic pertaining to an environment without oxygen

Analgesics drugs used to relieve pain

Anaphylaxis life-threatening allergic response that may cause cardiovascular shock and death

Androgens steroid sex hormones that promote the appearance of masculine characteristics

Anemia decreased oxygen-carrying capacity of the blood

Angina pectoris acute chest pain caused by myocardial ischemia

Angioedema rapid swelling of the throat, face, larynx, and tongue that can lead to airway obstruction and death

Angiogenesis the formation of new blood vessels

Angiotensin I a precursor to the formation of angiotensin II that is produced when angiotensinogen is split by the enzyme renin

Angiotensin II vasopressor substance released in response to falling blood pressure that causes vasoconstriction and release of aldosterone

Angiotensin-converting enzyme (ACE) inhibitor enzyme that blocks the formation of angiotensin II, decreasing blood pressure

Angiotensinogen protein synthesized by the liver that is continuously circulating in the bloodstream

Anorexiants drugs used to suppress appetite

Anovulatory cycles menstrual cycles without ovulation

Antacids inorganic compounds containing aluminum, magnesium, sodium, or calcium that neutralize gastric acid and inactivate pepsin

Antagonist agent that blocks the response of another drug

Antagonistic effect type of drug interaction in which adding a second drug results in a diminished pharmacologic response

Anterior pituitary gland (adenohypophysis) consists of glandular tissue that manufactures and secretes hormones that control major body functions and systems

Anterograde amnesia type of short-term memory loss where the user cannot remember events that occurred while under the influence of a drug

Anthrax an acute infectious disease that results from exposure to the spore-forming bacterium *Bacillus anthracis*

Antibiotic natural substance produced by a microorganism that can kill other microorganisms

Antibodies proteins produced by the body in response to an antigen; used interchangeably with the term immunoglobulin

Anticholinergic syndrome symptoms such as dry mouth, blurred vision, photophobia, visual changes, difficulty swallowing, agitation, and hallucinations, caused by an overdose of anticholinergic substances

Anticoagulants natural substances that inhibit the formation of blood clots

Antidepressants drugs used to enhance, elevate, or stabilize mood

Antidiuretic hormone (ADH) hormone released by the posterior pituitary gland when blood pressure falls or when the osmotic pressure of the blood increases; most important means the body uses to maintain fluid homeostasis

Antiflatulent agent that reduces gas

Antigens microbes and foreign substances that elicit an immune response

Anti-infective general term for any medication that is effective against pathogens

Antipyretics medications used to reduce body temperature

Antiretrovirals drugs that are effective against retroviruses

Antithrombin III (AT-III) protein that prevents abnormal clotting by inhibiting thrombin and other clotting factors

Antitussives medications that control cough

Anxiety state of apprehension, tension, or uneasiness that stems from the anticipation of danger, the source of which is largely unknown or recognized

Anxiolytic drugs that relieve anxiety

Apoprotein protein component of a lipoprotein

Apothecary system of measurement older system of measurement developed in ancient Greece; rarely used in modern medicine

Appetite a psychological response that drives food intake based on associations and memory

Aqueous humor fluid that fills the anterior and posterior chambers of the eye

Assessment appraisal of a patient's condition that involves gathering and interpreting subjective and objective data

Asthma chronic inflammatory disease of the lungs characterized by airway obstruction

Atherosclerosis condition characterized by the presence of plaque within the walls of arteries

Atonic seizures very short-lasting seizures during which the patient may stumble and fall for no apparent reason

Atrial natriuretic peptide (ANP) hormone secreted by specialized cells in the right atrium when large increases in blood volume produce excessive stretch on the atrial wall

Atrial reflex causes the heart rate and CO to increase until the backlog of venous blood (or IV fluid) is distributed throughout the body

Attention deficit/hyperactivity disorder (ADHD) disorder typically diagnosed in childhood characterized by hyperactivity as well as attention, organization, and behavior control issues

Attenuated organisms that have been rendered less able to cause disease through the application of heat or chemicals from which effective vaccines can be developed

Atypical antidepressants diverse class of drugs that act by mechanisms other than those of the selective serotonin reuptake inhibitors (SSRIs), tricyclic antidepressants, and monoamine oxidase inhibitors

Atypical mycobacterial infections (AMIs) nontuberculosis opportunistic diseases caused by mycobacteria

Auras sensory warnings such as flashing lights, visual blind spots, and arm or leg tingling that precede a migraine

Automaticity ability of certain myocardial cells to spontaneously generate an action potential

Automatisms repetitive arm movements, leg movements, head rolling, chewing, lip smacking, or swallowing that occur in complex partial seizures

Autonomic nervous system (ANS) portion of the peripheral nervous system that provides for the involuntary control of vital functions of the cardiovascular, digestive, respiratory, and genitourinary systems

Autonomic tone the background level of autonomic activity that occurs even in the absence of stimuli

Azole term for the major class of drugs used to treat mycoses

Azoospermia complete absence of sperm in an ejaculate

B

B cell lymphocyte responsible for humoral immunity

β-glucan an essential component that shapes and strengthens the cell walls of fungi

Bacteriocidal drug that kills bacteria

Bacteriostatic drug that inhibits the growth of bacteria

Bacteriuria uropathogens

Balanced anesthesia use of multiple medications to produce general anesthesia, provide sedation, rapid induction of unconsciousness, muscle relaxation, and analgesia

Baroreceptors receptors in the aorta and carotid artery that sense changes in blood pressure

Barrett's esophagus precancerous condition of the esophagus

Basal nuclei area of the brain responsible for starting and stopping synchronized motor activity such as leg and arm motions during walking; also called basal ganglia

Baseline data data gathered during the initial assessment that is compared with data gathered during later interactions

Beers criteria list of drugs compiled by physicians that have produced a high incidence of adverse effects in older adults

Belladonna natural source of alkaloids with anticholinergic activity acquired from the deadly nightshade plant, *Atropa belladonna*, which grows throughout the world

Benign prostatic hyperplasia (BPH) nonmalignant abnormal enlargement of the prostate gland

Best Pharmaceuticals for Children Act authorizes the FDA to contract for the testing of already approved pediatric drugs, or when the pharmaceutical company declines the option of exclusivity

Beta-adrenergic antagonists drugs that block beta-adrenergic receptors; may be nonselective or selective; also called beta blockers

Beta-lactam ring portion of the chemical structure of penicillin and some other antibiotics that is responsible for their antibacterial activity

Beta-lactamase enzyme produced by certain bacteria that are able to render certain antibiotics ineffective

Bioavailability the rate and extent to which the active ingredient is absorbed from a drug product and becomes available at the site of drug action to produce its effect

Biologic response modifiers natural cytokines that boost specific functions of the immune system

Bioterrorism intentional release of an infectious agent for the purpose of causing harm to a large number of people

Bipolar disorder syndrome characterized by extreme and opposite moods, such as euphoria and depression

Bisphosphonates class of drugs for treating osteoporosis that inhibit bone resorption by suppressing osteoclast activity

Black box warning in some drug inserts, a requirement by the FDA that warns prescribers that the drug carries a risk for serious or fatal adverse effects

Blood–brain barrier network of capillaries in the CNS that inhibits many chemicals and drugs from gaining access to the brain

Body mass index (BMI) measurement of obesity determined by dividing body weight (in kilograms) by the square of height (in meters)

Body surface area (BSA) method method of calculating pediatric dosages using an estimate of the child's BSA

Body weight method method of calculating pediatric dosages that requires a calculation of the number of milligrams of drug, based on the child's weight in kilograms (mg/kg)

Bolus feedings method of enteral feeding that typically delivers 250 to 400 mL of formula every 4 to 6 hours via a syringe or funnel

Bone deposition opposite of bone resorption; bone building

Bone resorption process of bone demineralization or the breaking down of bone into mineral components

Boosters follow-up doses of vaccines that are required to provide prolonged protection

Botanical plant extract used to treat or prevent illness

Botulism condition caused by *Clostridium botulinum*, an organism that secretes a potent toxin that paralyzes the muscles after a person is poisoned

Bradydysrhythmias disorders characterized by a heart rate of less than 60 beats/minute

Bradykinesia difficulty initiating movement and controlling fine muscle movements

Bradykinin chemical released by cells during inflammation that produces pain and side effects similar to those of histamine

Broad-spectrum antibiotic an anti-infective that is effective against a wide variety of different microbial species

Bronchospasm sudden contraction of the smooth muscle of the airways that causes acute dyspnea

Buffers chemicals that help maintain normal body pH by neutralizing strong acids or bases

C

Cachexia general wasting of muscle and other tissue

Calcineurin intracellular messenger enzyme that is activated when a T cell encounters an antigen

Calcitonin hormone secreted by the thyroid gland that decreases plasma levels of calcium by inhibiting resorption of calcium from bone and increasing excretion of calcium by the kidneys

Calcitriol the active form of vitamin D

Calcium channel type of voltage-gated channel in cardiac muscle and smooth muscles

Cancer malignant disease characterized by abnormal, uncontrolled cell division

Cannabinoid receptor (CB1) blockers class of antiobesity agents that block receptors in the brain

Capillary leak syndrome a serious condition in which plasma proteins and other substances leave the blood and enter the interstitial spaces because of porous capillaries

Capsid protein coat that surrounds a virus

Carbonic anhydrase enzyme that forms carbonic acid by combining carbon dioxide and water

Carcinogens agents that cause cancer

Cardiac output (CO) amount of blood pumped by a ventricle per minute

Cardiac remodeling change in the size, shape, and structure of the myocardial cells (myocytes) that occurs over time in heart failure

Cardiotonic drugs agents that increase the force of cardiac contraction; also called inotropic agents

Cardioversion electrical shock of the heart that under ideal conditions will allow the return to a normal heart rhythm; also called defibrillation

Cataplexy sudden loss of muscle strength manifested as slurred speech, sagging of the jaw, head nodding, or even complete collapse of the body

Catecholamine class of endogenous hormones involved in neurotransmission that include epinephrine (adrenalin), norepinephrine, and dopamine

Catechol-O-methyltransferase (COMT) enzyme that destroys catecholamines such as norepinephrine in kidney and liver cells

Cathartic substance that causes accelerated, stronger, and more complete bowel emptying

CD4 receptor protein that accepts HIV and allows entry of the virus into the T_4 lymphocyte

Cell-kill hypothesis theoretical model that predicts the ability of antineoplastic drugs to eliminate cancer cells

Central nervous system (CNS) stimulants agents that raise the general alertness level of the brain

Central vein total parenteral nutrition the administration of enteral feeding solution through a central vein

Cerumenolytics agents used to loosen and remove impacted cerumen from the ear canal

Chelation therapy use of agents to detoxify poisonous metals such as mercury, arsenic, and lead by converting them to a chemically inert form that can be easily excreted

Chemical names standard nomenclature for drugs assigned by the International Union of Pure and Applied Chemistry (IUPAC)

Chemoreceptors sensory receptors in the aorta and carotid artery that recognize levels of oxygen, pH, or carbon dioxide in the blood

Chemoreceptor trigger zone (CTZ) location in the cerebral cortex that sends sensory signals to the vomiting center

Chemotherapy pharmacotherapy of cancer

Chief cells cells located in the mucosa of the stomach that secrete pepsinogen, an inactive form of the enzyme pepsin that chemically breaks down proteins

Chloasma darkened pigmentation found on the forehead, temples, cheeks, and upper lips

Cholecalciferol inactive form of vitamin D

Cholestatic hepatitis type of liver inflammation caused by obstruction of the bile ducts

Cholinergic relating to neurons that release acetylcholine (Ach)

Cholinergic agonists drugs and chemicals that increase the action of acetylcholine (Ach) at a cholinergic receptor; also called parasympathomimetics

Cholinergic crisis caused by an overdosage with acetylcholinesterase (AchE) inhibitors or poisoning with organophosphate insecticides or toxic nerve gases; characterized by intense signs of parasympathetic stimulation such as miosis, nausea, vomiting, urinary incontinence, increased exocrine secretions, abdominal cramping, and diarrhea

Cholinesterase inhibitors the most widely prescribed drug class for treating Alzheimer's disease

Chronic bronchitis recurrent disease of the lungs characterized by excess mucus production, inflammation, and coughing

Chronic obstructive pulmonary disease (COPD) progressive pulmonary disorder characterized by chronic obstructive airflow

Chyme partly digested food that is passed from the stomach to the small intestine

Cinchonism syndrome with symptoms such as tinnitus, headache, diarrhea, blurred vision, hearing loss, and dysrhythmias, caused by high doses of quinidine

Circadian rhythm cyclic basis by which body temperature, blood pressure, hormone levels, and respiration all fluctuate throughout the 24-hour day

Climacteric the period of endocrine, somatic, and psychological changes occurring in the transition to menopause

Clinical phase trials the second stage of drug testing in a clinical investigation; involves the testing of a new drug in selected patients

Clonic spasms multiple, rapidly repeated muscular contractions

Closed-angle glaucoma acute glaucoma that is caused by obstruction of drainage of aqueous humor through the canal of Schlemm

Club drug a diverse group of abused substances taken by people at dance clubs, all-night parties, and raves

Coagulation formation of an insoluble clot

Colloids proteins, starches, or other large molecules that remain in the blood for a long time because they are too large to easily cross the capillary membranes

Colony-stimulating factors (CSFs) hormones that activate existing white blood cells to fight an infection and stimulate the growth and differentiation of one or more types of leukocytes

Combination drugs drug products with more than one active generic ingredient

Comedones types of acne lesions that develop just beneath the surface of the skin (whitehead) or as a result of a plugged oil gland (blackhead)

Complement system a cluster of 20 plasma proteins that combine in a specific sequence and order when an infection occurs

Complementary and alternative medicine (CAM) diverse set of therapies and healing systems that are considered to be outside of mainstream health care

Complex partial seizures seizures that originate from a single focus, usually in the temporal lobe of the brain, and involve sensory, motor, or autonomic symptoms with some degree of altered or impaired consciousness

COMT inhibitors drugs that prevent the destruction of catechol-O-methyltransferase (COMT) in peripheral tissues, thus increasing the amount of levodopa available to enter the brain

Conjugation the direct transfer of small pieces of DNA from one bacterium to another

Constipation infrequent passage of abnormally hard and dry stools

Continuous infusion feedings enteral feedings delivered by an infusion pump at a slow rate over a 16- to 24-hour period

Contraception the use of devices, drugs, or surgery to prevent pregnancy

Contractility the strength with which the myocardial fibers contract

Controlled substance in the United States, a drug whose use is restricted by the Comprehensive Drug Abuse Prevention and Control Act

Convulsions involuntary violent spasms of the face, neck, arms, and legs

Coronary artery disease (CAD) a narrowing or occlusion of one or more coronary arteries

Corpora cavernosa tissue in the penis that fills with blood during an erection

Corpus luteum endocrine tissue formed from a ruptured follicle that remains in the ovary after ovulation and secretes progesterone

Council for Responsible Nutrition (CRN) trade association representing ingredient suppliers and manufacturers in the dietary supplement industry

Cretinism condition marked by profound mental retardation and impaired growth that results from untreated congenital hypothyroidism

Cross-tolerance situation in which tolerance to one drug makes the patient tolerant to another drug

Crystalloids IV solutions that contain electrolytes and other agents in concentrations that mimic the body's extracellular fluid

Crystalluria crystals that form in the urine and potentially obstruct the kidneys or ureters

Cultural competence the ability of health care providers to care for people with diverse values, beliefs, and behaviors, including the ability to adapt delivery of care to meet the needs of these patients

Culture set of beliefs, values, religious rituals, language, customs, and behavioral expectations that provide meaning for an individual or group

Culture and sensitivity (C&S) testing a laboratory test used to identify bacteria and the most effective antibiotic

Curare the first neuromuscular blocker, which was initially extracted from several different plant species native to the rain forests of South America

Cushing's syndrome condition of high levels of corticosteroids in the body over a prolonged period of time

Cyclic feedings enteral feedings that are commonly infused over 8 to 16 hours daily (day or night)

Cyclic lipopeptides class of antibiotics that act on gram-positive pathogens

Cyclooxygenase (COX) key enzyme in the synthesis of prostaglandin that is blocked by aspirin and other NSAIDs

Cycloplegics drugs that relax or temporarily paralyze ciliary muscles and cause blurred vision

Cystitis bladder infection

Cysts protective capsules formed by some protozoa that allow the organisms to survive in harsh environments in a dormant state for prolonged time periods

Cytokine release syndrome an acute inflammatory response that occurs 30 to 60 minutes following the initial IV administration of muromonab due to massive cytokine release

Cytokines proteins produced by T cells, such as interleukins, leukotrienes, interferon, and tumor necrosis factor, that guide the immune response

D

Deep vein thrombosis (DVT) thrombosis that occurs in the legs

Defecation elimination of the indigestible substances from the body

Defibrillation electrical shock of the heart that under ideal conditions will allow the return to a normal heart rhythm; also called cardioversion

Delirium tremens a syndrome of intense agitation, confusion, terrifying hallucinations, uncontrollable tremors, panic attacks, and paranoia caused by alcohol withdrawal

Delusions false ideas and beliefs not founded in reality

Dementia degenerative disorder characterized by progressive memory loss, confusion, and the inability to think or communicate effectively

Dependence a powerful physiological or psychological need for a substance

Depolarization loss of membrane potential in a cell

Depression characterized by a sad or despondent mood that becomes out of proportion to actual life events

Dermatitis superficial inflammatory disorders of the skin characterized by redness, pain, and pruritus

Dermatomycosis fungal infections of the skin and hair

Diabetes insipidus (DI) disorder marked by production of large volumes of urine, usually accompanied by increased thirst

Diabetes mellitus metabolic disorder characterized by an imbalance between insulin availability and insulin need

Diabetic ketoacidosis (DKA) acute condition that occurs primarily in patients with type 1 diabetes characterized by hyperglycemia, metabolic acidosis, and osmotic diuresis

Diarrhea increase in the frequency and fluidity of bowel movements

Dietary supplements nondrug substances regulated by the DSHEA

Dietary Supplement and Nonprescription Drug Consumer Protection Act law that requires companies that market herbal and dietary supplements to include their address and phone number on the product labels so consumers can report adverse events

Dietary Supplement Health and Education Act of 1994 (DSHEA) primary law in the United States regulating herbal and dietary supplements

Diffusion the movement of a chemical from an area of higher concentration to an area of lower concentration

Digestion the mechanical and chemical breakdown of food into a form that may be absorbed into the systemic circulation

Digestive system body system consisting of the alimentary canal and the accessory organs

Digitalization procedure in which the dose of digoxin is gradually increased until tissues become saturated with the drug, and the symptoms of heart failure diminish

Dihydropyridines the largest class of CCBs that bind reversibly to closed-type (inactivated) calcium channels to make them unresponsive to depolarization

Directly observed therapy (DOT) requires that a health care provider directly observe the patient swallowing the pills, whether it is in the hospital, office, or home care setting

Disease-modifying antirheumatic drugs (DMARDs) drugs that slow or modify the progression of rheumatoid arthritis

Dissociative anesthesia a trance-like feeling of being separated from the environment produced by an anesthetic agent

Distribution the transport of drugs throughout the body after they are absorbed

Diuretic substance that increases the rate of urine flow

Diuretic resistance phenomenon in some patients who become less responsive as therapy continues with loop diuretics

DNA gyrase (topoisomerase II) in bacterial DNA replication, the enzyme that relaxes the supercoil

DNA helicase in bacterial DNA replication, the enzyme that unwinds the two DNA strands after the supercoil is relaxed

DNA polymerase in bacterial DNA replication, the enzyme that adds the precursor bases to replicate the original DNA and form new DNA strands

Dopamine chemical precursor in the synthesis of norepinephrine; classified as a catecholamine

Dopamine system stabilizers (DSS) drugs that exhibit both antagonist and partial agonist activities on dopamine receptors

Dopamine type 2 (D_2) receptors receptors for dopamine in the basal nuclei of the brain that are associated with schizophrenia and antipsychotic drugs

Dose–response relationship the way a patient responds to varying doses of a drug

Down-regulation the process by which cells make fewer receptors on their surface

Drug any substance that is taken to prevent, cure, or reduce symptoms of a medical condition

Drug allergies a hyperresponse of body defenses to a particular drug that may result in a diverse range of patient symptoms

Drug interaction occurs when a medication interacts with another substance such as another drug, a dietary supplement, an herbal product, or food that is taken concurrently with the medication, and the drug's actions are affected

Drug misuse improper use of drugs that includes overuse, underuse, or, in some cases, erratic use

Drug–protein complexes formed when a drug that binds reversibly to a plasma protein, particularly albumin, that makes the drug unavailable for distribution to its site of action

Dry powder inhaler (DPI) device used to convert a solid drug to a fine powder for the purpose of inhalation

Dumping syndrome the result of a sudden influx of enteral feeding into the GI tract and the creation of a high osmotic gradient within the small intestine

Dwarfism a growth hormone deficiency disorder in children associated with normal birth length followed by a slowing of the growth rate

Dysfunctional uterine bleeding hemorrhage that occurs on a noncyclic basis or in abnormal amounts

Dyslipidemia abnormal (excess or deficient) level of lipoproteins in the blood

Dysrhythmias disorders of cardiac rhythm characterized by an abnormal heart rate or irregular contractions

Dystonia chronic neurologic disorder that is characterized by involuntary muscle contraction that forces body parts into abnormal painful movements or postures

E

Eclampsia pregnancy-induced hypertensive disorder

Ectopic foci regions of the heart outside the normal cardiac conduction pathway that may send impulses across the myocardium

Ectopic pregnancy the development of the fetus elsewhere rather than in the uterus

Eczema chronic, inflammatory skin disorder

Efficacy the maximal response that can be produced from a particular drug

Electrocardiogram (ECG) graphic recording of the wave of electrical conduction across the myocardium

Electroconvulsive therapy (ECT) treatment used for serious and life-threatening mood disorders in patients who are unresponsive to pharmacotherapy and psychotherapy

Electrolyte charged substance in the blood such as sodium, potassium, calcium, chloride, and phosphate

Elemental (monomeric) formulas enteral products that are usually lactose free and contain only a small percentage of calories from fat

Emergency contraception (EC) the prevention of implantation following unprotected intercourse or contraceptive failure

Emergency preparedness the ability to respond quickly and effectively to an unexpected event that may impact human health

Emetic potential usually applied to antineoplastic agents; degree to which an agent is likely to trigger the vomiting center in the medulla, resulting in nausea and vomiting

Emetogenic potential the capacity of a chemotherapeutic drug to cause vomiting

Emphysema lung disease characterized by loss of bronchiolar elasticity and destruction of alveolar walls

Endocrine system body system that consists of various glands that secrete hormones

Endometriosis presence of endometrial tissue in nonuterine locations such as the pelvis and ovaries; a common cause of infertility

Endorphins a group of neurotransmitters that function as endogenous opioids or natural pain modifiers in the CNS

Endotoxins harmful nonproteins that are part of the normal cell wall of gram-negative bacteria

Enteral nutrition (EN) nutritional support used for patients with functioning GI tracts but who are unable to orally ingest adequate amounts of nutrients to meet their metabolic needs

Enteral route administration of drugs orally or through nasogastric or gastrostomy tubes

Enteric-coated tablets that have a hard, waxy coating designed to dissolve in the alkaline environment of the small intestine

Enteric nervous system (ENS) network of neurons in the submucosa of the alimentary canal that has sensory and motor functions that regulate the GI tract

Enteroendocrine cells cells that secrete hormones that modify the digestive processes

Enterohepatic recirculation recycling of drugs and other substances by the circulation of bile through the intestine and liver

Enzyme induction process by which a drug increases the activity of the hepatic microsomal enzymes

Ephedra plant species that originally provided the source of the noncatecholamine ephedrine, which activates both alpha and beta receptors

Epilepsy disruption of the activity of clusters of neurons in the brain that is characterized by two or more seizures

Erectile dysfunction (ED) consistent inability to either attain an erection or to sustain an erection long enough to achieve satisfactory sexual intercourse

Ergosterol lipid substance in fungal cell membranes

Erythema redness associated with skin irritation

Erythrocytic stage phase in malaria during which infected red blood cells rupture, releasing more merozoites and causing acute symptoms

Erythropoietin hormone secreted by the kidney that stimulates the body's production of erythrocytes (red blood cells)

Esters local anesthetics that act by decreasing the amount of sodium that enters the neuron

Estrogen general term that refers to several female sex hormones

Ethnicity groups of people with biologic and genetic similarities

Euphoria an intense sense of happiness and well-being

Evaluation systematic objective assessment of the effectiveness and impact of interventions

Evaluation criteria specific and measurable achievements that will be used to determine if a particular goal has been met

Evidence-based practice use of research, observations, nursing practice, and clinical judgment to determine care

Exclusivity after approval of a drug application by the U.S. Food and Drug Administration, a period of time when competing companies are not allowed to market generic versions of a drug

Excoriation scratches that break the skin surface and fill with blood or serous fluid to form crusty scales

Excretion the process of removing substances from the body

Exophthalmos an outward bulging of the eyes

Exotoxins proteins released by bacteria into surrounding tissues that have the ability to inactivate or kill host cells

Expectorants drugs used to increase bronchial secretions

Expiration date approximation of when a drug will begin to lose its effectiveness

Extended release tablets or capsules designed to dissolve very slowly, resulting in a longer duration of action for the medication; also called long-acting sustained release

External otitis an inflammation of the outer ear; commonly called swimmer's ear

Extracellular fluid (ECF) compartment of body fluid lying outside cells, which includes plasma and interstitial fluid

Extrapyramidal symptoms (EPS) symptoms of acute dystonia, akathisia, parkinsonism, and tardive dyskinesia often caused by antipsychotic drugs

Extrapyramidal system part of the CNS that controls locomotion, complex muscular movements, and posture

Extrinsic pathway activated in response to injury when blood leaks out of a vessel and enters tissue spaces; the pathway takes several seconds to complete

F

Fasting plasma glucose (FPG) test a primary blood test for diagnosing diabetes

Fat-soluble vitamins group of vitamins stored in the liver and fatty tissue that includes A, D, E, and K

Febrile seizures tonic–clonic motor activity lasting 1 to 2 minutes with rapid return of consciousness that occurs in conjunction with fever

Ferritin one of two protein complexes that maintain iron stores inside cells (hemosiderin is the other)

Fetal–placental barrier special anatomic barrier that inhibits many chemicals and drugs from entering the fetus

Fibrin an insoluble protein formed from fibrinogen by the action of thrombin in the blood clotting process

Fibrinogen blood protein that is converted to fibrin by the action of thrombin in the blood coagulation process

Fibrinolysis physiological process that limits clot formation and removes existing clots

Fight-or-flight response characteristic set of actions produced when the sympathetic nervous system is activated that prepares the body for heightened activity and for an immediate response to a threat

Filtrate fluid in the nephron that is filtered into the Bowman's capsule

First-dose phenomenon serious orthostatic hypotension that occurs with the initial doses of alpha$_1$-adrenergic blockers

First-pass effect mechanism whereby drugs are absorbed, enter into the hepatic portal circulation, and are inactivated by the liver before they reach the general circulation

Folic acid B vitamin that is essential for normal DNA and RNA synthesis; also called folate

Food and Drug Administration (FDA) U.S. agency responsible for the evaluation and approval of new drugs

Food and Drug Administration (FDA) Modernization Act act that gave financial incentives to pharmaceutical companies to conduct pediatric research in pharmacology; in exchange for providing pediatric labeling, the legislation gives drug companies the ability to exclusively market the drug for an additional 6 months with no competition

Formulary list of drug and drug recipes commonly used by pharmacists

Frequency distribution curve a graphic representation of the actual number of patients responding to a particular drug action at different doses

Fungi kingdom of organisms that includes mushrooms, yeasts, and molds

G

Gamma aminobutyric acid (GABA) neurotransmitter in the CNS

Ganglia collection of neuron cell bodies located outside the central nervous system

Ganglionic blockers drugs that inhibit transmission at the ganglia in the sympathetic and parasympathetic nervous systems

Gastroesophageal reflux disease (GERD) regurgitation of acidic stomach contents into the esophagus

Gate control theory proposes a gating mechanism for the transmission of pain in the spinal cord

General anesthesia medical procedure that produces unconsciousness and loss of sensation throughout the entire body

Generalized anxiety disorder (GAD) difficult-to-control, excessive anxiety that lasts for 6 months or longer

Generalized seizures seizures that travel throughout the entire brain

Generic name name assigned to a drug by the U.S. Adopted Name Council

Genetic polymorphism changes in enzyme structure and function due to mutation of the encoding gene

Gestational diabetes condition resulting from glucose intolerance with an onset, or first recognition, during pregnancy

Gigantism unusual tallness

Glaucoma condition that is characterized by optic neuropathy with gradual loss of peripheral vision and usually accompanied by increased intraocular pressure

Glomerular filtration rate (GFR) the volume of water filtered through the Bowman's capsules per minute

Glomerulus a specialized capillary in the Bowman's capsule of the kidney that filters the blood during urine formation

Glucocorticoids class of hormones secreted by the adrenal cortex that prepare the body for long-term stress; also called corticosteroids

Gluconeogenesis the production of new glucose from noncarbohydrate molecules

Glutamate amino acid that is the most common neurotransmitter in the CNS

Glycogenolysis the process of glycogen breaking down

Glycoprotein IIb/IIIa receptor found on the surface of platelets

Goal what the patient should be able to achieve and do, based on the problem or nursing diagnosis established from the assessment data

Goiter refers to an increase in the size of the thyroid gland

Gonadocorticoids sex hormones secreted by the adrenal cortex

Gout form of acute arthritis caused by an accumulation of uric acid (urate) crystals in the joints and other body tissues

Grading process that examines potential cancer cells under a microscope and compares their appearance to normal parent cells

Gram-negative bacteria that do not retain a purple stain because they have thinner cell walls

Gram-positive bacteria that contain a thick cell wall composed of peptidoglycan and retain the violet color after staining

Graves' disease syndrome caused by hypersecretion of thyroid hormone

Gray baby syndrome serious condition seen most often in premature or newborn infants, that occurs when the baby's liver is unable to metabolize or excrete chloramphenicol

Growth fraction the ratio of the number of replicating cells to resting cells in a tissue or tumor

Growth hormone (GH) hormone that is produced and secreted by the anterior pituitary gland; also called somatotropin or somatropin

H

H⁺, K⁺-ATPase enzyme secreting hydrochloride acid in the stomach

H₁ receptors histamine receptors that, when activated, produce allergy symptoms

H₂-receptor antagonists drugs that suppress gastric acid by blocking histamine receptors in the stomach

Hallucinations seeing, hearing, or feeling things that are not there

Hallucinogens chemicals that have the ability to produce an altered, dreamlike state of consciousness

Hashimoto's thyroiditis an autoimmune disorder that is the most common cause of hypothyroidism

Heart failure (HF) inability of the heart to pump enough blood to meet the body's metabolic needs

Helminths various species of multicell parasitic worms

Hemagglutinin an enzyme that facilitates the attachment of the virus to host cells

Hematopoiesis production and maturation of blood cells that occurs in red bone marrow; also called hemopoiesis

Hematopoietic growth factors drugs that promote the formation of specific blood cells and enhance the ability of the immune system to reduce some of the myelosuppression caused by antineoplastic medications

Hemoglobin A1C (HbA1C) a laboratory test used in diabetic management; also called glycosylated hemoglobin

Hemophilia series of coagulation disorders caused by genetic insufficiencies

Hemopoiesis production and maturation of blood cells which occurs in red bone marrow; also called hematopoiesis

Hemosiderin one of two protein complexes that maintain iron stores inside cells (ferritin is the other)

Hemostasis the slowing or stopping of blood flow

Hepatic microsomal enzyme system as it relates to pharmacotherapy, liver enzymes that metabolize drugs as well as nutrients and other endogenous substances; sometimes called the P-450 system

Hepatic portal system a network of venous vessels that collects blood draining from the stomach, small intestine, and most of the large intestine

Hepatitis inflammation of the liver

Herb plant with a soft stem that is used for healing or as a seasoning

High-density lipoprotein (HDL) lipid-carrying particle in the blood that transports excess cholesterol away from body tissues or back to the liver for metabolism

Highly active antiretroviral therapy (HAART) drug therapy for HIV infection that includes high doses of multiple medications given concurrently

Histamine chemical released by mast cells in response to foreign agents or injury that initiates the inflammatory response within seconds

HMG-CoA reductase primary enzyme in the biochemical pathway for the synthesis of cholesterol

Holistic treating a person as an integrated biologic, psychological, social, cultural, and spiritual whole, rather than treating just the symptoms of a disease

Home care nurse monitors the patient's condition, including medication adherence and reports any adverse effects, and works with the health care provider and pharmacist to achieve optimal therapeutic outcomes

Hormone replacement therapy (HRT) supplies physiological doses of estrogen, sometimes combined with progestin, to treat unpleasant symptoms of menopause and to prevent long-term consequences of estrogen loss

Hormones chemicals secreted by endocrine glands that act as chemical messengers to maintain homeostasis

Hospice nursing the care of terminally ill patients in their homes or in a health care facility that involves effective pain management

Host flora microorganisms that normally inhabit the human body

Household system of measurement older system of measurement that uses teaspoons, tablespoons, and cups

Human immunodeficiency virus (HIV) the causative agent for AIDS

Hyperaldosteronism excessive secretion of aldosterone

Hypercholesterolemia high levels of cholesterol in the blood

Hyperemesis gravidarum condition of continual vomiting during pregnancy

Hyperkalemia serum potassium level above 5 mEq/L

Hyperkinetic disorder (HKD) refers to the diagnosis of ADHD in Canada

Hyperlipidemia high levels of lipids in the blood

Hypernatremia high sodium level in the blood

Hyperosmolar hyperglycemic state (HHS) acute complication seen in persons with type 2 diabetes, that is characterized by extreme hyperglycemia, hyperosmolarity with dehydration, the absence of ketoacidosis, and CNS dysfunction

Hypertension (HTN) consistent elevation of systemic arterial blood pressure

Hypertensive emergency (HTN-E) a diastolic pressure of greater than 120 mmHg, with evidence of target-organ system damage; also called hypertensive crisis

Hypertensive urgency severe hypertension, but with no evidence of target-organ damage

Hypertrichosis the elongation, thickening, and increased pigmentation of body hair

Hypertriglyceridemia refers to an increase in triglyceride levels

Hyperuricemia serum uric acid level 7 mg/dL or higher

Hypervitaminosis intake of toxic levels of vitamins

Hypnagogic hallucinations vivid, fearful illusions that may be experienced at the onset of sleep or on awakening

Hypoaldosteronism lack of adequate aldosterone secretion

Hypogonadism lack of sufficient testosterone by the testes

Hypokalemia serum potassium level below 3.5 mEq/L

Hypomania characterized by the same symptoms as bipolar disorder, but they are less severe and do not cause impaired functioning

Hyponatremia low sodium level in the blood

Idiosyncratic response unpredictable and unexplained drug reaction

Immunity ability to resist injury and infections

Immunization process of disease prevention in which the body produces its own antibodies in response to initial exposure to antigens

Immunomodulator general term referring to any drug or therapy that affects body defenses

Immunostimulants drugs that increase the ability of the immune system to fight infection and disease

Immunosuppressants drugs that diminish the ability of the immune system to fight infection and disease

Implementation when the nurse applies the knowledge, skills, and principles of nursing care to help move the patient toward the desired goal and optimal wellness

Impotence inability to obtain or sustain an erection; also called erectile dysfunction

Incretins hormones released by the mucosa of the small intestine in response to meals

Incubation period following the first exposure to an antigen, the time needed for the body to process the antigen and mount an effective response

Indications the medical conditions for which a drug is approved

Infantile spasm usually occurs in the first year of life and is characterized by a sudden bending forward, body stiffening, or arching of the torso; also called West syndrome

Infertility inability to become pregnant after at least 1 year of frequent, unprotected intercourse

Inflammation nonspecific body defense that occurs in response to an injury or antigen

Inflammatory bowel disease (IBD) disease characterized by the presence of ulcers in the distal portion of the small intestine (Crohn's disease) or mucosal erosions in the large intestine (ulcerative colitis)

Influenza a viral infection characterized by acute symptoms that include sore throat, sneezing, coughing, fever, and chills; also called flu

Ingestion the process of taking food into the body by mouth

Innate body defenses those that are present even before an infection occurs and which provide the first line of protection from pathogens

Inoculation the placement of a foreign substance on or in an individual for the purpose of disease prevention using "live" virus particles obtained from an infected patient

Inotropic agents drugs or chemicals that increase the force of contraction of the heart; also called cardiotonic drugs

Insomnia inability to fall asleep or stay asleep

Insulin pancreatic hormone that acts to decrease blood glucose levels

Insulin resistance occurs in type 2 diabetes mellitus; cells become unresponsive to insulin due to a defect in insulin receptor function

Insulin-like growth factor (IGF) a family of peptides that promote cartilage and bone growth

Integrase an enzyme unique to HIV that incorporates the viral DNA into the host's chromosomes

Interferons (IFNs) type of cytokine secreted by T cells in response to antigens to protect uninfected cells

Interleukins (ILs) class of cytokines synthesized by lymphocytes, monocytes, macrophages, and certain other cells in response to antigen exposure

Intermittent claudication (IC) pain or cramping in the lower legs that worsens with walking or exercise

Intermittent feedings enteral feedings that are administered every 3 to 6 hours

Intervention nursing action that produces an effect or that is intended to alter the course of a disease or condition designed to move the patient toward the desired goal

Intracellular fluid (ICF) compartment contains water that is inside cells

Intracellular parasites infectious microbes that live inside host cells

Intrinsic activity the ability of a drug to bind to a receptor and produce a strong action

Intrinsic factor chemical substance secreted by stomach cells that is essential for the absorption of vitamin B_{12}

Intrinsic pathway coagulation pathway activated in response to injury; it takes several minutes to complete

Intrinsic sympathomimetic activity (ISA) low level of beta-agonist activity possessed by certain beta-adrenergic blockers

Invasiveness the ability of a pathogen to grow extremely rapidly and cause direct damage to surrounding tissues by virtue of sheer numbers

Investigational New Drug (IND) application to the FDA that contains all the animal and cell testing data

Iodism toxicity to Lugol's iodine solution therapy

Ion trapping phenomenon in which alkalinizing agents are used to aid in the renal excretion of toxic substances

Irritable bowel syndrome (IBS) disease of the lower GI tract, characterized by abdominal pain, bloating, gas, cramping, and alternating diarrhea and constipation

Irritative voiding symptoms cluster of complaints that accompanies cystitis

Isozymes multiple, similar forms of an enzyme that perform slightly different metabolic functions

J

Juxtaglomerular (JG) cells specialized smooth muscle cells found in the afferent arteriole that sense blood pressure and release rennin

K

Kappa receptors one of two major receptors in the CNS where opioids act

Keratolytic action that promotes shedding of the outer layer of the epidermis

Ketolides class of antibiotics that block bacterial protein synthesis by binding to two different sites on the 50S ribosomal subunit

L

Laxatives drugs that promote defecation

Lecithins phospholipids that are an important component of plasma membranes

Lennox-Gestaut syndrome mixed seizure that has characteristics of tonic–clonic, atonic, and atypical absence seizures

Leprosy a chronic infection caused by *Mycobacterium leprae*

Leptin hormone that regulates hunger and weight balance

Leucovorin rescue therapy drug therapy administered following chemotherapy with toxic folic acid analogs such as methotrexate to rescue normal cells

Leukotrienes chemical mediators of inflammation stored and released by mast cells

Leydig cells the primary cells in the testes that are responsible for androgen secretion

Libido interest in sexual activity

Limbic system area in the brain responsible for emotional expression, learning, and memory

Lipodystrophy a disorder in which fat is redistributed in specific areas in the body

Lipoproteins substances that carry lipids in the bloodstream that are composed of fat bound to carrier proteins

Loading dose relatively large dose of a drug given at the beginning of treatment to rapidly obtain a therapeutic response

Local anesthesia loss of sensation to a limited part of the body without loss of consciousness

Locus coeruleus within the brain stem, an area in the pons that has been associated with fear responses and panic attacks

Low-density lipoprotein (LDL) lipoprotein that carries the highest amount of cholesterol

Lymph nodes the principal lymphoid organs in the body

Lymphatic system consists of a network of cells, vessels, and tissues that provide immune surveillance

M

Macrominerals inorganic compound needed by the body in amounts of 100 mg or more daily

Macula densa specialized cells in the distal convoluted tubule of the nephron that sense the flow rate and osmolality in the filtrate and send a message to the juxtaglomerular cells to release more renin

Maintenance dose amount of drug that keeps the plasma drug concentration in the therapeutic range

Major depressive disorder a depressed mood lasting for a minimum of 2 weeks that is present for most of the day, every day, or almost every day

Malaria disease characterized by severe fever and chills caused by the protozoan *Plasmodium*

Malignant hyperthermia rare but potentially fatal condition that is an adverse effect of some general anesthetics characterized by a rapid onset of extremely high fever with muscle rigidity

Mania condition characterized by an inflated self-esteem, decreased need for sleep or food, distractibility, increased activity, excessive pursuit of pleasurable activities, increased talkativeness, delusions, paranoia, hallucinations, and bizarre behavior

Margin of safety (MOS) the amount of drug that is lethal to 1% of animals (LD_1) divided by the amount of drug that produces a therapeutic effect in 99% of the animals (ED_{99})

Mast cell stabilizers drugs that inhibit the release of inflammatory mediators from mast cells

Mastoiditis inflammation of the mastoid sinus

Median effective dose (ED_{50}) the dose of a drug required to produce a specific therapeutic response in 50% of a group of patients

Median lethal dose (LD_{50}) the dose of a drug that will kill 50% of a group of animals

Median toxicity dose (TD_{50}) the dose that will produce a given toxicity in 50% of a group of patients

Medication administration record (MAR) legal documentation of all pharmacotherapies received by the patient

Medication error any preventable event that may cause or lead to inappropriate medication use or patient harm while the medication is in the control of the health care provider, patient, or consumer

Medication error index categorization of medication errors according to the degree of harm an error can cause

Medication reconciliation the process of keeping track of a patient's medications as the patient's care proceeds from one health care provider to another

Menopause progressive decrease in estrogen secretion by the ovaries resulting in the permanent cessation of menses

Merozoites transformation of sporozoites carried by the blood to the liver inside the human host where they multiply into millions of progeny

Metabolic bone disease (MBD) refers to a cluster of disorders that have in common defects in the structure of bone

Metabolic syndrome a group of abnormalities that tend to occur together that places the patient at increased risk for developing diabetes and vascular complications

Metabolism the process used by the body to chemically change a drug molecule; also called biotransformation

Metastasis travel of cancer cells from their original site to a distant site

Metered-dose inhaler (MDI) inhaler device used to deliver a precise amount of medicine to the respiratory system

Methylxanthines chemical class for theophylline and caffeine and theobromine

Metric system of measurement the most common system of drug measurement that uses liters, milliliters, and grams

Microbial antagonism condition of various host flora in competition with each other for physical space and nutrients that helps protect the host from being overrun by pathogenic organisms

Microminerals inorganic compound needed by the body in amounts of 20 mg or less daily

Migraine severe headache preceded by auras and that may include nausea and vomiting

Milk-alkali syndrome syndrome caused by the administration of calcium carbonate antacids with milk or food containing vitamin D; symptoms include headache, urinary frequency, anorexia, nausea, and fatigue

Mineralocorticoids hormones secreted by the adrenal glands that affect the secretion of sodium and water

Minerals essential substances that constitute about 4% of a person's body weight and serve many diverse functions

Minimum alveolar concentration describes the potency of inhalation anesthetics

Minimum effective concentration amount of drug required to produce a therapeutic effect

Miosis constriction of the pupil

Mitochondrial toxicity specific type of adverse effects resulting from a drug's toxic actions on mitochondria

Modular formulas enteral feedings that contain nutrients that are designed to meet a specific nutrient deficiency or disease state

Monitored anesthesia care (MAC) use of sedatives, analgesics, and other low-dose drugs that allow patients to remain responsive and breathe without assistance

Monoamine oxidase (MAO) enzyme that destroys catecholamines such as norepinephrine in the nerve terminal

Monoamine oxidase inhibitor (MAOI) drug inhibiting monoamine oxidase, an enzyme that slows the destruction of norepinephrine, dopamine, and serotonin

Monoclonal antibody (MAB) antibody produced by a single B cell that targets a single type of cell or receptor

Mood disorder change in emotion that impairs the patient's ability to effectively deal with normal ADLs

Mood stabilizers drugs for bipolar disorder that can moderate extreme shifts in emotions and relieve symptoms of mania and depression during acute episodes

Motor end plate cholinergic synapse on skeletal muscle that allows for communication between the nervous system and skeletal muscle

Mu receptors one of two types of opioid receptors in the CNS

Mucolytics drugs used to remove mucus by loosening thick bronchial secretions

Mucositis inflammation of the epithelial lining of the digestive tract

Muscarinic type of cholinergic receptor found at postganglionic nerve endings in the parasympathetic nervous system that, when activated, result in stimulation

Muscarinic agonist drug that is selective for muscarinic receptors

Muscarinic antagonists drugs that block receptors at cholinergic synapses in the parasympathetic nervous system and at a few target organs in the sympathetic nervous system

Muscle rigidity stiffness occurring in Parkinson's disease that causes difficulty bending over and moving limbs, changes in facial expression, or a lack of facial expression

Muscle spasms involuntary contractions of muscles that cause sudden, intense pain, which slowly diminishes after a few minutes

Muscle spasticity condition caused by damage to the CNS in which certain muscle groups remain in a continuous state of contraction

Mutations errors made by bacteria while duplicating their genetic code

Myasthenia gravis (MG) muscular disorder caused by a destruction of nicotinic synapses on skeletal muscles and characterized by extreme fatigue, double vision, speech impairment, and difficulty chewing or swallowing

Myasthenic crisis extreme muscular weakness and symptoms similar to those of cholinergic crisis; caused by abrupt discontinuation of medication for myasthenia gravis

Mycobacterium avium complex (MAC) infection that usually arises as a secondary infection due to the immunosuppression caused by HIV-AIDS

Mycolic acid a complex lipid that covers the cell surfaces of the genus *Mycobacterium*, which protects them and makes them resistant to many disinfectants

Mycoses diseases caused by fungi

Mydriasis pupil dilation

Mydriatics drugs that cause pupil dilation

Myocardial infarctions (MIs) blood clots blocking a portion of a coronary artery that cause necrosis of cardiac muscle

Myocardial ischemia condition in which the heart is receiving an insufficient amount of oxygen to meet its metabolic needs

Myocardium the muscular layer of the heart, responsible for its physical pumping action

Myoclonic seizures seizures characterized by brief, sudden contractions of major muscle groups

Myxedema mucous type of edema caused by accumulation of hydrophilic substances in connective tissues

Myxedematous coma a life-threatening end-stage condition of hypothyroidism

N

Nadir lowest values of erythrocyte, leukocyte, and platelet counts caused by chemotherapy

Narcolepsy sleep disorder that is characterized by severe daytime sleepiness and inability to stay awake

Narcotic natural or synthetic drug related to morphine; may be used as a broader legal term referring to hallucinogens, CNS stimulants, marijuana, and other illegal drugs

Narrow-spectrum antibiotic an anti-infective that is effective against only one or a small number of organisms

Natriuresis sodium excretion in the urine

Natriuretic peptides substances secreted in response to increased pressure in the heart

Nausea unpleasant feeling of the need to vomit accompanied by weakness, diaphoresis, dizziness, and hyperproduction of saliva

Nebulizer machine that delivers medication as a fine mist for the purpose of inhalation; also called small-volume nebulizer

Negative chronotropic effect the property of slowing the speed of electrical conduction across the myocardium

Negative feedback controls secretion and release of hormones by signaling the endocrine system once homeostasis is restored

Negative inotropic effect the reduction in the force of myocardial contraction

Negative symptoms in schizophrenia, symptoms associated with a loss of normal functioning, including a lack of interest, motivation, responsiveness, or pleasure in daily activities

Neoadjuvant chemotherapy the administration of antineoplastic drugs before surgery or radiation therapy with the goal of shrinking a large tumor to a more manageable size

Neoplasm swelling, abnormal enlargement or mass; same as *tumor*

Nephrons structural and functional units of the kidney

Neuraminidase an enzyme that assists the virus in exiting the host cell

Neurodegenerative diseases degenerative diseases of the CNS that include a diverse set of disorders differing in their causes and outcomes

Neuroeffector junction specialized synapse where the postganglionic neuron terminates on smooth muscle, cardiac muscle, or a gland

Neurofibrillary tangles bundles of nerve fibers found in the brain of patients with Alzheimer's disease on autopsy

Neurolept analgesia type of general anesthesia that combines fentanyl with droperidol to produce a state in which patients are conscious though insensitive to pain and unconnected with surroundings

Neuroleptic malignant syndrome (NMS) potentially fatal condition caused by certain antipsychotic medications characterized by high fever, sweating, fluctuating blood pressure, tachycardia, and muscle rigidity

Neuromuscular blockers drugs that inhibit transmission at the neuromuscular junctions on skeletal muscles in the somatic nervous system

Neuron the primary functional cell in all portions of the nervous system; its purpose is to communicate messages through conduction of an action potential

Neuropathic pain is caused by injury or irritation to nerve tissue described as burning, shooting, or numbing pain

Neurotransmitters chemicals utilized in the communication of a message from one cell to another, or synaptic transmission

New Drug Application (NDA) application submitted to the FDA which signals that the pharmaceutical company is ready to sell the new drug

Nicotinic receptor for acetylcholine in the ganglia of both the sympathetic and parasympathetic nervous systems

Nicotinic agonist drug that selectively activates nicotinic receptors

Nicotinic antagonists drugs that block receptors at cholinergic synapses in the ganglia or in the somatic nervous system at the neuromuscular junction

Nitric oxide in vascular smooth muscle, an important cell signaling molecule and a potent vasodilator causing relaxation of both arterial and venous smooth muscle

Nits eggs of the louse parasite

Nociceptor pain pain produced by injury to body tissue

Nociceptors sensory nerve receptors located throughout the body that initiate pain transmission when stimulated

Nomogram chart used to plot a child's height and weight to determine body surface area

Nondepolarizing neuromuscular blocker class of nicotinic antagonists that bind to Ach receptors at motor end plates in skeletal muscle and prevent Ach from reaching its receptors

Nonopioid analgesics analgesics that have a peripheral site of action, no dependence potential, and provide the baseline pharmacotherapy for pain management; include NSAIDs, acetaminophen, and a few centrally acting agents

Non–rapid eye movement (NREM) sleep phase of sleep during which respirations slow, heart rate and blood pressure decrease, oxygen consumption by muscles decreases, and urine formation decreases

Norepinephrine (NE) primary neurotransmitter in the sympathetic and autonomic nervous systems

Nosocomial infections infections acquired in a health care setting

Nursing diagnoses list of problems that address the patient's responses to health and life processes

Nursing process five-part decision-making system that includes assessment, nursing diagnosis, planning, implementation, and evaluation

O

Obsessive–compulsive disorder (OCD) recurrent, intrusive thoughts or repetitive behaviors that interfere with normal activities or relationships

Occupational health nurse (OHN) addresses the health and safety of workers on the job

Oligospermia presence of less than 20 million sperm per mL of ejaculate

Oncology nurse nurse who has received special training to care for patients with cancer and to administer chemotherapy

On–off syndrome occurs when a patient with Parkinson's disease alternates between symptom-free periods (on) and times when the drugs stop working and symptoms abruptly reappear (off)

Onychomycosis the invasion of the nail plate by a fungus; also called tinea unguium

Open-angle glaucoma common form of glaucoma caused by the partial obstruction of the outflow of aqueous humor through the canal of Schlemm

Opiates natural substances obtained from opium, such as morphine and codeine

Opioid class of drugs that includes natural substances obtained from the seeds of the poppy plant such as opium, morphine, and codeine, and synthetic drugs such as meperidine, oxycodone, fentanyl, methadone, and heroin

Opium a milky substance extracted from the unripe seeds of the poppy plant that contains over 20 different chemicals having pharmacologic activity

Oral glucose tolerance test (OGTT) a primary blood test for diagnosing diabetes

Orphan disease serious, though rare, disease that affects less than 200,000 people in the United States

Orthostatic hypotension fall in blood pressure that occurs when changing position from recumbent to upright

Osmolality number of dissolved particles, or solutes, in 1 kg (1 L) of water

Osmosis process by which water moves from areas of low solute concentration (low osmolality) to areas of high solute concentration (high osmolality)

Osmotic pressure creates a force that moves substances between body compartments or across a membrane

Osteoarthritis (OA) progressive, degenerative joint disease caused by the breakdown of articular cartilage

Osteomalacia rickets in children; caused by vitamin D deficiency and characterized by softening of the bones without alteration of basic bone structure

Osteoporosis metabolic bone disease characterized by bone demineralization, decreased bone density, and subsequent fractures

Otitis interna condition that may occur as the result of chronic otitis media or as an upper respiratory infection; also called labyrinthitis

Otitis media inflammation of the middle ear

Outcome statement that includes specific measurable evaluation criteria

Ovarian hyperstimulation syndrome (OHS) serious complication of certain fertility drugs characterized by rapid, massive enlargement of the ovaries accompanied by physical symptoms

Ovulation release of an oocyte (egg) by the ovary

Ovulatory dysfunction the presence of abnormal, irregular, or absent ovulation

Oxazolidinones class of antibiotics that act by binding to a part of the bacterial 50S ribosome

Oxytocics drugs that stimulate uterine contractions and promote the induction of labor

P

Paget's disease chronic progressive condition characterized by accelerated remodeling of the bone, producing enlarged and softened bones; also called osteitis deformans

Palliation form of cancer chemotherapy intended to alleviate symptoms rather than cure the disease

Pancreatitis inflammation of the pancreas

Panic disorder anxiety disorder characterized by intense feelings of immediate apprehension, fearfulness, terror, or impending doom, accompanied by increased autonomic nervous system activity

Para-aminobenzoic acid (PABA) precursor molecule used by bacteria to make their own folic acid

Parasympathetic nervous system portion of the autonomic nervous system that is activated during nonstressful conditions and produces a set of symptoms known as the rest-and-digest response

Parenteral nutrition the administration of high-calorie nutrients via a central vein, such as the subclavian vein

Parietal cells cells in the stomach mucosa that secrete hydrochloric acid

Parish nursing refers to a specialty practice that emphasizes health and healing within a faith community

Parkinsonism having tremor, loss of fine motor skills, muscle rigidity, stooped posture, and a shuffling gait

Parkinson's disease (PD) degenerative disorder of the nervous system characterized by tremor, muscle rigidity, hypokinesia, masklike faces, and a slow, shuffling gait

Paroxysmal supraventricular tachycardia (PSVT) occurs when episodes of atrial tachycardia alternate with periods of normal rhythm; also called paroxysmal atrial tachycardia (PAT)

Partial agonist medication that produces a weaker, or less efficacious, response than an agonist

Partial fatty-acid oxidation inhibitors a class of drugs used in the treatment of CAD

Partial (focal) seizures seizures that start on one side of the brain and travel a short distance before stopping

Partial parenteral nutrition a parenteral solution that lacks an essential element, usually fats or lipids

Passive immunity immune defense that lasts 2 to 3 weeks; obtained by administering antibodies

Patent medicines in early America before drug regulation, products that contained an easily identified brand name that claimed to cure just about any symptom or disease

Pathogenicity ability of an organism to cause disease in humans

Pathogens microbes that are capable of causing disease

Pediatric Research Equity Act of 2003 act that authorizes the FDA to require research of pediatric uses for new drugs

Pediculicides drugs that kill lice

Pegylation process that attaches polyethylene glycol to a drug molecule to extend its duration of activity

Penicillinase enzyme present in certain bacteria that is able to make penicillin ineffective

Penicillin-binding proteins (PBPs) enzymes used by bacteria to build bacterial cell walls that are targets for penicillins and related antibiotics

Pepsin digestive enzyme that breaks down proteins from food

Peptic ulcer erosion of the mucosa in the stomach or small intestine

Peptidoglycan substance containing sugars bound to peptides that is only found in bacteria

Peripheral resistance amount of friction encountered by blood in the arteries

Peripheral vein total parenteral nutrition delivery system used when a central venous line cannot be accessed or when it is not appropriate for the patient

Peripherally inserted central catheter (PICC) line a central catheter that is threaded into the vena cava for administration of chemotherapy

Peristalsis contractions of layers of smooth muscle

Pernicious anemia type of anemia usually caused by a deficiency of vitamin B_{12}

Phagocytes cells that engulf and destroy pathogens and other foreign substances

Pharmacodynamics study of the mechanisms of drug action and how the body responds to drugs

Pharmacogenetics the study of genetic variations that alter patients' responses to medications; branch of pharmacology that examines the role of genetics in drug response

Pharmacokinetics study of drug movement throughout the body

Pharmacologic classification method of organizing drugs on the basis of their mechanisms of action

Pharmacology the study of medicines, ranging from how drugs are administered, to where they travel in the body, to the actual responses they produce

Pharmacopoeia a medical reference summarizing standards of drug purity, strength, and directions for synthesis

Pharmacotherapy the application of drugs for the purpose of disease prevention and treatment of suffering; also called pharmacotherapeutics

Pheochromocytoma a tumor, usually benign, arising from the adrenal medulla that is characterized by excessive secretion of catecholamines

Phobia fearful feeling attached to situations or objects such as snakes, spiders, crowds, or heights

Phosphodiesterase III enzyme in cardiac and smooth muscle; inhibition increases cardiac output due to an increase in myocardial contractility and a decrease in left ventricular afterload

Phospholipids type of lipid that contains two fatty acids, a phosphate group, and a chemical backbone of glycerol

Phototherapy therapy used for persons suffering from seasonal affective disorder that consists of artificial lighting approximately 5 to 20 times brighter than normal indoor lighting

Physical dependence condition of experiencing unpleasant withdrawal symptoms when a substance is discontinued after repeated use

Pill rolling common behavior in Parkinson's disease, in which patients rub the thumb and forefinger together in a circular motion, resembling the motion of rolling a tablet between two fingers

Placebo in drug testing, an inert substance that serves as a control "nontreatment" group used to compare the effectiveness of the new drug

Placenta organ that allows for nutrition and gas exchange between the mother and fetus

Planning phase of the nursing process in which appropriate goals and outcomes are developed and nursing interventions that will help the patient achieve them are determined

Plaque fibrous, fatty material that builds up in the walls of arteries

Plaques psoriatic lesions characterized by red, raised patches of skin covered with flaky, thick, silver scales

Plasma cells cells derived from B lymphocytes that secrete antibodies

Plasma half-life ($t_{1/2}$) the length of time required for the plasma concentration of a drug to decrease by one half after administration

Plasminogen inactive protein that is present in fibrin clot formation; precursor of plasmin

Pluripotent stem cell cell that is capable of maturing (differentiating) into any blood cell type

Pneumonic plague life-threatening infectious lung disease that occurs after breathing *Yersinia pestis*, a bacterium found on rodents and their fleas that is responsible for the bubonic plague

Polarized describes a cell that has negative membrane potential

Polyclonal antibodies contain a wide mixture of different antibodies that attack the T cells or T-cell receptors

Polycystic ovary syndrome a condition in which the ovaries are filled with follicular cysts and the patient has elevated levels of androgens and estrogen

Polydipsia excessive thirst

Polyherbacy use of multiple herbal and other supplements

Polymeric formulas solutions that contain various mixtures of proteins, lipids, and carbohydrates in high-molecular-weight form and are considered the most common enteral preparation

Polyphagia excessive appetite

Polypharmacy taking multiple drugs concurrently

Polyuria excessive urine production

Positive symptoms in schizophrenia, symptoms associated with an excess of distortion of normal function, including hallucinations, delusions, disorganized thought or speech patterns, and movement disorders

Postantibiotic effect antimicrobial activity that continues for a time after discontinuation of a drug

Posterior pituitary gland (neurohypophysis) consists of nervous tissue and is an extension of the hypothalamus that secretes antidiuretic hormone and oxytocin

Postherpetic neuralgia a serious form of the shingles in which the pain lasts for years

Postictal state period immediately following a seizure

Postmarketing surveillance stage 4 of the drug approval process during which testing is done to survey for harmful drug effects in a larger population

Postpartum onset depression major depression experienced by new mothers following delivery, which is related to hormonal shifts and situational stresses that occur during that period

Post-traumatic stress disorder (PTSD) type of anxiety that develops in response to reexperiencing a previous life event that was psychologically traumatic

Potency the strength of a drug at a specified concentration or dose

Potentially inappropriate medications (PIMs) medications that comprise the Beers criteria that are of special concern for older adults

Preclinical research first stage of drug development that involves extensive laboratory testing by the pharmaceutical company on human and microbial cells

Prediabetes condition in which serum glucose levels are elevated but are not high enough to be diagnosed as diabetes

Preeclampsia occurs during pregnancy when blood pressure increases to 140/90 mmHg or higher on two separate occasions, and 300 mg of protein is found in the urine over a 24-hour period

Pregnancy categories five classifications developed by the U.S. Food and Drug Administration (FDA) that rate medication risks during pregnancy

Preload degree of stretch of the cardiac muscle fibers just before they contract

Preterm labor the initiation of labor prior to week 37 of gestation

Primary hypertension hypertension having no identifiable cause

Procoagulants natural substances that promote the formation of blood clots

Prodrugs drugs that become more active after they are metabolized

Prodysrhythmics conditions that promote the formation of cardiac rhythm abnormalities

Progesterone a natural progestin secreted by the corpus luteum

Progestins synthetic hormones that have actions identical to natural endogenous progesterone

Prostaglandin E$_2$ hormone that stimulates the secretion of mucus and bicarbonate, promotes repair of damaged gastric mucosal cells, and increases blood flow to the mucosa to help maintain optimal mucosal conditions

Prostaglandins local hormones that have diverse functions depending on the location

Prostatitis bacterial infection of the prostate gland

Protease viral enzyme that is responsible for the final assembly of the HIV virions

Prothrombin blood clotting factor that is converted to the enzyme thrombin

Prothrombin time (PT) laboratory test used to measure blood coagulation

Proton pump inhibitors (PPIs) drugs that inhibit the enzyme H$^+$, K$^+$-ATPase

Prototype drug well-understood model drug to which other drugs in a pharmacologic class are compared

Protozoan single-celled organism that inhabits water, soil, and animal hosts

Provirus stage of a virus in which the viral DNA integrates into the host chromosome

Pruritus itching associated with dry, scaly skin or a parasite infection

Pseudocholinesterase enzyme that rapidly destroys certain drugs in the plasma

Pseudomembranous colitis (PMC) caused by *Clostridium difficile*, a rare though potentially severe disorder resulting from therapy with tetracyclines and other classes of antibiotics

Psoralens agents used along with phototherapy for the treatment of severe psoriasis

Psychological dependence desire to continue using a drug despite obvious negative economic, physical, or social consequences

Psychosis general term used in medicine to describe a loss of contact with reality

Psychosocial describes a person's psychological development in the context of one's social environment

Public health nurse has a primary focus on population-level outcomes to promote health and prevent disease for entire population groups

Pulmonary embolism condition that occurs when a venous clot dislodges, migrates to the pulmonary vessels, and blocks arterial circulation to the lungs

Pulmonary perfusion blood flow through the lung

Purified protein derivative (PPD) tuberculin skin test

Pyelonephritis an inflammation of the kidney, pelvis, and other renal cells

R

Radiation sickness occurs after exposure to ionizing radiation; symptoms include nausea, vomiting, and diarrhea, weight loss, anorexia, fatigue, and suppression of the bone marrow

Rapid eye movement (REM) sleep stage of sleep characterized by diminished muscle tone, movements of the eyes, and irregular heart rate and breathing

Raynaud's disease vasospasms of vessels serving the fingers and toes that can lead to intermittent pain and cyanosis of the digits

Reabsorption movement of filtered substances from the kidney tubule back into the blood

Rebound congestion adverse effect of intranasal decongestants; prolonged use causes hypersecretion of mucus and worsening nasal congestion once the drug effects wear off

Rebound effects symptoms of lethargy and fatigue caused by withdrawal of methamphetamine and other stimulants

Rebound insomnia increased sleeplessness that occurs when long-term sedative medication is discontinued abruptly

Receptor cellular molecule to which a drug binds to produce its effects

Recommended dietary allowances (RDAs) minimum amount of vitamins and minerals needed each day to prevent disease

Rectal route administration of drugs into the rectum for either local or systemic delivery

Refeeding syndrome metabolic complications that can occur when nutritional support, including enteral nutrition therapy, is introduced to severely malnourished patients

Reflex tachycardia temporary increase in heart rate that occurs when blood pressure falls

Refractory period time during which the myocardial cells rest and are not able to contract

Regional anesthesia similar to local anesthesia except that it encompasses a larger body area, such as an entire limb

Renal failure a condition characterized by a decrease in the kidneys' ability to maintain electrolyte and fluid balance and excrete waste products

Renin an enzyme that is synthesized, stored, and secreted by juxtaglomerular cells in the kidney

Renin-angiotensin-aldosterone system (RAAS) series of enzymatic steps by which the body raises blood pressure

Replacement therapy hormones administered to patients who are unable to secrete sufficient quantities of their own endogenous hormones

Repolarization return of a negative resting membrane potential to the cell

Rest-and-digest response signs and symptoms produced when the parasympathetic nervous system is activated that promote relaxation and maintenance activities

Reticular activating system (RAS) responsible for sleeping and wakefulness and performs an alerting function for the cerebral cortex

Reticular formation portion of the brain affecting awareness and wakefulness

Retinoids drug class related to vitamin A used in the treatment of inflammatory skin conditions, dermatologic malignancies, and acne

Reverse cholesterol transport the process by which cholesterol is transported away from body tissues to the liver

Reverse remodeling occurs after several months of therapy with beta-adrenergic antagonists, when heart size, shape, and function return to normal

Reverse transcriptase viral enzyme that converts RNA to DNA

Rhabdomyolysis breakdown of muscle fibers usually due to muscle trauma or ischemia

Rheumatoid arthritis (RA) chronic, progressive, autoimmune disease that causes inflammation of the joints

Rhinophyma reddened, bulbous, irregular swelling of the nose

Rifamycin derivatives include rifampin, rifabutin, and rifapentine, used in combination with other antituberculosis medications

Risk management system of reducing medication errors by modifying policies and procedures within the institution

Risk–benefit ratio determination of whether the risks from a drug outweigh the potential benefits received by taking the medication

Rosacea inflammatory skin disorder affecting mainly the face, characterized by small papules that swell, thicken, and become painful

S

Salicylates the chemical family to which aspirin belongs

Salicylism acute or chronic overdose of aspirin

Sarcolemma the muscle membrane

Sarcoplasmic reticula structures within cells that store the calcium ions that are released by depolarization

Satiety the psychological feeling of fullness or satisfaction following a meal

Satiety center region of the hypothalamus that recognizes satiety

Scabicides drugs that kill scabies mites

Scheduled drug in the United States, a term describing a drug placed into one of five categories based on its potential for misuse or abuse

Schizoaffective disorder psychosis with symptoms of both schizophrenia and mood disorders

Schizophrenia psychosis characterized by abnormal thoughts and thought processes, withdrawal from people and the outside environment, an inability to independently perform ADLs, and a high risk of suicide

Sclerosing abnormal tissue hardening of the veins

Seasonal affective disorder a type of depression experienced during the dark winter months

Seborrhea skin condition characterized by overproduction of sebum by the oil glands

Second messenger cascade of biochemical events that initiates a drug's action by either stimulating or inhibiting a normal activity of the cell

Secondary hypertension hypertension having a specific identifiable cause

Secretion in the kidney, movement of substances from the blood into the tubule after filtration has occurred

Sedatives substances that depress the CNS and cause drowsiness or sleep

Sedative–hypnotic drug with the ability to produce a calming effect at lower doses and sleep at higher doses

Seizure symptom of epilepsy characterized by abnormal neuronal discharges within the brain

Selective estrogen receptor modulators (SERMs) drugs that produce an action similar to estrogen in body tissues; used for the treatment of osteoporosis in postmenopausal women

Semielemental (oligomeric) formulas enteral solutions that contain larger molecules than elemental products and a higher percentage of fat

Serotonin a natural neurotransmitter that is found in high concentrations in the hypothalamus, limbic system, medulla, and spinal cord

Serotonin syndrome (SES) set of signs and symptoms associated with overmedication with antidepressants that includes altered mental status, fever, hypertension, tremors, sweating, and lack of muscular coordination

Shingles herpes zoster infection caused by reactivation of the varicella-zoster virus or chickenpox

Short stature height below the fifth percentile for age and gender, or more than two standard deviations below the mean (average) for age and gender

Side effects types of drug effects that are less serious than adverse effects, are predictable, and may occur even at therapeutic doses

Silent angina myocardial ischemia that occurs in the absence of pain

Simple partial seizures seizures that have an onset that may begin as a small, regional focus, and subsequently progress to a generalized seizure

Sinus rhythm number of beats per minute normally generated by the SA node

Situational anxiety anxiety experienced by people faced with a temporarily stressful environment

Sjögren's syndrome chronic autoimmune disorder characterized by excessive dryness of mucous membranes

Sleep attacks sudden bouts of sleep that last 10 to 30 minutes and may occur during the daytime without warning

Sleep paralysis the temporary inability to move after waking up from sleep

Small volume nebulizer machine that delivers medication as a fine mist for the purpose of inhalation; also called nebulizer

Smallpox serious, contagious potentially fatal disease that is caused by the variola virus

Social anxiety disorder unreasonable and persistent fear of crowds or of being judged, ridiculed, or embarrassed by others; also called social phobia

Somatic nervous system nerves that provide for voluntary control of the skeletal muscle

Somatostatin hormone released by the hypothalamus, stomach, intestine, and pancreas that inhibits the effects of growth hormone and lowers acid secretion; also known as growth hormone-inhibiting hormone

Specialty supplements nonherbal dietary products used to enhance a wide variety of body functions

Spermicides agents that kill sperm

Sporozoite mature and infective form of *Plasmodium* that resides in the gut of the female *Anopheles* mosquito

Stable angina type of angina that occurs in a predictable pattern of frequency, intensity, and duration, usually relieved by rest

Staging the process of determining where a cancer is located and the extent of its invasion

Status asthmaticus emergency situation in which acute asthma attacks are unresponsive to drug treatment; may lead to respiratory failure

Status epilepticus medical emergency that occurs when a seizure continues for more than 30 minutes or when two successive seizures occur without full recovery of consciousness between seizures

Steatorrhea the passing of bulky, foul-smelling fatty stools

Steroids types of lipids consisting of a ring structure

Sterol nucleus ring structure common to all steroids

Strategic National Stockpile (SNS) national repository of antibiotics, chemical antidotes, antitoxins, antiviral agents, and other essential medical supplies for use in a major health emergency

Streptogramins class of antibiotics that act by binding the 50S bacterial ribosome in a manner similar to that of the macrolides

Striatum location in the brain, where dopamine encounters its receptors and produces multiple actions

Stroke volume amount of blood pumped by a ventricle in a single contraction

Substance abuse self-administration of a drug that does not conform to the medical or social norms within the patient's given culture or society

Substantia nigra location in the brain where dopamine is produced that is responsible for regulation of unconscious muscle movement

Substrate drug that is metabolized by a CYP enzyme

Suicide the intentional act of ending one's life

Supercoil the highly twisted arrangement of the helix in bacterial DNA

Superinfections new infections caused when an antibiotic kills the host's normal flora, making additional space and nutrients available for pathogenic organisms to grow unchecked

Supplements additional vitamins or minerals that some people take to supplement their diets

Surgical anesthesia stage 3 of anesthesia, in which most major surgery occurs

Svedberg unit a unit of measurement represented by the letter "S" which indicates the size or sedimentation rate of the bacterial 70S ribosome

Sympathetic nervous system portion of the autonomic nervous system that is activated under emergency conditions or stress and produces a set of actions called the fight-or-flight response

Sympathomimetics drugs that activate adrenergic receptors in the sympathetic nervous system

Symporter a membrane protein that transports two molecules at the same time

Synapse a junction between two neurons or a neuron and a muscle

Synaptic cleft space where neurotransmitters enter that must be crossed for the impulse to reach the postganglionic neuron or organ

Syndrome of inappropriate antidiuretic hormone (SIADH) condition characterized by marked fluid retention, elevated urine osmolality, low serum osmolality, and sodium loss in the urine

Synergistic effect type of drug interaction in which two drugs produce an effect that is much greater than would be expected from simply adding the two individual drugs' responses

T

T cells types of lymphocytes that are essential for the cell-mediated immune response

Tachydysrhythmias disorders exhibiting a heart rate greater than 100 beats/minute

Tachyphylaxis the rapid development of tolerance to any action of a drug, either adverse or therapeutic effects

Tardive dyskinesia (TD) unusual tongue and face movements such as lip smacking, rapid eye blinking, and wormlike motions of the tongue that occur during pharmacotherapy with certain antipsychotics

Target cells cells affected by hormones

Targeted therapy drug that has been specifically engineered to attack cancer-specific antigens, such as those on cancer cells

Telomerase an enzyme contained in certain human stem cells that can lengthen the DNA chains and allow continued replication

Telomeres regions in chromosomes that prevent the vital sequences of DNA from being destroyed each time a cell divides

Tension headache common type of head pain caused by stress and relieved by OTC analgesics

Teratogen agent that causes birth defects

Tetrahydrocannabinol (THC) the active chemical in marijuana

Therapeutic classification method of organizing drugs on the basis of what condition is being treated by the drug

Therapeutic drug monitoring practice of monitoring plasma levels of drugs that have low safety profiles and using the data to predict drug action or toxicity

Therapeutic index (TI) the ratio of a drug's LD_{50} to its ED_{50}

Therapeutic range dosage that produces the desired effects of a drug

Threshold potential an action potential triggered by the membrane potential during myocardial electrical conduction

Thrombin enzyme that causes clotting by catalyzing the conversion of fibrinogen to fibrin

Thrombocytopenia coagulation disorder in which there is a deficiency of platelets

Thromboembolic disorder condition in which the body forms undesirable clots

Thrombopoietin hormone that promotes the formation of platelets in the blood

Thyroid crisis a rare, life-threatening form of thyrotoxicosis; also called thyroid storm

Thyroid storm a rare, life-threatening form of thyrotoxicosis; also called thyroid crisis

Thyroid-stimulating hormone (TSH) hormone secreted by the anterior pituitary when stimulated by thyrotropin-releasing hormone

Thyroid-stimulating immunoglobulins (TSIs) stimulate the thyroid gland in Graves' disease

Thyrotoxicosis an acute condition caused by very high levels of circulating thyroid hormone

Thyrotropin-releasing hormone (TRH) hormone secreted by the hypothalamus when blood levels of thyroid hormone are low

Thyroxine (T$_4$) thyroid hormone that is synthesized from the amino acid tyrosine and 4 atoms of iodine

Thyroxine-binding globulin (TBG) a plasma protein produced in the liver

Tocolytics drugs used to delay preterm labor

Tolerance process of adapting to a drug over a period of time and subsequently requiring higher doses to achieve the same effect

Tonic–clonic seizures seizures characterized by intense muscle contractions and loss of consciousness

Tonic spasm single, prolonged muscular contraction

Tonicity the ability of a solution to cause a change in water movement across a membrane owing to osmotic forces

Tonometry technique that tests for glaucoma by measuring intraocular pressure

Topical route medications applied to the skin or the membranous linings of the eye, ear, nose, respiratory tract, urinary tract, vagina, and rectum

Topoisomerase IV in DNA replication, the enzyme that frees the newly formed interlocked strands, allowing them to migrate into the two daughter cells

Torsades de pointe type of ventricular tachycardia that is characterized by rates between 200 and 250 beats/minute and "twisting of the points" of the QRS complex on the ECG

Total parenteral nutrition (TPN) nutrition provided through a peripheral or central vein

Toxic concentration level of drug that results in serious adverse effects

Toxoids type of vaccine that uses bacterial toxins that have been chemically modified to be incapable of causing disease

Trade name name assigned by the pharmaceutical company marketing a drug; sometimes called the proprietary, product, or brand name

Transdermal patches topical delivery method that uses patches that contain a specified amount of medication that is released over a specified time period

Transferrin protein complex that transports iron to sites in the body where it is needed

Translation basic steps in protein synthesis

Transplant rejection recognition by the immune system of a transplanted tissue as foreign and subsequent attack on the tissue

Tricyclic antidepressants (TCAs) class of drugs used in the pharmacotherapy of depression

Triglycerides types of lipids that contain three fatty acids attached to a chemical backbone of glycerol

Tri-iodothyronine (T_3) thyroid hormone that is synthesized from the amino acid tyrosine and 3 atoms of iodine

Troches drugs in lozenge format formulated to slowly dissolve in the mouth

Trophozoite the active, growing stage during which a protozoan organism feeds, often at the expense of its host

Tropic hormones ability of the anterior pituitary gland hormones to regulate the secretory actions of other endocrine glands

Tubercles cavity-like lesions in the lung characteristic of infection by *Mycobacterium tuberculosis*

Tuberculosis (TB) a highly contagious infection caused by the organism *Mycobacterium tuberculosis*

Tularemia serious infectious disease found in rodents, rabbits, and hares that is caused by the organism *Francisella tularensis*

Tumor abnormal swelling, enlargement, or mass; also called neoplasm

Type 1 diabetes metabolic disorder characterized by hyperglycemia caused by a lack of secretion of insulin by the pancreas in which glucose cannot enter cells and fatty acids are used as the primary energy source

Type 2 diabetes chronic metabolic disease characterized by hyperglycemia and insulin resistance

Tyramine form of the amino acid tyrosine that is found in foods such as cheese, beer, wine, and yeast products

U

Unstable angina angina that occurs suddenly, has added intensity, and occurs during periods of rest

Up-regulation process by which cells create more receptors on their surface to capture hormone molecules

Urethritis infection of the urethra

Uricosurics drugs that increase the rate of excretion of uric acid by blocking its reabsorption in the kidney

Uropathogens harmful microorganisms that invade the urinary system

Urticaria hypersensitivity response that is characterized by hives and is often accompanied by pruritus (itching)

U.S. Food and Drug Administration (FDA) U.S. regulatory agency responsible for ensuring that drugs and medical devices are safe and effective

USP verification program mark on the label of a dietary supplement that indicates to consumers that the product has been manufactured under acceptable standards of purity, has been tested for active ingredients stated on the label, and is free of harmful contaminants

V

Vaccination process of introducing foreign proteins or inactive cells (vaccines) into the body to trigger immune activation before the patient is exposed to the real pathogen

Vaginal route administration of drugs into the vagina to treat local conditions such as infections, pain, and itching

Vasomotor center cluster of neurons in the medulla that controls baseline blood pressure

Vasospastic (Prinzmetal's) angina type of angina in which the decreased myocardial blood flow is caused by spasms of the coronary arteries

Vectors organisms that harbor pathogens and spread several major protozoan infections by carrying them from one host to another

Venous return the volume of blood returning to the heart from the veins

Venous thromboembolism (VTE) occurs when blood flow through a vein is very slow (stasis)

Ventilation process of moving air into and out of the lungs

Very low-density lipoprotein (VLDL) primary carrier of triglycerides in the blood that is converted to LDL in the liver

Vesicants agents that can cause serious tissue injury if they escape from an artery or vein during an infusion or injection; many antineoplastics are vesicants

Viral load a measurement of HIV RNA levels in the blood that provides an estimate of how rapidly the virus is replicating

Virilization appearance of the male sex characteristics

Virion mature infective virus particle

Virulence quantitative measure of an organism's pathogenicity

Viruses nonliving agents that do not contain any of the cellular organelles that are present in living organisms that are able to cause disease

Vitamins organic nutrient substances required for the health of the human body

Vomiting emesis in which the stomach contents are forced upward into the esophagus and out of the mouth

Vomiting center area in the medulla that controls the vomiting reflex

von Willebrand's disease (vWD) decrease in quantity or quality of von Willebrand factor

W

Water-soluble vitamins group of vitamins stored briefly in the body and then excreted in the urine, including the C and B-complex vitamins

Wearing-off effect appears gradually near the end of a dosing interval; symptoms become worse because the concentration of the drug has fallen below the therapeutic level

Withdrawal syndrome symptoms that result when a patient discontinues taking a substance on which he or she was dependent

X

Xanthine oxidase enzyme responsible for the formation of uric acid

Xerostomia dry mouth

Z

Zollinger-Ellison syndrome (ZES) disorder of excess acid secretion in the stomach resulting in peptic ulcer disease

Index